Neurological Clinical Pharmacology

Neurological Clinical Pharmacology

Mervyn J. Eadie, M.D., Ph.D (Queensland), F.R.A.C.P.
Professor of Clinical Neurology and Neuropharmacology, University of Queensland;
Neurologist, Royal Brisbane Hospital

John H. Tyrer, M.D. (Sydney), F.R.C.P. (London), F.R.C.P. (Edinburgh), F.R.A.C.P.
Professor of Medicine, University of Queensland; Senior Neurologist, Royal Brisbane
Hospital; Consultant Physician, Mater Misericordiae Hospital, Brisbane; Membre
d'Honneur de la Societe Francaise de Neurologie

MTPPRESS LIMITED *International Medical Publishers*

Neurological Clinical Pharmacology

Published in UK, Europe and Middle East
by MTP Press Limited
Falcon House
Lancaster
England

ISBN-13: 978-94-011-6283-8   e-ISBN-13: 978-94-011-6281-4
DOI: 10.1007/978-94-011-6281-4

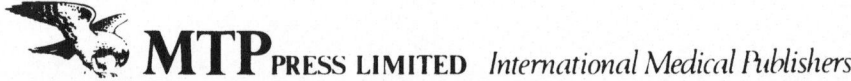

MTPPRESS LIMITED *International Medical Publishers*

Printed by Shanghai Printing Press Ltd.

Preface

In recent years there has been much interest in clinical pharmacology and its application to the treatment of disease, including disease of the nervous system. At the same time there have been major advances in basic neuropharmacology. The aim of this book is to integrate clinical pharmacology with basic neuropharmacology and clinical neurology. The book discusses, in the light of clinical pharmacology, and particularly pharmacokinetics, the treatment of those disorders of the nervous system that are conventionally managed by the clinical neurologist. Matters pertaining to psychopharmacology have been deliberately excluded except in so far as they impinge on ordinary clinical neurological practice. The extent to which various disorders have been considered has depended partly on their importance to the clinical neurologist practising in non-tropical areas, and partly on the amount of data available relating to the relevant drug treatment. Thus the book is directed at clinical neurologists and those intending to practise clinical neurology. However it also contains material of interest to the general physician, paediatrician, psychiatrist and clinical pharmacologist.

Although the emphasis in this book is on drug treatment, to preserve balance it has seemed desirable to discuss briefly certain non-pharmacological aspects of therapeutics. The orderly methodical approach used in the book offers two possible advantages: first, once the reader is familiar with the approach (see Guide to the Use of This Book, p.ix) he can find his way to particular topics without as frequent consultation of the index as might otherwise have been necessary; secondly, the ordered type of presentation reveals gaps in knowledge which might be missed in a less structured consideration of the available material.

In such a book as this there will inevitably be argument about what should have been included and what omitted. Since the neurologist is often called upon to diagnose pituitary tumours, should endocrine replacement therapy have been considered?

Since hypertension is intimately related to the pathogenesis of 'stroke', should antihypertensive therapy have been dealt with? We have included only those matters that are usually managed in both the short and the long term by the neurologist, and have tended to exclude those matters which will usually be managed in the long term by other specialists.

It is hoped that this book will provide a pharmacokinetically orientated source of drug information and interpretation of therapeutic practice for the clinical neurologist. It is also hoped that the book may serve as a basis for improved treatment in a speciality which has, in the past, sometimes been regarded as chiefly diagnostic in its aspiration.

Mervyn J. Eadie
John H. Tyrer

Contents

Preface v

Guide to the Use of This Book ix

Section 1: General Principles

Chapter I
    General Principles of Clinical Neuropharmacology 1

Section 2: Treatment of Neurological Disorders of Function

Chapter II
    Raised Intracranial Pressure 25

Chapter III
    Disorders of Motor Function, I: Voluntary Movement Disorders 46

Chapter IV
    Disorders of Motor Function, II: Involuntary Movement Disorders 81

Chapter V
    Vertigo, Nausea and Vomiting 153

Chapter VI
    Paroxysmal Disorders 163

Chapter VII
    Pain 230

Chapter VIII
    Disorders of Sleep 289

Chapter IX
    Sphincter Disturbances 298

Section 3: Treatment of Underlying Neurological Diseases

Chapter X
    Vascular Disease 306

Chapter XI
    Demyelinating and Autoimmune Disease 327

Chapter XII
    Infections 342

Chapter XIII
    Toxic and Deficiency Disorders 383

Chapter XIV
    Neoplasms 399

References 402

Section 4: Appendices

I. Concise Drug Data 450

II. Synonyms and Proprietary Names of Drugs 454

Subject Index 457

Guide to Use of This Book

Following an introductory section on certain major concepts of clinical pharmacology and their application to the nervous system, this book attempts to deal with the more common disorders of neurological function and then with certain broad categories of neurological disease.

The sequence in which these disorders is discussed has to some extent been determined by the convenience of considering drugs with multiple neurological uses early in the book (to facilitate subsequent reference) and the desirability of dealing in detail with a drug in relation to that neurological disorder for which it is mainly used. Thus raised intracranial pressure is discussed early in the book because this is probably the major disorder for which steroids are used in contemporary neurology, though steroids have many other uses and therefore need repeated mention throughout the book. The reader may find the list of principal disorders and drugs discussed, which heads each chapter, an aid to quick reference; where a drug is dealt with in detail elsewhere in the book, this is indicated.

With a few minor exceptions, each of the conditions considered has been dealt with in the same order. For a given disorder or disease, pathogenesis has first been outlined chiefly in terms of abnormal physiological and biochemical mechanisms. Then the therapeutic possibilities for correcting these abnormal mechanisms are considered. The drugs used in treatment of the disorders are next dealt with in systematic fashion *viz* uses, chemistry, pharmacology (biochemical pharmacology, pharmacodynamics, pharmacokinetics, interactions) and toxicity. Lastly the practical treatment of the various disorders is discussed.

In order to limit the bibliography, we have tended not to supply references to questions of pathogenesis which are likely to be familiar to clinical neurologists, or to points of pharmacology which are well established and documented in widely available texts such as 'The Pharmacological Basis of Therapeutics' (Goodman & Gilman, 1975). Major sources of information are indicated in the text. Unless specifically referenced, details of drug interactions are found in Hansten (1973) or the American Pharmaceutical Association's evaluations (1973 and 1974). Values for pharmacokinetic parameters, where no reference is given, are taken from Avery (1976). Official British Pharmacopoeal names are used throughout and details of drug chemistry are as contained in the Merck Index (1976 edition) except where other sources of information are indicated.

Except where otherwise indicated, drug dosages refer to average adults, and should be taken as a guide only. Dosage may need to be modified in relation to the individual clinical situation.

Chapter I

General Principles of Clinical Neuropharmacology

Principles Discussed

Pharmacokinetic concepts

The entry of drugs into the nervous system

Mechanism of drug action in the nervous system

Pharmacological possibilities in treating neurological disease

---

Drugs for treating neurological disease are usually given by mouth. Less often these drugs are given parenterally (and rarely they are given intrathecally). Therefore, in the great majority of instances, drugs that reach the nervous system are carried there via the circulation. Unless drugs are injected directly into the circulation, they must be absorbed from their administration sites before they enter the circulation. Once within the circulation drugs are rapidly distributed through the body. They pass out again from the capillaries to interstitial fluid, and then may enter tissue cells or remain confined to extracellular fluid. The exit of drugs from cerebral capillaries into the brain substance involves factors which do not apply to the same extent to the egress of drugs from the capillary beds of other organs. This particular aspect of drug distribution, *viz* the entry of drugs into the brain, will be considered in greater detail later (see p.16). Those drug molecules which come into contact with, or enter the nervous tissue are responsible for the neurological actions of the drug. The various known mechanisms of action of drugs on neural tissues are considered in some detail on page 18. Within the body drugs are often distributed to, and may be concentrated in, regions where they produce no apparent pharmacological action. These regions serve as storage sites for the drug.

Once a drug has been absorbed and reached its sites of action its effects will continue indefinitely unless something occurs to terminate its action. The action of a drug continues until all that drug is *eliminated* from the body, by *excretion* (usually mainly in urine) and/or by *biotransformation* (to pharmacologically less active, or pharmacologically inactive, molecules). A few drugs bond irreversibly to tissue molecules at their sites of action. The action of these drugs continues, irrespective of how rapidly the drug is eliminated, until biochemical processes reform or replace the altered tissue molecules at the site of action. In a very much more common situation, reversible bonding of the drugs to its site of action initiates drug action. In this circumstance the duration and extent of the action of a drug parallels the time course of the drug's concentration around its sites of action (in the 'biophase'). Drug molecules in the biophase are in dynamic equilibrium with drug molecules elsewhere in intracellular and/or extracellular fluid. Therefore drug concentrations in the plasma compartment of extracellular fluid parallel the extent and course of drug action for the great majority of drugs, *viz* those that bond reversibly to their receptors. The major events the drug undergoes are schematised in figure 1.1.

The term *pharmacokinetics* is used to embrace the absorption, distribution and elimination of drugs, although the word is sometimes applied in a more restricted sense to the mathematical analysis of these processes. The term *pharmacodynamics* refers to processes immediately involved in the pharmacological action of drugs.

Pharmacokinetic Concepts

Drug Absorption

Oral Administration
In clinical neurological practice most drug therapy is given by mouth, commonly in tablet form, sometimes in capsules, and occasionally as solutions or suspensions. Rarely (e.g. ergotamine), the drug may be given with the intention that it should be absorbed across the buccal and sublingual mucosae. Nearly always drugs given by mouth are intended for swallowing and subsequent absorption lower in the alimen-

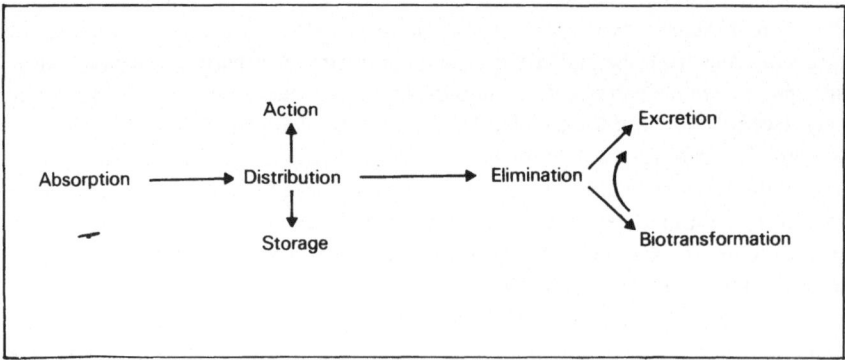

Fig. 1.1. Schematic version of major events undergone by a drug in the body.

tary tract. For solid dosage forms and for suspensions the drug must go into solution in the fluids of the alimentary tract prior to absorption. Prior to dissolution tablets and capsules first need to disintegrate, releasing particles containing the drug (and perhaps components of the various excipients in the preparations). Drug molecules separate from the disintegrating particles and go into true solution. The rate of disintegration of solid preparations can to some extent be controlled pharmaceutically. Preparations can be designed to disintegrate quickly or slowly, or to disintegrate when they encounter particular pH conditions e.g. the acid environment of the stomach or, for enteric coated preparations, the more neutral or mildly basic environment of the upper small intestine. As well as depending on factors which can be controlled by the pharmaceutical manufacturer, disintegration of solid dosage forms depends on biological factors (e.g. local pH, motility of the alimentary tract).

Dissolution of the drug in the fluids of the alimentary tract also depends on physicochemical factors such as the particle size of the products resulting from tablet disintegration and the solubility of the drug under the prevailing local pH conditions. After the drug molecules are in solution in the alimentary fluids they can undergo absorption across the alimentary mucosa. Absorption is almost always a passive process; very few of the drugs used in neurology undergo active absorption. However levodopa, for instance, is actively absorbed by the specific amino acid absorption mechanisms present in the wall of the small intestine. Passive drug absorption occurs by means of diffusion, and depends on the following factors:

1) The solubility of the drug in chemical components of the alimentary mucosa. The lipid solubility of a drug generally provides a good measure of its ability to pass through cell membranes and cells. However, local pH may influence the ionisation of a drug, and ionised molecules are almost always too polar to be lipid soluble. Therefore only non-ionised drug molecules are likely to be absorbed

2) The area of the absorptive surface, which is relatively enormous in the case of the small intestine

3) The concentration gradient of drug molecules between the alimentary lumen and the plasma in the submucosal capillaries

4) The time of contact with the absorptive surface. This varies with alimentary motility and is usually a matter of several hours.

Passive absorption is a first-order process. In a first-order process, reaction rate is proportional to the concentration of one of the reactants.
Thus

$$V = k [S] \text{ where } V = \text{reaction velocity}$$
$$k = \text{rate constant}$$
$$[S] = \text{concentration of the reaction substrate}$$

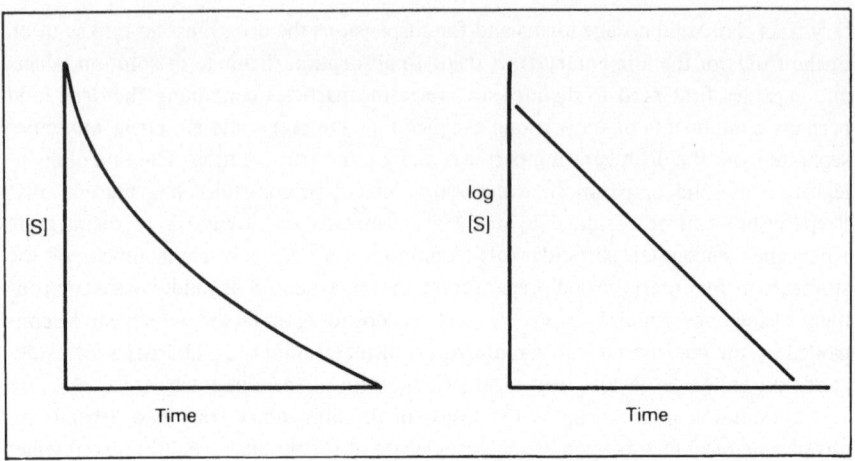

Fig. 1.2. Linear and semilogarithmic plots of substrate concentration against time.

The rate of fall in concentration of S as the reaction proceeds can be expressed algebraically:

$$[S]_t = [S]_o e^{-kt}$$
where $[S]_t$ = concentration of S at time t
$[S]_o$ = concentration of S at the start of the reaction
e = basis of natural logarithms
k = rate constant

The concentration of S follows a time course as shown graphically in figure 1.2.

Passive absorption may sometimes appear rate-limited simply because drug dissolution, though also a passive process, may sometimes be so slow that the amount of the drug in solution at any time limits the amount available for absorption. Active (enzyme-mediated) drug absorption, as applies for levodopa, is a rate-limited process obeying Michaelis-Menten kinetics. Michaelis-Menten kinetics describe the kinetics of a reaction which achieves a maximum velocity as substrate concentration increases.

$$V = \frac{V_{max}\,[S]}{K_m + [S]}$$

where K_m = the Michaelis constant (the substrate concentration at which the reaction achieves half its maximum velocity), V_{max} = the maximum velocity of the reaction and the other symbols have meanings as above. For such a process the time course of S is as in figure 1.3.

Rectal Administration

Drugs used in neurology are rarely given rectally. Rectal absorption is a passive process, involving the same physicochemical factors that are important in absorption from higher levels of the alimentary tract. For a drug to be absorbed from the rectum, drug molecules must first dissolve in the aqueous fluids within the rectum. For drugs given in suppositories, dissolution may not be very rapid. Drug absorption from the rectum has usually proved relatively inefficient, probably mainly because of the comparatively small absorptive surface of the rectal mucosa. In neurology, drugs are likely to be given by rectum when vomiting precludes oral drug administration and when injection is not practicable (e.g. ergotamine for self-administration to a patient vomiting during a migraine attack).

Injection

Drugs may be injected subcutaneously, intramuscularly or intravenously when, for various reasons, they cannot be given by mouth, when it is essential that a known drug dose be received by the patient, and/or when it is hoped that a more rapid action will be obtained than if the drug is given orally. Drug absorption from subcutaneous and intramuscular injection sites is a passive process. High drug concentration gradients across the absorptive surface are possible if the local circulation is swift. However absorption from injection sites may be an inefficient process because of a com-

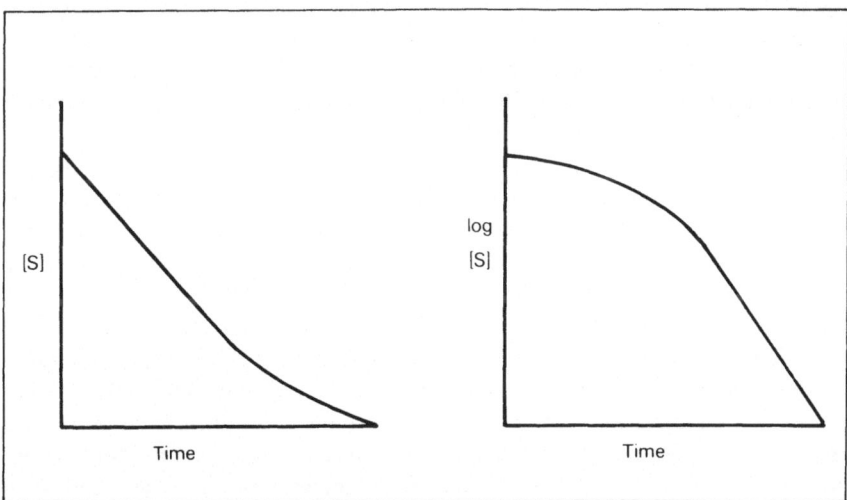

Fig. 1.3. Linear and semilogarithmic plots of concentration against time for a substance which obeys Michaelis-Menten kinetics.

paratively small absorptive surface relative to the volume of material injected. A number of recent quantitative studies have shown that several drugs, for instance digoxin and diazepam, are absorbed more slowly after intramuscular injection than after oral administration. If rapidity of action is required, intravenous injection of a suitable drug dose is more reliable and efficient than injection of the same dose into the tissues for subsequent absorption. Although the parenteral route is employed when reliable drug intake is essential, or when the drug in question cannot be given by mouth, it should be remembered that with subcutaneous or intramuscular injection rapid entry of the drug into the circulation will not necessarily be achieved.

Drug Inhalation

The only drug in common use in neurology which is given by inhalation is ergotamine. No data are available as to efficiency for the absorption of ergotamine given in this way. The aim of using inhaled ergotamine is for the particles of drug to reach the alveoli, where there is an extensive potential absorptive surface and a rich blood supply to carry away any absorbed drug.

Drug Distribution

Within the bloodstream drugs are present in solution in plasma water. Drug molecules may also be bound to plasma proteins, principally albumin, though a few drugs bind specifically to other plasma protein subfractions. Drugs generally bind reversibly to plasma proteins, so that drug molecules in plasma water are in equilibrium with drug molecules bound to plasma protein. Depending on their solubility in lipids (which enables them to enter blood cells) and their binding to proteins and other molecules within cells, drug molecules may also be present at various concentrations in blood cells. The drug in blood cells is generally in dynamic equilibrium with drug molecules in plasma water.

Some drug molecules in plasma water may be present in ionised form, depending on the pK_a of the drug relative to the pH of plasma (7.4). The ionised drug molecules are nearly always too polar to pass through endothelial cell membranes to leave the bloodstream. However, non-ionised drug molecules are often sufficiently non-polar to pass through capillary endothelium to enter extravascular interstitial fluid or other fluid collections within the body e.g. CSF, milk, tears, sweat, saliva, bile and urine. Entry of drugs into these fluids is usually a passive process, depending on the factors which influence passive diffusion, as already discussed (viz lipid solubility, concentration gradient, area of surface through which diffusion occurs, and time of contact with the surface through which diffusion occurs). Non-ionised drug (i.e. diffusable drug) comes into a dynamic equilibrium across the membranes separating plasma from other body fluids so that the ratios of drug concentrations in the various fluids are constant so long as pH in the various fluids does not change.

However, particularly in the kidneys, drugs may also be actively secreted into a collection of body fluid. In this case there may no longer be a constant ratio between drug concentrations in plasma and urine.

Drug that has entered interstitial fluid may or may not be able to make its way through cell membranes to enter intracellular fluid. Within intracellular fluid, drugs may or may not bind to various intracellular proteins or to organelles, and at times may become selectively concentrated in these intracellular sites. Entry of nearly all drugs into cells is a passive process.

Thus in most cases drug distribution within the body involves a number of dynamic equilibria, which may include those in figure 1.4.

Most drugs act after combining with, and thereby altering the properties of, certain tissue molecules (drug 'receptors'). These molecules are usually situated on the surface of cells, or within cells. If the receptors are on the cell surface any drug which escapes from the vascular compartment is likely to gain access to them. However, if drug receptors are intracellular, only drugs which enter intracellular fluid can reach their receptors to exert their actions. A drug may act at receptors on the cell surface even though it is distributed through total body water i.e. it also enters intracellular fluid. Most binding of drugs to receptors involves the formation of reversible chemical bonds, and drug concentration around receptors (in the 'biophase') determines the

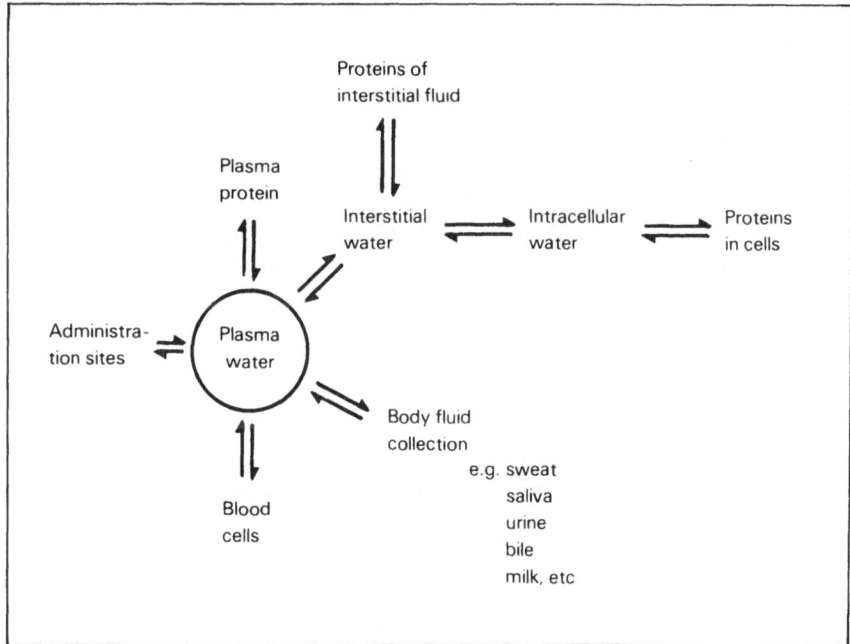

Fig. 1.4. Dynamic equilibria involved in drug distribution within the body.

number of drug-receptor combinations, and hence the extent of drug action. Thus drug action is proportional to drug concentration in the biophase, and drug concentration here, through one or more of the series of equilibria shown above, is proportional to drug concentration in plasma water. For drugs bound to plasma proteins, drug in plasma water is also in equilibrium with drug bound to plasma protein. Hence total drug concentration in whole plasma is usually proportional to the pharmacological action of the drug. *This is the rationale for measuring plasma concentrations of drugs and attempting to correlate these with clinical events. As mentioned earlier, this rationale does not apply for drugs which bond irreversibly to receptors.*

Drug Elimination

As previously indicated, drug elimination is the consequence of two processes, drug biotransformation and drug excretion. In a strict sense, once a drug has been biotransformed it has also been eliminated. However, if drug metabolites are pharmacologically active, drug action may appear to continue after the unchanged drug is no longer present in the body. Thus the clinician may tend to consider that the drug is not eliminated not only till all the unchanged drug has been excreted, but also till its pharmacologically active metabolites have been excreted. If the disappearance of the drug from the body is measured (drug elimination in a strict sense, since drug assay methods are now generally specific enough to distinguish a drug from its metabolites) the time course of this elimination may not parallel the time course of the decline in drug action. The clinician may have regarded this decline as a measure of drug elimination. Often the decay in drug action does parallel the disappearance of unchanged drug from the body, simply because the drug's biotransformation products, even though they may be pharmacologically active, are eliminated faster than the drug itself. However one should realise that measurements of drug elimination relate to elimination of the drug itself, and may not necessarily be applicable to the rate of decay in drug action.

Drug Biotransformation

Most drug biotransformation occurs in the liver, but drugs can undergo biotransformation reactions in other sites (e.g. the gut wall, skin, adrenals and bloodstream). There are 4 main types of chemical reaction involved in drug biotransformation:

1) Oxidation
2) Reduction
3) Hydrolysis
4) Conjugation.

The overall effect of drug biotransformation in most instances is to convert drugs into more polar molecules which are less pharmacologically active and which are more readily excreted than the parent drug molecules.

Most drug oxidation occurs in the liver in the so-called microsomal mixed oxidase system. This group of enzymes appears to have the physiological function of oxidising and thereby inactivating endogenous substances such as steroids. Such oxidation can lead to:

1) Formation of hydroxyl derivatives from acyclic and cyclic carbon compounds, and particularly from the benzene rings which often occur in drug molecules
2) Formation of oxides at nitrogen and sulphur atoms within drug molecules
3) Molecular cleavage (so that oxidative dealkylation and deamination may occur).

Apart from these nonspecific oxidations, certain drugs may undergo oxidation by specific enzymes in the liver and other sites (e.g. monoamine oxidase, alcohol dehydrogenase, aldehyde dehydrogenase).

Certain chemical groups in drug molecules [e.g. nitro groups, ($-NO_2$)] may be reduced enzymatically. Esters (R-O-R^1) and to some extent amides (R-CONH$_2$) may undergo enzymatic hydrolytic cleavage. Parent drug molecules, or their first stage biotransformation products [e.g. those containing hydroxyl ($-OH$) groups] may undergo conjugation reactions, mainly in the liver. Most conjugation of drugs involves linkage to glucuronic acid, producing various types of glucuronide. However sulphate, glycine, methyl and acetyl conjugates may also be formed from certain drugs.

Because these various biotransformation reactions are enzymatically mediated they are rate-limited and therefore follow Michaelis-Menten kinetics. Despite this, at the drug concentrations encountered in human therapeutics the body's biotransformation capacity for most drugs is far from saturated. Hence the biotransformation process for most drugs can be adequately described mathematically by the simpler first-order kinetics. However, at therapeutic concentrations a few drugs (e.g. phenytoin) clearly follow Michaelis-Menten kinetics. First-order kinetics will not adequately describe what happens to these drugs in the body.

Excretion

Drugs and drug biotransformation products may be excreted from the body in urine, faeces, sweat, saliva, milk, tears and expired air. Most drug excretion occurs in urine.

Excretion in urine: Compared to capillary endothelium elsewhere in the body the renal glomerular capillary endothelium is relatively permeable to small molecules (MW $<$ 69000). All drug molecules free in plasma water, whether or not they are ionised, are likely to be filtered from plasma water into glomerular fluid. As glomerular filtrate passes down the renal tubules there is resorption of water and resorption and secretion of ions, with consequent pH changes. As water is absorbed from tubular urine, raising drug concentration in this fluid, lipid soluble drug molecules are likely to be resorbed passively into extracellular fluid. Drug molecules in ionised form are generally too polar to be resorbed across the renal tubular epithelium and remain behind in the tubular lumen. However, tubular fluid pH is adjusted, particularly in the distal tubules, so that it is usually lower than the pH at which drug molecules are filtered into glomerular fluid. As tubular fluid pH changes, there are concomitant alterations in the proportion of drug molecules in tubular fluid that are ionised. This in turn alters the extent of drug resorption from tubular fluid. The extent to which many drugs are excreted in urine depends on urine pH. Acid urine, by increasing the ionisation of basic drugs, diminishes their resorption and therefore facilitates their excretion. Conversely, alkaline urine favours the excretion of acid drugs.

As well as being resorbed from tubular urine, drugs may be actively secreted into the renal tubular lumen. This occurs particularly in the proximal renal tubules, where there are specific enzymatic mechanisms for secreting acidic or basic molecules and glucuronide conjugates. Molecules secreted into the proximal tubular lumen may still undergo passive resorption further along the renal tubular system, depending on the influence of the various factors discussed above.

Excretion in bile: Drugs and drug metabolites may enter bile from liver cells by passive diffusion along concentration gradients. There are also enzymatic mechanisms for active secretion of certain acid and basic molecules into bile. When bile reaches the small intestine some of the drug or drug metabolite that has been present in the bile may be absorbed into the bloodstream across the extensive mucosal absorptive surface of the intestine. Thus drug molecules may undergo an enterohepatic circulation. Glucuronide conjugates of the drug that have been present in bile may undergo hydrolytic cleavage in the small intestine, owing to the presence of the enzyme β-glucuronidase in the intestinal lining, and in intestinal bacteria. This hydrolysis releases drug or drug metabolite molecules which are less polar than the glucuronide conjugates. These products of hydrolysis are more likely to be resorbed across the intestinal mucosa than are the glucuronide conjugates.

Excretion in faeces: Drugs which have not been absorbed after oral administration, and drugs and drug metabolites which have been secreted into bile after absorption, may be lost from the body in the faeces.

Other routes of excretion: Volatile drugs (for practical purposes gaseous anaesthetics) are excreted in expired air, and small quantities of drug may be lost from the body in sweat, saliva, tears, etc. Appreciable drug loss in milk may occur in lactating women. In general, drugs enter all these various fluids by passive diffusion, and drug concentrations in these fluids tend to be similar to drug concentrations in plasma water. However, if drugs bind to proteins, drug concentrations in the fluids with appreciable protein content (e.g. whole milk) may be higher than drug concentrations in plasma water.

Although the excretion of some drugs involves an element of active, enzyme-mediated secretion, for the most part drug excretion is a passive process following first-order kinetics. Thus, overall, drug elimination involves:

1) Michaelis-Menten kinetically determined biotransformation, which often occurs at such low substrate concentrations in man that simple first-order kinetics may describe the process adequately

2) Excretion, largely a passive process, which can be described adequately by first-order kinetics.

Therefore, in many instances, the whole process of drug elimination can be accounted for in terms of first-order kinetics.

Therapeutic Ranges

For most drugs, certain ranges of plasma drug concentration are associated with the best chance of controlling the disorder for which the drug is given, without producing an undue incidence of unwanted effects. These ranges are the 'therapeutic ranges' for the drugs in question. Plasma levels above these ranges are often referred to as 'toxic', in that the incidence and/or the severity of unwanted effects in patients has become unacceptable in relation to the benefit derived from the drugs. However toxicity, particularly of an idiosyncratic type, can be associated with 'therapeutic' or even 'subtherapeutic' plasma drug levels.

It should be realised that the values for therapeutic ranges have often not been determined by rigorous statistical procedures. Rather, the ranges have been defined by clinicians' impressions of the ranges of plasma drug level that offer the best therapeutic results.

Interactions

When a patient is given two drugs simultaneously, it is possible that the drugs may interact. If drug A alters the absorption, distribution or elimination of drug B, (previously taken by the patient) the amount of drug B in his body may be changed. Accordingly, the concentration of drug B in plasma water will be changed and its pharmacological effect will increase or decrease correspondingly. Interactions which occur during drug absorption, distribution or elimination are *pharmacokinetic interactions*. They alter plasma drug concentrations.

An interaction may also occur when drug A acts at the receptors of drug B to increase or decrease the effect of previously administered drug B. Such *pharma-*

codynamic interactions e.g. drug agonism, antagonism, do not alter the plasma concentrations of the interacting drugs.

Quantitative Aspects of Pharmacokinetics

Some mention has already been made of the various kinetic processes involved in drug absorption, distribution and elimination. This was intended to provide a background to the mathematical expression of pharmacokinetic data. While the pharmacokinetics of drugs can usefully be described purely in qualitative terms, expressions of pharmacokinetic data in numerical terms are appearing increasingly often in the literature. Therefore the clinician needs some acquaintance with the quantitative implications of pharmacokinetic parameters to make use of a considerable amount of data that is already available. It is proposed to discuss pharmacokinetics here only in a simple way, emphasising the implications for the clinician of the various pharmacokinetic parameters that are commonly measured, and for which values will be quoted, where possible, later in this book when specific drugs are discussed.

Time Course of Plasma Drug Levels

When a drug is given by mouth, after an interval (the lag time) the drug appears in plasma in measurable quantities as absorption proceeds. After a variable time (T_{max}) the plasma drug level reaches its peak. Thereafter the plasma drug level begins to decline as elimination rate exceeds absorption rate. If the logarithms of plasma drug concentration are plotted against time, both the phase of rising plasma drug levels (the absorption phase) and the phase of declining drug levels (the elimination phase) often appear as straight lines, connected by a curved phase around the time of the peak level (fig. 1.5).

This is so because, as indicated earlier, in most instances both absorption and elimination are first-order processes. To some extent the T_{max} is an indication of the speed of drug absorption, though it is really more a measure of the time when elimination begins to exceed absorption. Clinically it is useful to have an indication of when maximum drug action is likely to occur after each dose. The slope of the elimination phase determines the elimination rate constant, i.e. the fraction of the drug dose eliminated in unit time. The elimination rate constant (k) is often converted into half-life ($T_{1/2}$), another measure of elimination rate. This quantity is perhaps more easily appreciated by clinicians than is the elimination rate constant. The half-life is the time in which the plasma drug level falls by half. It is related to the elimination rate constant as follows:

$$T_{1/2} = \frac{\log_e 2}{k} = \frac{.693}{k}$$

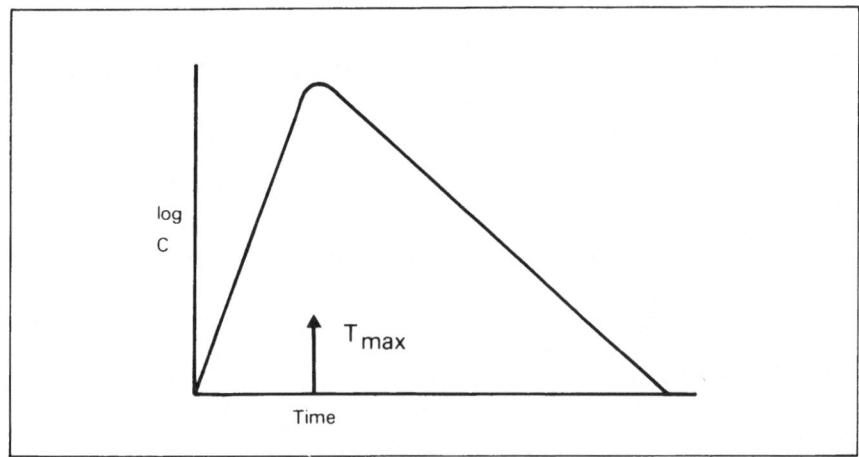

Fig. 1.5. Semilogarithmic plot of the time-course of plasma concentrations of a drug. The time to achieve maximum concentration (T_{max}) is shown.

By subtracting the values on the absorption phase of the plasma level curve from the values at the corresponding times on the elimination phase extrapolated back towards the *y* axis of the plasma level plot against time, one obtains a plot of the amount of the drug still to be absorbed at each time. From this an absorption rate constant, and absorption half-time, analogous to the elimination parameters discussed above, can be calculated.

In some circumstances, (e.g. after intravenous administration, and for certain drugs given orally) the plot of the logarithm of plasma drug level against time may show two linear phases during elimination (the α and β phases). This occurs because the drug is first distributed through a relatively small portion of the body (the 'central compartment') and then is more slowly distributed through a 'peripheral compartment' as well. For many drugs the α phase is not seen, as it occurs while drug absorption is going on and is concealed by this. In this two compartment situation the slope of the β phase defines the half-life.

The area under the plasma level curve (expressed in mg per litre hours, or other concentration $\times$ time units) is proportional to the amount of drug absorbed. If it is assumed there is 100% absorption, as there is after intravenous administration, the dose, divided by the area under the plasma level curve (the AUC), defines the volume of the body cleared of drug each unit of time.

$$\text{i.e. Clearance} \ = \ \frac{\text{dose}}{\text{AUC}}$$

The clearance, divided by the elimination rate constant (k) defines the apparent volume through which the drug is distributed in the body (the V_D).

Hence $V_D \times k$ = clearance.

Should the full dose of the drug not be absorbed when the drug is given by mouth, the AUC after the drug is given orally will be less than the AUC when the same dose of drug is given intravenously. The ratio:

$$\frac{\text{AUC oral}}{\text{AUC intravenous}}$$

defines the bioavailability of the drug, the extent to which the drug gains entry to the systemic circulation after oral administration. Impaired bioavailability may be due to orally administered drug disintegrating, dissolving and/or being absorbed slowly, so that the full dose does not have time to be absorbed before the drug is excreted from the alimentary tract. However, the appearance of impaired bioavailability can occur for a drug which is fully absorbed but is very rapidly metabolised on its first passage through the intestinal wall and/or the liver after entering the portal circulation. Because of this 'first-pass' effect the full dose does not reach the systemic circulation unmetabolised. The presence of significant first-pass metabolism can be suspected if bioavailability is impaired and yet a drug is rapidly absorbed, and if the clearance of the drug is high. For a drug that undergoes extensive first-pass metabolism the clearance of the drug will approximate to the expected value of total portal blood flow, *viz* 96 litres per hour.

Pharmacokinetic analysis can be very much more complex than the above, particularly if the elimination phase follows mixed Michaelis-Menten (biotransformation) and first-order (excretion) processes. However the simple parameters discussed are the most generally useful ones, and from them the clinician can draw useful conclusions.

Inferences to be Drawn From Pharmacokinetic Parameters

The half-life: The faster a drug is eliminated, the shorter is its half-life. If a drug is given regularly and repetitively, as most drugs are, so that each dose is given before the previous dose has disappeared from the body, the drug accumulates. As it accumulates the elimination rate increases till finally, in ordinary therapeutic circumstances, a steady-state is reached at which the amount of drug absorbed over a dosage interval equals the amount eliminated over this same interval. Plasma drug levels will still rise, peak and then fall across each dosage interval, but the mean level will be the same over each successive dosage interval. It can be shown that a) plasma drug levels achieve 97% of their final steady-state values by the time 5 drug half-lives have elapsed, and 99% after 7 half-lives; and b) the steady-state mean plasma drug concentration (C_{ss}) is

$$C_{ss} = \frac{Dose}{V_D \cdot k \cdot r}$$

where V_D = apparent volume of distribution
k = elimination rate constant = $\dfrac{\log_e 2}{T_{1/2}} = \dfrac{.693}{T_{1/2}}$
r = the dosage interval

These inferences depend on the elimination rate constant and V_D not altering as the drug is given repetitively. With repeated administration the rate of biotransformation by the hepatic drug oxidising enzymes may increase due to enzyme induction, and the $T_{1/2}$ will then shorten.

Most statements about plasma drug levels refer to levels in the steady-state unless something to the contrary is indicated.

Absorption half-time: The faster a drug is absorbed the more likely it is that it will have time to be absorbed during its passage along the alimentary tract, and thus be completely (100%) bioavailable. Conversely, the slower a drug is absorbed the less likely it is to be 100% bioavailable. Drug preparations with a poor bioavailability often have an unpredictable and variable bioavailability because of variability in alimentary transit time. Thus the pharmacological effects of such preparations are quantitatively variable in relation to their dose.

The T_{max}: The time at which peak plasma levels occur (T_{max}) provides some indication of absorption rate, though this parameter is also influenced by the elimination rate. T_{max} determines the time of maximum drug action, which is important in many clinical situations. Maximum drug action may coincide with, or follow, T_{max}.

The V_D (apparent volume of distribution): The V_D value provides an indication of the portion of the body in which a drug is distributed. Thus a V_D of 0.05L/kg suggests that a drug is present in plasma water only (plasma water occupying about 5% of body weight). Similarly a V_D of 0.15L/kg suggests the distribution is throughout extracellular water, while a V_D of around 0.5L/kg suggests a distribution throughout total body water. Values of V_D well in excess of 0.5L/kg may occur, e.g. 20L/kg. This can happen because the drug is selectively concentrated in some component of body water, generally the intracellular compartment.

Clearance: Clearance is a more meaningful indicator of the extent of drug elimination than is the $T_{1/2}$ (the elimination rate constant), since it involves both k and V_D and thus relates to the amount of drug removed from the body. Taken in conjunction with the amount of unchanged drug excreted in urine (which can easily be measured if drug in the plasma can be measured), clearance values provide a good deal of information as to how a drug is eliminated. If the greater part of a drug dose is excreted unchanged, clearances of around 120ml/m (i.e. 7L/h or 0.1L kg^{-1}h^{-1}) suggest the drug is eliminated simply by glomerular filtration. Lower values suggest that there is tubular resorption as well. Higher values, up to 650ml/m (40L/h or about 0.6L kg^{-1}h^{-1}, i.e. renal plasma flow) suggest that there is also active tubular secretion of the drug. If little of the drug is excreted unchanged in the urine, so that biotransformation is probably the chief means of elimination of the drug, the value of the clearance gives some indication of the activity of hepatic metabolism of the drug. It is possible to obtain values as high as 96L/h (1.4L kg^{-1}h^{-1}) for a drug which is completely cleared from plasma and blood cells during a single passage through the liver.

Thus the numerical values of simple pharmacokinetic parameters, which can be expressed in a comparatively small space, can provide a considerable amount of information about what happens to a drug in the body.

A number of accounts of pharmacokinetics are available. These range from reasonably elementary works written for clinicians, e.g. Smith and Rawlings (1973), to advanced mathematical descriptions of the subject, e.g. Gibaldi and Perrier (1975) and Wagner (1975).

The Entry of Drugs into the Nervous System

This is a special facet of drug distribution which is important in determining drug action in the nervous system. Most drugs leave the plasma water in cerebral capillaries and enter the brain substance by means of the same passive filtration processes which enable drugs to leave capillaries and enter other tissues. Rarely (e.g. levodopa), drugs enter the brain substance by means of specific transfer mechanisms. Certain drugs which enter most tissues readily do not enter the brain, except at a few special locations. Carbon particles and certain dyestuffs, which diffuse freely from capillaries into most tissues, also do not enter the brain substance readily. There appears to be a 'blood-brain barrier' effect. Previously it was thought that the anatomical basis for the blood-brain barrier might lie in the layer of astrocytic processes which wrap around cerebral capillaries. However, electron microscopic studies (Pappas, 1970) indicate that the chief factor in producing this blood-brain barrier effect is the tightness of the junctions between endothelial cells in cerebral capillaries. These junctions are tighter than those between endothelial cells elsewhere in the body. This tightness of the junctions prevents molecules which are just small enough, or just low enough in polarity to penetrate capillaries elsewhere, from diffusing through the brain capillary endothelium. In a few brain regions the blood-brain barrier effect does not occur. These regions include the anterior perforated substance and the area postrema in the floor of the fourth ventricle. In the latter region the absence of a blood-brain barrier may have a protective effect, allowing noxious substances more ready access to the chemoreceptor trigger zone for vomiting in the floor of the fourth ventricle, than to the brain generally. If these noxious molecules induce early vomiting, and the substance has been taken by mouth, its harmful effects may be reduced.

The blood-brain barrier prevents several drugs with systemic effects on certain chemical processes from affecting these processes within the brain. Thus a number of anticholinergic drugs containing a quaternary nitrogen atom, which makes them rather polar, have no action on acetylcholine within the central nervous system but antagonise the actions of acetylcholine on the peripheral nervous system. Certain inhibitors of the enzyme L-aromatic amino acid decarboxylase (DOPA decarboxylase) e.g. carbidopa and benserazide, block the conversion of levodopa to dopamine in peripheral tissues, but do not impair the conversion of levodopa in the brain because the inhibitors do not cross the blood-brain barrier.

The integrity of the blood-brain barrier may be impaired in brain disease (e.g. hypoxia, infarction, infection or neoplasm of the brain). In these circumstances it is possible that certain drugs which do not ordinarily enter the brain substance may gain access to it. The antibiotic penicillin, which is a convulsant, does not ordinarily cross the blood-brain barrier. However in uraemia it has been suggested that the integrity of the blood-brain barrier may be compromised so that, if penicillin is given, the drug may be able to enter the brain substance in sufficient concentration to produce convulsions. When the blood-brain barrier is intact massive intravenous doses of penicillin do not cause convulsions.

The blood-brain barrier determines which drugs enter the brain substance, and also influences the rate of entry of these drugs. However, drug distribution in brain is not determined solely by the blood-brain barrier: the affinity of drug molecules for various tissue molecules in brain is also involved. Further, in the period immediately following the administration of a dose of a drug, the pattern of regional blood flow in the brain helps determine drug distribution in that organ.

Entry of Drugs into the CSF

Drugs enter the CSF from the bloodstream by means of the same passive diffusion mechanisms which determine the entry of drugs into other collections of body fluid. The protein content of normal CSF is relatively low so that the concentrations of most drugs in CSF is very similar to their concentrations in plasma water. In fact, drug concentrations in CSF are sometimes measured and compared with drug concentrations in whole plasma as an indication of the extent of plasma protein binding of the drug. However, CSF concentrations of certain drugs (e.g. the antibiotic penicillin), are much lower than would be expected from their simultaneous concentrations in plasma water. Such observations have raised the question of a selective blood-CSF barrier. In the case of penicillin the explanation appears to be that, rather than there being selective entry of drug into the CSF, there is active secretion of penicillin out of CSF (Fishman, 1966). This secretory mechanism transports certain molecules, including amino acids and some organic acids (e.g. penicillin), from CSF to blood through the cells of the choroid plexus. When the choroid plexus is damaged, as in meningitis, the CSF concentrations of these substances may rise, not because they more readily enter CSF but because they are less readily excreted from it.

Drugs leave the CSF not only by passive diffusion and active secretion, as described above, they are also carried with the bulk flow of CSF which passes through the arachnoid villi into the cerebral venous sinuses.

Mechanisms of Drug Action in the Nervous System (Pharmacodynamics)

I. Drugs may relieve the manifestations of neurological disease because they correct the underlying disease processes which have affected brain function. Thus cerebral swelling may be reduced by osmotic brain dehydrating agents, bacterial infection of the nervous system may be treated with antibiotics and brain tumours sometimes may be reduced in size by the use of various antineoplastic agents. Such mechanisms of drug action would apply for analogous disease processes wherever they are situated in the body.

II. Disordered neurological function may also be restored in a different way, by the use of drugs which directly modify nervous system function without altering underlying disease processes. Some of the mechanisms involved in these latter modifying actions are discussed below.

Drugs may act by influencing neurochemical mechanisms. In the nervous system, energy, in the form of high energy phosphate, is produced from the oxidative metabolism of glucose. This energy has three main uses:

1) The synthesis of molecules required for the maintenance of neural structure, which is essential for the continuity of neurological function. In the nervous system, function is highly dependent on anatomical factors such as patterns of neuronal interconnexion

2) The maintenance and restoration of ionic concentration gradients across the cell membranes of neurones. These gradients are required to keep neurones in

a state of excitation which makes nerve impulse production and conduction possible

3) The maintenance of the various facets of the synaptic transmission process. which permits the activity of one neurone to be transmitted to others.

Drugs which decrease the available supply of brain energy may have a general depressant effect on all aspects of brain function. Certain barbiturates (e.g. amylobarbitone) may act in this way by inhibiting stages of mitochondrial electron transfer. There would be little prospect of much specificity of action within neurones or between neurones from drugs which act in this way.

Apart from noxious chemicals applied locally to alter neural function by damaging cell structure (e.g. phenol injected around nerve roots) there do not seem to be any drugs which can correct neurological disorder by altering the structure of neurones or their component organelles selectively. The ionic concentration gradients across neuronal cell membranes (responsible for neural excitability) are maintained by the actions of the enzyme Na^+, K^+-linked adenosine triphosphatase. the 'sodium pump' (Skou, 1965). The anticonvulsant phenytoin activates this enzyme. Such an activation would be expected to increase the Na^+ and K^+ concentration gradient across the neuronal membrane and thereby increase the polarisation of the membrane. making it less able to transmit action potentials or to discharge spontaneously. Such a drug effect might be expected to involve nerve tissue diffusely. However there is evidence that the enzyme-activating effect of phenytoin may be restricted to adenosine triphosphatase in injured rather than in normal neurones (Escueta and Appel, 1972). thus providing an element of selectivity to the actions of this drug.

Because the biochemical mechanisms involved in energy production. formation of structural components and maintenance of ionic concentration gradients across cell membranes are probably similar throughout the nervous system. there is relatively little prospect of a selective effect on one particular facet of regional brain function if systemically administered drugs exert their effects on any of the three mechanisms considered above. *However, there is the possibility of a selectivity of drug action on the nervous system if drugs are given which affect synaptic transmission. Synaptic transmission in specific pathways mediating particular functions utilises specific transmitter chemicals. Therefore drugs which alter the formation, storage, release, action, re-uptake or degradation of synaptic transmitter chemicals may selectively alter particular facets of neural function.* Neuropharmacology is very much the pharmacology of synaptic transmission.

Drug-induced Modification of Synaptic Function

Synthesis of Transmitter Molecules

Synaptic transmitter molecules are synthesised within neurones, often in axon terminals. The rate of synthesis may be increased by supplying precursors of the transmitter molecules. (It is often not practicable to supply the transmitter itself in human therapeutics, since several transmitters are too polar to cross the blood-brain barrier). Levodopa (*l*-dihydroxyphenylalanine) is given orally, for enzymatic decarboxylation to dopamine within certain neurones. This dopamine may remedy to some extent the striatal dopamine deficiency state in Parkinsonism. There are reports of the use of tryptophan or 5-hydroxytryptophan in an attempt to increase the amounts of 5-hydroxytryptamine present in brain, with the aim of treating depression or the movements of action myoclonus.

Storage and Release of Synaptic Transmitters

After synthesis, synaptic transmitters are stored in granules in axon terminals, to be released into the synaptic cleft when nerve impulses reach the axon terminal. Within storage granules transmitter molecules are protected from enzymatic degradation. Drugs which bear a structural resemblance to a synaptic transmitter molecule may, if given in sufficient amount, competitively displace the synaptic transmitter from its storage granules. Thus amphetamine causes release of stored noradrenaline. This release produces the postsynaptic action of noradrenaline leading for instance to increased alertness, an action useful in treating narcolepsy. The released noradrenaline can be taken up again into storage sites, for subsequent re-release. Thus there is no net deficiency of noradrenaline.

Storage of such catecholamines is blocked by agents such as reserpine and tetrabenazine. Since released catecholamines are inactivated enzymatically, the net effect of reserpine and tetrabenazine is to produce a basal ganglia dopamine and noradrenaline deficiency state, resembling Parkinsonism. Reserpine or tetrabenazine may correct states of excessive basal ganglia dopamine action, e.g. chorea.

Synaptic Transmitter Action at Receptors

Certain drugs mimic the action of synaptic transmitters at their postsynaptic receptors. Thus apomorphine mimics the actions of dopamine, and lysergic acid diethylamine mimics the actions of 5-hydroxytryptamine. Specific receptor-blocking agents are known (e.g. atropine for acetylcholine, haloperidol and certain phenothiazines for dopamine receptors).

Transmitter Re-uptake

The actions of synaptic transmitters may be terminated by enzymatic degradation of transmitter molecules. However the actions of catecholamines, 5-hydroxytryptamine and amino acid transmitters (e.g. γ-aminobutyric acid), but not acetylcholine, are also terminated by active re-uptake of the released transmitters into axon terminals. Re-uptake may be blocked, and transmitter action thereby prolonged and increased, by the use of certain drugs (e.g. the various tricyclic antidepressants used to block noradrenaline re-uptake).

Transmitter Molecule Degradation

Enzymatic mechanisms exist in the synaptic region for the degradation of synaptic transmitter molecules. Agents which inhibit these enzymes are used to increase and prolong transmitter action. Inhibition of monoamine oxidase can increase concentrations of dopamine, noradrenaline and 5-hydroxytryptamine. Such monoamine oxidase inhibition is occasionally utilised in the treatment of depression. In the peripheral nervous system, anticholinesterase agents (which reversibly inhibit the enzyme which degrades acetylcholine) are used to prolong the action of acetylcholine at the myoneural junction. This is of therapeutic benefit in myasthenia gravis (page 49).

The chemical modulation of synaptic function has been extensively studied experimentally (Cooper et al., 1978), but the application of this knowledge to human disease still lags to some extent. Future prospects for the chemical modulation of brain function appear to reside chiefly in an increased understanding of synaptic function.

Pharmacological Possibilities in Treating Neurological Disease

Treatment of Underlying Disease

Some of the disease processes which affect the nervous system may be treated by pharmacological means. Thus drug treatment may help overcome infective processes (e.g. meningitis), may lead to the resolution of cerebral oedema by restoring the integrity of the blood-brain barrier (e.g. by using glucocorticoids) or may prevent further cerebral embolism by anticoagulant action. In such cases the subsequent improvement in neurological function depends on the recuperative powers of those neural elements which have been damaged, but not destroyed, by the disease process (since neurones in postnatal life cannot reproduce). When drugs are used to treat an underlying disease process the pharmacological possibilities thus depend on:

1) The responsiveness of the disease process to the drug
2) The extent of nerve tissue destruction before the disease process is controlled
3) The potential for recovery in surviving, but damaged, nerve tissue.

The use of drugs to treat an underlying disease process is a fundamental method of treatment which involves principles applicable throughout medicine, though to some extent modified in the nervous system by local circumstances of anatomy, biochemistry and function. Such drug use will not be considered further in this section.

Drugs may also be used for symptomatic treatment. If so, drugs are given to modify neurological function directly, and not to influence the underlying disease process. This symptomatic use of drugs is a special neurological matter; some possibilities will be discussed below.

Symptomatic Treatment

Motor Function
Disorders of motor function within the nervous system involve an increase or decrease in the activity of the final common motor pathway, the lower motor neurone. However this changed activity in the lower motor neurone often arises from alteration in function at other levels in the nervous system. When disorder of motor function arises at the myoneural junctions, appropriate drug treatment can often produce an almost complete restoration to normal function, as in myasthenia gravis (page 57). This is so because the intricate spatio-temporal pattern of nerve impulses associated with willed movement is intact, and the defect in the transmission of this information from nerve endings to muscle cells can be made good by increasing the available acetylcholine at the synapse. However, with more central lesions of the lower motor neurone, and with disease of the upper motor neurone, there is interference with the spatio-temporal patterns of nerve impulses. If motor neurones are dead, no drug can make them function. No disorders are known involving simple transmission failure between upper and lower motor neurones (when the upper and lower motor neurones are functioning normally). It is difficult to conceive how any practicable method of drug administration could deliver exactly the right quantities of a synaptic transmitter substance, its agonist or antagonist, at exactly the right instant and selectively to the dendrites of appropriate motor neurones to restore the spatio-temporal patterns of nerve impulses necessary for each particular pattern of willed movement. Therefore there seems little prospect of employing pharmacological means to restore defective motor function in upper or lower motor neurone lesions. However, if motor function is disordered because of damage to one or more of the systems modulating activity in the lower motor neurone, there are better prospects for drug treatment.

Spasticity (when due to damage at higher neuronal levels releasing excessive activity in the γ-motor neurone and thereby, indirectly, in the α lower motor neurone). may be relieved by a drug such as baclofen (page 72). This drug is an antagonist to γ-aminobutyric acid (GABA), a synaptic transmitter in the γ loop. Such spasticity may also be relieved by applying chemicals which damage nerve tissue (e.g. ethyl alcohol, phenol) in proximity to nerve roots. Here these noxious agents are more likely to penetrate into, and damage, the thinly myelinated γ-motor neurone axons than the more thickly myelinated α motor neurone fibres or proprioceptive afferent fibres. In practice, lesions which cause spasticity nearly always damage the corticospinal fibres also, reducing the prospect for full restoration of normal voluntary motor function.

In recent years it has become possible to use drugs to treat disorders of the basal ganglia which alter the modulating effects of these regions on corticospinal motor function. Deficiency of the striatal synaptic transmitter dopamine can be relieved by supplying dihydroxyphenylalanine (DOPA), the precursor of dopamine. A relative excess of striatal dopaminergic activity, as in chorea, can be reversed by using agents (e.g. haloperidol) which deny dopamine access to its receptors in the striatum.

Up to the present time, disorder of cerebellar function has not proved amenable to drug therapy. Cerebellar disease, whatever its nature, leads to a decreased outflow of cerebellar impulses. When one considers the relatively uniform pattern of the microscopic anatomy of the cerebellar efferent system it seems likely that only one or two synaptic transmitters will prove to be involved in cerebellar efferent modulation of the corticospinal system. Once these transmitters are identified there may be prospects for remedying the effects of deficient cerebellar function.

Sensory Function

As with motor function, normal sensory function depends largely on the spatio-temporal pattern of impulses in the first, second and third sensory neurones. The relevant synaptic transmitters in the sensory pathway are not yet identified with certainty. Unless it is demonstrated that sensory disturbance can be due to a failure of synaptic transmission in the sensory pathways, it seems unlikely that drug treatment would be able to restore sensory function, even if the relevant synaptic transmitters were known. To do this it would be necessary to provide exactly the right quantity of transmitter at the right instant at each appropriate synapse, and yet not at other synapses which might be activated by the transmitter. In the present state of knowledge it is difficult to conceive how this could be done. If sensory neurones are dead, no drug therapy will be able to make them function.

Autonomic Function

Our understanding of autonomic pharmacology is more advanced than our understanding of many other aspects of neuropharmacology. The terminal autonomic transmitters in the effector organs are well known, and autonomic function often does not appear to involve such fine temporal and spatial patterns of control as do voluntary motor and somatic sensory function. Therefore it is sometimes possible to achieve reasonably adequate correction of disturbed autonomic function by giving autonomic synaptic transmitter agents, or their agonists or antagonists.

Intellectual Function

Comparatively little is known of the anatomical and biochemical backgrounds of various aspects of intellectual function. Excluding certain deficiency states, attempts to treat disorders of intellectual function by pharmacological means have so far met with little consistent success. However, despite an almost equal ignorance of the presumably complex anatomical and chemical background of mood and thought disorder, pharmacological agents have been found which will alleviate anxiety, depression and schizophrenia. Therefore, in time, it may also prove possible to improve some intellectual functions by prescribing drugs.

As judged by past experience, prospects for the restoration of deranged neurological function by pharmacological means will be governed by an increased understanding of the synaptic transmitter chemistry of the nervous system. Unless the underlying disease processes can be cured before they produce irreparable damage to the nervous system, it seems unlikely that every disturbance of neurological function will prove amenable to pharmacological means, simply because of the difficulty of delivering appropriate quantities of drugs where and when they are wanted, to mimic the exquisitely fine spatio-temporal patterns of normal neural activity.

Chapter II

Raised Intracranial Pressure

Disorders and Drugs Discussed

Raised intracranial pressure

Mannitol and glycerol
Corticosteroids
(also corticotrophin and tetracosactrin)

A variety of intracranial disorders, and sometimes even primarily extracranial conditions, may cause the contents of the skull to be under increased pressure. Sometimes a primary causative condition may be treatable in its own right but, whether or not this is so, it may still be possible to reduce the intracranial pressure and improve the patient's clinical state by using measures which do not directly affect the primary cause of the raised pressure. The rational treatment of raised intracranial pressure requires an understanding of the mechanisms that may be involved in raising or lowering the intracranial pressure.

Disordered Mechanisms

Except in the young child, the normal skull is a relatively inexpandable box. Its main contents are brain tissue, blood and CSF. Increase in the bulk of any one, or more, of these three major components will raise the intracranial pressure unless there is a corresponding reduction in bulk of another component. The presence of a raised intracranial (and therefore CSF) pressure is often inferred from the clinical features rather than from actual measurement of the CSF pressure. In fact a raised intracranial pressure may not be transmitted to the lumbar CSF if there is obstruction to the CSF circulation at the tentorial orifice or foramen magnum. Measurement of a raised intracranial pressure may be dangerous if removal of CSF during the measurement leads to altered CSF hydrodynamics and brain displacement.

Table I. Causes of raised intracranial pressure resulting from increased bulk of the brain

---

Neoplasm, primary or secondary

Abscess

Haematoma related to:
  hypertensive vascular disease
  ruptured aneurysm or vascular malformation
  haemorrhagic disorders
  trauma

Brain oedema related to:
  trauma
  infection, e.g. encephalitis
  ischaemia and/or infarction
  venous obstruction
  neoplasm

Table II. Causes of raised intracranial pressure resulting from an increase in the amount of blood within the skull

---

Extravascular blood (haematoma)
  within the brain[1]
  outside the brain, e.g. subdural or extradural haematomas

Intravascular blood
  extracranial venous obstruction, e.g. from a mediastinal mass
  intracranial venous obstruction[2] e.g. lateral sinus thrombosis causing benign intracranial hypertension

---

1   See under Haematoma, table I.
2   This will also cause cerebral oedema, see table I.

Table III. Causes of raised intracranial pressure resulting from increased CSF volume within the skull (hydrocephalus)

Increased CSF production
  meningitis
  subarachnoid haemorrhage
  choroid plexus papilloma

Obstructed CSF circulation at various sites, and from various causes

Diminished CSF absorption
  obstructed arachnoid villi from protein, exudate, malignant cells
  superior sagittal sinus thrombosis

The more important causes of raised intracranial pressure arising from increases in brain bulk, amount of blood and amount of CSF within the skull are shown in tables I, II and III respectively.

Once there is sufficient increase in the bulk of some intracranial component to raise the intracranial pressure there is compression of thin-walled intracranial veins, increased intracranial venous pressure and displacement of some intracranial venous blood to the extracranial venous system (Prokop, 1976). When venous drainage of the brain, locally or generally, is impeded by an abnormal intracranial mass, this venous obstruction is likely to cause brain oedema. This oedema further increases the bulk of abnormal intracranial contents, and the intracranial pressure. Pre-existing ischaemia, or ischaemia from reduced cerebral blood flow due to impaired venous drainage, may cause anoxia and impair the integrity of the cerebral capillary endothelium. This causes increased capillary permeability, fluid and protein transudation, with consequent cerebral oedema. Inflammation, and the histologically abnormal endothelium that is often seen in the newly formed capillaries within the more malignant gliomas, also favour increased capillary endothelial permeability, and the occurrence of cerebral oedema. The effects of a local abnormal intracranial mass, with or without associated cerebral oedema, may have further consequences, e.g.:

1) Obstruction of the CSF circulation, as by blocking an interventricular foramen
2) Brain displacement
   a) under the falx cerebri
   b) through the tentorial orifice
   c) through the foramen magnum.

The latter displacement may kink or stretch veins or arteries, causing further venous or arterial obstruction and oedema, often at a distance from the site of the original lesion. Altered blood flow in the brain stem may lead to depressed consciousness and cardiorespiratory function, with consequent further brain hypoxia and acidosis.

Basically, once there is an increase of intracranial mass, it is likely that a series of secondary events will follow (fig. 2.1), including some vicious circle mechanisms. Intracranial pressure will then increase progressively, especially if there is not time for compensatory alterations in brain water content, CSF absorption and blood flow to stabilise the situation.

Correction of Disordered Mechanisms

The therapeutic possibilities in raised intracranial pressure comprise the treatment of the primary causative process and the interruption of various secondary (vicious circle) mechanisms, particularly at the stage of brain oedema.

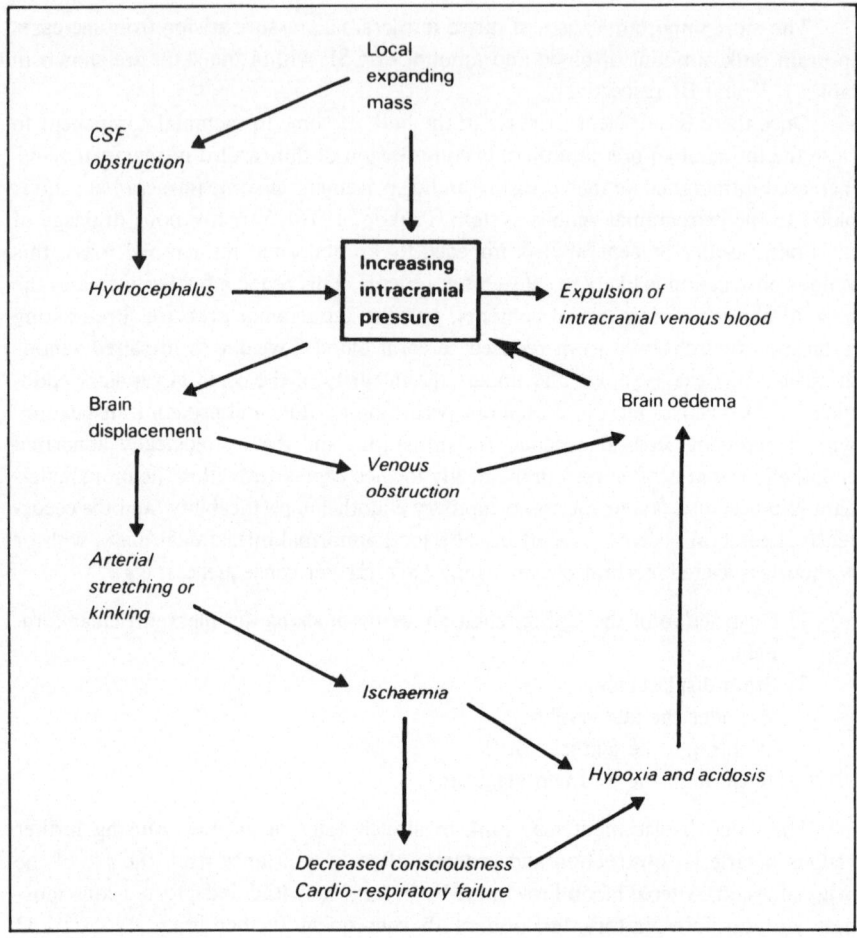

Fig. 2.1. Scheme of possible events and vicious circle mechanisms which may occur when a rise of intracranial pressure is initiated by a local expanding mass. Other primary causes of raised intracranial pressure may enter the scheme at appropriate points e.g. CSF obstruction caused by aqueduct stenosis. Brain oedema is the main target in the pharmacological treatment of raised intracranial pressure.

Treatment of the Primary Causative Process

The treatment of various disorders which may raise intracranial pressure will be considered in detail when the individual disorders are dealt with in other chapters. Here it will suffice to indicate that a neoplasm may be resected, totally or subtotally, and/or shrunken by radiotherapy, or in certain circumstances by chemotherapy, while an abscess or haematoma may be drained surgically. In cerebral abscess the infection is also treated with antibiotics.

Interruption of Secondary Mechanisms

Figure 2.1 indicates that several of the secondary pressure raising mechanisms act by producing cerebral oedema. Drug treatment of raised intracranial pressure is largely an attempt to relieve cerebral oedema by:

1) Using cerebral dehydrating agents, particularly osmotically active agents, to shrink swollen brain (though actually the effect may occur largely by shrinking normal brain tissue).

2) Using adrenal steroids to restore to normal the increased permeability of cerebral capillary endothelium which may be due to ischaemia or other causes of hypoxia, to toxins from infection or to abnormal capillary development (in glioma). Exudation of protein and fluid from capillaries may thus be lessened.

Where intracranial pressure is primarily raised due to an increased mass of CSF (i.e. in obstructive hydrocephalus) the brain is, if anything, compressed. Thus there is no cerebral oedema and indeed cerebral water content may be reduced. Hence drug treatment is unlikely to decrease intracranial pressure significantly in these circumstances.

It should be noted that Klatzko (1967) considered that there are two types of cerebral oedema. In 'vasogenic' oedema, alterations in the blood-brain barrier allow fluid and protein from capillaries to escape into the brain substance, predominantly into the white matter. There is increased fluid in the brain extracellular space and in astrocyte cytoplasm. In 'cytotoxic' oedema, injury to neural elements causes them to swell but there may be no alteration in cerebral capillary permeability. The rational treatment of 'vasogenic' oedema would be the use of steroids, while the use of dehydrating agents may be preferable for 'cytotoxic' oedema. However, it is far from certain that 'cytotoxic' cerebral oedema is of much importance clinically, if it occurs at all.

Non-pharmacological measures which may help relieve secondary mechanisms involved in raising intracranial pressure include:

1) Maintaining the venous drainage and oxygenation of the brain by:
   a) ensuring patency of the airway and promoting respiration
   b) maintaining the circulation and the chemical composition of the internal environment
   c) sitting the patient up to improve cerebral venous drainage (unless this posture endangers the airway)
   d) avoiding, if possible, drugs which may depress respiration, e.g. morphine, which might otherwise be used to relieve pain, as in head-injured patients with multiple injuries
2) Relieving hydrocephalus surgically, e.g. by ventricular drainage.

Drugs Used to Lower Intracranial Pressure

Osmotically Active Cerebral Dehydrating Agents

Over the past half-century a variety of agents has been administered intra-venously in hypertonic solution with the aim of decreasing intracranial pressure by dehydrating the brain. These agents include hypertonic solutions of sodium salts, glucose, sucrose, urea, mannitol and glycerol. The action of these substances depends on their not crossing the blood-brain barrier, or crossing it only slowly, so that for a time they maintain the osmotic pressure of the plasma circulating through cerebral capillaries at a higher level than the osmotic pressure within the brain substance. Hence water is transferred from brain to plasma, thus dehydrating the brain to achieve iso-osmolarity. An osmotic gradient of at least 35m osmol/L is needed to move water from the brain to plasma (Guisado and Arieff, 1975). The agents used to dehydrate brain also function as osmotic diuretics. They are filtered through the renal glomeruli and either are not resorbed from the renal tubular fluid (e.g. mannitol) or else are resorbed incompletely (e.g. urea, or glucose if sufficient is given to saturate the enzymatic mechanisms transporting glucose from the tubular lumen to plasma). The presence of these molecules in renal tubular fluid leads to diminished renal water resorption and hence diuresis. However, the diuretic action of these substances does not appear to play any major role in reducing intracranial pressure. Clinically, highly efficient diuretics, e.g. intravenous frusemide, do not appear particularly effective in alleviating the manifestations of raised intracranial pressure. Conversely, preventing the diuretic effect of mannitol and urea had little effect on their capacities to reduce intracranial pressure in dogs (Wise and Chater, 1961).

The efficiency of these osmotic cerebral dehydrating agents is related to their relative inability to cross the blood-brain barrier. Substances such as sucrose and mannitol have little tendency to enter brain tissue, so that their osmotic action tends to persist till they disappear from the circulation. On the other hand, urea is a molecule small enough to pass through the blood-brain barrier, as are electrolytes such as Na^+ which can be given in hypertonic solution to dehydrate brain. Glucose is a larger molecule than urea or the electrolytes, but there is a specific enzymatic mechanism for glucose uptake into brain. Hence glucose will move progressively from plasma water to brain tissue. The entry of these osmotically active molecules into the brain may not only terminate the osmotic dehydrating effect, but may lead to a rebound rise in CSF pressure which, experimentally, may occur after the agents have been used for some 4 to 6 hours (Clark and Einsbruch, 1962). This risk of a secondary rise of pressure is less with agents which pass less readily through the blood-brain barrier, e.g. mannitol (Wise and Chater, 1961) and glycerol. Meyer et al. (1971) did not encounter the phenomenon over a 24-hour period in 10 subjects given glycerol.

However, the blood-brain barrier may not be intact within tumours, or in regions of cerebral oedema, ischaemia or congestion. In such regions the osmotic dehydrating agent may enter abnormal brain tissue though it does not enter the surrounding normal brain tissue. Glycerol appears to pass through damaged capillary endothelium and then to enter the CSF *via* the damaged brain tissue. The osmotic effect of glycerol in the CSF and in the damaged portions of the brain contributes to the rebound rise in CSF pressure which may occur even though the brain as a whole remains dehydrated (Guisado et al., 1976). A local breakdown of the blood-brain barrier also means that there may be less efficient osmotic dehydration where it is required, *viz* in the lesion itself, than in normal brain. A reduction in intracranial pressure may thus be achieved by shrinking normal brain rather than by shrinking the lesion itself. This is known to be the case experimentally when cerebral oedema is produced by local freezing of brain (Clasen et al., 1965; Guisado et al., 1976). If such preferential osmotic shrinking of normal brain occurred to a significant extent in man it might have the paradoxical effect of causing a tumour or other local mass to enlarge further at the expense of nearby normal brain. In certain circumstances this might make the patient worse, rather than better. In theory, the risk should be least with those agents (e.g. glycerol and mannitol) which, because of their physical properties and lack of active transport systems, are least able to traverse cerebral capillary endothelium.

The use of hypertonic sucrose has led to renal damage (Anderson and Bethea, 1940). Because of this, and because of the various physicochemical considerations discussed above, mannitol and glycerol are at the present time the most commonly used osmotically active cerebral dehydrating agents.

Mannitol and Glycerol

Both substances are used as osmotically active cerebral dehydrating agents, mannitol tending to be used in more acute situations than glycerol. The history of the use of glycerol for this purpose is given by Tourtelotte et al. (1972). Mannitol is also used as an osmotic diuretic, and glycerol is present in preparations intended for local application to the skin and mucosae of the alimentary tract.

Chemistry

Mannitol and glycerol are polyhydric alcohols. Both are neutral polar molecules and soluble in water. Their molecular weights are 182.17 and 92.09 respectively.

Pharmacology

Biochemical Pharmacology
The action of these substances is physical, i.e. osmotic, rather than chemical.

Pharmacodynamics

Both substances are osmotically active cerebral dehydrating agents, as explained above.

Pharmacokinetics

Absorption and bioavailability: Given intravenously, both mannitol and glycerol are completely bioavailable. The molecule of mannitol is a little too large (diameter about 4 Å) in relation to its polarity for it to be absorbed in adequate quantities when given by mouth (Wagner, 1971). If a large enough dose of mannitol is given orally, the amount not absorbed may have a sufficient osmotic effect to produce diarrhoea.

Glycerol is a smaller molecule than mannitol and, despite its polarity, it would appear that after oral administration enough can be absorbed to effect a useful degree of cerebral dehydration.

Distribution: After intravenous administration mannitol, in normal man, is distributed throughout the extracellular fluid. The apparent volume of distribution of mannitol averages 0.159L/kg (Schwartz et al., 1950), i.e. about 11 litres for a 70kg adult.

To some extent glycerol enters cells where it undergoes metabolic transformation, though it does not appear to penetrate the normal blood-brain barrier in significant quantities. Tourtelotte et al. (1972) stated that glycerol's V_D is that of extracellular fluid.

Elimination: Mannitol does not appear to undergo appreciable biotransformation in man (Parke, 1968). It is eliminated from the body by renal excretion. There is no tubular resorption and its renal handling is similar to that of inulin. Knowing that its elimination is entirely by glomerular filtration, and that its volume of distribution corresponds to that of extracellular water, one can calculate that the elimination half-life of mannitol should be about 1.1 hours.

The half-life of plasma glycerol is 30 minutes (Senior and Loridan, 1968). Glycerol is phosphorylated by glyceryl kinase in the liver, and as glycerol-3-phosphate enters the anaerobic glycolytic pathway and Krebs cycle, or else may be transformed to amino acids, e.g. serine. Glycerol may yield energy to the extent of 4.32cals/g. However, it is likely that part of a therapeutic intravenous glycerol load would be excreted unchanged in urine. Once its plasma levels exceed 1mg/ml, glycerol appears in urine (Zilversmit and McCandless, 1957). It is unlikely that much glycerol would be metabolised in the brain even if it crossed the blood-brain barrier, as the required enzyme (α-glycerophosphate dehydrogenase) is poorly developed (Guisado and Arieff, 1975).

Plasma level correlations: Plasma level data for mannitol are not available.

Brain dehydration from glycerol is said to begin within 30 minutes of commencing an intravenous infusion, and to last for up to 9 hours after the infusion ceases.

Tourtelotte et al. (1972) considered that a plasma glycerol level above 10mmol/L was necessary to lower intracranial pressure, while for this purpose Prockop (1976) advised giving sufficient glycerol to maintain plasma osmolarity above 320m osmol/kg.

Interactions
None are known.

Toxicity

Idiosyncratic Toxicity
No idiosyncratic reactions are known.

Dose-related Toxicity
Excessive diuresis from intravenous mannitol or glycerol could lead to electrolyte disturbance e.g. hypokalaemia, hyponatraemia and to hypovolaemic shock. In patients with cardiac failure, rapid infusion of these hyperosmolar agents, with attendant temporary transfer of interstitial water to plasma, may worsen the cardiac decompensation. The use of mannitol may cause uricosuria (Skeith, 1967).

With glycerol concentrations greater than 10% in 0.45% saline, infused at a rate greater than 4.5ml/m, there is some risk of haemolysis (Reinglass, 1974).

In patients with mature onset diabetes mellitus or prediabetes, continued glycerol therapy has been reported to cause non-ketotic hyperosmolar hyperglycaemia which can lead to coma. This coma could be confused with coma due to raised intracranial pressure. The effect appears to occur because glycerol can be utilised as a substrate in glycolysis and it has a gluconeogenic effect, and also an antiketotic effect. The resultant hyperglycaemia can lead to exhaustion of insulin stores in predisposed persons and thus to hyperosmotic hyperglycaemic coma without ketosis (Sears, 1976).

Dysmorphogenicity
No information is available. In the circumstances in which these agents are used in neurology, dysmorphogenicity would rarely be a relevant consideration.

Corticosteroids

The corticosteroids in clinical use in contemporary neurology comprise cortisone itself, its biologically active metabolite hydrocortisone (cortisol), and various synthetic steroids which can be broadly classified as mineralocorticoids or glucocorticoids, according to their predominant patterns of action.

In neurology, cortisone and cortisol are used relatively little — chiefly as replacement therapy in patients with diminished adrenal cortical function secondary to pituitary disease. The mineralocorticoid, fludrocortisone, is also little used in neurology, though it finds a role in retaining salt and raising blood pressure in patients with sufficiently troublesome postural hypotension (e.g. from autonomic neuropathies) when this cannot be treated effectively by other means. On the other hand the synthetic glucocorticoids are among the most important drugs used by the neurologist. They are employed for several purposes:

1) To diminish cerebral oedema, probably by restoring to normal the permeability of the cerebral capillary endothelial layer (Eisenberg et al., 1970)
2) As anti-inflammatory agents (e.g. in meningitis) to prevent the formation of adhesions, and in primary demyelinating disorders, (e.g. multiple sclerosis, though all might not agree that the mechanism of action in the latter is purely an anti-inflammatory one)
3) To suppress immune reactions, as in the Guillain-Barre syndrome, polyarteritis nodosa, polymyositis and myasthenia gravis
4) In hypsarrythmia, where the mode of action is obscure.

The monograph of Cope (1972) provides a great deal of information concerning the corticosteroids.

Chemistry

The corticosteroids have a common molecular structure, cyclopentenoperhydrophenanthrene, as shown in figure 2.2. Relatively small chemical modifications can

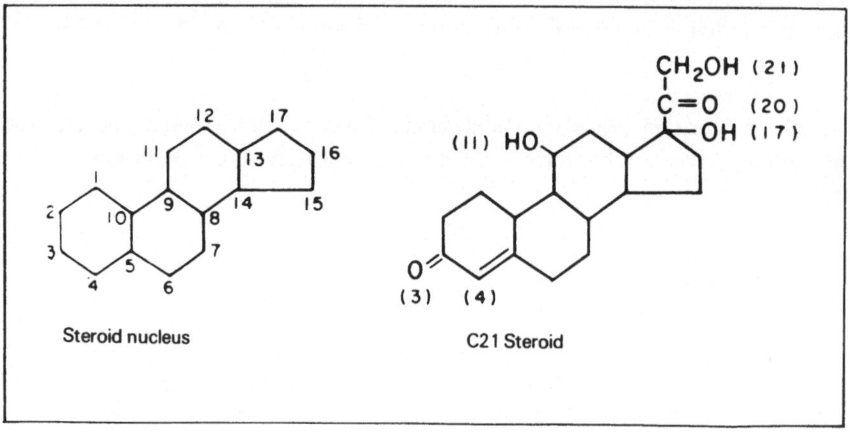

Steroid nucleus   C21 Steroid

Fig. 2.2. Basic steroidal structure.

Table IV. Some corticosteroids

Cortisol i.e. hydrocortisone (MW362.47): the major natural hormone, with mineralocorticoid and
   glucocorticoid activity
Cortisone (MW360.46): the 11-keto derivative of cortisol

Mineralocorticoid
Fludrocortisone (MW380.46): 9α fluorocortisol

Glucocorticoids
Prednisone (MW355.44): Δ^1 Cortisone, i.e. prednisone has the same structure as cortisone except
   for a double bond linking C atoms in the 1 and 2 positions.
Prednisolone (MW360.44): Δ^1 Cortisol, i.e. prednisolone is the 11-hydroxy derivative of prednisone,
   just as cortisol is the 11-hydroxy derivative of cortisone
Methylprednisolone (MW374.46): the 6-methyl derivative of prednisolone
Dexamethasone (MW392.45): 16α methyl-9α fluoro-prednisolone
Betamethasone (MW392.45): 16β methyl-9α fluoro-prednisolone (i.e. dexamethasone and beta-
   methasone are stereo-isomers)
Paramethasone (MW392.45): 16α methyl-6α fluoro-prednisolone

---

selectively and profoundly alter certain pharmacological properties of the molecule.
Some of the more commonly used analogues are listed in table IV.

In terms of therapeutic efficacy (as glucocorticoids) the following doses of the
various steroids appear approximately equal:

cortisone	30mg
cortisol	25mg
prednisone	5mg
prednisolone	5mg
betamethasone and dexamethasone	0.75mg
paramethasone	2.0mg

As a simplification, glucocorticoid and anti-inflammatory activity is increased by
adding a fluorine atom at C_9, and by the presence of a double bond at the C_1 position,
in the basic corticosteroid molecule. The presence of the carbonyl oxygen at C_3, the
C_{4-5} double bond, the --OH group at C_{11}, and the unaltered side chain at C_{17} appear
essential for biological activity. The necessity for a hydroxyl group at the C_{11} position
correlates with the belief that neither cortisone nor prednisone is biologically active
till it undergoes metabolism to cortisol, or prednisolone, respectively.

Pharmacology

Biochemical Pharmacology
Although corticosteroids may have some action on cell membranes and certain
enzymes, the best available evidence suggests that corticosteroids have one dominant

mode of action in vetebrates, irrespective of their target organs and the changes they produce in these organs. It is believed that steroids penetrate into their target cells and bind to high affinity receptors. The steroid-receptor complexes become active and attach to chromatin. These attachments lead to the induction of RNA and protein (enzyme) synthesis. The (enzyme) proteins so formed are responsible for the diverse actions of steroids in the different organs which they affect (Edelman, 1975).

Pharmacodynamics

Mineralocorticoid functions: Mineralocorticoids enhance Na^+ resorption by the cells of the distal renal tubule, and increase the excretion of K^+ and H^+ from these cells into the urine. They have similar actions on cation transport across cell membranes in other tissues. They produce salt and water retention in the body with expansion of extracellular fluid volume, and a degree of hypernatraemia, hypokalaemia and alkalosis.

Glucocorticoid and associated functions: Glucocorticoids act by:

1) Increasing glucose formation and its storage as glycogen. Proteins in various tissues are broken down and their amino acid products are metabolised to glucose in the liver. There is thus a tendency to hyperglycaemia, glycosuria and an increased insulin requirement. The tendency to protein breakdown may affect:

   a) skeletal muscle, causing wasting and myopathy;
   b) lymphoid tissue, which is reduced in bulk. This can have immunosuppressive consequences (see 3 below);
   c) bone, leading to osteoporosis.

2) Decreasing formation of DNA in many tissues. This can delay growth and wound healing.

3) Preventing or suppressing inflammation. Oedema formation lessens (probably owing to decreased capillary permeability) and fibrin formation, capillary dilatation, leucocyte and phagocyte reaction are lessened. At later stages in the inflammatory process collagen formation and scarring lessen. To some extent this anti-inflammatory action may depend on the steroid decreasing DNA formation (see 2 above). This anti-inflammatory action may be responsible for dexamethasone inhibiting the expansion of experimental subdural haematomas in rats (Glover and Labadie, 1976).

4) Diminishing immune responses (actions 1, 2 and 3 are also likely to contribute to this effect).

5) Altering subcutaneous fat distribution (e.g. producing the 'moon' face and 'buffalo hump' of Cushing's syndrome).

6) Altering mood and personality. The mechanisms involved in these effects are uncertain.

7) Improving the hypsarrhythmic type of infantile epilepsy. Here the mode of action of steroids is obscure.

8) There is now some evidence that high doses of steroids may inhibit the growth of experimental gliomas (Gurcay et al., 1971) and reduce thymidine incorporation into such tumours (Shapiro and Posner, 1974).

The main use of steroids in neurology is in connection with their anti-inflammatory and/or immunosuppressive effects, and their effects on glioma growth.

Pharmacokinetics

Absorption and bioavailability: When given *by mouth* cortisone is said to be fully absorbed, though its congener, the more biologically active natural hormone cortisol, is less well absorbed from the alimentary tract. There is some clinical circumstantial evidence that the bioavailabilities of prednisone and prednisolone after oral intake may be variable and incomplete (Sugita and Niebergall, 1973). The drugs are usually absorbed rapidly, and after oral administration peak plasma levels occur in approximately 1 hour (English et al., 1975). Because of faster dissolution, bioavailability problems might be a little less likely with the rather more water-soluble prednisolone than with prednisone.

Dexamethasone appears to be absorbed reasonably well. Duggan et al. (1975) showed that oral dexamethasone tablets had a 78.0 ± 12.1% bioavailability as compared with an 82.6 ± 17.7% bioavailability of the drug when given as an elixir. Peak plasma levels occurred 1 to 3 hours after oral administration.

Intramuscular cortisone acetate is absorbed more slowly than oral cortisone. In consequence its action is more delayed and lasts longer. For up to 8 hours after administration, intramuscular cortisol produces lower plasma cortisol levels than does the same drug dose given orally. For practical purposes a single intramuscular injection of 200mg cortisol might easily have no neurologically useful action for 8 hours after its administration.

Intravenous steroid is immediately available for distribution throughout the circulation. The more water-soluble steroid esters, e.g. the succinates, should be injected intravenously. The esters appear to be rapidly hydrolysed after injection, releasing the active drug. Hare et al. (1975) have shown that dexamethasone phosphate injected intravenously into man results in peak levels of the biologically active free alcohol in 10 minutes. They showed an overall hydrolysis of 90% of the dose of the phosphate, with the rate of the reaction so fast that the conversion seemed likely to occur within cells and not simply within the circulation.

Steroids are administered *intrathecally* to obtain high local concentrations and/or prolonged local actions of the drugs. Systemic absorption is undesirable in these instances (e.g. spinal arachnoiditis) though there is evidence that some absorption does occur (Seghal et al., 1963; Lehrer et al., 1973). Preparations with a low water solubility, e.g. acetates, are used since there are suggestions that the more water-soluble steroids may ionise too rapidly, and set up a chemical meningitis (Irvine, 1975). However, there has been a report (Bernat et al., 1976) that polyethylene glycol, the vehicle in one commercial preparation of methylprednisolone acetate, is itself an irritant which can produce a sclerosing pachymeningitis. Given intrathecally, methylprednisolone acetate produces very high local steroid concentrations in brain and cord near the injection site (Lehrer et al., 1973). One day after methylprednisolone acetate is injected into the lumbar theca, local CSF steroid levels are very much higher than cisternal CSF steroid levels (Sehgal and Gardner, 1963).

Distribution: Apart from plasma protein binding little is known of corticosteroid distribution in man. The V_D of cortisol corresponds to that of extracellular water (Peterson, 1959). The V_D of prednisolone (54-90 litres) and the V_D of prednisone both increase with increasing drug dose (Meikle et al., 1972; Tanner et al., 1979). The calculated apparent volume of distribution of methylprednisolone (1.5L/kg i.e. 105 litres for a 70kg adult) is greater than the actual volume of body water, suggesting that the drug is concentrated at some site in the body, possibly intracellularly.

In plasma the various corticosteroids are carried bound to a specific cortisol-binding α-globulin, though some cortisol also binds to albumin. The percentage of steroid bound to plasma protein tends to fall as steroid concentration rises. At 37°C, 93% of endogenous plasma cortisol (normal range 6 to 16µg/100ml) is protein-bound. At total cortisol levels of 10µg/100ml, 95% of the hormone is bound. At levels of 100µg/100ml only 75% is bound. At concentrations greater than 70µg/100ml prednisolone is approximately 60% bound, but the percentage bound is higher at lower steroid plasma levels. Dexamethasone is said to be about 77% bound, and fludrocortisone 70 to 79% bound. The various corticosteroids may compete with each other or with other drugs for plasma protein-binding sites. Levels of cortisol-binding globulin rise in late pregnancy. In states of hypoalbuminaemia, plasma water prednisolone levels, and biological effects, are increased relative to prednisone dose (Lewis et al., 1971).

Cortisol concentrations in CSF are similar to those in plasma water. Even after high dosage, little cortisol or prednisolone is present in milk (McKenzie et al., 1975).

In cats after intrathecal administration of methylprednisolone acetate, steroid levels are higher in white than in grey matter (Lehrer et al., 1973).

Elimination: Corticosteroids are eliminated by biotransformation and excretion. The approximate elimination half-lives are shown in table V.

The half-lives of the biological effects of these steroids are a good deal longer than their plasma half-lives. Thus prednisone has a biological half-life of 12 to 36 hours, and dexamethasone a biological half-life of 36 to 52 hours (Dobkin, 1977).

Corticosteroid biotransformation occurs mainly in the liver, but some biotransformation is extrahepatic. The 11-oxy compounds (cortisone and prednisone) are thought to be biologically inactive. They are rapidly reduced in the healthy liver by the enzyme 11-β hydroxysteroid dehydrogenase, forming respectively their pharmacologically active counterparts cortisol and prednisolone. These reactions are bi-

Table V. Corticosteroid elimination half-lives

Corticosteroid	Half-life (hours)
Cortisone	0.5-2.0 (or 23-35m)[1]
Cortisol	1.5-2.0[2]
Fludrocortisone	0.5
Prednisone	1.0
Prednisolone	**3.5**[3,4]
Methylprednisolone	3.5
Dexamethasone	3.0-4.5, or 3.2-5.4[5]

1 Peterson et al., 1957.
2 Peterson, 1959.
3 Leclercq and Copinschi, 1974.
4 Tanner et al., 1979.
5 Hichens and Hogans, 1974.

directional. However, for the above drugs and derivatives, in dogs the dominant corticosteroid in plasma is the drug given (Colburn et al., 1976). There is some evidence that the steroid reduction reaction may be less efficient in patients with liver disease (Powell and Axelsen, 1972). If steroids are to be used in patients with liver disease, cortisol or prednisolone may thus be preferable to cortisone or prednisone.

The basic steroid molecule may undergo a number of further hepatic biotransformations, which have been worked out in some detail for cortisol and which may apply to its congeners. The reactions decrease the biological activity of the steroid. These reactions comprise:

oxidation at C_2, forming a hydroxy derivative
reduction at C_3, forming a hydroxy derivative
reduction of the C_{4-5} double bond
oxidation at C_6, forming a hydroxy derivative
reduction at C_{20}, forming 2 isometric hydroxy derivatives
reversible oxidation at the C_{11} position.

The various derivatives are excreted in urine, largely in conjugated form, as glucuronides and sulphates. Conjugation occurs at the C_1 position. These conjugations occur mainly in the liver but to a minor extent in the kidneys. Little cortisol metabolite is excreted in bile or faeces. About 90% of the metabolite appears in the urine.

Some 10 to 30% of a prednisolone dose is excreted unchanged in urine. Prednisone in urine accounts for 1 to 10% of the prednisolone dose; 3 to 12% is excreted as 20α-hydroxy prednisolone and 3 to 10% as 20β-hydroxy prednisolone, while 2 to

6 % of the dose is excreted as 20-hydroxy prednisone derivatives. From 20 to 40 % of metabolites are excreted unconjugated.

Plasma level correlations: Data are not available correlating plasma steroid levels with their pharmacological effects when used to treat neurological disease. Because of the biochemical mechanism of action of steroid hormones, *viz* formation of new intracellular protein with specific functions, it might be anticipated that the time course of their pharmacological effects might not parallel the concentrations of the drugs in plasma.

Plasma prednisolone levels show a wide scatter when plotted against dose, and the levels are generally similar to those obtained when the same doses of prednisone are used (Wilson et al., 1975).

Interactions

Pharmacodynamic interactions: The gluconeogenic action of the corticosteroids tends to antagonise the antidiabetic actions of insulin and of the various oral hypoglycaemic agents. The mineralocorticoid effects that lead to sodium retention and hypokalaemia can allow steroids to augment the potassium-losing effects of amphotericin B (Chung and Koenig, 1971), or of diuretics such as frusemide or ethacrynic acid (Thorn, 1966).

Pharmacokinetic interactions: These are of 2 types: consequences of hepatic enzyme microsomal induction and competition for plasma binding sites.

1) Prior or concurrent administration of drugs e.g. phenobarbitone, butobarbitone and phenytoin, which induce the hepatic microsomal mixed oxidase system, can increase the metabolism of corticosteroids and diminish their pharmacological effects. The interaction between phenytoin and dexamethasone is well documented (Jubiz et al., 1970).

2) The various corticosteroids may compete with each other for attachment sites on cortisol-binding globulin. Anti-inflammatory agents such as salicylates and phenylbutazone may compete with corticosteroids for plasma protein-binding sites and increase the amount of steroid free in plasma water.

Toxicity

Idiosyncratic Toxicity
Idiosyncratic side effects of corticosteroids are rare.

Dose-related Toxicity
Corticosteroid therapy may produce a number of dose-related side effects which are listed in table VI.

Table VI. The dose-related side effects of glucocorticoids

Suppression of function of the adrenal-pituitary axis, with consequent decreased ability to resist stress (e.g. in relation to acute infections, trauma and surgery)

Cushing's syndrome with its moon face, buffalo hump, obesity, livid striae, acne, tendency to ecchymoses and hirsutism

Hyperglycaemia and glycosuria

Salt and water retention causing oedema

Hypokalaemic alkalosis

Peptic ulceration

Myopathy

Psychological disorders and sometimes psychoses

Osteoporosis

Decreased resistance to infection

Growth suppression in children

Delayed wound healing

Cataracts and glaucoma

Benign intracranial hypertension, occasionally recurring on steroid withdrawal[1]

---

1 Levine and Leopold, 1973

Dysmorphogenicity

Steroids are teratogenic in mice and rabbits. There is some evidence that steroid therapy given to women in the first trimester of pregnancy may lead to an increased risk of cleft palate in the offspring. Fetal adrenal disturbance does not seem to be a major risk (Cope, 1972).

Corticotrophin (ACTH) and Tetracosactrin

It is convenient to consider these substances with the corticosteroids. Corticotrophin (adrenocorticotrophic hormone: MW 4,500) is a coiled chain polypeptide containing 39 amino acids. It is a natural hormonal secretion of the anterior pituitary and stimulates the adrenal cortex to synthesise and secrete cortisol, aldosterone and related hormones. Tetracosactrin is a synthetic polypeptide which comprises the first 24 amino acids of the corticotrophin molecule in correct sequence. It possesses similar biological activity to the natural hormone.

As far as is known, the value of both substances in neurology depends on their ability to stimulate the formation of adrenal cortical hormones. The therapeutic effects are due to these corticosteroids. ACTH and tetracosactrin have the theoretical advantage over corticosteroids in that they do not suppress adrenal function. However, their use leads to the secretion of steroids with mineralocorticoid and androgenic effects (which are rarely desired in treating neurological disease), as well as to the secretion of steroids with the desired anti-inflammatory effects which appear to be inseparable from glucocorticoid functions. Further, very high doses of cortico-steroids are often needed to treat neurological conditions. Even though large doses of ACTH or tetracosactrin may be given, there can be no certainty that the adrenals will produce a glucocorticoid response comparable to the exogenous dose that can be given; if they do so, the mineralocorticoid effects may be prohibitive. Because of these considerations, and the availability of oral and parenteral corticosteroids with relatively little mineralocorticoid effect, ACTH and tetracosactrin would seem to have little place in clinical neurology. The use of them could be regarded as an incon-venient and quantitatively imprecise way of giving glucocorticoids as well as being more likely to produce unwanted effects. Admittedly, there are some who believe that ACTH and tetracosactrin may have a specific place in treating primary demyelinating disease and hypsarrhythmia. However this belief might be based on a failure to com-pare equivalent doses and a lack of awareness that there may be bioavailability problems with certain prednisone preparations.

If corticotrophin or tetracosactrin is used it has the disadvantage that it must be injected since both polypeptides are destroyed by peptidase enzymes in the alimentary tract. ACTH has a plasma half-life of 15 minutes and its biological effect is deter-mined by the peculiarities of individual adrenal response. Tetracosactrin is said to have a longer duration of action than ACTH. Tetracosactrin and ACTH are usually injected intramuscularly. To delay their absorption, and thus to prolong their action so that they are likely to maintain an adrenal-stimulating effect for 24 hours, they are often provided in gel preparations. Their undesirable effects are those of glucocor-ticoids, with the exception that they do not cause adrenal suppression. Occasionally serious allergic reactions may occur with tetracosactrin (Mohr, 1975). With prolonged use an acquired resistance to ACTH may develop.

Treatment of Raised Intracranial Pressure

Indications

There are two major situations in which raised intracranial pressure will require symptomatic medical treatment. In the first, more acute, situation the aim of short term treatment is either to reduce intracranial pressure for a few hours or days while investigations are done to clarify the diagnosis, permitting specific treatment (e.g. surgery) or to allow time for an intrinsically self-limiting process to resolve (e.g. oedema around a brain infarct or area of trauma). In the second, more chronic, situa-tion long term medical measures must be used for weeks or months to reduce in-tracranial pressure which cannot otherwise be relieved (e.g. inoperable tumour, benign intracranial hypertension).

Short Term Treatment of Raised Intracranial Pressure

Clinically apparent benefit from corticosteroids usually takes 24 to 48 hours to appear in patients with raised intracranial pressure. If a more rapid therapeutic effect is needed intravenous glycerol or mannitol should be used initially. Even so it would be logical to prescribe corticosteroids concurrently so that they could take over the pressure reduction after a day or two. It is possible that the corticosteroids might tend to restore the integrity of the blood-brain barrier if this was defective locally. This might reduce the risk of rebound rise in CSF pressure, and differential expansion of the abnormal area of brain at the expense of its surroundings during use of the osmotic dehydrating agent.

Osmotically Active Agents

For rapid reduction of intracranial pressure intravenous mannitol in a 20% or 25% solution is infused (to a total dose of 1.5 to 2.0g/kg) over approximately 30 minutes i.e. approximately 500 to 700ml of a 20% solution for a 70kg adult. By this time benefit may have begun to appear. The pressure reduction is likely to last several hours, and the procedure may then be repeated. During infusion the patient should be watched for evidence of circulatory overload. Appropriate nursing care should be available, the patient's airway maintained and respiration assisted if necessary. Venous congestion of the head is reduced if the head can be kept at a higher level than the chest. The hyperosmotic infusion is likely to produce a diuresis, and in unconscious patients or persons with micturation difficulties catheterisation is advisable.

As an alternative to mannitol, 10% glycerol in glucose solution or in saline may be given intravenously. The total daily dose of glycerol is approximately 1.2g/kg, i.e. about 850ml of a 10% solution for a 70kg adult. If the rate of infusion of the 10% solution does not exceed 250ml/h there should be little risk of haemolysis (Reinglass, 1974). Such an infusion rate used initially is slowed after 0.5 to 1 hour, by which stage intracranial pressure should have begun to fall. Considerations as to general care of the patient are as for intravenous mannitol.

Steroids

If the patient can swallow, and is unlikely to vomit, corticosteroids can be given by mouth in the expectation that they will achieve peak plasma levels 1 to 2 hours after administration. Prednisone or prednisolone in doses of 100 to 250mg/day may be used for an adult, and smaller doses for a child. It should be remembered that, in general, children metabolise drugs faster than adults, hence, relative to adults, children usually require higher doses of drugs than might be expected on the basis of body weight. Equal fractions of the steroid dose may be given 6-hourly. Alternatively dexamethasone or betamethasone can be used in a dose of 4 to 8mg 3 or 4 times daily. In patients with raised intracranial pressure it is preferable to err rather on the side of too large a dose of steroid than too small a dose.

If the patient cannot swallow, steroids are often injected intramuscularly. It may prove hazardous to rely on a therapeutic effect occurring within a few hours of the first intramuscular injection of a corticosteroid. Adequate data are not available as to how rapidly glucocorticoids enter the circulation after intramuscular injection, but for a number of important drugs (e.g. phenytoin, diazepam, digoxin) it has now been shown that absorption is appreciably slower after intramuscular than after oral administration in people with normal alimentary function. At least for cortisone acetate, it is known that intramuscular injection leads to slow absorption. Therefore, in a situation in which rapid systemic availability of steroid may be of decisive importance, it seems reasonable to suggest that if steroids cannot be swallowed they should be injected intravenously in the same dosage, and at the same intervals, as if given by mouth (at least for the first day of therapy). Oral and intravenous doses are similar since the various steroids seem to have reasonably complete bioavailabilities when given orally. If the patient is unable to swallow, a sufficient steroid dose may be given intravenously for 24 hours and the same dose also given intramuscularly in divided doses 2 or 3 times a day from the outset. It seems likely that after 24 hours enough steroid will be entering the circulation from the intramuscular injection sites to allow the intravenous use of steroid to cease, if desired, while the intramuscular therapy is continued. However, in general, once the patient can swallow, orally administered steroids are usually more reliable than steroids given by intramuscular injection.

Long Term Treatment of Raised Intracranial Pressure

If definitive action to remedy the situation (e.g. removal of a space-occupying lesion) is not possible within a few days after the above measures have brought raised intracranial pressure under control, continued medical treatment for weeks or months may be required. In these circumstances parenteral therapy is rarely practicable.

Osmotically Active Agents

To avoid steroid side effects it is possible to use oral glycerol, mixed with orange, lemon or tomato juice to make the taste more acceptable. The initial glycerol dose is 1.5g/kg/day (e.g. approximately 100g of glycerol per day for a 70kg adult), but the dose should be varied according to the clinical response and the patient's acceptance of the treatment. Some patients may be able to take such therapy with benefit for many weeks (Newkirk et al., 1972) until a self-limiting condition, such as benign intracranial hypertension, resolves. If glycerol is to be used for more than a day or so, it is wise to keep checking plasma electrolyte and glucose concentrations, perhaps initially at intervals of 2 to 3 days, in case it is necessary to correct electrolyte imbalance or hyperglycaemia.

Steroids

Often patients find long term orally administered glycerol unacceptable (mainly because of its taste) and steroids have to be used. In the great majority of instances chronically raised intracranial pressure is due to inoperable primary or secondary brain tumours. Here the side effects of continued use of high dose glucocorticoids are often an acceptable price to pay for comfortable survival for weeks and months beyond the time at which the patient might otherwise have been expected to die. In such long term use of steroids the clinician should reduce the dose progressively once intracranial pressure is controlled. e.g. dexamethasone to perhaps 4mg per day. He should prescribe the lowest dose that keeps the patient comfortable. adjusting the dose as needed every few weeks and dealing with treatable steroid side effects as they occur (e.g. dyspepsia).

While the medical measures discussed above offer no complete answer to the problems of raised intracranial pressure. they often afford temporary relief and thus give the neurologist or neurosurgeon time to investigate the patient. and to organise treatment. These measures can also greatly improve the quality and duration of survival in patients with chronically raised intracranial pressure due to incurable tumours.

Recently there has been interest in producing barbiturate coma to lower the intracranial pressure (Rockoff et al., 1979). Cerebral metabolism decreases, cerebral blood flow falls, and the intracranial pressure is reduced. The procedure has not yet come into routine use.

Chapter III

Disorders of Motor Function, I:
Voluntary Movement Disorders

Principal Disorders and Drugs Discussed

Myasthenia

    Corticosteroids, see also chapter II
    Anticholinesterases
    Guanidine

Myotonia

    Quinine
    Procainamide
    Phenytoin, see also chapter VI
    Corticosteroids, see also chapter II

Spasticity

    Baclofen
    Diazepam, see also chapter VI
    Dantrolene

Bell's Palsy

    Corticosteroids, see also chapter II

Periodic paralysis

    Acetazolamide

There are a number of voluntary movement disorders which are, to different degrees, amenable to drug treatment. These treatable disorders will be considered in the following order:

myasthenia
myotonia
spasticity
facial palsy
periodic paralysis.
The involuntary movement disorders will be discussed in chapter IV.

Myasthenia

Disordered Mechanisms

The term myasthenia implies pathological fatigability and weakness in voluntary muscle following use, with at least partial recovery after rest. In myasthenia it appears that too little acetylcholine activity is present at the myoneural junction to maintain normal muscle contraction. Whether the primary fault is pre-junctional or post-junctional is arguable (Drachman et al., 1976). Because of a reduced amplitude of miniature end plate potentials (Elmquist et al., 1964) it has been suggested that, in myasthenia gravis, individual 'quanta' of acetylcholine (collections of acetylcholine molecules released when a storage granule discharges from an axon terminal) are of smaller than normal size, though they are normal in number. In the less common myasthenic syndrome (Eaton-Lambert syndrome), often but not always associated with malignant disease elsewhere in the body, the acetylcholine quanta appear of normal size (Brown and Johns, 1974), though fewer than the normal number of quanta are released by each action potential reaching the nerve terminal (Lambert and Elmquist, 1971). The physiological defect of the myasthenic syndrome appears similar to that of botulism, though the defects in the two conditions are not quite identical (Gutmann, 1976). In both myasthenia gravis and the myasthenic syndrome, the response of muscle to each nerve impulse is reduced, with consequent weakness.

As well as the above evidence favouring a pre-junctional site for the defect in myasthenia gravis, there is evidence for a post-junctional defect. Circulating antibodies to the acetylcholine receptor are formed in myasthenia gravis (Almon and Appel, 1976). It is thought that these antibodies may compete with acetylcholine for the receptors at neuromuscular junctions in myasthenia gravis. Thus the response to the available acetylcholine is reduced. In myasthenia gravis antibodies may also form against proteins in the terminal axon. These antibodies could have pre-junctional effects.

In myasthenia gravis Simpson (1960) suggested that the relevant antibodies may be synthesised in the thymus (in some 10% of cases there are thymic tumours) and, particularly at later stages of the disorder, also in the lymphocyte collections (lymphorrhages) which develop in muscle. The event that initiates the abnormal antibody production remains obscure, though at times it may be associated with emotional factors. In some instances abnormal antibody production may not be directed solely against the acetylcholine receptor or other proteins found in the myoneural junction region. There is also an association between myasthenia gravis and certain autoimmune conditions such as thyroid disorder, diabetes mellitus and polymyositis.

The events involved in myasthenia gravis may be schematised as in figure 3.1.

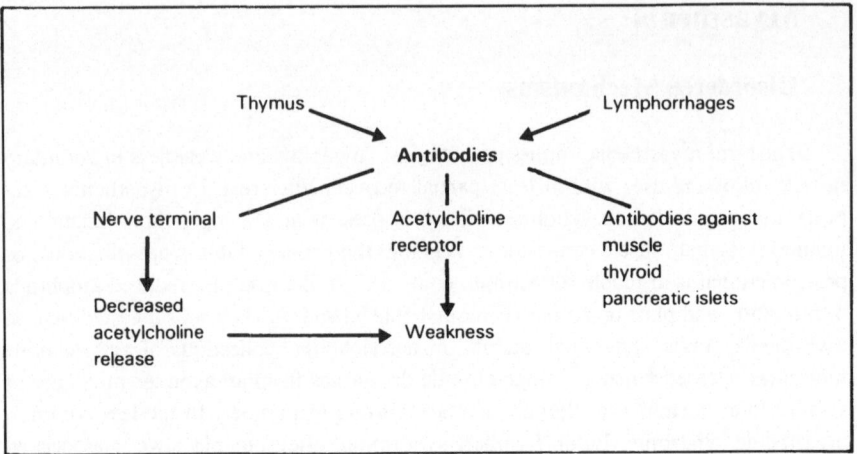

Fig. 3.1. Schematic representation of the events involved in myasthenia gravis.

Correction of Disordered Mechanisms

There are two main therapeutic possibilities in myasthenia: preventing the formation of abnormal antibodies and increasing the amount of acetylcholine present at myoneural junctions, to enhance the activation of post-junctional membrane receptors. Plasmapheresis may remove enough antibody to give temporary benefit.

Preventing Antibody Production

In the early stages of myasthenia gravis most of the abnormal antibody production is thought to occur in the thymus. Thymectomy (also indicated if there is a thymoma), possibly thymic irradiation, and surgical removal of non-thymic tumours causing the myasthenic syndrome, may therefore improve or cure myasthenia if lymphorrhages in muscle are not making a major contribution to antibody production.

Once there are multiple areas of antibody formation throughout the body, chemotherapy is required to suppress antibody production. Various types of immunosuppressive agent may be used, but at the time of writing high dosage synthetic adrenal corticosteroids are the chief agents employed. There is much current interest in using steroids in bolus doses every second day, given in an attempt to achieve immunosuppression while minimising steroid side effects (e.g. adrenal cortical suppression). This mode of steroid administration may permit continued therapy for many months or years, without prohibitive consequences.

Increasing Acetylcholine Concentrations at Myoneural Junctions

In axon terminals, acetylcholine is synthesised from choline and acetyl groups in the presence of the enzyme choline acetylase (choline acetyl transferase). After release from storage granules in axon terminals, and before or after attachment to post-junctional receptors, acetylcholine is inactivated by hydrolysis — acetyl groups and choline forming again. This hydrolysis is catalysed by the enzyme acetylcholinesterase. In theory acetylcholine concentrations at the motor end plate could be increased by:

1) Increasing acetylcholine synthesis and increasing acetylcholine release
2) Decreasing acetylcholine inactivation.

At present there is no known practicable method of increasing acetylcholine synthesis in man. A drug such as carbamylcholine may displace preformed acetylcholine from storage granules or normal axon terminals, though this action does not appear useful in treating myasthenia gravis. The drug guanidine appears to increase the number of acetylcholine quanta per nerve impulse released from axon terminals, and symptomatically may benefit the Eaton-Lambert syndrome, and botulism (Cherington, 1974).

The enzymatic hydrolysis of released acetylcholine can be decreased by various acetylcholinesterase inhibitors. These drugs are the chief therapeutic agents used in treating myasthenia gravis. The main classes of anti-acetylcholinesterase are:

1) Certain carbamyl esters (physostigmine, neostigmine, pyridostigmine, ambenonium and edrophonium)
2) Organophosphorus derivatives.

Only the carbamyl esters are used to treat myasthenia. The action of the organophosphorus anti-acetylcholinesterases persists so long that these substances were at first regarded as irreversible inhibitors of the enzyme. The organophosphorus derivatives are used as insecticides. Because of their prolonged action and consequent risks if given in overdosage they are unsafe for use in human myasthenia.

The sympathomimetic drug ephedrine, potassium salts, and spironolactone (to retain K^+) have been used as adjuvants in treating myasthenia. Whether they are really of benefit is open to doubt.

Drugs Used in Myasthenia

Corticosteroids

These drugs have been considered in detail in chapter II (pages 33-41). They are used in myasthenia for their immunosuppressive effect. It has been found that

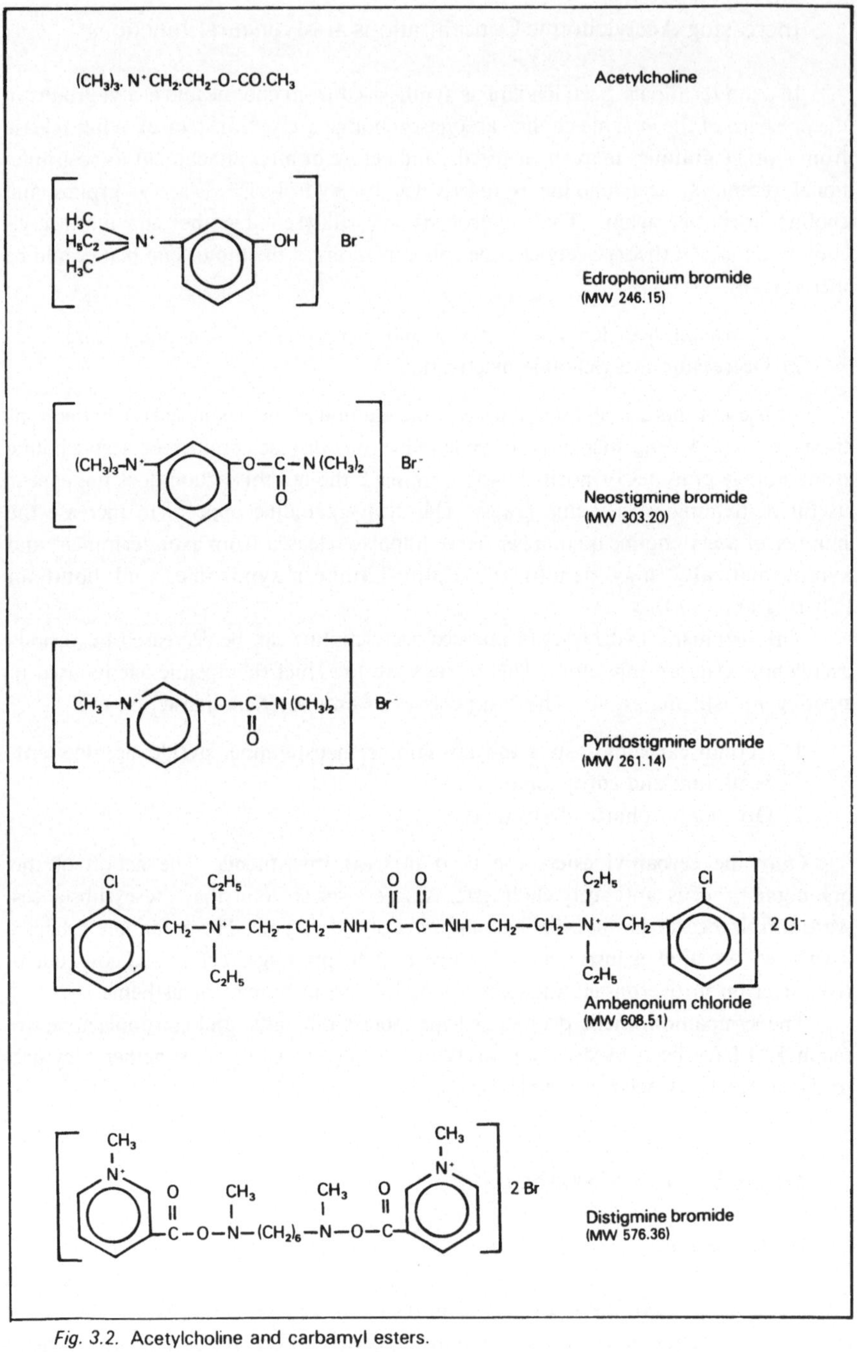

$(CH_3)_3.\,N^+CH_2.CH_2\text{-}O\text{-}CO.CH_3$ Acetylcholine

Edrophonium bromide
(MW 246.15)

Neostigmine bromide
(MW 303.20)

Pyridostigmine bromide
(MW 261.14)

Ambenonium chloride
(MW 608.51)

Distigmine bromide
(MW 576.36)

Fig. 3.2. Acetylcholine and carbamyl esters.

this effect can be achieved by a single large oral steroid dose given once every 48 hours. The elimination half-life of most synthetic glucocorticoids is no more than 2 or 3 hours. Allowing 4 hours for the absorptive phase after oral dosage, within 20 hours of steroid dosage drug concentrations in the body should be negligible, even though the biological effects of the drug may persist for longer. Thus with bolus steroid use, 1 day in 2 is left during which it is hoped endogenous ACTH secretion will not be suppressed by the raised steroid levels in plasma. Consequently the risk of adrenal cortical atrophy may be reduced. This pattern of intermittent high dosage use of steroids also reduces the severity of the side effects associated with excess glucocorticoid (Axelrod, 1976; Dobkin, 1977) while apparently maintaining immunosuppression. Such therapy has been continued for 2 years or more without serious side effects.

Anticholinesterases

The main use of anticholinesterases in human therapeutics is in the diagnosis and treatment of myasthenia.

The carbamyl ester types of anticholinesterase bear structural resemblances to the molecule of acetylcholine (fig. 3.2). All these drugs, except pyridostigmine, are quaternary ammonium derivatives. The synthetic derivatives are set out in figure 3.2 in order of increasing duration of action. They are polar, water-soluble, basic molecules, generally administered as their halogen salts.

Pharmacology

Biochemical pharmacology

Detailed accounts of the biochemical actions of the anticholinesterases are available (Michelson and Danilov, 1971). The enzyme acetylcholinesterase contains two active sites, an anionic one and an esteratic one. The positively charged quaternary nitrogen atom of acetylcholine, or of one of the carbamate types of anticholinesterase, is attracted electrostatically to negative charges in the anionic site of the enzyme. At the esteratic site a covalent bond forms with the carbonyl C atom of acetylcholine. The acetylcholine molecule then cleaves, releasing free choline and leaving the acetyl group bound to the enzyme. The acetyl group then reacts with water to form an acetic acid molecule, which is released from the enzyme molecule (fig. 3.3).

Edrophonium, a potent reversible acetylcholinesterase inhibitor with a short duration of action, competes with acetylcholine for both sites on the enzyme. Thus it prolongs the mean life of acetylcholine molecules at the myoneural junction. Longer acting carbamate inhibitors (neostigmine and pyridostigmine) are also electrostatically attracted to both sites on the active surface of acetylcholinesterase, but

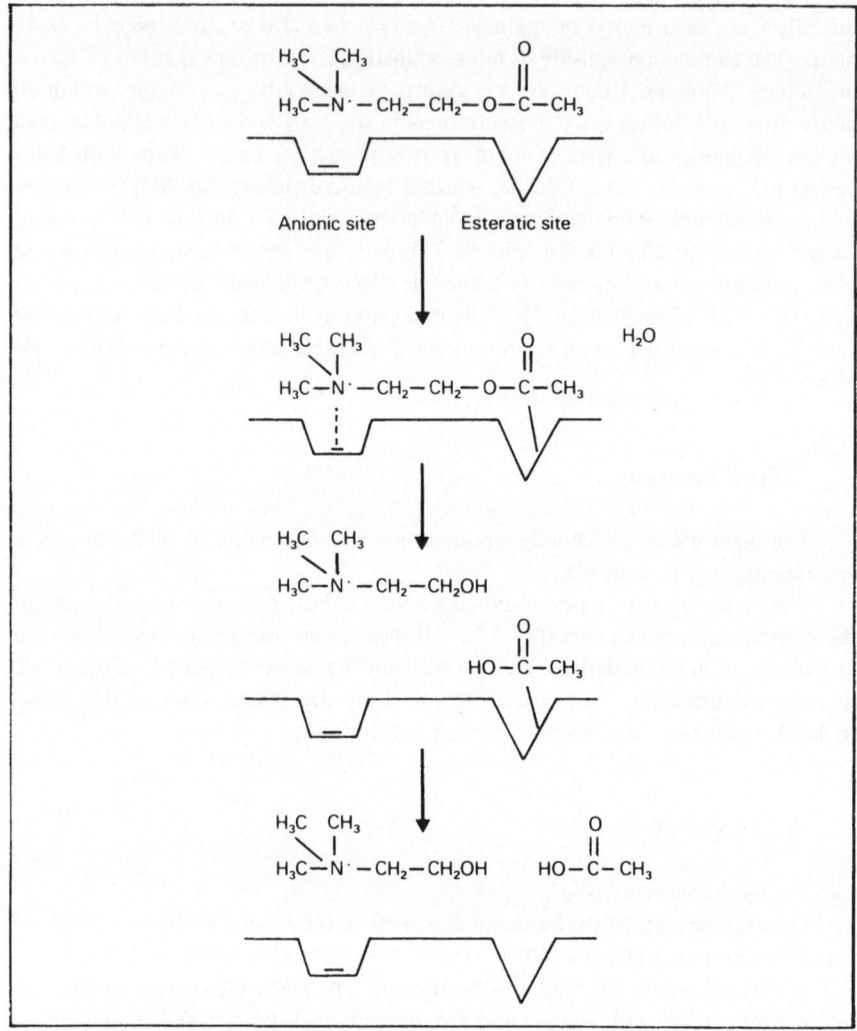

Fig. 3.3. Sequence of reactions undergone by acetylcholine at the acetylcholinesterase receptor.

are not competitively displaced by acetylcholine. Rather they remain bound till they
are slowly hydrolysed by the enzyme. Thus they deny acetylcholine access to the active sites on the enzyme and therefore prolong the presence and increase the concentration of acetylcholine at the myoneural junction, hence increasing the action of
acetylcholine.

The structure of the active sites on the muscle cholinoreceptor is reasonably
similar to that of the active sites on the acetylcholinesterase receptor. Hence the

quaternary nitrogen-containing anticholinesterase drugs may also fit into the cholinoreceptors, and activate them. Therefore a minor portion of the action of these drugs comes about through direct receptor stimulation. This direct effect is least developed in pyridostigmine, in which the charged nitrogen is not a quaternary one, but forms part of a pyridine ring.

Pharmacodynamics

The anticholinesterases used in treating myasthenia enhance the local actions of acetylcholine wherever they gain access to sites of acetylcholinesterase activity. The carbamate esters have their main effects at myoneural junctions. They appear to have some action at autonomic cholinergic sites, but relatively less action on autonomic ganglia. Their lipid solubility is too low for them to enter the central nervous system so that they have no central effects. Their actions on autonomic effector cells and autonomic ganglia, but not on myoneural junctions, are blocked by atropine. Administration of anticholinesterases may cause:

1) Pupil constriction
2) Increased sweating and increased tear production
3) Bradycardia and hypotension
4) Increased motor activity of the stomach, small and large intestine, and urinary bladder
5) In normal persons, increased voluntary muscle contraction, muscle fasciculation and, in overdosage, depolarisation block of myoneural junctions with consequent paralysis
6) Bronchoconstriction.

Pharmacokinetics

Absorption and bioavailability: The quaternary nitrogen-containing anticholinesterases, and pyridostigmine with its charged pyridine ring, are polar water-soluble compounds. One would expect them to be poorly soluble in lipid and hence to be poorly absorbed if given by mouth. The fact that their parenteral dose is less than 10% of their oral dose is consistent with this suggestion, though the possibility of their first-pass metabolism in the liver and gut wall needs clarification. Cohan et al.(1977) obtained direct evidence of impaired bioavailability of pyridostigmine in man. From their physicochemical characteristics one would anticipate that these anticholinesterase agents would be better absorbed from the intestine than from the stomach, where the acid environment would tend to keep the drug molecules ionised.

The greater part of a pyridostigmine dose is thought to remain in the alimentary tract without being absorbed. Therefore it is difficult to see the justification for marketing a sustained release preparation of the drug, unless the unabsorbed drug in the gut is fairly rapidly inactivated after its release from the drug preparation.

Cohan et al. (1976) showed that, in man, orally administered pyridostigmine appeared in blood 0.5 to 1 hour after dosing, and achieved peak plasma levels 1.5 to 2 hours after dosing.

Edrophonium is only given intravenously. As will be explained later, its brief action may depend on its pattern of distribution.

The rate and extent of absorption of anticholinesterases after intramuscular injection is not known with accuracy. Clinically, effects may be seen within 15 minutes. After intravenous injection the effect of edrophonium is apparent within 1 minute.

Distribution: No detailed data are available. Because the drug molecules are polar one would expect them to be distributed mainly in extracellular water and not to cross the blood-brain barrier. In fact, the anticholinesterases do not affect acetylcholine activity within the central nervous system, though they must reach extracellular water to affect myoneural and autonomic ganglionic transmission.

Figures for plasma protein binding of these drugs are not available.

Elimination: After intravenous administration edrophonium has an α phase half-life of 0.54 to 1.92 minutes, and a β phase half-life of 24.23 to 45.00 minutes (Calvey et al., 1976). The short biological action of edrophonium is probably due to its pattern of distribution rather than to fast elimination. The drug is taken up from the circulation by the kidneys and liver, and in the latter organ is converted to an inactive 3-oxo-glucuronide metabolite.

There is no detailed information on the half-lives of the other drugs.

The mode of action of neostigmine and pyridostigmine leads to their cleavage by the enzyme acetylcholinesterase, forming aromatic hydroxy derivatives and substituted carbamic acids. Other cholinesterases might contribute to hydrolysis of these drugs. The hydrolysis products appear in urine. Some 9.4% of a pyridostigmine dose is excreted unchanged in urine (Somani et al., 1972), and 2.5% is excreted as 3-hydroxy-N-methylpyridinium. In the rat the main metabolite of neostigmine is m-hydroxyphenyltrimethylammonium (Robert et al., 1966).

Plasma level correlations: No plasma level data are available, except for pyridostigmine. In a small group of patients, Cohan et al. (1976) appeared to find optimal therapeutic effects with plasma drug concentrations around 4×10^{-8} moles/L, and cholinergic weakness by the time the concentrations were about 6 to 7×10^{-8} moles/L. The nature of myasthenia is such that the clinical response to therapy is usually relatively easy to quantitate. On the basis of clinical observation it may be said that the effects of conventional doses of edrophonium last some 5 to 10 minutes, those of neostigmine last 2 to 4 hours, and those of pyridostigmine and ambenonium 3 to 6 hours.

Interactions

Pharmacodynamic interactions: Atropine antagonises the effects of anticholinesterases on autonomic ganglia and autonomic effector organs. However atropine does not antagonise anticholinesterase effects at skeletal neuromuscular junctions. Thus atropine is useful in preventing certain undesired effects of anticholinesterases.

Non-depolarising neuromuscular blocking agents (e.g. tubocurarine) and aminoglycoside antibiotics (e.g. streptomycin, kanamycin, gentamicin) [Hokkanen, 1964] are pharmacological antagonists to anticholinesterases at the neuromuscular junction. Depolarising neuromuscular blocking agents (e.g. succinylcholine) will also prevent anticholinesterases from acting in myasthenia.

Procainamide stabilises muscle membranes, decreases acetylcholine release at nerve terminals and blocks the action of administered acetylcholine (Drachman and Skom, 1965). Procainamide therefore antagonises anticholinesterases.

Pharmacokinetic interactions: No data are available.

Toxicity

Idiosyncratic Toxicity

We have been unable to trace reports of idiosyncratic side effects of anticholinesterase therapy, though theoretically there might be an increased risk of overdosage in patients with pseudocholinesterase deficiency.

Dose-related Toxicity

Excessive dosage with anticholinesterases may lead to manifestations of excess cholinergic activity, e.g.

miosis
increased salivation
sweating
urinary urgency
gastrointestinal pain and cramps
hypotension
bronchospasm
skeletal muscle fasciculation
cholinergic paresis of skeletal muscle.

Dysmorphogenicity

Dysmorphogenicity from anticholinesterases has not been reported.

Guanidine

Guanidine is used to treat the Eaton-Lambert myasthenic syndrome, and botulism. It has also been used to treat amyotrophic lateral sclerosis, and is said to slow the downhill course of this disorder for several months (Norris et al., 1974).

Chemistry

Guanidine (iminourea, MW 59.07) is a strong base which is freely soluble in water and in ethanol. For pharmaceutical use it is usually supplied as the hydrochloride.

Pharmacology

Biochemical Pharmacology
Guanidine increases the number of acetylcholine quanta released at nerve terminals in response to a single motor nerve action potential (Kamenskaya et al., 1975). It does not alter the postsynaptic response to acetylcholine.

Pharmacodynamics
Guanidine improves voluntary muscle power in the Eaton-Lambert syndrome and in botulism.

Pharmacokinetics
No information is available.

Interactions
No information is available.

Toxicity

Unwanted effects include (Norris et al., 1974):
skin rashes
dry mouth
hypotension, atrial fibrillation
dose-related distal paraesthesiae, irritability, ataxia, confusion
acute paralysis
hypocalcaemia
chronic interstitial nephritis and renal tubular necrosis
bone marrow depression [in 3 of 150 cases (Norris et al., 1974)].

Management of Myasthenia

Localised (Ocular) Myasthenia

In about one-third of patients with myasthenia gravis the disorder remains localised to the external eye muscles. The possibility of underlying disease requiring treatment in its own right e.g. thymoma, should be considered. At least over the first year or two of the disorder, the clinician should remain alert to the possibility that the myasthenia might become generalised. For patients with localised ocular myasthenia an anticholinesterase agent (e.g. pyridostigmine 60mg 3 times a day for an adult, proportionately less for a child) may be prescribed and the response in the affected muscles observed. If the dose at its time of maximum action (usually about 1 to 2 hours after oral administration) does not produce a satisfactory correction of eye muscle paresis, a larger dose is required. If the response at the time of peak action is satisfactory, but does not persist throughout the dosage interval, the dosage interval should be shortened so that the next dose is given about half to one hour before the patient again becomes troubled by his symptoms. Alternatively, if the duration of effect of pyridostigmine is 2 or 3 hours less than that desired, a dose of a shorter acting drug (e.g. neostigmine) can be added about 30 minutes before diplopia or ptosis troubles the patient. Anticholinesterase side effects due to excess autonomic stimulation (abdominal cramps, urinary urgency, excessive sweating and salivation) can be relieved by the oral use of atropine (e.g. 0.6mg 3 times a day) or of a synthetic anticholinergic (e.g. propantheline 15mg 3 times a day).

Ocular myasthenia is sometimes unresponsive to anticholinesterases for weeks or months, then may become responsive. If responsive, the anticholinesterase requirement may vary from time to time. These facts should be borne in mind when ocular myasthenia is treated, and it should be recognised that overdosage with anticholinesterases can produce weakness. Therefore, if an initial anticholinergic dose does not produce an adequate effect, rather than simply increasing the dose, it may first be preferable to give an intravenous injection of the very short-acting anticholinesterase, edrophonium, at the time of expected maximum action of oral anticholinesterase therapy. Edrophonium is given at a rate of about 2mg per minute to a maximum of 10mg unless power in the affected muscles increases, or decreases, at a lesser dosage. A preliminary injection of atropine is sometimes given to prevent autonomic effects of the anticholinesterase. If edrophonium increases power in the affected muscle, a larger dose of pyridostigmine or neostigmine is required. If edrophonium weakens the affected muscles, the patient has already been overdosed, or at the least has attained his maximal response so that a larger dose of pyridostigmine can offer him no benefit and may increase muscle weakness. Judiciously timed test injections of edrophonium can often allow optimal anticholinesterase doses to be found more quickly and more safely than is possible by simply adjusting the dose on the basis of the patient's clinical response. However the fact that the brief action of edrophonium is due to its pattern of distribution after intravenous dosage, rather than to rapid elimination, raises the possibility that the effects of edrophonium overdosage might persist much longer than would be suggested by its duration of action when used as a diagnostic agent. No matter how carefully anticholinesterase dosage is adjusted it may occasionally be impossible to control ocular myasthenia completely. The clinician may then have to decide whether to attempt to reduce autoantibody production if the patient's symptoms are sufficiently troublesome. As experience with immunosuppression grows, clinicians may be increasingly willing to use steroids in these circumstances (Mann et al., 1976).

Generalised Myasthenia

As in the case of localised myasthenia the possibility of underlying disease e.g. thymoma, should be considered not only when therapy is instituted but throughout the course of the disorder.

Anticholinesterase Therapy

At the present time most clinicians would probably begin treatment of myasthenia gravis with anticholinesterases. The mode of prescribing these drugs, and of adjusting dosages, perhaps with the aid of edrophonium injections, is as described above for the treatment of localised (ocular) myasthenia. The clinician needs to be aware that anticholinesterase requirement in some patients is not static during the earlier months of their myasthenia, so that doses may need repeated adjustment. Doses that may allow a myasthenic patient adequate power when he is living quietly in hospital may prove quite inadequate a few days later when he attempts to resume his normal activities. Not all muscles have the same requirement for anticholinesterase in the myasthenic. Often the external eye muscles require more anticholinesterase than the rest of the musculature. Diplopia may continue to trouble the patient until enough drug is given to correct the paresis in his external eye muscle completely. However the doses required to produce an optimal response in the eye muscles may produce cholinergic weakness from overdosage in other muscles, including the respiratory muscles. The myasthenic may then have to accept a less than perfect response in some muscles in order to preserve adequate function in more vital ones.

Cholinergic crisis and its differential diagnosis: Cholinergic crisis is always a danger in treating myasthenia with anticholinesterases. Often the story of a cholinergic crisis is that the patient has felt weak after his usual doses of anticholinesterase. Consequently increasing doses have been prescribed, or have been taken without prescription. However, power may not have improved, and may have deteriorated further. Typically the pupils are small and the palms sweaty, unless the patient is also taking an anticholinergic agent to relieve anticholinesterase effects on his alimentary tract, or elsewhere. If weakness increases briefly after edrophonium is injected intravenously, the patient has cholinergic weakness. (It is advisable to have atropine ready for intravenous use in case autonomic effects of edrophonium distress the patient). Reduced anticholinesterase dosage may then lead to improvement. If power increases after edrophonium is given, the patient is underdosed. If the response to edrophonium is equivocal, as it may be, it is wise to assume that the patient has cholinergic weakness, and to reduce the anticholinesterase dose. Whenever the anticholinesterase dose is reduced in a patient who is already weak, facilities for assisted respiration should be available.

To obtain an optimal response from anticholinesterase therapy in myasthenia it may be necessary to organise critically timed dosage with one or two anticholinesterases with different durations of action. Such therapy may make great demands on the endurance and courage of the patient, and on the patience and skill of the physician. However, as time passes, myasthenia in the patient often becomes more stable and anticholinesterase therapy is correspondingly easier to manage.

Adjuvants: The uses of potassium salts, spironolactone, or triamterene (Satoyoshi et al., 1964) to raise intracellular K^+ levels, or the use of ephedrine, have been suggested as adjuvants in treating myasthenia. The usefulness of these measures is open to question. Suppression of ovulation by hormonal means has been reported to help relieve premenstrual exacerbations of myasthenia (Frankel, 1964).

Suppression of Antibody Production

Thymectomy: Till quite recently the only serious attempt to suppress autoantibody production in myasthenia gravis was by thymectomy, though in the past it was not realised that the operation removed a major source of antibody formation. Following Simpson's (1958) investigations, thymectomy was thought to yield best results in females under the age of 35 years who had suffered from myasthenia for less than 5 years, and who did not have a thymoma. However, it was fairly generally accepted that thymectomy might benefit any patient, irrespective of age, sex or duration of disorder. In practice, the operation was restricted to patients in whom medical treatment failed, and to patients found to have a thymoma (which might or might not have been irradiated prior to surgery). If myasthenia did benefit from thymectomy the improvement often did not develop till weeks or months after operation. The postoperative course was often stormy, requiring careful attention to anticholinesterase dose, and sometimes assisted respiration.

Now that thymectomy is seen as removing a major site of autoantibody production the argument is being advanced that the operation should be considered early in the course of generalised myasthenia, before the lymphorrhages take over a significant role in antibody formation. Anticholinesterase treatment may still be required, but there is the hope that early thymectomy, with or without immunosuppressive chemotherapy, may reduce the severity of the disorder, perhaps let it become inactive sooner and avoid the secondary myopathy which often develops later in the disease. At least in younger people with severe myasthenia of recent onset, there may now be a reasonably strong argument for early thymectomy, plus immunosuppression, though possibly immunosuppression alone might suffice. Thus Mann et al. (1976) advocate the use of steroids to achieve immunosuppression, with anticholinesterases as necessary to control weakness, in all cases except for instances of mild ocular myasthenia. Once maximum improvement occurs thymectomy is considered.

Steroids: Over the years since Simon's (1935) report, occasional patients with myasthenia have been treated with ACTH, often when they were in myasthenic crisis. Initially their weakness might worsen, even to a dangerous degree, but after several days there was sometimes a period of useful improvement lasting perhaps for weeks or months (Liversedge et al., 1974). Continued high dosage corticosteroids (e.g. 60mg methylprednisolone daily) proved to have similar benefits after a short initial delay (Brunner et al., 1972). However, long term continuous ACTH therapy tended to be precluded because of steroid side effects. At about the time when cortico-steroids were seen to fulfil a possible immunosuppressive role in myasthenia gravis, it was also recognised that steroids might still produce immunosuppression in myasthenia gravis if given in high dosage once each 48 hours (Warmoults et al., 1970). Such bolus dosage considerably reduced steroid side effects (Pinelli et al., 1974). Unfortunately this technique of steroid use is not invariably successful (Howard et al., 1976).

In myasthenia gravis, oral prednisone or prenisolone may be given in a bolus dose of 100mg every second morning, and this regime can be continued for months or years. Sometimes, but not always, myasthenia may worsen for the first few days of such treatment (Brunner et al., 1976), so that it is desirable to observe the patient closely over this time. Seybold and Drachman (1974) claimed that this deterioration could be avoided by beginning prednisone in a dose of 25mg every second day, with a gradual dose increase to 100mg on alternate days. When improvement begins, and this may not happen for several weeks, the patient often feels stronger on the after-noon of his steroid dose, and worse again the next day. Occasionally the peak benefit is on the second morning. As time passes the period of improvement over each steroid dosage interval often lengthens and the requirement for anticholinesterases drops. If this is not appreciated it is possible that the patient's weakness may worsen, because of cholinergic intoxication.

After 1 or 2 years of full steroid dosage it may prove possible to reduce slowly the size of the individual steroid bolus. Ultimately the patient may be left taking con-siderably lower doses of prednisone (e.g. 25mg every second or third day). He may then take small amounts of anticholinesterase once or twice a day, or perhaps no anti-cholinesterase at all, while leading a moderately active life. Steroid side effects are relatively slight, and sometimes not clinically detectable, even after more than 2 years of high dosage bolus steroid therapy. Sufficient time has not yet passed for it to be known whether such steroid therapy can be stopped, with permanent cure. After 2.5 years of treatment one of the author's patients was able to omit steroids for 3 months, but then resumed therapy as she began to find she was becoming fatigued again in her occupation as a shopkeeper.

Prednisone or prednisolone may be replaced by other steroids, such as dexamethasone or betamethasone, used in this way (Brunner et al., 1976). The use of bolus high dosage steroids has proved a major advance in the treatment of myasthenia and may become the treatment of choice for all but the mildest cases. In older people with reasonably stable but troublesome myasthenia gravis, such use of steroids may be effective in producing considerable sustained improvement in strength, without the necessity for thymectomy.

Other immunosuppressants: If corticosteroids and thymectomy fail, there may be a place for the use of other immunosuppressants e.g. azathioprine.

The Eaton-Lambert Myasthenic Syndrome

In this condition the treatment appropriate to any underlying malignancy is given where possible. The myasthenia often does not respond fully to anticholinesterases and the response lessens with time; guanidine is said to be a more satisfactory treatment. The initial dose of guanidine recommended is 250mg 3 times a day orally, but the dose may be increased to 2 or 3 times this amount, if necessary, to help control the condition. The expected pattern of side effects from excess cholinergic action may occur, together with other unwanted effects as listed on page 56). Caffeine has an action similar to guanidine at the terminal motor axon, and may be of some help (Takamori, 1972).

Neonatal Myasthenia

Some children born to myasthenic mothers have temporary myasthenia which wears off after a few days. Affected children suck and swallow poorly and their breathing movements may be weak. If the diagnosis of neonatal myasthenia is confirmed by the intravenous injection of a low dose of edrophonium (0.5-1.5mg), oral or parenteral anticholinesterase therapy is required for a few days till the condition passes off.

Drugs to be Avoided in Myasthenics

A number of drugs can make myasthenic weakness worse and should be avoided where possible. These include aminoglycoside antibiotics, colistin sulphomethate (colistimethate) [Decker and Fincham, 1971], drugs which benefit myotonia, such as phenytoin, procainamide, quinine or quinidine (Drachman and Skom, 1965), and chlorpromazine (McQuiller et al., 1963).

Myotonia

Myotonia is an abnormally slow relaxation of voluntary muscle after contraction. Recent work suggests that myotonia may be associated with an inherited defect in cell membranes which affects muscle cells more conspicuously than other body cells (Roses and Appel, 1974). Experimentally, reduced membrane conductance for Cl^- ions can produce a state electrically resembling myotonia (Bretag, 1973). Myotonia occurs in the following disorders:

1) Dystrophia myotonica, where myotonia is accompanied by muscle dystrophy and certain endocrine and ocular changes
2) Myotonia congenita, where myotonia occurs alone
3) Paramyotonia congenita, where myotonia is provoked by cold, and where there may be an associated periodic paralysis syndrome related to altered K^+ metabolism.

Disordered Mechanisms

The details of the cell membrane disorder responsible for myotonia are somewhat uncertain. Myotonia persists even though peripheral motor nerves or neuromuscular junctions are blocked by local anaesthetics. Hence myotonia clearly originates in muscle. The resting potential of the muscle cell membrane appears normal but the electrical resistance of the membrane is increased, due to a reduced permeability to Cl^- ions (Barchi, 1975).

Correction of Disordered Mechanisms

Since the disordered mechanism responsible for myotonia is imperfectly understood it is difficult to devise logical methods of correcting the disorder. Empirically, it is known that drugs which 'stabilise' cell membranes tend to correct myotonia, though the mechanisms involved in the 'stabilisation' are not well understood. Possibly altered membrane Na^+ transport or permeability to Na^+ is involved (Barchi, 1975). Procaine and other membrane-stabilising agents inhibit the Na^+ currents that develop in response to abrupt depolarisation. This effect may offset the reduced membrane Cl^- currents in myotonia. Phenytoin increases net Na^+ influx rate during muscle excitation without altering Na^+ flux in the resting membrane. The effects of an increased Na^+ influx tend to balance the effects of reduced Cl^- permeability of the membrane. Thus myotonia, apparently due to decreased membrane permeability to Cl^- ions, may be corrected by a variety of pharmacological agents which alter the passage of Na^+ ions through membranes.

Drugs Used in Treating Myotonia

Quinine

Quinine is still used as an antimalarial, particularly in chloroquine-resistant cases, and is widely employed to treat nocturnal cramps. It may be used to relieve myotonia.

Chemistry

Quinine is a basic substance (MW 324.41) with a very bitter taste and is relatively poorly soluble in water. It is the chief alkaloid extracted from the bark of the cinchona tree. Quinine has pK_a values of 5.07 and 9.7. Quinidine is the d-isomer of quinine.

Pharmacology

Biochemical Pharmacology
It has been suggested that quinidine, and probably quinine, reduces the availability of the Na^+ carrier mechanism in cell membranes, and so alters membrane properties.

Pharmacodynamics
Quinine has the following actions:

1) Antimalarial schizontocide
2) It increases muscle tension in response to a single supramaximal stimulus, increases the refractory period of muscle, and has a curare-like effect on the motor end plate
3) Local anaesthetic
4) Local (e.g. gastric) irritant
5) Analgesic and antipyretic
6) Oxytocic
7) It acts like quinidine on the heart, depressing myocardial excitability, conduction velocity and contractility, and also blocks vagal effects on the heart
8) It has a mild hypoprothrombinaemic effect.

Pharmacokinetics
Less pharmacokinetic information is available for quinine than for quinidine.

Absorption and bioavailability: Quinine, given orally, is rapidly absorbed from the upper small intestine. Peak plasma levels occur within 1 to 3 hours of oral dosage.

Distribution: Quinine is extensively bound (90%) to plasma protein. CSF concentrations of the drug are only 2 to 5% of concentrations in whole plasma.

Elimination: Quinine undergoes extensive biotransformation, mainly to hydroxy derivatives (Brodie et al., 1951). The 2-hydroxy derivative is the chief metabolic product though oxidative scission also occurs (Parke, 1968). Only about 5% of a dose is excreted unchanged. The plasma half-life is about 8.5 hours.

Plasma level correlations: No data are available correlating plasma quinine concentrations with therapeutic effect in myotonia.

Interactions
Pharmacodynamic interactions: The actions of quinine on muscle cell membranes allow it to augment the effects of neuromuscular blocking agents. It may be dangerous to use quinine in patients with myasthenia, in whom there is already a degree of neuromuscular block.

The effect of quinine in decreasing prothrombin synthesis in the liver can increase the effects of coumarin anticoagulants.

Pharmacokinetic interactions: Quinine may compete with the anti-malarial pyrimethamine for plasma protein binding sites, so that the use of either drug may increase the effect of the other by increasing its concentrations free in the biophase.

Quinine, a base, may react with acidic groups on the heparin molecule, diminishing the anticoagulant action of heparin.

Toxicity

Idiosyncratic Toxicity
The following unwanted effects may occur:

1) Thrombocytopenic purpura
2) Agranulocytosis
3) Haemolytic anaemia, which occurs only in pregnant women and persons with malaria.

Table I. The dose-related toxic effects of quinine

Affected system	Consequence
Hearing	Tinnitus, deafness
Vision	Blurring, photophobia, diplopia, visual field defects, ischaemic optic atrophy
Gastrointestinal	Nausea, vomiting, abdominal pain, diarrhoea
Nervous	Headache, confusion, delirium, coma
Liver	Hypoprothrombinaemia
Uterus	Abortion
Heart	Ventricular tachycardia

Dose-related Toxicity

Quinine overdosage (cinchonism) may affect many organ systems, with the consequences listed in table I.

Dysmorphogenicity

The oxytocic effect of quinine raises the possibility that, if the drug is taken in overdosage in pregnancy, it might cause fetal malformation by disturbing the placenta.

Procainamide

The chief use of procainamide is in treating cardiac arrhythmias, but it may be used to relieve myotonia.

Chemistry

Procainamide is *p*-amino-*N*-(2-diethylaminoethyl) benzamide (MW 271.79). Structurally it is very similar to procaine, which contains an ester rather than an amide link between the benzene ring and nitrogen-containing aliphatic portion of the molecule. Procainamide is a basic drug with a pKa of 9.2. It is fairly soluble in water.

Pharmacology

Biochemical Pharmacology

The effects of procainamide, like those of procaine, are probably related to the drug's ability to impair the passage of anions (Na^+, K^+) through cell membranes.

Pharmacodynamics

Procainamide has the following actions:

1) It depresses conductivity and excitability in the myocardium and decreases myocardial contractility
2) It produces peripheral vasodilatation and large doses may cause hypotension
3) It has quinine-like effects on skeletal muscle
4) It has local anaesthetic effects.

Pharmacokinetics

Pharmacokinetic data for the drug are given by Giardina et al. (1976).

Absorption and bioavailability: Absorption of procainamide from the alimentary tract is rapid and reasonably complete. Koch-Weser (1971) quoted a 75 to 100% bioavailability for the drug, given orally. Peak plasma levels occur 1 to 2 hours after oral dosage.

Distribution: About 15% of the procainamide in plasma is protein-bound. The apparent volume of distribution of the drug is 184 ± 24 litres (Galeazzi et al., 1976) or 1.7 to 2.2L/kg (Koch-Weser, 1971), suggesting that is is concentrated in tissues. Except for the brain, procainamide concentrations in most organs are higher than those in plasma. Salivary procainamide levels are higher than plasma levels, suggesting active secretion of the drug into saliva (Galeazzi et al., 1976).

Elimination: The plasma half-life of procainamide in normal persons has been shown by various workers to be: 2.2 to 3.2 hours (Dreyfuss et al., 1972); 2.85 ± 0.25 hours (Weily and Genton, 1972); 2.9 hours (Galeazzi et al., 1976); and 3.5 hours (Koch-Weser and Klein, 1971). The plasma clearance of the drug is 396 to 680ml/m (Koch-Weser, 1971) or 828ml/m (Galeazzi et al., 1976). The proportion of a procainamide dose excreted unchanged in urine has been reported as 40 to 54% (Koch-Weser and Klein, 1971) and 73 to 91% (Giardina et al., 1976). The latter authors found that 7 to 25% of the dose was present in urine as *N*-acetyl-procainamide, 6 to 10% as an unknown metabolite, and less than 0.2% as free or conjugated *p*-aminobenzoic acid, formed by hydrolysis catalysed by plasma esterases. *N*-acetylprocainamide has antiarrhythmic properties (Frislid et al., 1976). Peak plasma levels of this metabolite occur 3 to 8 hours after procainamide dosage. The metabolic products of procainamide are shown in figure 3.4.

Plasma level correlations: Correlations between plasma procainamide levels and effects in myotonia are not available. In treating cardiac arrhythmias, plasma levels of 2 to 8µg/ml are likely to be effective, and levels above 8µg/ml are likely to be associated with toxic effects.

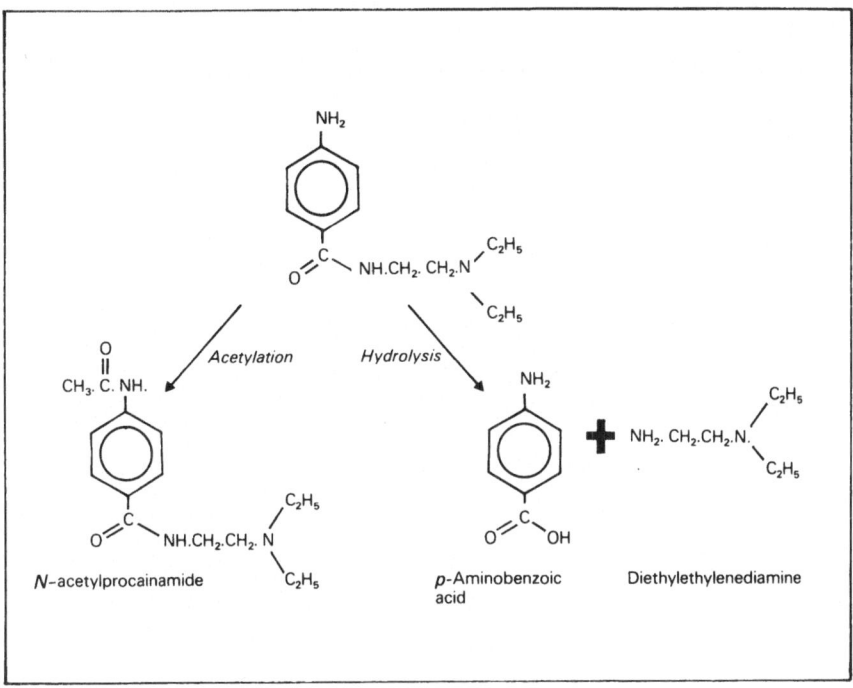

Fig. 3.4. Metabolism of procainamide.

Interactions

Pharmacodynamic interactions: Procainamide may increase the hypotensive effect of antihypertensive agents and possibly increase the effects of neuromuscular junction blocking agents.

Pharmacokinetic interactions: No pharmacokinetic interactions can be traced.

Toxicity

Idiosyncratic Toxicity

Rapid acetylators appear to have an increased risk of developing lupus erythematosus if they are given procainamide (McQueen, 1976). Seemingly the acetamido metabolite of the drug is responsible for this effect. Frislid et al. (1976) found 9 of 20 subjects tested were fast acetylators of the drug.

Hypersensitivity reactions (fever, arthralgia, itching, urticaria and other skin rashes) may occur, and agranulocytosis has been reported.

Dose-related Toxicity
Procainamide overdosage may cause:

1) Anorexia, nausea and vomiting, diarrhoea
2) Giddiness
3) Psychosis
4) Cardiac arrhythmia.

Dysmorphogenicity
No information is available.

Phenytoin

This drug is discussed in detail in chapter VI, in connection with its use as an anticonvulsant.

Glucocorticoids

These drugs are discussed in chapter II.

Treatment of Myotonia

Treatment of myotonia is not always necessary, nor always helpful to the patient. In dystrophia myotonica the patient's problem is nearly always weakness, and treating his myotonia often does not improve his capacity for physical activity or the quality of his life. In the rare paramyotonia congenita the myotonia is often too mild to bother the patient. However, in myotonia congenita, the presence of myotonia may interfere with the patient's physical performance by preventing his stopping one movement quickly in order to undertake another. Here the myotonia is worth treating. Ordinarily oral quinine (0.3g 3 times a day) or procainamide (0.25g 4 times a day) may be used initially, with higher doses later if necessary, depending on the therapeutic response and the presence of side effects. When using quinine it is prudent to give a single test dose, to detect idiosyncrasy, before beginning the course of treatment. As patients with myotonia congenita grow older and tend to undertake less physical activity, some find their myotonia less of a handicap. They may then prefer to use therapy intermittently, reserving their drugs for occasions when they wish to undertake more physical activity than usual.

Although prednisone is said to be effective in relieving myotonia, it seems unlikely that many would regard continuous glucocorticoid therapy, with its attendant side effects, as an acceptable price for relief of myotonia. While phenytoin would provide a safer alternative therapy. there is uncertainty about its effectiveness in relieving myotonia. Munsat (1967) claimed its therapeutic effect was equal to that of procainamide.

Patients with myotonia should be warned of the need to indicate this diagnosis to any doctor who proposes to give them an anaesthetic. Depolarising neuromuscular blocking agents (e.g. succinylcholine) given to produce laryngeal relaxation to permit endotracheal intubation. in some persons with myotonia can trigger severe laryngeal spasm. The blocking agent causes initial firing of acetylcholine receptors on muscle. thus initiating myotonia, before these receptors are blockaded. Competitive non-depolarising neuromuscular blocking agents (e.g. tubocurarine) obviate this risk. Patients with myotonic dystrophy may face an additional anaesthetic hazard: occasionally they show great sensitivity to the anaesthetic effects of thiopentone (Lodge. 1958).

There has been a report that the anti-spasticity agent baclofen (page 72) will relieve myotonia (Karli and Bergstrom, 1974).

Spasticity

Spasticity is a particular form of hypertonus in which increasing muscle contraction develops involuntarily during muscle stretch. With further stretch. relaxation may ensue. Spasticity is conventionally regarded as a cardinal feature of upper motor neurone lesions. though Bucy (1951) pointed out that a pure corticospinal tract lesion will not produce spasticity. Involvement of cortico-reticulo-spinal pathways running close to the corticospinal tracts. seems required for the production of spasticity. In practice spasticity is commonly associated with weakness. since the corticospinal tract and its associated cortico-reticulo-spinal pathways are often involved simultaneously by disease processes (e.g. infarction. neoplasia. primary demyelination).

Disordered Mechanisms

Spasticity arises when the peripheral mechanisms for maintaining muscle tone are released from the overall dampening influence of descending cortico-reticulo-spinal pathways. or when these peripheral mechanisms are facilitated through other pathways such as the vestibulo-spinal pathways. These latter pathways are dominantly facilitatory and their discharging activates γ-motoneurones in the lateral part of the anterior horns of the spinal cord. The descending reticulo-spinal and vestibulo-spinal systems are normally kept in a state of inhibition by cerebral cortical and basal ganglia influences. though they are activated by the cerebellum. Lesions of the cortico-reticulo-spinal system above the medulla disinhibit the reticular formation. thus causing increased activation of γ-motoneurones. Lesions of the cortico-reticulo-spinal system below the medulla remove both inhibitory influences and facilitatory (cerebellar) ones, and allow the γ-motoneurones to take up their own inherent pattern of activity. The final effect of lesions at these various sites is to increase the discharging of γ-motoneurones. This increased firing of the γ-motoneurones causes increased contraction of intrafusal fibres within muscle. The tension on the annulo-spiral sensory endings around the muscle spindles is thereby increased. The firing rate of the Ia afferent fibres from these annulo-spiral endings then increases. These Ia fibres discharge on the α-motoneurones in the anterior horn. In consequence, there is increased firing of the α-motoneurones, leading to contraction of the general body of extrafusal muscle fibres, with consequent tightening of muscle (fig. 3.5). Thus loss of descending inhibitory influences leads to spasticity from unrestrained overactivity in the γ-loop mechanism. The characteristic clasp-knife response to muscle stretch is also due to overactivity in this mechanism. The reflex extrafusal muscle contraction initiated

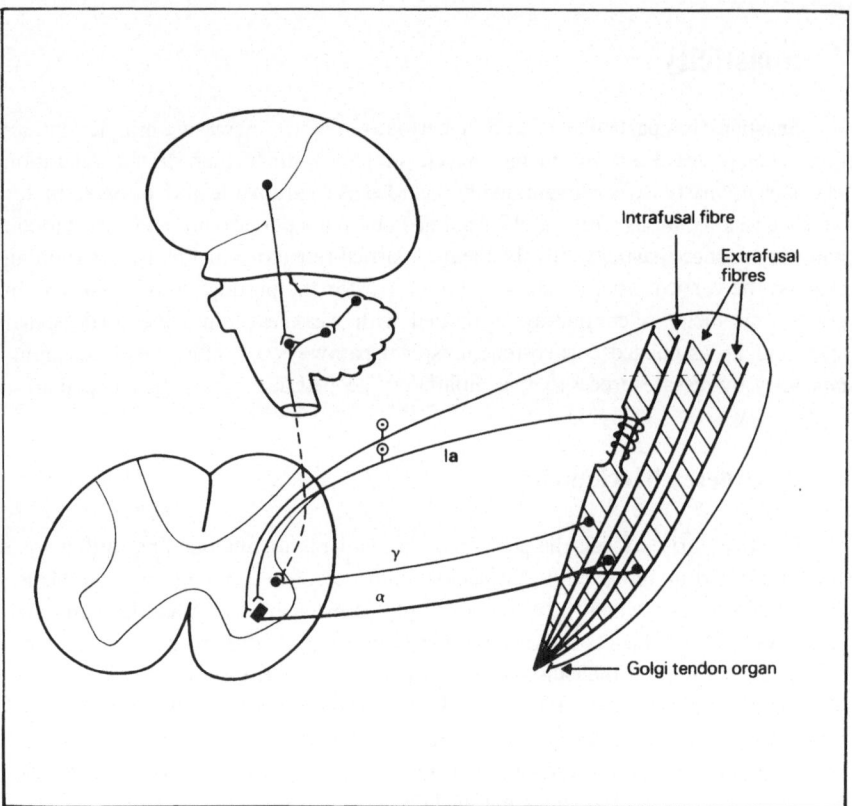

Fig. 3.5. Diagrammatic representation of spinal reflex and gamma loop.

by this stretch of annulo-spiral endings produces considerable tension on the Golgi tendon organs and at the same time the tension on the intrafusal fibres relaxes as the extrafusal fibres contract. An exaggerated heightening in muscle tension is therefore followed by sudden relaxation as Golgi tendon organ firing increases rapidly just as spindle afferent discharging lessens.

It is also possible to obtain spasticity by direct activation of α-motoneurones (Rushworth, 1962). Such α-spasticity is less common than the γ-spasticity described above.

Correction of Disordered Mechanisms

The following theoretical possibilities for relieving spasticity exist:

1) Augmenting the residual descending inhibitory impulses acting on the γ-motoneurones. Unless correcting the causative process has this effect, no way has yet been found of achieving this, either pharmacologically or surgically.

2) Diminishing the descending excitatory impulses playing on the γ-motoneurones. This can be achieved surgically by interrupting the cerebellar outflow by stereotaxic operations on the dentate nuclei or thalamus.

3) Diminishing activity in the γ-motoneurone. This can be done by depositing certain substances locally around the appropriate γ-motoneurones and their axons. These substances (e.g. ethyl alcohol, phenol) tend to damage γ-motoneurones rather selectively, because of their thinly myelinated axons. Near their motor end plates γ-motoneurones are vulnerable to the effects of dilute local anaesthetics (e.g. 0.1 % procaine). Injury confined to the γ-motoneurone will reduce muscle tone without decreasing voluntary power, which is mediated through the larger, more thickly myelinated axons of α-motoneurones. Gamma motoneurone activity is also diminished by the oral or parenteral use of the drug baclofen.

4) Diminishing the activity of the spinal reflex arcs connecting Ia fibres with the α-motoneurone. Several drugs (e.g. baclofen, diazepam) appear to act in this way.

5) Damaging the large Ia afferent fibres at appropriate levels. This may be achieved by surgical operations on posterior nerve roots. Diminishing the afferent inflow to the α-motoneurones will diminish reflex muscle contraction, without reducing voluntary power.

6) Damaging the α-motoneurones, partly blocking the myoneural junctions, diminishing the contractility of skeletal muscle (believed to be the mode of action of the drug dantrolene), or directly damaging the affected muscles or their tendons. These latter measures can diminish spasticity only at the cost of producing weakness of voluntary movement. In practice the only measure that has so far been much used is partial section of the tendons of spastic muscles. This is a simple peripheral procedure which can be restricted to only the most affected muscles.

Drugs Used in Spasticity

Though several drugs are currently used in the attempt to relieve spasticity, none is completely effective.

Baclofen

The only recognised use of this drug is to relieve spasticity (Jones et al., 1970).

Chemistry

Baclofen is β-(p-chlorophenyl)-γ aminobutyric acid. Its structure resembles that of γ-aminobutyric acid (GABA), and also noradrenaline (fig. 3.6).

Baclofen is a colourless, tasteless and odourless amphoteric substance, with pK_a values of 3.85 and 9.25. At pH 7.4 it exists as a zwitterion. It has a relatively low solubility in water at neutral pH, but is more soluble at pH values below 4 or above 8.

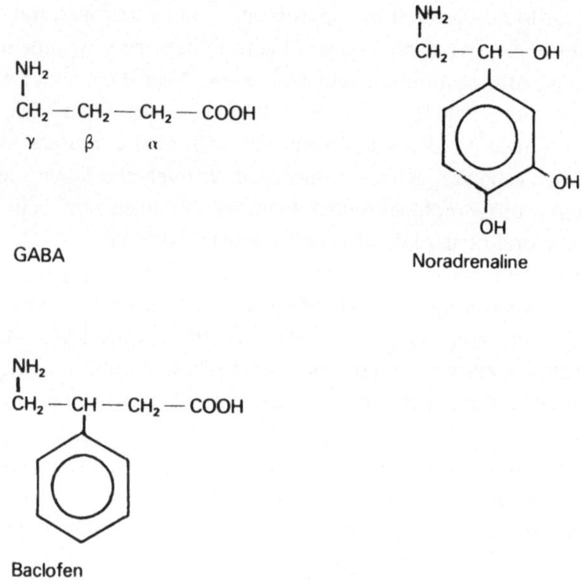

Fig. 3.6. Baclofen.

Baclofen is also somewhat soluble in lipids. Its lipophilicity is greater than that of GABA, and suffices for it to be absorbed from the intestine and to cross the blood-brain barrier, unlike GABA.

Pharmacology

The pharmacology of baclofen has been reviewed by Brogden et al. (1974).

Biochemical Pharmacology

Although baclofen was synthesised in attempts to find GABA analogues which would cross the blood-brain barrier, there is some evidence that its action may not depend on its structural resemblance to GABA. Baclofen does inhibit the enzyme GABA transaminase so that it could be expected to increase brain GABA levels. However, the electro-physiological effects of baclofen are not reduced by bicuculline, a specific blocking agent at GABA receptors (Curtis et al., 1974). The latter authors pointed out that the structure of baclofen also resembles that of catecholamines, raising the possibility that the drug may act on biogenic amine mechanisms.

Pharmacodynamics

Baclofen has no effect on neuromuscular transmission or on the afferent input to the cord from de-efferented muscle spindles (Fehr and Bein, 1974). In anaesthetised cats baclofen depresses the firing of spinal interneurones, pyramidal tract neurones and Purkinje cells (Curtis et al., 1974). It inhibits both monosynaptic and polysynaptic reflex transmission at spinal level and reduces the activity of γ-motoneurones (Bein, 1972). These actions at spinal level should help correct spasticity by diminishing the number of impulses impinging on α-motoneurones.

Pharmacokinetics

Absorption and bioavailability: Unlike GABA, baclofen is sufficiently lipid-soluble to be absorbed from the alimentary tract. It is said to be rapidly and almost completely absorbed after oral administration in man, with peak plasma levels reported at 1 to 2 hours (McLellan, 1977) and 2 hours (Knuttson et al., 1974).

Distribution: Autoradiographic studies show that baclofen is fairly uniformly distributed throughout the internal organs of mice, though concentrations are lower in the brain and spinal cord than in other organs. Plasma baclofen levels are said to be more than 10 times CSF levels of the drug (Knuttson et al., 1974). 30% of the drug in plasma is protein-bound.

Elimination: The plasma half-life of the drug in man is 3 to 4 hours (Knuttson et al., 1974). 80% of the dose is excreted in the urine in 24 hours. Only about 15% of the dose is biotransformed, mainly to β-(p-chlorophenyl)-γ-hydroxybutyric acid. The remainder is excreted unchanged (Faigle and Keberle, 1973).

Plasma level correlations: In the individual, plasma baclofen concentrations do not increase in proportion to drug dose (Faigle and Keberle, 1972). Plasma baclofen levels that improve γ-spasticity are not effective in α-spasticity (Knuttson et al., 1974).

Interactions
Pharmacodynamic interactions: Baclofen may interact additively with diazepam to relieve spasticity.

Pharmacokinetic interactions: No information is available.

Toxicity

Idiosyncratic Toxicity
No information is available.

Dose-related Toxicity
Nausea, vomiting, sedation, hypotonia, fatigue and weakness may occur. The drug is said to activate epilepsy.

Dysmorphogenicity
No information is available.

Diazepam

Diazepam is considered in chapter VI, in relation to its use as an anticonvulsant.

Dantrolene

Dantrolene is a recently introduced agent used to relieve skeletal muscle spasm and spasticity (Gelenberg and Poskanzer, 1973; Ladd et al., 1974). Its properties and pharmacology have been reviewed by Pinder et al. (1977a).

Chemistry

Dantrolene (MW 314.26) is an acidic drug which is used as the sodium salt.

Pharmacology

Biochemical Pharmacology

Dantrolene relaxes voluntary muscle by preventing the depolarisation of the muscle cell membrane from causing muscle contraction. It probably does this by interfering with the release of Ca^{++} from the sarcoplasmic reticulum (Ellis and Carpenter, 1974). This action appears to be reasonably specific for skeletal muscle (Ellis et al., 1976).

Pharmacodynamics

Dantrolene relaxes skeletal muscle and may cause weakness by a direct action on the muscle. It does not alter neuromuscular transmission, or the membrane potential of skeletal muscle. The drug has some depressant action on the central nervous system.

Pharmacokinetics

Absorption and bioavailability: Dantrolene is slowly and incompletely absorbed after oral administration — about 70%, according to Dykes (1975). After a 150mg dose the T_{max} is 3 to 6 hours (Monster et al., 1973).

Distribution: Adequate data are not available, but from published figures the V_D can be calculated to be about 1.5L/kg. The drug does bind to plasma albumin, though the extent of the binding is not known.

Elimination: The mean half-life of dantrolene in adults is 8.7 hours (Dykes, 1975). Only 1% of a dose is excreted unchanged in urine, with 20 to 25% of a dose being found as urinary metabolites, particularly the 5-hydroxy, the 5-amino and the acetamido derivatives (Dykes, 1975).

Plasma level correlations: It is said that plasma dantrolene levels are related to the drug dose. In normal persons blood levels of about 1μg/ml are associated with decreased muscle tone.

Interactions

Pharmacodynamic interactions: It appears likely that dantrolene would interact additively if given with more centrally acting muscle relaxants e.g. diazepam.

Pharmacokinetic interactions: Data are not available.

Toxicity

Idiosyncratic Toxicity

No information is available.

Dose-related Toxicity

Dantrolene can cause skeletal muscle weakness which limits the benefit of the drug in relieving spasticity. Some patients experience dizziness, euphoria and fatigue. Diarrhoea may occur and there have been reports of hepatotoxicity. Some 1% of patients develop raised alkaline phosphatase and transaminase levels, which usually return to normal when dantrolene therapy ceases. Occasional instances of fatal hepatitis have occurred following the use of dantrolene.

Dysmorphogenicity

No information is available.

Treatment of Spasticity

It may not be possible to correct the disease process which causes spasticity in a patient and, even if it can be corrected, there may be so much residual damage to the descending motor pathways that spasticity persists. In these circumstances, the spasticity may produce sufficient handicap to justify symptomatic treatment. However, the disease process causing spasticity usually involves the corticospinal pathways also, and the resulting weakness is often a greater handicap to the patient than his spasticity. Relief of spasticity will not relieve weakness, though sometimes a reduction in spasticity may enable a patient to make greater use of his residual power. Conversely, at times reduction of spasticity in the lower limbs may decrease a patient's capacity to walk. In the presence of weakness, spasticity may have been tending to splint a patient's knee joints, thus permitting walking. Spasticity requires treatment only when it troubles the patient because of pain or because it prevents full use of residual motor capacity. At times the treatment of spasticity may be justified because nursing is made easier. Landau (1974) has further discussed the philosophy of treating spasticity.

Baclofen Therapy

Baclofen is probably the most effective drug available for spasticity, though it is very much more useful in spasticity of spinal origin than in spasticity arising at higher levels (Jones and Lance, 1976). It is given orally, beginning with low dosage, e.g. 5mg 3 times a day. Because the drug has a relatively short elimination half-life (3 to 4 hours), with regular dosage steady-state conditions are likely to apply after 1 to 2 days' therapy. It would therefore appear reasonable to increase the dose as often as every second or third day, in an attempt to find the dosage which gives optimal relief of spasticity in the individual patient. However, a more gradual introduction of the drug may reduce the incidence and severity of side effects, and usually control of spasticity is not a matter of urgency. Ultimately, the patient may be given baclofen at a dose of 100mg or more, each day, if this quantity is necessary to reduce spasticity and if the patient can tolerate such a dose. It is unlikely that baclofen would need to be taken more often than 3 or 4 times a day, when one allows 1 or 2 hours after dosage before plasma levels reach a peak, and then 3 or 4 hours for a 50% decline. So long as the underlying disease is not progressive, the antispastic effect of baclofen does not diminish with time (Jones and Lance, 1976).

Diazepam Therapy

Should baclofen fail, or not be tolerated, diazepam may be used. Cartlidge et al. (1974) found that the beneficial effect of baclofen and diazepam on spasticity tended to be similar at the lower dosage levels; in higher doses baclofen was superior. In general the biological effects of the benzodiazepines do not correlate particularly well with their plasma levels. Since diazepam has a half-life of about 24 hours, and its biologically active metabolite desmethyldiazepam has a half-life that is twice as long, or longer, it seems unlikely that diazepam would need to be given more often than once a day. It would seem logical to give the whole day's dose of diazepam on going to bed so that, if drowsiness develops during the phase of rising plasma and tissue drug levels, this occurs when the patient is in bed. Many patients tolerate an initial dose of 5mg. The long half-life of desmethyldiazepam implies that it would take about 2 weeks after a diazepam dosage change for a new steady-state to be achieved. Thus if diazepam dose is increased more frequently than once a fortnight, there is a possibility that a patient will be given an unnecessarily large dose in order to attain a desired therapeutic effect. Despite these pharmacokinetic considerations diazepam is often given 2 or 3 times a day. Subject to the presence of side effects (often drowsiness, weakness or faintness), diazepam dose can be increased as necessary to reduce spasticity. The upper limit of dose is reached when side effects of diazepam outweigh the benefits obtained from the drug.

If either baclofen or diazepam proves useful in relieving a patient's spasticity, the drug can be continued long term. Should both drugs fail, dantrolene might be tried. The writers have no personal experience with this agent, but reports suggest its efficacy is similar to that of diazepam (Schmidt et al., 1976). The potential hepatotoxicity of dantrolene should be borne in mind.

The drug is begun in low dosage (e.g. 12.5mg twice daily). Once or twice a week dosage is increased, the drug being given 2 or 3 times daily until a useful clinical response occurs or adverse effects preclude any further dosage increase. Typical reported doses in adults are 200 to 400mg per day.

Other Procedures

If drug therapy of spasticity fails, various other procedures might be considered.

1) For lower limb spasticity, an intrathecal injection of local anaesthetic at the appropriate vertebral level, e.g. L2,3 for adductor spasm, may be tried. If the injec-

tion is successful in relieving the spasticity for a short time, more permanent relief may be sought by intrathecal injection of phenol at this level (Nathan, 1959). This procedure carries some hazards for control of bladder function and therefore may tend to be restricted to those patients with unimpaired bladder control or to those patients who already have no bladder control.

2) For spasticity in upper or lower limbs selective tenotomy for the most severely affected muscles may sometimes be considered.

3) Occasionally posterior rhizotomy at the appropriate level may be worth consideration though there may be some sensory loss. In special centres stereotaxic surgery on the facilitatory pathways which influence the cortico-reticulo-spinal motor system (e.g. the cerebello-dentato-thalamic connections) may be possible.

Bell's Palsy

The great majority of instances of peripheral facial palsy are due to a compression neuropathy of the facial nerve within its canal in the temporal bone (Bell's palsy). The aetiology is uncertain. Apart from Bell's palsy compression neuropathies in man usually involve sensory or mixed nerves, and their main symptoms are sensory. They have therefore been discussed in chapter VII (p.286) of this book. However Bell's palsy warrants separate consideration because it is dominantly a motor neuropathy with an aetiology and prognosis that appear different from those of the other compression neuropathies. There is a variety of relatively uncommon brain stem and peripheral nerve lesions that can also cause a lower motor neurone facial palsy. Here only idiopathic Bell's palsy will be dealt with.

Disordered Mechanisms

Possibly as a result of viral infection a facial nerve may become inflamed and swollen within the confines of its canal in the temporal bone. The vascular supply to the affected segment of the nerve may be impaired if the swelling causes compression against the bony wall of the facial canal. Nerve function is then interrupted and the muscles of facial expression become weakened or paralysed on the affected side. In severe cases the facial nerve may also be involved central to the origin of the chorda tympani branch, in which case taste is affected ipsilaterally. Often the tension within the facial canal causes local pain in the mastoid region and this may trigger unilateral posterior neck muscle spasm with consequent contraction headache (see chapter VII, p.247).

Correction of Disordered Mechanisms

Since the aetiology of Bell's palsy is uncertain. no treatment can be directed against the aetiological agent. Corticosteroids (or ACTH to augment endogenous corticosteroid production) might be expected to help by reducing the inflammatory response in the affected nerve. The use of steroids does improve the prognosis for recovery (Taverner et al., 1967; Wolf et al., 1978). Alternatively the facial canal has been enlarged surgically to allow room for the inflamed nerve to expand. In practice such surgery does not appear of benefit (Mechelse et al., 1971). Korkis (1961) advocated cervical sympathetic block for Bell's palsy, on the basis that the procedure would improve the blood supply of the compressed facial nerve. In a controlled trial, Fearnley et al. (1964) found that cervical sympathectomy did not improve the outcome in Bell's palsy. Analgesics and measures to treat contraction headache (see chapter VII, p.232, 249), may also be required.

Drugs Used in Bell's Palsy

Corticosteroids are discussed in chapter II, (p.33) and analgesics in chapter VII (p.232).

Treatment of Bell's Palsy

Bell's palsy usually has a good prognosis for full spontaneous recovery. If the facial paralysis is incomplete when the patient is seen in the first 2 or 3 days of illness. and the paresis does not progress during the first week. there is no need to take any therapeutic action apart from prescribing analgesics when required and warning the patient to protect his eye from the accidental entry of dust. Full recovery is highly likely. When the face is very severely or fully paralysed the outlook is uncertain but some patients will still recover fully without treatment. Loss of taste sensation on the anterior two-thirds of the tongue on the same side as the affected nerve. and loss of responsiveness of the nerve to electrical stimulation. suggest a bad prognosis. If these features are present. and perhaps in all cases of total facial palsy, so long as the patient is seen within the first 2 weeks of onset, corticosteroids should be used immediately. Oral prednisolone or prednisone. 60 to 75mg per day in divided doses for 1 week, and then in reducing dosage over the next 1 or 2 weeks, often suffices. Taverner et al. (1971) showed that prednisolone in an initial dose of 80mg per day was superior to ACTH in an initial dose of 60 units per day in improving the outcome in Bell's palsy.

In the past. surgical decompression was advocated whenever the facial nerve was electrically unresponsive (Cawthorne and Haynes. 1956). As mentioned above. it seems doubtful if such surgery improves the prognosis.

Traditionally physiotherapy and electrical stimulation of the facial nerve have been used to promote recovery but Mosforth and Taverner (1958) showed that electrical stimulation did not improve the outcome.

Where permanent paralysis occurs, often with subsequent contracture, various plastic surgical operations may improve the function of local portions of the face. Hypoglossal-facial nerve anastomosis may permit the return of some motor function in the face. Should hemifacial spasm occur, no medical treatment appears of any consistent benefit — as in other varieties of this distressing disorder.

Periodic Paralysis

In patients with familial hypokalaemic periodic paralysis, attacks of weakness are associated with a fall in serum potassium because K^+ ions enter cells. While such attacks can be treated by administering potassium salts, the hazards of inducing hyperkalaemia should be appreciated. Jarell et al. (1976) reported that oral acetazolamide e.g. 250mg 3 or 4 times a day, taken regularly, would prevent attacks developing. The drug produces a metabolic acidosis, which slows the rate of entry of K^+ into muscle (Vroom et al., 1975).

In patients with hyperkalaemic periodic paralysis (as occurs in paramyotonia congenita and adynamia episodica hereditaria) the regular intake of diuretics which cause K^+ loss may tend to prevent attacks. Thiazide diuretics may be used. McArdle (1962) obtained satisfactory results with acetazolamide.

Chapter IV

Disorders of Motor Function, II:
Involuntary Movement Disorders

Principal Disorders and Drugs Discussed

Parkinsonism
  Levodopa, dopa-decarboxylase inhibitors
  Amantadine
  Anticholinergics

Dystonias
  Penicillamine
  Dimercaprol

Chorea
  Tetrabenazine
  Phenothiazines
  Haloperidol
  Metoclopramide

Myoclonus
  Anticonvulsants
  (see also chapter VI)

Tardive dyskinesia
  Phenothiazines, haloperidol,
  tetrabenazine

Tremor
  Propranolol, pindolol
  Diazepam (see also chapter VI)

There are several types of abnormality of involuntary movement. The precise pathological basis of these various disorders is incompletely understood, as is their biochemical background. However, sufficient knowledge is available to suggest that most, if not all, of the disorders arise from disturbed function of the basal ganglia, and that many of the disorders are related to altered dopamine action in these regions of the brain.

The term dyskinesia embraces these various disorders of involuntary movement. Within the dyskinesias are a number of long-recognised clinical syndromes which have their own generally accepted names. The term sometimes tends to be applied mainly to disorders of involuntary movement which are not easily classified, or which have been widely recognised only in recent times.

It is possible to divide the dyskinesias into two broad groups. In the first group there is a reduction of involuntary movements normally present, as occurs in Parkinsonism and, rarely, in rigid forms of Huntington's disease. In the second group, involuntary movements are present in excess. There are a number of different patterns of such non-Parkinsonian dyskinesias. Parkinsonian dyskinesia is associated with reduced dopaminic activity in the striatum and at least some varieties of non-Parkinsonian dyskinesia are related to increased basal ganglia dopaminic activity.

The dyskinesias will be considered in the following order:

Parkinsonism
non-Parkinsonian dyskinesias
chorea and hemiballismus
athetosis
tardive dyskinesia
dystonias — generalised and localised
myoclonus
tremor
asterixis, tics, paroxysmal choreoathetosis.

A number of accounts of the pharmacology of these disorders are available, including the monograph of Klawans (1973b).

Parkinsonism: Striatal Dopamine Deficiency

The Parkinsonism syndrome is the most common basal ganglia disorder. At the present time the majority of cases are probably of the idiopathic type (paralysis agitans); post-encephalitic Parkinsonism has become rare as the years have passed since the encephalitis lethargica pandemic of 1917 to 1926. It is becoming increasingly accepted that cerebral arteriosclerosis is not a common cause of Parkinsonism (Eadie and Sutherland, 1964). Drug-induced Parkinsonism is comparatively frequent, though for the most part reversible. Uncommon causes of Parkinsonism include carbon monoxide poisoning, manganese poisoning, olivo-ponto-cerebellar atrophy, striato-nigral degeneration, progressive supranuclear palsy and the Shy-Drager syndrome, and the Parkinsonism-dementia complex of Guam.

Disordered Mechanisms

The essential features of Parkinsonism are explicable in terms of rigidity and bradykinesis which together cause a poverty of normal involuntary movements.

Rigidity and bradykinesis to some extent behave as independent variables, though Walshe (1955) regarded bradykinesis simply as a consequence of rigidity. A characteristic resting tremor is commonly present, particularly in idiopathic paralysis agitans. Neuropathological study over many years failed to provide any precise and consistent correlations between sites of disease in the basal ganglia and various manifestations of the Parkinsonian syndrome. The substantia nigra appears to be the most frequently affected structure within the brain (Greenfield and Bosanquet, 1953). However Denny-Brown (1962) was reluctant to accept it as the essential pathological locus of Parkinsonism, and Alvord (1958) found it necessary to speak of nigral and extra-nigral Parkinsonism. This failure of neuropathologists over many years to agree that the substantia nigra was the essential site of Parkinsonian pathology should not be forgotten when one comes to consider modern concepts of the pathogenesis of the disorder, with their ready acceptance of a nigral location for the essential pathological changes.

For many years dopamine was regarded simply as a metabolic intermediary in the formation of noradrenaline and adrenaline in the brain:

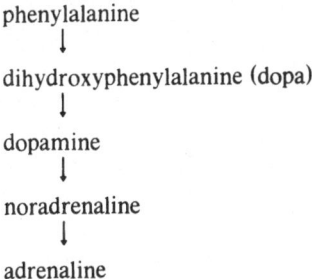

phenylalanine
↓
dihydroxyphenylalanine (dopa)
↓
dopamine
↓
noradrenaline
↓
adrenaline

However, Carlsson (1959) recognised that dopamine concentrations in the normal striatum (caudate nucleus and putamen) were so high relative to noradrenaline concentrations that dopamine might play a primary role in neurotransmission. Ehringer and Hornykiewicz (1960) found reduced striatal dopamine concentrations in Parkinsonian brains. By means of fluorescence histochemistry, a dopaminergic pathway was traced from the substantia nigra to the striatum on each side (Anden et al., 1964). Birkmayer and Hornykiewicz (1961) demonstrated that administration of levodopa, the precursor of dopamine, in sufficient dosage reversed many of the manifestations of Parkinsonism. When these observations were considered in relation to the neurosurgically established fact that lesions in the inner part of the globus pallidus, the ansa lenticularis or the ventero-lateral nucleus of the thalamus tended to relieve Parkinsonism on the contralateral side, and the known benefit of anticholinergic drugs in the disorder, it became possible to construct a schema of events involved in the pathogenesis of Parkinsonism.

It is thought that various forms of disease process, as yet not adequately under-stood, cause a failure of dopamine production in the nigral neurones which provide the axons of the nigro-striatal dopaminergic pathway. Consequently there is a relative deficiency of dopamine at the axon terminals in the striatum and reduced concentra-tions of the dopamine metabolite homovanillic acid (HVA) in the CSF (Curzon, 1973). This dopamine deficiency leads to a relative over-action of the cholinergic fibres which appear to arise in the neocortex and which synapse onto striatal neurones. The net effect of this dopamine-acetylcholine imbalance (in favour of the latter) at the cell surfaces of striatal neurones is to cause increased activity in the neurones of the globus pallidus. These neurones discharge onto the ventero-lateral nucleus of the thalamus and thence to the cortex. From the cortex impulses pass through the internal capsule with the corticospinal tracts to influence activity of lower motor neurones (fig. 4.1). Increased activity in this pallido-thalamo-corticospinal cir-cuit appears to be responsible for Parkinsonian rigidity and bradykinesis. Evidence from the effects of neurosurgical lesions at various sites suggests that Parkinsonian tremor may be mediated by abnormal activity in a pathway that runs from the den-tate nucleus of the cerebellum to the ventro-lateral thalamic nucleus and thence to the cortex in common with the pallido-thalamic outflow. Pathological evidence of damage to this 'tremorgenic' pathway in Parkinsonism is not well established but it must be remembered that widespread and variably sited neurological lesions have long been described in Parkinsonism. There have been suggestions that Parkinsonian tremor may be mediated through a 5-hydroxytryptaminic (i.e. serotoninergic) path-way rather than a catecholaminergic one. However the use of tryptophan (a precursor of 5-hydroxytryptamine) which crosses the blood-brain barrier, does not relieve Parkinsonian tremor (Coppen et al., 1972). There has been a recent report that methysergide, a 5-hydroxytryptamine antagonist, relieves the type of Parkinsonism present in progressive supranuclear palsy (Rafal et al., 1977). It is difficult to recon-cile this observation with current ideas of the pathogenesis of Parkinsonism.

There is a rather widespread deficiency of the enzyme glutamic acid decarboxyl-ase in Parkinsonian brains (McGeer et al., 1971; Pinne et al., 1974). The relation of this finding to the pathogenesis of Parkinsonism is obscure.

The above account not only provides a simplified statement of contemporary views of the pathogenesis of Parkinsonism but may also serve as a basis for the un-derstanding of the pharmacology of the basal ganglia disorders. Except for dopamine in the nigro-striatal pathway, and acetylcholine in the cortico-striatal axons, the syn-aptic transmitters in the relevant pathways are uncertain.

Correction of Disordered Mechanisms

Because the pathophysiology of Parkinsonism involves dysfunction in a number of neural circuits, with their synapses, there are several points at which a therapeutic attack might in theory be directed.

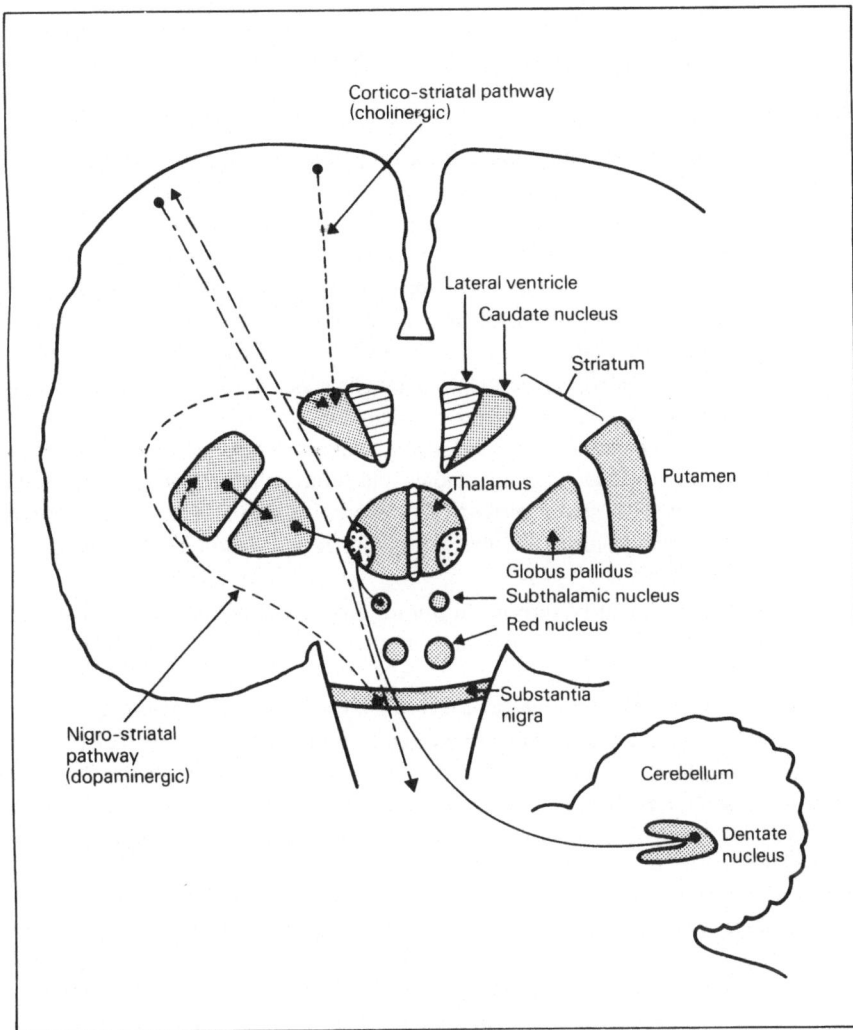

Fig. 4.1. Nigro-striatal (dopaminergic) and cortico-striatal (cholinergic) pathways of the brain.

1) Treatment might be aimed at correcting the disease process which has caused Parkinsonism. Drug-induced Parkinsonism can be treated by withdrawing the offending drug. which is usually reserpine or a phenothiazine. However in the great majority of instances the nature of the disease process causing Parkinsonism is not understood. No rational treatment directed at the causative process is then possible.

2) Treatment might be aimed at restoring optimal dopamine concentrations or dopamine effects at neuronal receptors in the striatum. This might be achieved in 3 ways:

a) By supplying a dopamine precursor (1-dihydroxyphenylalanine i.e. levodopa or l-dopa), since dopamine itself will not cross the blood-brain barrier. The success of this therapeutic manoeuvre would depend on the decarboxylase enzymatic mechanisms remaining functional in the nigro-striatal pathway, or in the striatum, so that the levodopa may be converted to dopamine.

b) By inhibiting the metabolic breakdown of dopamine. This breakdown involves the enzymes monoamine oxidase and catechol-O-methyltransferase. Inhibition of monoamine oxidase may have potentially dangerous effects (p.270). Inhibition of catechol-O-methyl transferase (by N-butyl gallate) is said to improve the results of treating Parkinsonism with levodopa by reducing dyskinesia due to relative levodopa overdosage (Ericsson, 1971). Catechol-O-methyl transferase inhibitors have not yet come into general clinical use, possibly because of their toxicity.

c) By supplying drugs which are dopamine agonists and which will cross the blood-brain barrier (e.g. amantadine and bromocriptine) and the still partly experimental substance piribedil. Apomorphine also is a dopamine agonist but its potential for producing vomiting makes it unsuitable for therapy of Parkinsonism.

3) Treatment might be directed at diminishing acetylcholine effects on striatal neurones e.g. by administering anticholinergic agents which cross the blood-brain barrier.

4) Treatment might be aimed at decreasing the overall inflow of discharges from the inner part of the globus pallidus to the ventro-lateral nucleus of the thalamus *via* the ansa lenticularis. No chemotherapeutic attack is yet possible in this region. The relevant synaptic transmitters are unknown. However, surgical lesions made in the region of the ansa can be moderately effective in relieving Parkinsonism.

Modifying neural activity in the ways listed above (1 to 4) tends to correct the manifestations of rigidity and bradykinesis in patients with Parkinsonism, but has rather less effect on tremor, if this is present.

5) Treatment might diminish neural activity in the ventro-lateral nucleus of the thalamus. Stereotaxic lesions made in this structure may relieve Parkinsonian tremor as well as rigidity though they are not very effective in easing bradykinesis. Lesions which interrupt the relevant efferent pathways in the internal capsule, cerebral peduncles or lateral funiculus of the spinal cord also relieve Parkinsonism to some extent, but are likely to produce weakness due to a corticospinal tract deficit as well.

The benefits that can be derived from the surgical treatment of Parkinsonism tend to be limited by the uncertainties of producing a lesion of exactly the right dimensions and site to rectify the condition. Even if a lesion completely corrects the disorder for a time, the natural progression of the disease process may later make the surgical lesion inadequate.

In practice, stereotaxic thalamotomy proves the most effective way of treating severe Parkinsonian tremor. For Parkinsonian rigidity and bradykinesis, particularly the latter, treatment with levodopa or, in milder cases, with dopamine agonists, generally offers the best results.

Drugs Used in Parkinsonism

Levodopa

The only common use of levodopa is in the treatment of Parkinsonism. Since levodopa is a precursor of noradrenaline, as well as of dopamine, the use of levodopa has been suggested where increased noradrenaline activity is desired e.g. in persisting postural hypotension, possibly in migraine prophylaxis. Levodopa has also been used to treat torsion dystonia, progressive supranuclear palsy, striato-nigral degeneration, the rigid form of Huntington's disease, depression, and hepatic coma; however in these conditions results have often been equivocal. It is of no benefit in the stiff-man syndrome (Guilleminault et al., 1973). There have been several major reviews of the properties and uses of levodopa (Barbeau, 1963; Brogden et al., 1971; Calne, 1973).

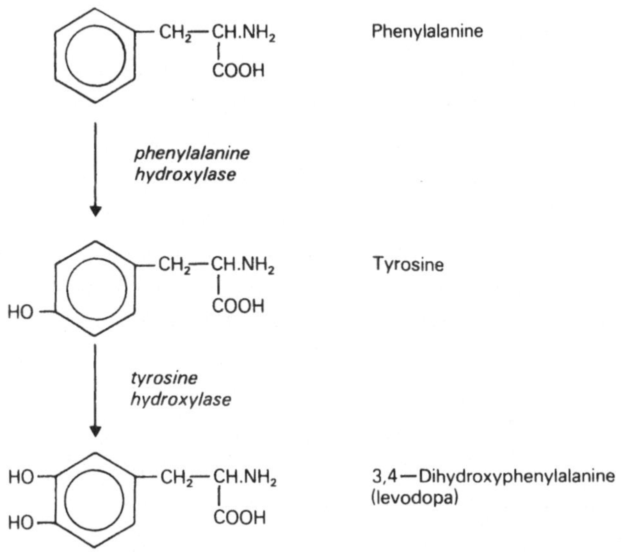

Fig. 4.2. The synthesis of levodopa from phenylalanine.

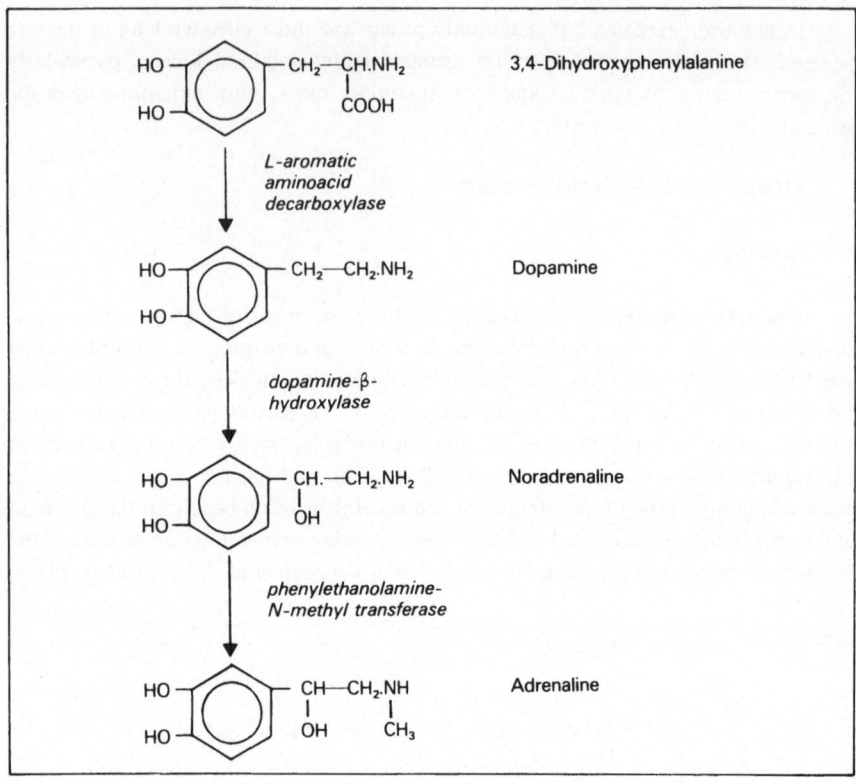

Fig. 4.3. Steps in the biotransformation of levodopa to adrenaline.

Chemistry

Levodopa (L-dopa) is l-3,4-dihydroxyphenylalanine (MW 197.19). It is a naturally occurring neutral amino acid with pK_a values of 2.3, 8.7 and 9.9. The molecule is a zwitterion at physiological pH: Despite its polarity levodopa can cross cell membranes by utilising the specific enzymatic uptake mechanisms which exist for neutral amino acids. In the body levodopa is synthesised enzymatically from phenylalanine (fig. 4.2).

Pharmacology

Biochemical Pharmacology

The beneficial effects of levodopa are believed to be due to dopamine which is formed from it by enzymatic decarboxylation in various tissues, including the brain.

The enzyme involved in the decarboxylation is L-aromatic amino acid decarboxylase, often called dopa-decarboxylase (Lovenberg et al., 1962). Details of its distribution in the human brain are given by Lloyd and Hornykiewicz (1972). In various tissues, and in many regions of the brain, though not in the striatum, the dopamine that is formed in the decarboxylation is further enzymatically biotransformed to noradrenaline and adrenaline (fig. 4.3). The biological effects of levodopa are mediated through the various catecholamines derived from it, especially dopamine.

For dopamine to be formed from levodopa and for this dopamine to restore function in the Parkinsonian striatum, it is necessary for dopa-decarboxylase to be present in nigro-striatal neurones, or at least in the region of dopamine receptors on striatal neurones. It is possible that dopamine formation may be reduced in nigro-striatal neurones at an early stage of Parkinsonism even though some dopa-decarboxylase activity persists in these neurones. In these circumstances if a high local concentration of levodopa were produced by medication this would lead to dopamine formation in nigro-striatal neurones and restoration of dopamine function in the striatum. However, at later stages of Parkinson's disease there is degeneration of the substantia nigra and atrophy of the nigro-striatal pathway. In such circumstances it is difficult to conceive that there would be sufficient dopa-decarboxylase activity in the nigro-striatal neurones to form enough dopamine to restore striatal function, yet clinically levodopa may still be effective. However, the normal striatum contains serotoninergic axon terminals as well as dopaminergic ones, and serotonin is also said to be formed in these terminals from 5-hydroxytryptophan by the enzyme L-aromatic amino acid decarboxylase (dopa-decarboxylase). It has been suggested that levodopa which enters the striatum in Parkinsonism may be taken up by serotoninergic axon terminals. In these terminals it may be decarboxylated and the resulting dopamine released near the cell bodies of striatal neurones. Administered in this way levodopa might bypass the degenerating or degenerated nigro-striatal terminals to produce dopamine which then acts directly in the striatum. It should be pointed out that some workers e.g. Sims et al. (1973) have suggested that, in rat brain, levodopa and 5-hydroxytryptophan are decarboxylated by different enzymes. If this finding applies to man, the explanation of the biochemical mode of action of levodopa will require modification.

Levodopa therapy causes a fall in brain serotonin levels (Miller and Neiburg, 1974). After 8 to 12 months of levodopa therapy the previously depleted levels of glutamic acid decarboxylase in the striatum and substantia nigra rise towards normal (Lloyd and Hornykiewicz, 1973). Prolonged high dose therapy with levodopa causes a decrease in the activities of the enzymes tyrosine hydroxylase, aromatic L-amino acid decarboxylase, and catechol-O-methyltransferase, and increased activity of monoamine oxidase (Weiss et al., 1971).

Dopa undergoes rather extensive metabolism in nervous tissue, and it has been suggested that various metabolic products of dopa may have an anti-Parkinsonian effect. It has also been suggested that levodopa may be methylated to form 3-methoxydopa in nervous tissue. The methoxydopa may later be demethylated to levodopa again and thus may serve as a store for levodopa within neural tissue. The further metabolism of methoxydopa was described by Kuruma et al. (1971). Additional metabolic pathways for 3-methoxydopa were mentioned by Bartholini et al. (1972).

Pharmacodynamics

The effects of levodopa on muscle tone and movement are not usually seen in normal persons but only in persons with basal ganglia disorders. In patients with Parkinsonism the extrapyramidal type of rigidity may disappear and voluntary movement may become more rapid and free. The normal semi-automatic, associated and emotional expressive movements reappear and bradykinesis may lessen. There may sometimes be a reduction in tremor but if this takes place it often occurs later than the relief of rigidity and bradykinesis. As the levodopa dose is increased, rigidity may be replaced by hypotonia, and choreic types of involuntary movement and other dyskinesias may appear.

Levodopa action on neural pathways and catecholaminergic transmission outside the basal ganglia may have a mood-elevating and alerting effect. However the drug does not improve defective cognitive function in Parkinsonism (Bowen et al., 1975). Levodopa therapy may alter certain aspects of hypothalamic function. This may be the explanation of the orthostatic hypotension that may follow levodopa therapy. The drug increases growth hormone production. Sebum secretion is decreased in Parkinsonism, perhaps through an endocrine-mediated mechanism (Burton and Shuster, 1970) which may be influenced by levodopa. Increased peripheral formation of catecholamines from levodopa may cause cardiac stimulation. Circulating dopamine levels are increased. Dopamine is able to traverse the blood-brain barrier in the area where the barrier is relatively defective, in the neighbourhood of the chemoreceptor trigger zone in the floor of the fourth ventricle. Here the dopamine may cause nausea and vomiting. Other peripheral effects mediated by increased plasma dopamine levels include increased glomerular filtration, increased renal plasma flow and increased Na^+ and K^+ excretion.

Pharmacokinetics

Bianchine and Shaw (1976) have provided a major review of the pharmacokinetics of levodopa.

Absorption and bioavailability: Levodopa is a relatively polar molecule but it is absorbed from the alimentary tract by means of the specific neutral amino acid uptake mechanism in the wall of the small intestine. This is a capacity-limited mechanism and dietary amino acids may compete for the mechanism with levodopa. Consequently the extent of absorption of a dose of levodopa tends to be determined by how close to a meal it is taken, and by the protein content of that meal. Plasma levodopa levels are said to be increased by a low protein diet (Sweet and McDowell, 1974). The extent of absorption of a levodopa dose is also determined by the time the drug spends in the stomach before it reaches the intestine. Within the stomach levodopa is enzymatically decarboxylated and the resultant dopamine is too polar to be absorbed passively from the alimentary tract and it lacks a specific uptake mechanism. Therefore, delay in gastric emptying is likely to reduce the amount of a levodopa dose that is available for absorption. Such delay in gastric emptying may be due to food or milk intake (Morgan et al., 1971) or an acid gastric pH (Rivera-Calimlim et al., 1970). Antacid intake speeds gastric emptying and increases the absorption of a levodopa dose (Bianchine et al., 1971). Because intragastric destruction of levodopa is avoided, the drug may be better absorbed from enteric-coated preparations so that its dose can be reduced (Gilligan and Hancock, 1975).

Absorption of levodopa from the intestine is a fairly rapid process, maximum plasma levels of the drug often occurring 1 to 3 hours after dosage (Hare et al., 1973; Imai et al., 1971; Morris et al., 1976). Slowly absorbed preparations of levodopa are available. Laitinen (1973) showed that one such preparation containing radioactive drug kept plasma radioactivity (i.e. the sum of activities of levodopa and its metabolites) fairly constant over 24 hours. However another sustained release preparation produced very similar plasma levodopa concentration curves to an ordinary preparation of the drug given in the same dosage (Curzon et al., 1973). Morris et al. (1976) obtained some evidence that levodopa is absorbed over only a restricted area of the small intestine. If this is the case there would be little point in producing sustained release preparations of the drug. This matter is discussed in some detail by Sandler et al. (1974).

Distribution: More than 90% of the levodopa in plasma is free in plasma water. The remainder is in red blood cells (Hinterberg, 1971). There does not appear to be significant binding of levodopa to plasma proteins.

Levodopa is widely distributed throughout the body. In mice the drug accumulates in pancreas, liver, kidney, gut and skin. There is also evidence of substantial uptake in skeletal and smooth muscle, which contains little dopa-decarboxylase or catechol-*O*-methyl transferase (Ordonez et al., 1974). In Parkinsonian brains after levodopa intake there are increased levels of dopamine, and the dopamine metabolite homovanillic acid, in the basal ganglia, hypothalamus, thalamus and cerebral and cerebellar cortices. The entry of levodopa from plasma into the various organs is dependent on active uptake through cell membranes, including those of the cerebral capillary endothelium. Thus levodopa uptake is a process that may well vary from tissue to tissue and to some extent be independent of plasma levodopa concentrations. In rats, Daniel et al. (1976) showed that certain circulating aromatic amino acids competed with levodopa for entry into brain. Levodopa enters the CSF slowly. In Parkinsonism it has been noted that the highest CSF dopa levels (and levels of the dopamine metabolite homovanillic acid) tend to occur after levodopa dosage in those patients who respond least to the drug (Ericsson et al., 1970; Godwin-Austen et al., 1971). It is suggested that homovanillic acid entry into CSF depends on a 'spill-over'

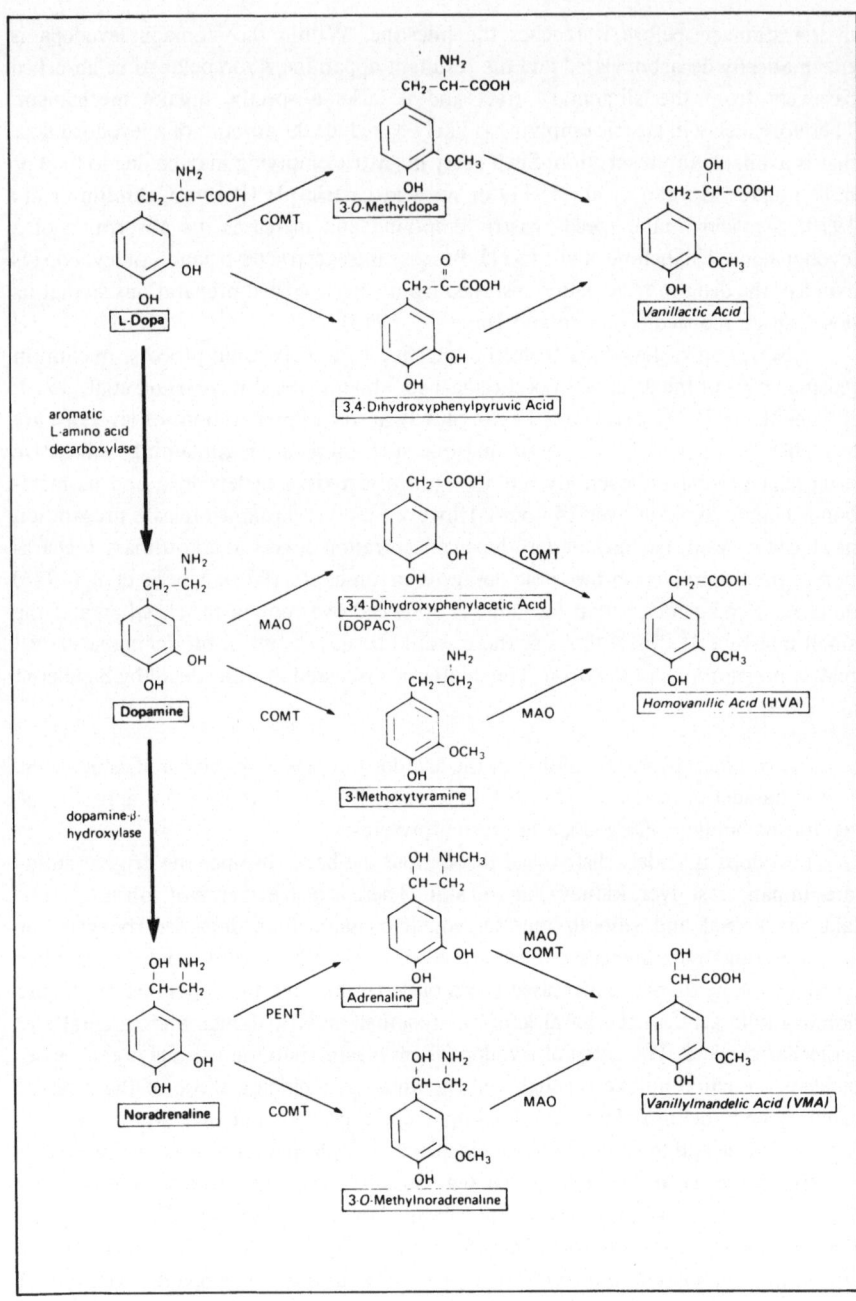

Fig. 4.4. Important metabolic pathways of levodopa (COMT = catechol O-methyl transferase; MAO = monoamine oxidase; PENT = phenylethanolamine N-methyl transferase).

of dopamine from the brain and its metabolism in capillary walls (Goodwin et al., 1971).

Elimination: Levodopa undergoes extensive biotransformation in the brain and in peripheral tissues. The extent of peripheral metabolism is so great that only 1% or so of a levodopa dose is available for entry into the brain. The major known metabolic pathways are indicated in figure 4.4. However levodopa can undergo other patterns of biotransformation (e.g. to form melanin). The major final metabolic product in man after large doses of levodopa is homovanillic acid.

Very little of a dose of radioactive levodopa is found in faeces or in expired air and less than 1% of a dose is excreted in urine as unchanged drug (Morgan et al., 1971). The drug is excreted chiefly as free and conjugated dopamine, as homovanillic acid and as 3,4-dihydroxyphenylacetic acid. In Parkinsonian patients, up to 59% of a levodopa dose may be excreted as homovanillic acid. Cotzias et al. (1969) found a linear relation between levodopa dose and homovanillic acid excretion in Parkinsonian patients. Approximately 24% of the levodopa dose was excreted as homovanillic acid, 0.1 to 0.7% as unchanged levodopa and up to 5% as dopamine. However there is a good deal of individual variation in the relative proportions of the various metabolites.

Thus the elimination of levodopa is almost entirely by biotransformation. The plasma half-life of the drug is 1 to 3 hours (Rinne et al., 1973). Since in man the biological half-life of 3-methoxydopa is 15 hours, and this metabolite forms reversibly from levodopa, 3-methoxydopa may serve as a reservoir for levodopa.

Plasma level correlations: There is disagreement as to how closely plasma levodopa concentration is related to oral dosage of the drug. Meunter and Tyce (1971) found the two were related whereas Hare et al. (1973) and Pilling et al. (1975) did not.

Although there might be some quantitative relationship between plasma concentrations of levodopa and its therapeutic effects in Parkinsonism one would not expect this relationship to be a close one since:

1) There are two rate-limited processes intervening between levodopa in plasma and the action of dopamine in the striatum, *viz* active transport of levodopa through cerebral capillary endothelium and into neurones, and enzymatic decarboxylation of levodopa.

2) There may be an effect of the reserve of levodopa within the brain, stored as 3-methoxydopa.

In fact, the time course of the anti-Parkinsonian effect of administered levodopa does not appear to parallel closely the plasma concentrations of this substance.

Rinne et al. (1973) found, with chronic administration of levodopa, that plasma levels of the drug correlated with vomiting and dystonia, but not with capacity for voluntary movement. Tolosa et al. (1975) noted that Parkinsonism tended to worsen about 2 hours after plasma levodopa level fell below the threshold value which was peculiar to each individual patient; in some, but not all patients, high plasma levodopa levels correlated with the presence of dyskinesia. On the other hand Reid et al. (1974) found that in a given individual there was a consistent plasma levodopa level which was associated with the onset of involuntary movements. While Pilling et al. (1975) found no close correlation between plasma concentration of levodopa and improvement in patients with Parkinsonism, they found there was a closer correlation between plasma 3-methoxydopa levels and clinical improvement. However Bergmann et al. (1974) could not relate plasma levels of 3-methoxydopa to either the therapeutic or the toxic effects of levodopa.

Attempts to correlate CSF concentrations of levodopa and its metabolites (e.g. homovanillic acid) with therapeutic response in Parkinsonism have generally been rather unsuccessful, again in part because the entry of drug and metabolite into the brain depends on active transport processes. If anything, there is an inverse relationship between CSF levels of levodopa and homovanillic acid and response to treatment, as pointed out above.

Interactions

Levodopa is a pro-drug which exerts its biological action after being metabolised to dopamine. In a strict sense the receptor for levodopa is the enzyme L-aromatic amino acid decarboxylase (dopa decarboxylase). However, in practice it is more useful to consider the interactions of levodopa in relation to the dopamine receptor.

Pharmacodynamic interactions

In theory the catecholamines formed from levodopa might increase the effects of directly acting sympathomimetics (e.g. adrenaline, isoprenaline) and indirectly acting ones (e.g. ephedrine, amphetamine). Phenothiazines and butyrophenones block striatal dopamine receptors and prevent the effects of dopamine formed from levodopa, thus aggravating Parkinsonism.

Amantadine and centrally acting anticholinergics increase the anti-Parkinsonian effect of levodopa. This effect of amantadine has been shown not to be due to a pharmacokinetic interaction (Bergmann et al., 1974).

Gibberd and Small (1973) reported a possible pharmacodynamic interaction between levodopa and α-methyldopa which enhanced the antihypertensive effect of the latter.

Pharmacokinetic interactions: Pharmacokinetic interactions of levodopa may occur at several levels:

1) During absorption from the alimentary tract

Drugs which delay gastric emptying (e.g. anticholinergics and imipramine) according to Messiha and Morgan (1974) reduce the amount of levodopa available for absorption as they increase the time the drug is exposed to enzymatic degradation in the stomach. Drugs e.g. antacids, which expedite gastric emptying have the opposite effect (Bianchine et al., 1971). Dietary amino acids may compete with levodopa for absorption from the alimentary tract. Thus a low protein diet may raise plasma levels of levodopa (Sweet and McDowell, 1974).

2) During distribution

The pattern of distribution of levodopa is altered by administering pyridoxine, from which pyridoxal phosphate is derived. Pyridoxine (or its phosphate) appears to cross the blood-brain barrier. Pyridoxal phosphate is the co-enzyme for dopa-decar-boxylase. Hence pyridoxine therapy increases the peripheral decarboxylation of levodopa and leaves less available for entry into the nervous system. Johnston (1971) suggested that pyridoxal-5-phosphate might inactivate levodopa by forming a tetrahydro-isoquinoline derivative.

Conversely dopa-decarboxylase inhibitors, particularly those which do not pass through the blood-brain barrier (e.g. carbidopa, benserazide; p.97-101) diminish the peripheral decarboxylation of levodopa and make more available for entry into ner-vous tissue. The antihypertensive agent α-methyldopa also acts as a dopa-decarbox-ylase inhibitor (Sweet et al., 1972) but as α-methyldopa penetrates the blood-brain barrier this drug also decreases the formation of dopamine from levodopa in the brain. However, these actions of α-methyldopa are relatively weak.

The capacity of neurones to store dopamine is reduced by the drug reserpine. This action of reserpine leads to striatal dopamine deficiency and aggravates Parkin-sonism.

3) During elimination

The elimination of dopamine, the biologically active product of levodopa, de-pends on the activities of the enzymes monoamine oxidase and catechol-O-methyl transferase. Inhibitors of the latter enzyme are not used in human therapeutics but monoamine oxidase inhibitors interact with levodopa to produce excess peripheral and central catecholamine action. Since many monoamine oxidase inhibitors act ir-reversibly their effects may persist for 2 weeks or more after the drugs are stopped and they may interact with dopamine formed from levodopa over this period.

Toxicity

Idiosyncratic Toxicity
Idiosyncratic side effects of levodopa are rare.

Dose-related Toxicity
The dose-related side effects of levodopa are essentially due to formation of ex-cessive amounts of dopamine and possibly other biotransformation products. These side effects include the production of:

1) Hypotonia, choreiform and dystonic involuntary movements and myoclonus. These dyskinesias are relieved by reducing the dose of levodopa. They are said to be relieved by increasing acetylcholine activity in the brain. This might be done by giving the centrally acting anticholinesterase physostigmine (Tarsy et al., 1974), or deanol, the dimethylaminoethanol salt of p-acetaminobenzoic acid (Miller, 1974). Relief of the dyskinesia by physostigmine is associated with an increase in Parkinsonism but it was claimed that this did not occur with deanol. However Jenkins and Groh (1970), Klawans et al. (1975) and Laterre and Fortemps (1975) could not substantiate these claims for the beneficial effects of deanol. Myoclonic jerks from long term levodopa therapy may be due to dopamine re-uptake into serotoninergic axon terminals altering serotonin function in the striatum. This myoclonus can be relieved by the serotonin antagonist methysergide (Klawans et al., 1975).

2) Hallucinations and delusions, mainly in older persons with a degree of pre-existing dementia or with post-encephalitic Parkinsonism (Celesia and Barr, 1970). These mental disturbances usually settle when treatment with levodopa is discontinued.

3) Mood alterations: euphoria or depression.

4) Increased libido, at least in males.

5) Anorexia, nausea, vomiting.

6) Weight loss after prolonged use of the drug. Competition between dietary amino acids and levodopa for the specific intestinal absorption mechanism might contribute to this weight loss. However Vardi et al. (1976) have suggested that levodopa therapy may cause high plasma insulin levels which may have a lipolytic effect.

7) Cardiac arrhythmia (occasionally).

8) Postural hypotension.

9) Mydriasis or miosis; exacerbation of glaucoma.

10) Reappearance of oculogyric crises in cases of post-encephalitic Parkinsonism.

11) Positive direct and indirect Coombs' tests.

12) Change in urine colour — urine turning dark on exposure to alkali e.g. on contact with detergent.

13) Increased growth in malignant melanomas (Lieberman and Shupack, 1974).

After treatment with levodopa the increased mobility of patients with Parkinsonism may occasionally lead to complications (e.g. fractures of bones affected by disease such as osteoporosis).

Dysmorphogenicity

Parkinsonism rarely occurs during the reproductive years so that the question of dysmorphogenicity from levodopa rarely arises in practice. There is little evidence of dysmorphogenicity in laboratory animals.

Dopa-decarboxylase Inhibitors

Although the antihypertensive agent α-methyldopa is a weak inhibitor of dopa-decarboxylase (L-aromatic amino acid decarboxylase) and crosses the blood-brain barrier (Sweet et al., 1972), only two drugs (carbidopa and benserazide) are in common use for the specific purpose of inhibiting this enzyme. Neither drug has any other known use in human therapeutics. Since both drugs are almost always used in combination with levodopa they are usually marketed in fixed dose combinations with it. These combinations reduce the extracerebral side effects of levodopa and permit a satisfactory therapeutic effect to be achieved much more rapidly. Pinder et al. (1976) have provided a major source of data concerning these drugs.

Chemistry

Carbidopa [(-)-L-α-hydrazino-3,4-dihydroxy-α methylbenzene proprionic acid-MW 244.25] bears a structural resemblance to levodopa, as does benserazide [(± -DL-seryl-2-(2,3,4-trihydroxybenzyl) hydrazine-MW 257.25] (fig. 4.5).

Pharmacology

Biochemical Pharmacology
Carbidopa and benserazide inhibit the enzyme L-aromatic amino acid decarboxylase in peripheral tissues. They have relatively little effect on this enzyme in the central nervous system, since neither drug crosses the blood-brain barrier readily.

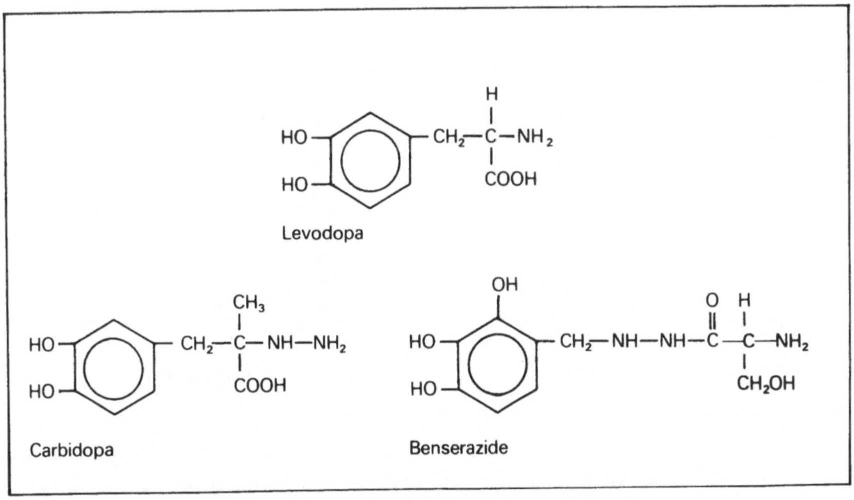

Fig. 4.5. Structural formulae of levodopa, carbidopa and benserazide.

Given alone, they decrease the urinary excretion of tryptamine, 5-hydroxy indole-acetic acid and 3-methoxy-4-hydroxyphenol glycol and produce raised plasma levels of prolactin and glucagon. They do not alter plasma levels of growth hormone, cortisol, thyroid stimulating hormone or insulin (Garfinkel et al., 1977). When the inhibitors are given with levodopa the diminished peripheral decarboxylation of levodopa allows a greater proportion of a levodopa dose to be available for entry into the central nervous system. This increases the neurological actions of levodopa relative to its dose and simultaneously would be expected to reduce the unwanted consequences of peripheral formation of dopamine e.g. nausea, vomiting (Leiberman et al., 1975). However, Liebowitz and Lieberman (1975) found that dopa-decarboxylase inhibitor combinations did not reduce the incidence of hypotension and ventricular arrhythmias in patients with Parkinsonism.

Inhibition of dopa-decarboxylase activity in the alimentary tract increases the bioavailability of levodopa given orally. Diminished decarboxylation in extraneural tissues means that levodopa doses may be reduced by 80 % without decrease in anti-Parkinsonian effect when carbidopa or benserazide is added to levodopa therapy (Cotzias, 1969). The qualitative effects of levodopa on the central nervous system are not altered by dopa-decarboxylase inhibitors but pyridoxine therapy no longer reduces the effect of levodopa (as the peripheral potentiation of levodopa decarboxylation by pyridoxine is blocked by the inhibitor). In fact, in the presence of a peripheral dopa-decarboxylase inhibitor pyridoxine may increase the central effects of levodopa, as it now increases the formation of dopamine in the brain (fig. 4.6).

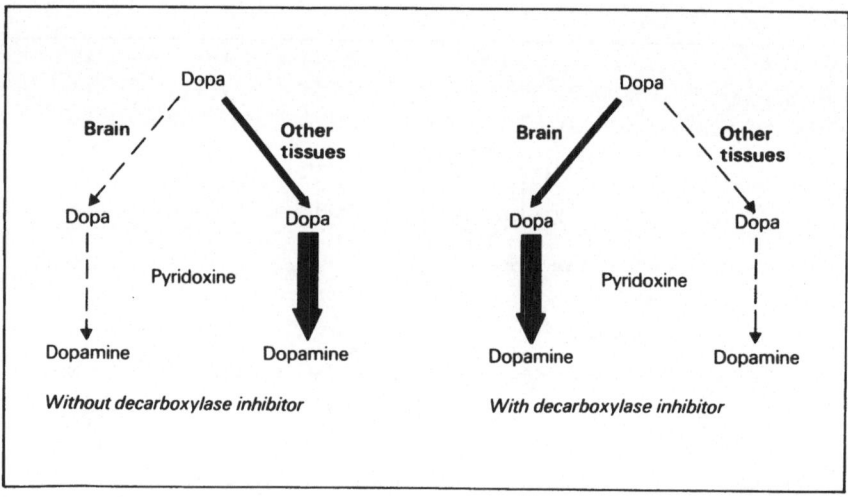

Fig. 4.6. Schematic representation of the effect on brain dopamine levels of adding a decarboxylase inhibitor and pyridoxine to levodopa.

Benserazide is also a partial competitive inhibitor of the enzyme catechol-*O*-methyl transferase and a weak inhibitor of monoamine oxidase (Baldessarini and Greiner, 1973). If blood-brain barrier permeability increased so that benserazide gained access to the brain these actions would theoretically tend to increase dopamine concentrations. However any benefit from this would be more than offset by decreased dopamine formation due to inhibition of brain dopa decarboxylation.

Pharmacodynamics

Carbidopa and benserazide, at ordinary doses, have no pharmacodynamic effects of their own though they alter quantitatively the effects of simultaneously administered levodopa.

Pharmacokinetics

Absorption and bioavailability: In man 40 to 70 % of an oral dose of carbidopa (Vickers 1974, 1975) and 66 to 74 % of an oral dose of benserazide (Schwartz, 1974) are absorbed. At intestinal pH some benserazide is oxidised to quinone derivatives. Maximum plasma levels of carbidopa occur 0.5 to 5 hours after dosage in persons with Parkinsonism whereas peak levels of benserazide occur within 1 hour.

Plasma levodopa levels are increased by a factor of 5 to 7 when dopa-decarboxylase inhibitors are given with levodopa. Peak plasma levodopa levels then occur 1 to 2 hours after administration.

Distribution: Carbidopa and benserazide tend to be concentrated in the kidneys, lungs, small intestine and liver of laboratory animals and to a lesser extent in the heart and other peripheral organs. Very little of either drug is found in brain where concentrations are only about 6 % of those in plasma. Thus when given in ordinary doses neither drug penetrates the blood-brain barrier readily. Carbidopa readily crosses the placenta of the rat and also appears in the breast milk of rats at about one-twelfth of its plasma concentration.

Elimination: About 40 to 55 % of a carbidopa dose is excreted in faeces. Nearly all the remainder is excreted in urine where about 15 % of the dose appears as unchanged drug. Carbidopa biotransformation patterns are shown in figure 4.7. The acid metabolites are excreted in urine as glucuronide conjugates. The plasma half-life of carbidopa is about 2 hours.

Benserazide is thought to be extensively metabolised. Its elimination is said not to follow first-order kinetics. At first benserazide is rapidly excreted in urine but later the rate of excretion slows so that 60 % of an oral dose is not excreted till 6 to 7 days have elapsed. A substantial portion of a benserazide dose is excreted in faeces, even after intravenous administration. Details of the metabolites of benserazide are not known; its plasma half-life appears to be less than 2 hours.

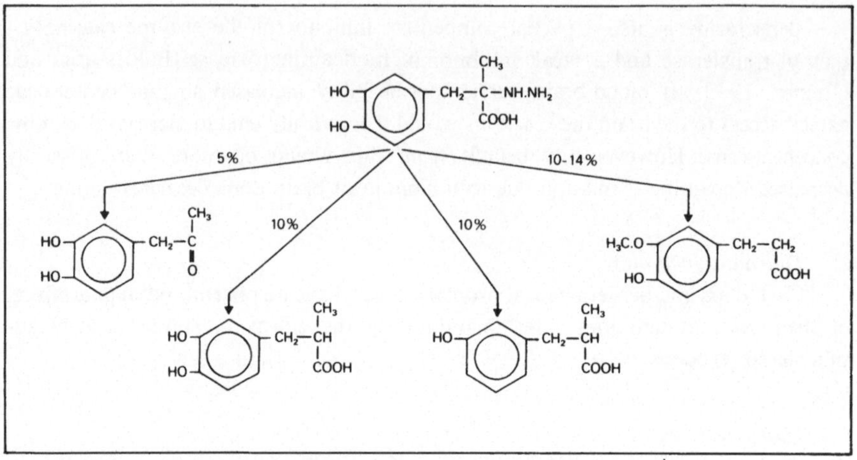

Fig. 4.7. Biotransformation patterns of carbidopa.

As might be expected, use of these dopa-decarboxylase inhibitors slows the elimination of levodopa and increases its plasma half-life. The prolongation of half-life may be by only about 30 minutes (possibly because levodopa is still biotransformed in the brain and in peripheral tissues by pathways which do not involve decarboxylation).

Plasma level correlations: Data correlating carbidopa or benserazide plasma levels with biological effects are not available. These effects, of course, depend on the dose of levodopa which is being taken.

Interactions
Pharmacodynamic interactions: No interactions are known.

Pharmacokinetic interactions: The therapeutic effect of the decarboxylase inhibitors depends on their interaction with levodopa.

There is some experimental evidence that these inhibitors, taken with levodopa, may slow the metabolism of other drugs in man (e.g. antipyrine). It is not yet clear whether this effect will prove important in human therapeutics.

It should be remembered that the enzyme inhibited by these inhibitors is L-aromatic amino acid decarboxylase and that this enzyme also catalyses the decarboxylation of amino acids other than levodopa (e.g. tryptophan and 5-hydroxytryptophan). Should these latter substances come to be used in therapeutics, as is probable (p.144), dopa-decarboxylase inhibitors are likely to be involved in interactions with these drugs.

Toxicity

Since these drugs are given with levodopa, the side effects of dopa-decarboxylase inhibitors in practice are the side effects of levodopa, though modified by a reduction in those peripheral effects of levodopa which are due to excess catecholamine production. The central nervous system side effects of levodopa are basically unaltered.

Amantadine

Amantadine was first marketed as an anti-influenzal agent and is still used for this purpose. Although it is also occasionally used against other viruses the evidence is that the drug is only effective against influenza A_2 virus. The anti-Parkinsonian actions of amantadine were discovered fortuitously during studies of its anti-influenzal effects (Schwab et al., 1969). Its chief use is now in the treatment of Parkinsonism. Parkes (1974) has provided a major review of the drug.

Chemistry

Amantadine (1-adamantanamine) [fig. 4.8] is a crystalline primary amine with a cyclic structure (MW 151.26). Amantadine itself is sparingly soluble in water and the drug is usually supplied as the hydrochloride.

Pharmacology

Biochemical Pharmacology
Amantadine causes the release of dopamine from neuronal storage sites in the peripheral nervous system and seems to have a similar action in the central nervous

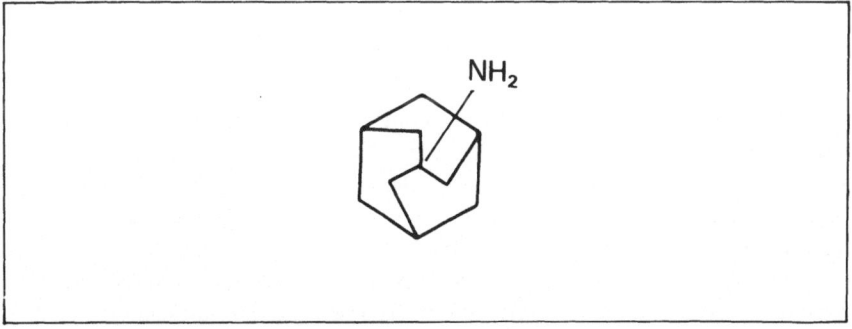

Fig. 4.8. Structural formula of amantadine.

system (Scatton et al., 1970). If this suggested central mode of action is correct the presence of some residual dopamine in nigro-striatal axon terminals would be necessary for the action of amantadine in Parkinsonism. That this may be so is suggested by the clinical observation that relatively low doses of levodopa augment the effects of amantadine. Experimentally, amantadine also causes release of 5-hydroxytryptamine from isolated nerve endings and inhibits 5-hydroxytryptamine uptake (Sturm et al., 1975). In the first few days of amantadine therapy in Parkinsonian patients there is increased urine excretion of 5-hydroxy-indole acetic acid, a metabolite of 5-hydroxytryptamine, and some tendency to increased excretion of dopamine and its metabolite homovanillic acid (Jones et al., 1972). These findings are consistent with amantadine's action in displacing dopamine and serotonin from nerve terminals.

Pharmacodynamics

Amantadine relieves the manifestations of Parkinsonism, particularly rigidity and tremor, though in this regard it is not as effective as levodopa given in full dosage. There have been suggestions that benefits from amantadine diminish after a few months of treatment, though measurable improvement in Parkinsonism can still be detected after a year of therapy (Butzer et al., 1975). It has no clinical effects on normal persons if given in usual doses.

Amantadine will prevent infection of experimental animals with different strains of type A_2 influenza. In man, if given within 20 hours of the onset of illness, it reduces the severity of influenzal manifestations. In some patients it produces peripheral vasoconstriction (Pearce et al., 1974).

Pharmacokinetics

Some details are given by Bleidner et al. (1965).

Absorption and bioavailability: Amantadine is said to be completely absorbed from the alimentary tract (Parkes, 1974). Since the drug is chemically a base, it is probably absorbed from the intestine rather than the stomach. Maximum plasma levels occur 1 to 4 hours after oral dosage.

Distribution: In a single patient Rizzo et al. (1973) estimated a V_D of 6.2L/kg.

Elimination: Bleidner et al. (1965) found an amantadine half-life of 9 to 15 hours, and Rizzo et al. (1973) a half-life of 21 hours. In elderly men the half-life averaged 34 hours (Montanari et al., 1975). There is no evidence that amantadine undergoes biotransformation in man. Some 86% of an oral dose is excreted unchanged in urine, 50% being lost in the first 20 hours. Since the drug is eliminated almost exclusively by renal excretion, dosage reduction may be necessary in the presence of renal insufficiency. In the rat only 20% of the dose is excreted unchanged. A 3-hydroxymethyl metabolite is formed (Sturm et al., 1975).

Plasma level correlations: In 4 subjects given 300mg of amantadine daily, steady-state plasma levels of the drug varied between 0.68 and 1.01µg/ml (Rizzo et al., 1973).

Interactions

Pharmacodynamic interactions: Levodopa and dopamine agonists (e.g. apomorphine) may produce additional relief if combined with amantadine in the treatment of patients with Parkinsonism (Fahn and Isgreen, 1975).

Dopamine antagonists (e.g. phenothiazines and butyrophenones) tend to block the actions of amantadine.

Pharmacokinetic interactions: No pharmacokinetic interactions involving amantadine are known. O'Malley et al. (1972) showed that amantadine did not have a statistically significant effect on the elimination of antipyrine. Therefore amantadine may not induce the hepatic mixed-oxidase system.

Toxicity

Idiosyncratic Toxicity

No clearcut idiosyncratic side effects of amantadine are known.

Dose-related Toxicity

In general, the dose-related side effects of amantadine are not severe. Ankle oedema and livedo reticularis, particularly of the thighs, are not uncommon. Mild postural hypotension occurs in a moderate number of patients taking the drug. Psychiatric disorders, confusion and hallucinations may occur in the elderly or in persons with a degree of dementia. Approximately 24 hours after sudden cessation of amantadine intake in Parkinsonian patients who are not receiving reasonably full doses of levodopa, an acute Parkinsonian crisis may occur, with intense rigidity, immobility, dysphagia, drooling and dysarthria. The immobility and dysphagia may lead to dehydration, and inability to take medication by mouth. Therefore temporary parenteral fluid therapy or tube feeding may be necessary though an intravenous dose of atropine may permit a loading dose of amantadine to be swallowed shortly afterwards, thus relieving the patient's problem.

Dysmorphogenicity

There is no good evidence that amantadine is dysmorphogenetic in man. However, Nora et al. (1975) reported the birth of an infant with congenital heart disease to a mother who took amantadine in the first trimester of pregnancy.

Centrally Acting Anticholinergics

For many years atropine and related alkaloids were the main medical treatments for Parkinsonism. In more recent times they were for the most part replaced by a number of synthetic anticholinergic agents which were capable of crossing the blood-brain barrier. Since the advent of levodopa and amantadine the anticholinergic agents have been used mainly as adjuvants to these more effective drugs, though anticholinergics may be used alone in mild cases of Parkinsonism and in drug-induced cases.

Chemistry

The anticholinergic agents used in recent times for treating Parkinsonism fall into several chemical groups as shown in figures 4.9a-d.

Pharmacology

Biochemical Pharmacology

In Parkinsonism the centrally acting anticholinergics are believed to block striatal acetylcholine receptors, thus diminishing the effect of cholinergic impulses in the excitatory cortico-striatal pathways. The effects of activity in these cortico-striatal pathways is normally damped by dopaminergic inhibitory nigro-striatal impulses. It is thought that the effects of reduction of this nigro-striatal inflow in Parkinsonism can to some extent be counterbalanced by reducing the cortico-striatal inflow. However Coyle and Snyder (1969) observed that anticholinergic drugs can also block dopamine re-uptake by axon terminals in the striatum. This action would tend to increase dopamine concentrations near its striatal receptors. Such an action might be expected to improve the striatal dopamine deficiency state of Parkinsonism. Benztropine has a similar action on synaptosomes from the rat nucleus accumbens and olfactory tubercule (Horn et al. 1974). *In vitro*, atropine is a competitive inhibitor of monoamine oxidase (Mohammed and Mahfouz, 1977).

Pharmacodynamics

It is convenient to discuss separately the central and peripheral actions of the anticholinergic drugs.

Central actions: Atropine and the centrally acting synthetic anticholinergics reduce to some extent the rigidity and tremor of Parkinsonism but have little action on the bradykinesis. In clinical doses atropine is a mild central vagal stimulant. Larger doses cause higher level excitation with restlessness, irritability, hallucina-

Atropine and congeners

Atropine (dl-hyoscyamine) MW 289.38

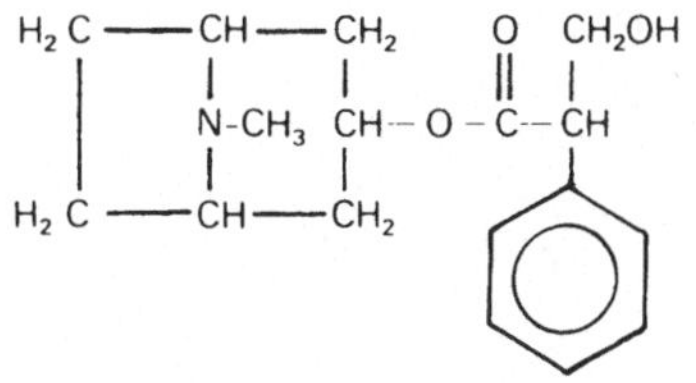

Hyoscine (scopolamine) MW 303.35

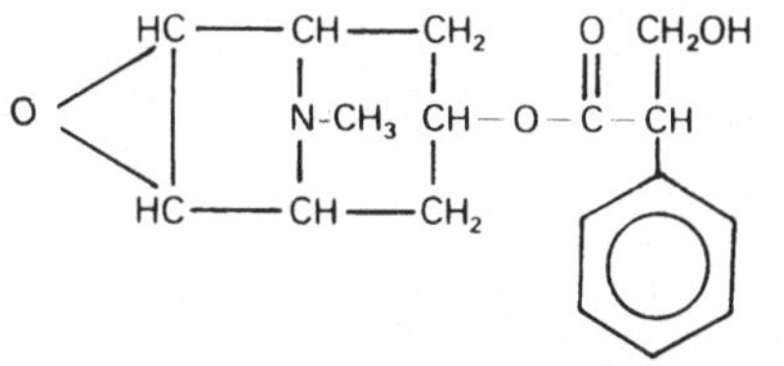

Benztropine methanesulphonate MW 403.53

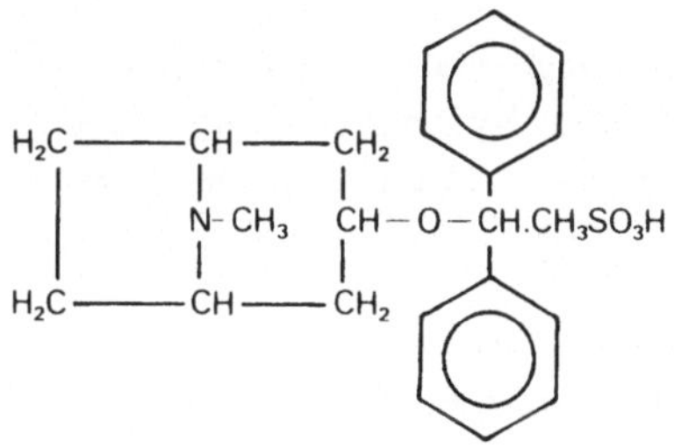

Benzehexol and congeners

Benzhexol MW 337.92

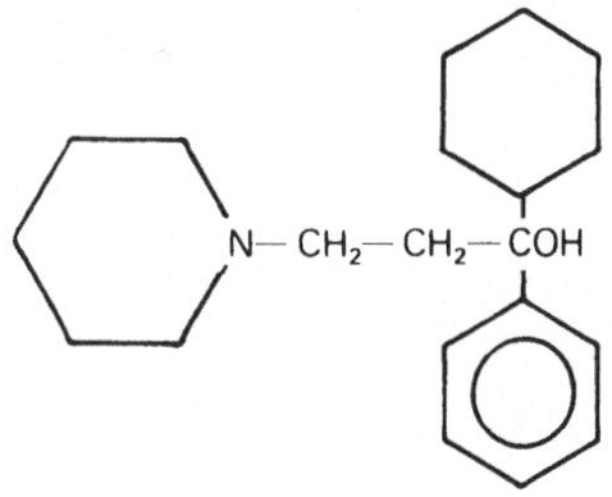

Cycrimine hydrochloride MW 323.90

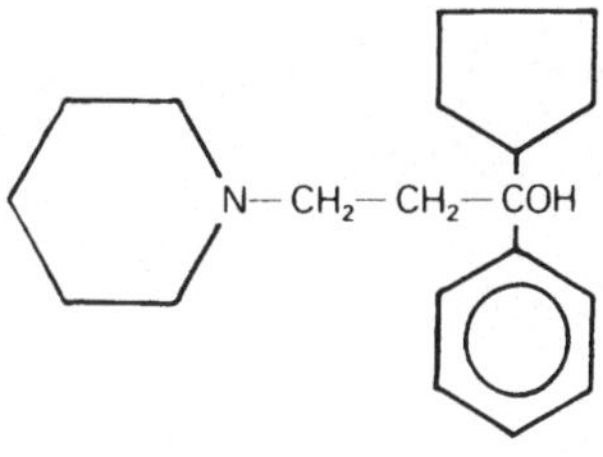

Procyclidine MW 287.43

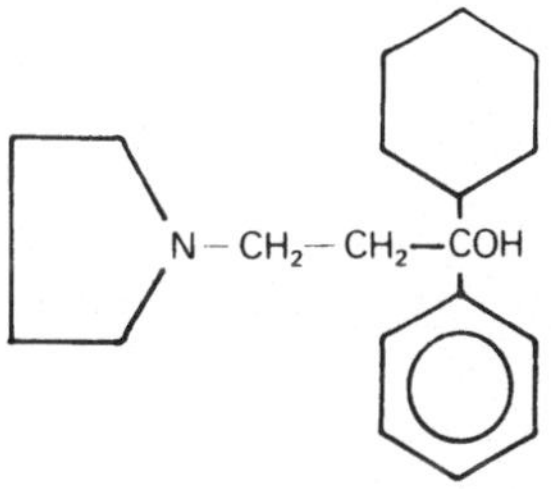

Biperiden MW 311.45

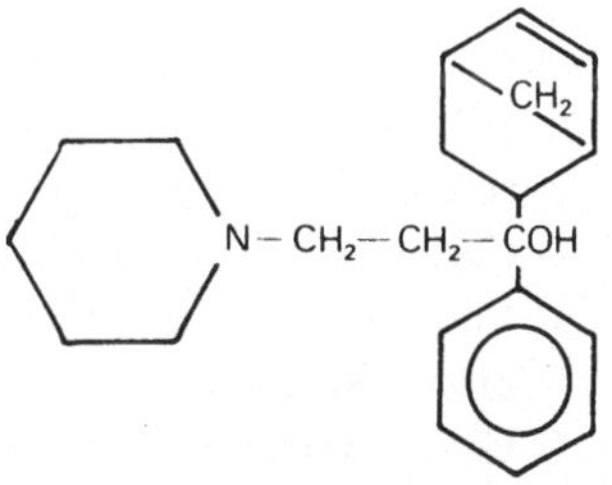

9a   b

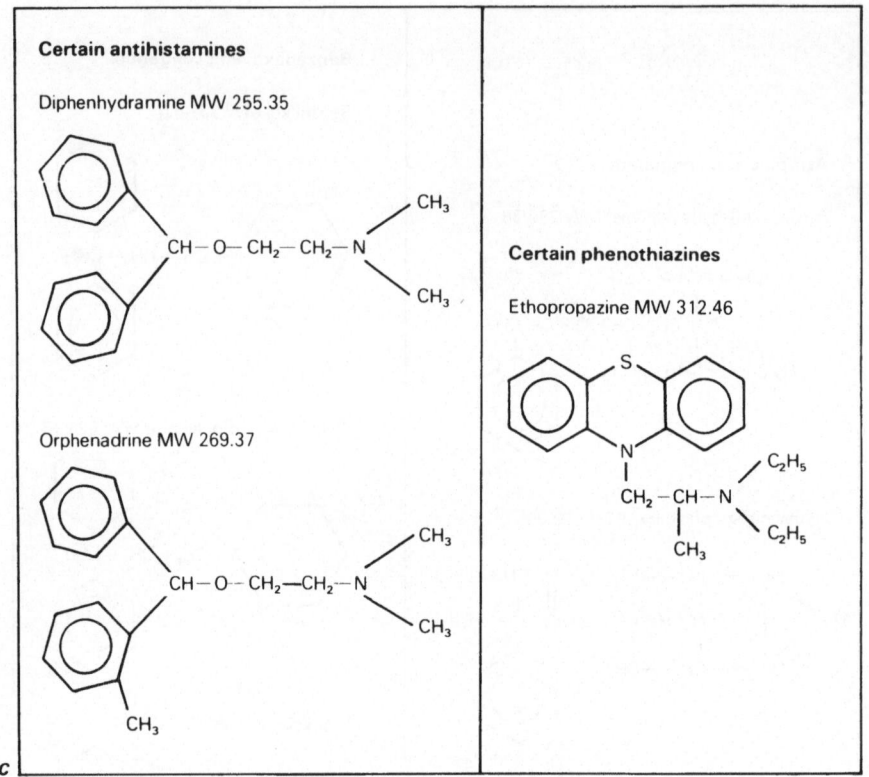

Certain antihistamines

Diphenhydramine MW 255.35

Certain phenothiazines

Ethopropazine MW 312.46

Orphenadrine MW 269.37

Fig. 4.9a-d. Centrally acting anticholinergics grouped by chemical type.

tions, confusion and delirium. With still higher doses there may be coma and paralysis of medullary function, causing death. Hyoscine is a central depressant. In therapeutic doses it causes drowsiness, amnesia and sleep. In higher doses its central effects resemble those of atropine.

Peripheral actions: These may be summarised:
1) Eye: pupillary dilatation; paralysis of accommodation, causing blurred vision; risk of increasing intraocular pressure in persons with narrow angle glaucoma
2) Cardiovascular system: tendency to tachycardia
3) Respiratory system: decreased secretion at all levels of the respiratory tract; bronchodilatation
4) Gastrointestinal system: decreased salivary secretion causing dry mouth; tendency to decreased gastric secretion of fluid and acid; tendency to inhibit motility of the alimentary tract

5) Urinary tract: decreased motility, leading to a risk of urinary retention in patients with a degree of urethral obstruction

6) Sweat glands: diminished sweat production.

Pharmacokinetics

Relatively little pharmacokinetic information is available about these drugs, many of which are declining in use.

Absorption and bioavailability: Since the centrally acting anticholinergics cross the blood-brain barrier they are likely to possess sufficient lipophilicity to be absorbed reasonably well from the alimentary tract. The fact that their oral and intravenous doses are similar suggests that they usually have fairly complete bioavailability. Being bases they are probably absorbed from the small intestine. Beermann et al. (1971) showed that orally administered atropine had at least a 90 % bioavailability. The data of Ellison et al. (1971) suggest that orphenadrine has a greater than 90 % bioavailability. After oral dosage, plasma diphenhydramine levels achieve peak values in 2 to 4 hours (Glazko et al., 1974). The bioavailability of the drug is about 50 % due to first-pass metabolism rather than poor absorption (Albert et al., 1975).

Distribution: Data for apparent volumes of distribution of these drugs are not available. Atropine is said to be distributed throughout the body, as might be expected for a drug lipophilic enough to cross the blood-brain barrier. It seems likely that a similar widespread distribution would apply for the other anticholinergic drugs.

Atropine enters various body secretions, including milk. About 50 % of the atropine in plasma is protein-bound. Less than 2 % of the diphenhydramine in plasma is free in plasma water (Albert et al., 1975).

Elimination: Atropine is excreted in urine, some 13 to 50 % being unchanged and the remainder being in the form of as yet unidentified metabolites. Its plasma half-life is 13 to 38 hours (Kalser, 1971). Hyoscine is more extensively metabolised.

Ellison et al., (1971) found that the half-life of orphenadrine was 14 hours. Only 8 % of an administered dose of orphenadrine was excreted unchanged in the urine of man.

Diphenhydramine has a half-life in man of 7 hours (Glazko et al., 1974). It forms mono and di-*N*-desalkylated metabolites as well as diphenylmethoxyacetic acid (Chang et al., 1974).

Plasma level correlations: No data are available correlating anti-Parkinsonian effects of these drugs with their plasma concentrations.

Interactions

Pharmacodynamic interactions: In the past, two or more centrally acting anticholinergic drugs were often combined in the attempt to obtain additive effects. Drugs used for other purposes (e.g. tricyclic antidepressants) may have central anti-cholinergic actions which reinforce those of the anticholinergic anti-Parkinsonian agents.

The additional anti-Parkinsonian effect of combining centrally acting anti-cholinergics with amantadine or levodopa probably is not so much an additive interaction as an effect at two different classes of receptor on the same neurones.

Centrally acting dopamine antagonists, particularly phenothiazines, have certain of their central toxic effects (e.g. Parkinsonism) reversed by anticholinergics such as benzhexol. However there are data suggesting that this anti-Parkinsonian action may involve a pharmacokinetic effect decreasing the absorption of the phenothiazine (Rivera-Calimlim et al., 1973).

There have been suggestions of an interaction between orphenadrine and the analgesic dextropropoxyphene. However this may not be an interaction but the summation of similar effects of two drugs.

Pharmacokinetic interactions: There are no well documented pharmacokinetic interactions affecting the centrally acting anticholinergics. This is scarcely surprising when there have been so few measurements made of plasma levels. Benzhexol may delay gastric emptying and thus increase the intragastric breakdown of levodopa, so diminishing its plasma concentrations (Morgan et al., 1975). Orphenadrine therapy may cause a fall in plasma chlorpromazine levels (Loga et al., 1975).

It is said that monoamine oxidase inhibitors enhance the effects of centrally acting anticholinergics. While the mechanism of this interaction is not established it might be anticipated that those anticholinergics which are tertiary amines might undergo deamination as part of their biotransformation (as does orphenadrine). Monoamine oxidase might be involved in the further oxidation of some of these deaminated products and the inhibition of this enzyme conceivably might allow accumulation of biologically active metabolic intermediates of the anticholinergics.

Toxicity

Idiosyncratic Toxicity
Skin rashes may occur in occasional patients given these drugs.

Dose-related Toxicity
Therapeutic doses of the centrally acting anticholinergics often produce dryness of the mouth and blurred vision. Anticholinergics tend to cause constipation and difficulty with micturition. Palpitation may occur and, particularly in the elderly, there may be confusion, disorientation and hallucinations.

In very hot weather, Parkinsonian patients treated with high doses of anti-cholinergics are at risk of heat stroke, due to anticholinergic blockade of sweating mechanisms.

Rarely, anticholinergics cause reversible dyskinetic movements of the limbs, face and mouth (Birket-Smith, 1974).

Dysmorphogenicity

No data are available. Dysmorphogenicity is unlikely to be an important consideration when these agents are used to treat Parkinsonism, which is largely a disorder of middle and later life.

Treatment of Parkinsonism

In practice it is rarely possible to treat Parkinsonism by correcting its cause but the clinician should ensure the patient is not taking drugs which could worsen the condition e.g. phenothiazines, butyrophenones, reserpine, and that he is not still exposed to the causative factor e.g. manganese poisoning.

The advent of levodopa and amantadine about a decade ago virtually revolutionised the medical treatment of Parkinsonism. In particular, levodopa has displaced stereotaxic surgery as the treatment of choice for severely affected patients. It was suggested that levodopa should be given as early as possible in the disorder, in the hope that the fundamental biochemical disturbance would be corrected by the replacement therapy, and the progress of the condition thereby halted. Accumulating experience has shown that this hope was ill-founded and it now appears clear that the basic process of idiopathic Parkinsonism progresses despite treatment. The medical treatment of Parkinsonism is still evolving. What appears optimal treatment at the time of writing may not do so a short time hence.

On the whole the aetiology of Parkinsonism is not a major determinant of response to therapy, though some of the symptomatic varieties of the disorder do not seem to respond as well as others. The diagnosis of Parkinsonism, and hence its treatment, may be delayed in certain symptomatic varieties because of the confusing effects of associated corticospinal, cerebellar and other deficits (as in olivo-ponto-cerebellar atrophy and progressive supranuclear palsy). In such disorders striatal damage may have already become too severe for a good response to therapy before the presence of Parkinsonism is recognised.

The Management of Mild Parkinsonism

When Parkinsonism is mild, either because the patient is seen early in the evolution of the disorder or because the disorder is only slowly progressive, the benefits of therapy with levodopa may be more than counterbalanced by the side effects. In these circumstances amantadine or centrally acting anticholinergics will often suffice. Levodopa is reserved for the patients who do not receive adequate benefit from these lesser drugs or who develop unacceptable side effects. In general amantadine is more effective than the anticholinergics and produces fewer side effects. It is therefore usually the initial treatment of choice in mild Parkinsonism.

Amantadine Therapy

Amantadine is often given initially in a dose of 100mg morning and midday. There seems no particular pharmacokinetic rationale for this timing of dosage. Amantadine has a half-life of about 12 hours or longer and is intended for long term use in Parkinsonism. Therefore there seems little point in giving the drug more frequently than 12-hourly. Possibly giving amantadine at approximately 7am and 1pm might produce peak drug levels in the afternoon when the patient might be tiring and require maximum help from his treatment. The half-life of amantadine suggests that, with regular drug intake, a steady-state should be reached 3 or 4 days after treatment starts. Clinical improvement is sometimes detectable within a few hours of a patient's beginning amantadine but maximum improvement often seems to require 1 or 2 weeks of therapy at constant dosage, and sometimes as long as 2 months or more. Generally rigidity and akinesia respond better than does tremor.

If, after 1 month of treatment with 200mg of amantadine per day, there is inadequate relief, the dose should be increased to 300mg per day. While this is customarily given as 100mg 3 times a day the pharmacokinetic data suggest twice daily dosage should suffice. At approximately monthly intervals further dosage increases may be made but, although doses as high as 800mg per day have been used, it seems to be fairly general experience that relatively little additional advantage is likely to accrue from doses exceeding 300mg per day (Parkes et al. 1970). This relatively narrow optimal daily dosage range (200 to 300mg) is not surprising for a drug which is eliminated almost entirely by renal excretion, since renal function in the normal person is much less variable than hepatic biotransformation capacity, which is the main avenue of elimination of so many drugs. This pattern of elimination of amantadine suggests that reduced dosage might be necessary in patients with renal insufficiency.

Side effects from amantadine are generally slight and often negligible. Early in the course of treatment postural hypotension causes some patients to experience faintness but this generally lessens with time. Livedo reticularis may worry some patients till its nature is explained to them. Oedema of the feet and ankles is probably more common in patients who are inactive, whether by virtue of inadequately treated disease or the patient's occupation or temperament. If necessary the oedema may be treated with diuretics. Some older patients, particularly those with evidence of pre-existing blunting of intellect, may become confused and hallucinated when treated with amantadine. This may be sufficiently troublesome to make withdrawal of treatment necessary. Unfortunately, if amantadine upsets cerebral function there is a risk that levodopa and anticholinergics will do likewise. Further, it can be dangerous to stop amantadine treatment *abruptly*. Even if the patient's Parkinsonism does not seem to have responded well to amantadine, *sudden* cessation of the drug may provoke a

Parkinsonian crisis. The patient may become virtually unable to move or swallow. It may then be necessary to administer intravenous fluids to correct dehydration and intravenous atropine to relieve the Parkinsonism sufficiently to permit the patient to swallow amantadine again.

Centrally Acting Anticholinergic Therapy

If amantadine does not afford sufficient relief to the patient with mild Parkinsonism, or if he is troubled by excess saliva, one of the centrally acting anticholinergics may be given also. Benztropine, which is reputed to be long acting, is usually given once a day and the other drugs 3 times a day (sometimes twice). In general the pharmacokinetic data which would provide a rational basis for using these drugs are lacking. However, the half-lives of atropine and orphenadrine suggest that it would be adequate to give these 2 drugs twice daily. In the past, when anticholinergics were the only moderately effective drugs available for Parkinsonism, several different agents were often combined. There was really no good evidence that these combinations were more effective or less prone to produce side effects than a single drug with the dose taken to the patient's limit of tolerance. At present, when anticholinergics are simply providing a supplementary attack on the biochemical disturbance of Parkinsonism, with the main attack at the striatal dopamine receptors, it should rarely be necessary to use more than one anticholinergic agent at once. There is probably little to choose between the various anticholinergic agents. Orphenadrine appears the least likely to cause confusion and there are more pharmacokinetic data available about it than the other anticholinergic drugs. Therefore orphenadrine might be the preferred anticholinergic. Doses of the order of 50 to 100mg twice daily are usual. With such doses side effects are uncommon, apart from blurred vision and a dry mouth. When higher doses of anticholinergics are used constipation may become a problem and higher cerebral functions may become disturbed.

The Management of More Severe Parkinsonism

Levodopa Therapy

If Parkinsonism is already severe when the patient presents and/or if amantadine and anticholinergics have proved inadequate, levodopa should be used. With its use higher cerebral function may worsen, particularly in elderly patients who already have confusion or dementia. It may then be necessary to reduce the dose or stop the drug. There is no contraindication to continuing amantadine and/or anticholinergics when levodopa is used. In fact the combination of levodopa and anticholinergics may confer additional minor benefits (Whyte et al., 1971; Horrocks et al., 1973). In particular, sialorrhoea is better controlled (Hughes et al., 1971). It is said that if a maximum tolerated dose of levodopa is used amantadine may not offer additional advantages (Godwin-Austen et al., 1970).

It appears worth trying levodopa regardless of the aetiology of Parkinsonism. On the whole the idiopathic and the post-encephalitic types respond best, the latter tending to require lower doses of levodopa than the former (Duvoisin et al., 1972). Even in a rare entity such as pallido-pyramidal degeneration the Parkinsonism may respond to levodopa (Horowitz and Greenberg, 1975).

It seems unlikely that many patients will now start therapy with levodopa alone rather than combined with a decarboxylase inhibitor. If levodopa alone is used, the patient usually begins taking a low dose e.g. 250mg once or twice a day for an average adult and perhaps 100mg once or twice daily after meals, for a frail elderly person. At weekly or fortnightly intervals the dose may be increased by 100 or 250mg daily, on a 3 times a day routine basis, till an optimal response is attained or side effects limit dose increase. An average levodopa dose is 3 to 5 grams per day. Side effects are reduced by the very gradual introduction of the drug; benefit may not appear for weeks or months, though it may be noticed within a few days. In contrast, benefit from the levodopa-decarboxylase inhibitor combinations may be apparent after a single dose. Patients taking levodopa alone (i.e. not combined with decarboxylase inhibitor) should be instructed to avoid preparations containing pyridoxine (notably multiple vitamin preparations). Despite the gradual build-up in levodopa dose, and despite taking the drug after food, such patients will often require antiemetics (e.g. meclozine, cyclizine) and antacids, to reduce nausea. Should patients become overdosed and develop dyskinesia, treatment with pyridoxine e.g. 50mg 3 times a day, will speed the destruction of levodopa peripherally, and hasten recovery from the overdosage. However pyridoxine therapy would not have a dyskinesia-reducing effect in overdosed patients taking a levodopa-decarboxylase inhibitor. Giving pyridoxine might then even worsen the dyskinesia as, in theory, it might increase the central decarboxylation of levodopa to dopamine (Mars, 1974).

Levodopa-Decarboxylase Inhibitor Combination Therapy

If levodopa-dopa decarboxylase inhibitor combinations are available many would now prefer them to levodopa alone as initial therapy for severe Parkinsonism. The combinations minimise the peripheral side effects of levodopa. Because of this, and particularly because of the reduced incidence of nausea and vomiting, the levodopa dose can be built up much more rapidly. Thus the patient obtains benefit a good deal more quickly than if levodopa is used alone. With the combinations, the average adult patient takes an initial dose of 100mg levodopa (plus inhibitor) 3 or 4 times a day, the dose being increased once or twice a week by 100 to 150mg per day till an optimum response occurs. It does not appear necessary to give the combination more often than 3 or 4 times a day. An average levodopa dose (in combination) to achieve an optimum response is likely to be 750 to 1000mg per day. As the levodopa dose is increased dyskinesia may occur. The advent of dyskinesia is usually taken as indicating that the optimum dose has been exceeded, so that some dose reduction is indicated. The concurrent administration of anticholinergics may worsen dyskinesia

(Birket-Smith, 1975). However, some patients may prefer to have some dyskinesia rather than to be free from these involuntary movements but limited by residual Parkinsonian rigidity. The levodopa-inhibitor combinations do not always prevent dopamine-induced nausea and an antinauseant (e.g. meclozine 12.5 to 25mg 2 or 3 times a day) may be necessary. Phenothiazines and butyrophenones are contraindicated as they increase Parkinsonism (Klawans and Weiner, 1974, 1974a), but metoclopramide, despite its action as a dopamine antagonist, apparently does not (Tarsy et al., 1975). Whenever levodopa is used it is desirable to review the patient every few months as a previously satisfactory dose may subsequently prove too great (or too small) for the patient.

Many patients with severe Parkinsonism were treated with levodopa alone before the levodopa-decarboxylase inhibitor combinations became available. If these patients have achieved a completely satisfactory therapeutic response with negligible side effects there is little point in changing their treatment to the levodopa-inhibitor combination therapy. If, however, the response of their Parkinsonism has been unsatisfactory or if the peripheral types of side effect have been troublesome, the use of levodopa combined with a decarboxylase inhibitor should be considered.

Addition of a Decarboxylase Inhibitor to Levodopa Therapy

When a patient's therapy is changed from levodopa alone to a levodopa-decarboxylase inhibitor combination, all levodopa should first be discontinued for 12 to 24 hours, though it is not necessary to discontinue amantadine or anticholinergics. This allows plasma and tissue levodopa levels time to fall (so that the decarboxylase inhibitors do not inhibit the peripheral breakdown of accumulated levodopa and cause a greatly increased, though temporary, central action). If levodopa-carbidopa is to be used, 20% (Cotzias, 1969) or if levodopa-benserazine, 40% (Miller and Wiener, 1974) of the previous daily levodopa dose is then given in 3 or 4 divided doses over 24 hours. Thereafter dosage is increased or decreased as necessary every few days to achieve an optimal response.

Levodopa Failure

There appear to be a number of causes of an inadequate response to levodopa:

1) The Parkinsonism may be of a type that does not respond well to levodopa e.g. the Shy-Drager syndrome (Aminoff et al., 1973), striato-nigral degeneration (Rajput et al., 1972).

2) An insufficient dose of levodopa is given because:

   a) too little is prescribed, or

   b) no more can be tolerated because of unwanted central or peripheral effects.

3) A potentially sufficient oral dose of levodopa is not absorbed adequately, possibly because of delayed gastric emptying, allowing increased intragastric destruction of the drug.

4) The actions of a sufficient dose of levodopa may be blocked by concurrently administered dopamine receptor blocking agents (e.g. phenothiazines, mistakenly given to counteract nausea due to levodopa). Levodopa effects may be reduced by pyridoxine (taken by some patients who are vitamin enthusiasts, or prescribed unwittingly when one of the antihistamine-pyridoxine combinations used for morning sickness of pregnancy is given to treat levodopa-induced nausea and vomiting). While pyridoxine will reduce the central actions of levodopa in patients with Parkinsonism, it does not have this effect if the patient is also taking a dopa-decarboxylase inhibitor (Mars, 1974).

5) After several years of successful levodopa therapy periods of apparent refractoriness to the drug may occur, lasting minutes to hours, and alternating with periods of responsiveness and sometimes with periods of dyskinesia i.e. an apparent excessive responsiveness. The mechanism of this 'on-off' phenomenon is not fully understood. In some patients the periods of apparent refractoriness are associated with low plasma levels of levodopa. This raises the question of temporarily impaired drug absorption (which may be improved by a low protein diet), or of altered peripheral handling of the drug (Sweet and McDowell, 1974). However, poor absorption is unlikely to be the full explanation of the 'on-off' phenomenon. Replacement of levodopa by a dopa-decarboxylase inhibitor combination does not influence the 'on-off' effect according to Fahn (1974) though Sweet et al. (1975) found the combination did lessen the 'on-off' effect in 13 of 20 patients studied. CSF levels of homovanillic acid and hydroxy-indoleacetic acid do not correlate with the 'on-off' phenomenon. This suggests that alterations in brain dopamine and serotonin metabolism are not responsible for the effect (Sweet and McDowell, 1974). There have been suggestions that certain levodopa metabolites e.g. tetrahydropapaveroline (Sourkes, 1971) may be responsible for the 'on-off' effect by temporarily blockading dopamine receptors (Dougan et al., 1975). The fact that Parkinsonism may sometimes worsen at times of peak plasma levels of levodopa (Claveria et al., 1973) would be consistent with the 'off' periods being due to a toxic effect of levodopa or one of its metabolites. This type of 'off' effect may be relieved by giving the drug in smaller, more frequent, doses. The observation of Kartzinel and Calne (1976) that substitution of the centrally acting dopaminergic agent bromocriptine for levodopa did not cure the 'on-off' effect raises the possibility that fluctuation in receptor sensitivity may be responsible.

Marsden and Parkes (1976) have provided a useful review of the 'on-off' phenomenon. They believe that more than one mechanism is involved. To some extent the phenomenon is due to progression of the basic pathology of Parkinsonism and to some extent to a shortened duration of action of levodopa. 'Off' periods at the end of a dosage interval may be relieved by more frequent drug dosage. Rapid fluctuations between 'on' and 'off' periods may be helped by gradual reduction in levodopa dosage and adjustments in its frequency of administration. However, no available therapy produces a satisfactory outcome in every instance of the 'on-off' phenomenon.

Measurement of the plasma concentration of levodopa might help differentiate between certain of these five possible explanations of failure of levodopa therapy but facilities for these measurements are not available to most clinicians. Therefore when the response to levodopa is unsatisfactory, except when this is due to the overdosage type of unwanted 'on' effect, the clinician is often forced to try a larger dose of the drug or to improve the availability to the brain of the dose already given. He should exclude the intake of drugs which might reduce the effect of levodopa. Prescribing levodopa before meals, and/or with a dose of antacid, may speed the drug's entry into the small intestine but preprandial dosage unfortunately often increases drug-induced nausea. Replacing levodopa with levodopa-decarboxylase inhibitor combinations reduces the problems arising from gastric stasis and also those of dosage limitation due to peripheral side effects (e.g. nausea and vomiting). Thus the use of the levodopa-decarboxylase inhibitor combinations can improve control of Parkinsonism in patients with drug absorption problems (probably including some instances of the 'on-off' phenomenon) and in patients whose dosage has been limited by the peripheral type of side effect. The combinations do not improve the control of Parkinsonism in patients whose disease is intrinsically refractory or in patients whose dosage is limited by the occurrence of the central type of side effect. Such side effects worsen if more levodopa enters cerebral tissues.

Therapy with levodopa has revolutionised the treatment of Parkinsonism. The improvement in rigidity and bradykinesis and the restoration of speech, freedom of movement and facial expression is sometimes almost complete, and far greater than could be achieved with previous therapies. The response of tremor is less and develops more slowly than the response of the other manifestations. Useful improvement in tremor can occur in the 6 to 9 months after therapy is instituted but rigidity and bradykinesis usually responds within days or weeks.

Other Drug Therapies

With recognition of the role of striatal dopamine deficiency in Parkinsonism there has been a search for dopamine agonists which will cross the blood-brain barrier. Such substances might have an advantage over levodopa in that they would influence striatal efferent neurones directly. They would not depend on an enzymatic mechanism, which might be altered by disease, to produce the pharmacologically active substance (dopamine).

Apomorphine is a dopamine agonist but the amount of vomiting it induces makes its use unacceptable in practice. Indeed, it is used as an emetic. Duby et al. (1972) showed that apomorphine does not benefit Parkinsonism in the same way that levodopa does. For instance apomorphine has a rapid effect on Parkinsonian tremor, but little effect on akinesia.

Piribedil (Sweet et al., 1974; Chase et al., 1974) and *bromocriptine* (2-bromo-alpha-ergocryptine) (Gerlach, 1976) have rather more tolerable side effects than apomorphine. They appear at least comparable with amantadine in anti-Parkinsonian effect. Piribedil may produce psychiatric disturbance (Engel et al., 1975) and dyskinesia (Chase et al., 1974). Bromocriptine may also cause dyskinesia and hallucinations, suppresses lactation and causes increased plasma growth hormone levels. It may be used to replace levodopa if the latter causes unacceptable side effects or excessive swings in response (Parkes, 1979).

Other agents that have been used include *elantrine*, which acts more on tremor than on rigidity or bradykinesis (Blonsky et al., 1974); *lergotrile*, an inhibitor of prolactin secretion which relieves Parkinsonism but which may produce orthostatic hypotension, vomiting and altered behaviour (Lieberman et al., 1975); and *nomifensine* (Teychenne et al., 1976).

β-Adrenergic blocking agents (e.g. *propranolol, oxprenolol*) have been used to relieve Parkinsonian tremor but their efficacy seems doubtful (Sandler et al., 1975). Chase (1974) claimed that *desipramine* reduced Parkinsonian tremor and Loeb and Priano (1977) claimed the anticonvulsant *clonazepam* was of benefit. Intravenous melanocyte-stimulating-hormone release inhibiting factor (MIF) i.e. L-prolyl-L-leucyl-glycine amide, is said to improve Parkinsonian tremor slightly (Fischer et al., 1974).

Surgery

If Parkinsonian tremor is the patient's main handicap after medical treatment has been taken to its limit for a sufficient time, stereotaxic destruction of the venterolateral nucleus of the thalamus (on the side opposite to the tremor) may still offer prospects of considerable improvement. In patients with severe typical Parkinsonism the combination of stereotaxic thalamotomy and levodopa therapy appears to offer the maximum prospect for restoration of function. However treatment with levodopa alone often provides the patient with sufficient benefit. Levodopa is said to work less well in previously thalamectomised patients than in unoperated patients (Laitinen, 1973).

Other Therapeutic Measures

Long before effective drugs became available it was apparent that patients with Parkinsonism remained mobile much longer if they undertook as much physical activity as possible. The more physical work the patient did the longer he seemed to remain able to do physical work. Now that a highly effective therapy in the form of levodopa is available the importance of physical activity should not be neglected.

It is becoming increasingly clear that the fundamental brain degeneration in idiopathic Parkinsonism continues despite levodopa therapy. Therefore it is conceivable that patients may ultimately become refractory to levodopa. However there may still be a place in therapy for dopamine agonists, anticholinergics and surgery.

Chorea

In a pharmacological sense as well as to some extent in a clinical sense, chorea is in many ways the antithesis of Parkinsonism. Chorea appears to be a result of a relative excess of striatal dopamine activity.

Disordered Mechanisms

In contrast to Parkinsonism, chorea involves a state of widespread muscle hypotonia and a hyperkinesis with exaggeration of associated movements. The causes of chorea are:

1) Rheumatic fever (Sydenham's chorea)
2) Huntington's disease
3) Senile chorea
4) Overdosage with levodopa given for the treatment of Parkinsonism
5) Rarely, the intake of oral contraceptives (Lewis and Harrison, 1969) or phenytoin (Chadwick et al., 1976).

The existence of senile chorea is perhaps arguable and a rigid form of Huntington's disease occurs as well as the more common choreic type. The rigidity in Huntington's disease may respond to levodopa therapy. Chorea in pregnancy may or may not be related to previous Sydenham's chorea. A pharmacological and biochemical classification of basal ganglia disorders may not correspond completely with the traditional clinical and pathological classification of these conditions.

In cases of chorea histological changes are found in the basal ganglia (and elsewhere in the nervous system) but no precise correlation has been established between disorders of function and sites of lesions. However, shrinkage of the head of the caudate nucleus, and to a lesser extent the putamen and globus pallidus, is conspicuous in Huntington's disease. In hemiballismus, which may be regarded as a form of violent hemichorea, any pathological changes which are found are situated in the contralateral subthalamic nucleus where the abnormality is nearly always a focal haemorrhage or infarct (Martin, 1959).

The striatum of patients with chorea has a normal concentration of dopamine, despite local neuronal loss, so that there is a local excess of dopamine relative to the number of surviving striatal neurones. In patients with Parkinsonism, if levodopa dose is increased sufficiently, choreic manifestations appear, possibly because too much dopamine is then formed in the striatum. While chorea may be due to a local excess of dopamine in the striatum, it is also possible that in chorea striatal dopamine receptors are in a state of denervation hypersensitivity (Klawans, 1970). There may be other biochemical alterations in chorea. For instance in Huntington's chorea concentrations of the enzyme glutamic acid decarboxylase are reduced in the striatum and substantia nigra. This reduction is more than can be accounted for by cell loss (Bird et al., 1973). Glutamic acid decarboxylase is responsible for the formation of the inhibitory synaptic transmitter γ-aminobutyric acid (GABA) from glutamic acid and local basal ganglia GABA concentrations are reduced in Huntington's chorea (Perry et al., 1973). It is possible that decreased GABA activity in the striatum also plays a role in chorea. However, administration of valproic acid (which raises brain GABA concentrations by inhibiting its metabolic breakdown) does not improve Huntington's chorea (Shoulson et al., 1976).

It is possible to give a coherent account of the altered physiology and biochemistry of chorea in terms of altered regional dopamine function. Loss of neurones in the caudate nucleus and putamen, with an intact nigro-striatal dopaminic inflow, leads to a relative dopamine overaction in the striatum. This alters the inflow to the globus pallidus and thence to the ventro-lateral thalamic nuclei. Regulatory impulses from the subthalamic nuclei also discharge upon the ventro-lateral thalamic nuclei. Loss of these impulses, or increased dopaminic action in the striatum, lead to an altered pattern of discharging of the ventro-lateral thalamic nuclei on the cortex, and this produces the movement disorder of chorea.

Correction of Disordered Mechanisms

Correction of the Causative Process

The most fundamental therapeutic approach to chorea would be to correct the underlying disease process. The natural history of rheumatic chorea is for spontaneous recovery to occur, though there may be later relapses e.g. in pregnancy. Therefore if further infection with β-haemolytic streptococci is prevented by prophylactic antibiotics (e.g. phenoxymethylpenicillin) spontaneous recovery of rheumatic chorea is very likely as the disease process resolves. Symptomatic relief of the chorea is also desirable while recovery is taking place.

The nature of the underlying genetic process in Huntington's disease is not understood and it cannot be corrected by any known therapeutic measure. Similar considerations apply to the process underlying senile chorea, which is sometimes suspected of being a late-onset form of Huntington's disease. Chorea due to excess levodopa dosage in Parkinsonism can be relieved, if judged desirable, by reducing the levodopa dose. The infarction or haemorrhage responsible for hemiballismus often tends to produce the chorea only during its acute phase, so that the condition may be self-limiting. Chorea due to oral contraceptives can be relieved by withdrawing the causative agent (Gamboa et al., 1971).

Relief of Chorea

Chorea and hemiballism can be relieved by:
1) Decreasing the amount of dopamine present in nigro-striatal axon terminals
2) Blocking the action of dopamine on striatal receptors
3) Blocking the passage of impulses through the ventro-lateral thalamic nuclei by stereotaxic destruction of these regions.

Drugs such as reserpine and tetrabenazine cause release of dopamine from nigro-striatal axon terminals and block its re-uptake. The released transmitter amine is degraded enzymatically. Thus a state of local dopamine deficiency supervenes. Phenothiazines and butyrophenones block dopaminic receptors on striatal neurones. These chemotherapeutic measures are usually quite effective in relieving chorea and thalamotomy is hardly ever necessary.

Agents Altering Dopamine Release

Although reserpine is still sometimes used as an antihypertensive agent, it is a drug which is being superseded by newer and more effective agents. There is some suspicion that its chronic use may cause breast malignancy. Therefore it seems unnecessary to consider reserpine further for use in neurology.

Tetrabenazine

The main use of tetrabenazine is in the treatment of chorea though it has been used in schizophrenia. It is of occasional benefit in torsion dystonia and spasmodic torticollis (Swash et al., 1972).

Chemistry

Tetrabenazine (MW 317.41) is a derivative of 1,2,3,4,6,7-hexahydro-11b H-benzo(a)quinolizine (fig. 4.10), usually used as the hydrochloride or methanesulphonate.

Pharmacology

Biochemical Pharmacology
Tetrabenazine acts like reserpine (Pletscher et al., 1962) to release biogenic amines from axon terminals and block their re-uptake. It also blocks the action of a

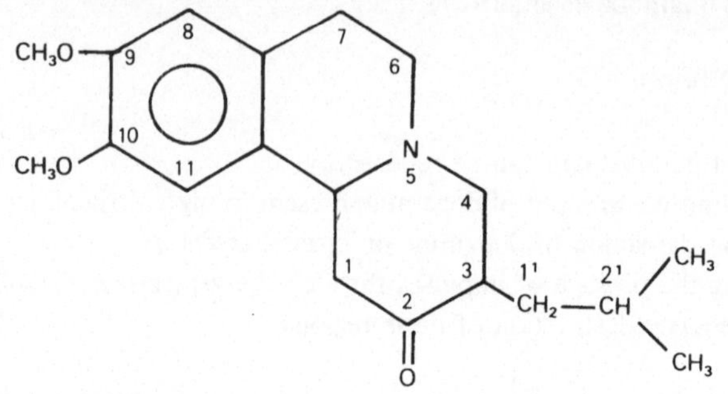

Fig. 4.10. Structural formula of tetrabenazine.

soluble factor in rat brain which inhibits the enzyme adenosine triphosphatase (Schaefer et al., 1973). The central actions of tetrabenazine relative to its peripheral actions are more developed than those of reserpine. The use of tetrabenazine leads to decreased brain concentrations of dopamine, noradrenaline and 5-hydroxy-tryptamine.

Pharmacodynamics

The drug may have beneficial actions in schizophrenia. In high dosage it produces Parkinsonian rigidity and bradykinesis, the converse of chorea.

Pharmacokinetics

Very little information is available as to the pharmacokinetics of tetrabenazine in man. The drug is known to undergo the following biotransformation reactions in man:

i) reduction of the keto group at the 2 position
ii) oxidation at the carbon atom at position 2 on the isobutyl side-chain
iii) ether cleavage of the methoxy group attached to the 9 position.

The resulting hydroxyl derivatives may form conjugates with glucuronic acid prior to excretion (Schwartz et al., 1966).

Interactions

Pharmacodynamic interactions: Additive interactions with phenothiazines and butyrophenones, and antagonism to levodopa, might be anticipated.

Pharmacokinetic interactions: None are known.

Toxicity

Tetrabenazine overdose may cause Parkinsonism and might be expected to cause depression and hypotension (by analogy with the effects of reserpine). Tetrabenazine may cause drowsiness, or insomnia. Snaith and Warren (1974) reported that the drug, in controlling chorea, might produce dysphagia and choking.

Dopamine Receptor Blocking Agents

Phenothiazines

The phenothiazines are used in psychiatry as antipsychotic agents and major tranquillisers. Some are also used as antiemetics and as premedication for certain neuro-radiological investigations. Some phenothiazines are used for their antihistamine actions e.g. promethazines, and one is used as an anticholinergic anti-Parkinsonian agent (ethopropazine).

Chemistry

The basic phenothiazine structure is shown in figure 4.11. The various phenothiazine derivatives used in therapeutics are substituted at the 2 and 10 positions. The substituent groups of some of the more commonly used phenothiazines are also shown. Phenothiazine bases are often used as their corresponding hydrochlorides.

Pharmacology

Biochemical Pharmacology

The phenothiazines inhibit re-uptake of noradrenaline and 5-hydroxy-tryptamine released from storage granules in axon terminals, thus decreasing brain concentrations of these amines. However the most important action of these drugs from the neurological point of view is their capacity to block dopamine receptors in the basal ganglia, hypothalamus and chemoreceptor trigger zone in the floor of the fourth ventricle. Chlorpromazine also inhibits brain uptake of GABA (Iversen and Johnston, 1971). Chlorpromazine is a potent competitive inhibitor of the enzyme adenylcyclase which can be isolated from the rat caudate nucleus (Kebabian et al., 1972). Possibly this enzyme is the striatal dopamine receptor. In the rat chlorpromazine also inhibits the increase in cyclic adenosine monophosphate formation which is produced by dopamine deficiency in the nucleus accumbens and

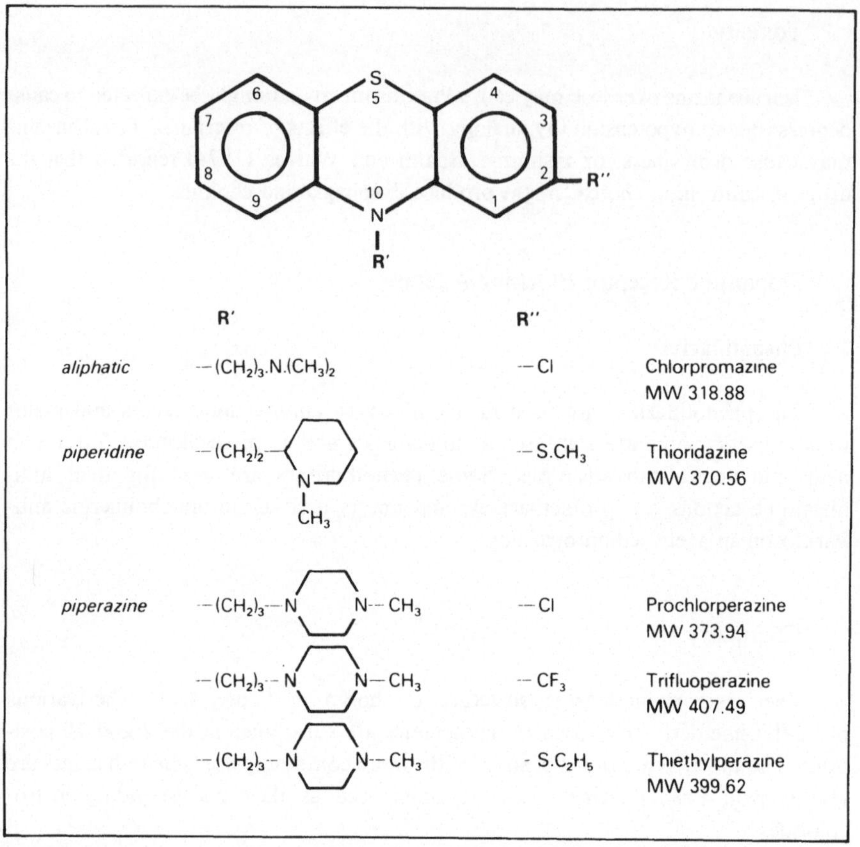

Fig. 4.11. The chemical formulae of phenothiazine and some of its most commonly used derivatives.

olfactory tubercule (Horn et al., 1974). Phenothiazines alter the protein structure of membranes from brain cells (Leterrier et al., 1973). They inhibit the mitochondrial enzyme Mg^{++}-linked adenosine triphosphatase and also flavine nucleotide co-enzymes (Guth and Spirtes, 1964). Either chlorpromazine (Schaefer et al., 1973) or a free radicle formed from it by ultraviolet irradiation or through enzymatic oxidation with peroxidase (Gubitz et al., 1973), inhibits Na^+, K^+-linked adenosine triphosphatase. Phenothiazines also inhibit acetylcholinesterase and nonspecific cholinesterase (Michalek, 1973).

Pharmacodynamics

Central effects: The phenothiazines act at many levels of the central nervous system. They produce sedation, relieve anxiety, reduce spontaneous motor activity and tend to cause affective indifference. They may reduce the seizure threshold. They depress central vasomotor reflexes, causing hypotension, and block the action of certain emetics on the chemoreceptor trigger zone for vomiting in the medulla. In man they reduce the responsiveness of the vestibular system to vertigo-producing stimuli (Johnson and Ireland, 1965). Chlorpromazine is a potent local anaesthetic. It acts in the hypothalamus to cause decreased growth hormone release and antagonises prolactin-release-inhibiting hormone (occasionally causing galactorrhoea in females). Corticotrophin and antidiuretic hormone secretion may be reduced. Phenothiazines deplete rat pituitary melanocyte-stimulating-hormone (MSH), possibly by inhibiting MSH-inhibiting factor (Robins, 1973).

Peripheral effects: The phenothiazines have some antihistamine and antiserotonin actions. They are weak acetylcholine blocking agents. Whilst they are *a*-adrenergic blocking agents, phenothiazines also have adrenergic effects because they block the re-uptake of catecholamines released from nerve terminals.

Chlorpromazine may have a diuretic effect, perhaps partly due to decreased antidiuretic hormone secretion and partly due to a direct effect on renal tubules.

Pharmacokinetics

Absorption and bioavailability: The absorption of chlorpromazine depends on its dosage form (Hollister et al., 1970). Higher plasma levels of the drug are achieved if chlorpromazine is given as the elixir rather than as tablets. However plasma thioridazine levels are reasonably similar, relative to dose, whether this drug is given in ordinary tablets, in slow release tablets, or in a suspension (Viukari and Salminies, 1973). Plasma chlorpromazine levels are much higher if the drug is given intramuscularly rather than orally in the same dose. This may be due to 'first-pass' metabolism of the drug in the intestinal wall (Curry et al., 1970a). Peak plasma chlorpromazine levels occur 2 to 4 hours after oral dosage (Curry et al., 1970b).

Distribution: After intravenous injection in dogs, chlorpromazine was shown to be highly bound to brain where its level became 70 times that in plasma (Salzman and Brodie, 1956). The drug was also concentrated in the kidneys, spleen, liver and lungs, and to a lesser extent in fat, skeletal muscle and myocardium. Data for other phenothiazines, reviewed by Saunders (1974), suggest that this class of drug generally tends to be highly concentrated in cerebral tissues. The apparent volume of distribution of chlorpromazine, reflecting its considerable tissue binding, is 20L/kg.

Chlorpromazine in plasma is 95 to 98% protein bound (Curry et al., 1970b). Data are not readily available for the protein binding of the other phenothiazines listed.

Elimination: The plasma half-life of chlorpromazine averages 1.29 days (Maxwell et al., 1972). The mean half-life of thioridazine is 24 hours and that of prochlor-

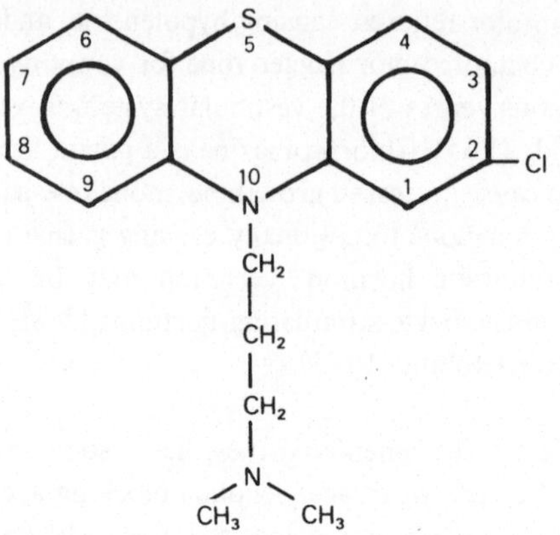

1) Mono- and di-N desmethylation at the terminal N atom of the aliphatic side-chain attached to the 10 position of the phenothiazine ring

2) N-oxide formation at the terminal N atom on this side-chain

3) Sulphoxidation at the 5 position

4) Hydroxylation, and then glucuronide conjugation, at the C atom at the 7 position

5) Elimination of the N10 side-chain

Fig. 4.12. Chlorpromazine and its major patterns of biotransformation.

perazine is 23 hours. With prolonged use the plasma half-life of chlorpromazine is said to shorten (Kaul et al., 1976).

The elimination of chlorpromazine is almost entirely by biotransformation, negligible quantities of unchanged drug being found in human urine during chlorpromazine treatment. It is estimated that chlorpromazine might yield as many as 150 different metabolites, over 50 of which have been detected (Curry, 1973). There are still traces of metabolites in urine 6 months after the phenothiazine intake has ceased. Chlorpromazine undergoes the major patterns of biotransformation shown in figure 4.12 (Parke, 1968). The various metabolites are more polar than chlorpromazine but some possess biological activity. For instance chlorpromazine sulphoxide has about 1/8th of the sedative effect on the parent drug in man.

Other phenothiazines undergo analogous biotransformation reactions of their phenothiazine rings and are likely to undergo side-chain dealkylation. The piperazine ring in the side-chain of certain phenothiazines may undergo ring opening followed by a series of dealkylations of the side-chain (Breyer et al., 1974). This process can produce metabolites similar to those formed from phenothiazines with aliphatic side-chains. The S atom at the 2 position on the molecule of thioridazine can undergo sulphoxidation (Parke, 1968), forming a sulphoxide (mesoridazine). Further details of thioridazine biotransformation are given by Dinovo et al. (1976).

The observation that steady-state chlorpromazine plasma levels fall progressively for a time after a constant daily drug dose is given to man for about 2 weeks raises the possibility that the drug can induce the enzymes involved in its own biotransformation (Curry, 1973). There is some evidence that chlorpromazine may be metabolised in the intestinal wall as well as in the liver.

Plasma level correlations: There is a limited correlation between plasma chlorpromazine levels and biological effects of the drug when first given. As time passes, steady-state plasma drug levels fall but biological effect may remain unaltered (Curry, 1973). It is possible that biologically active metabolites are in part responsible for the actions of the drug and that their concentrations increase as more chlorpromazine is biotransformed. In the steady-state, plasma chlorpromazine levels tend to reach a peak about 2 hours after dosage and then decline to reach baseline values about 10 hours after the peak.

Plasma chlorpromazine levels vary widely in patients taking the same dose. For example in subjects taking 100mg of the drug 3 times a day, after one week plasma drug levels ranged between 26 and 193ng/ml (Sakalis et al., 1972). Rivera-Calimlim et al. (1973) cited a therapeutic range of plasma chlorpromazine levels of 150-300ng/ml in treating schizophrenia and stated that tremors and convulsions occurred at plasma chlorpromazine levels of 750 to 1000ng/ml.

Interactions

Pharmacodynamic interactions: Phenothiazines may react additively with alcohol, barbiturates and various analgesics (e.g. morphine) to depress central neural function. They block catecholamine re-uptake at nerve terminals and thus may prevent the action of amphetamine which can no longer be taken up by terminals to exert its effects by displacing noradrenaline from its storage sites. A similar interaction may occur with guanethidine. Phenothiazines may reinforce the anticholinergic effects of tricyclic antidepressants.

Phenothiazines antagonise the effects of amantadine and levodopa in treating Parkinsonism.

Pharmacokinetic interactions: Antacids, or drugs which delay gastric emptying, such as anticholinergics (e.g. benzhexol), diminish the absorption of chlorpromazine and lower its plasma levels (Rivera-Calimlim et al., 1973).

Phenothiazines appear to decrease the biotransformation of phenytoin. There is evidence that continued phenothiazine intake induces the hepatic drug-metabolising enzymes of man (Kolakowska et al., 1975).

Barbiturates and orphenadrine (Loga et al., 1975) induce the enzyme systems which biotransform chlorpromazine and thereby decrease plasma chlorpromazine levels.

Monoamine oxidase inhibitors appear to increase the actions of phenothiazines, possibly because they prevent the further breakdown of some primary amine meta-bolites of certain phenothiazines.

Toxicity

Idiosyncratic Toxicity
The following manifestations have been described:

a) Blood dyscrasias — leucopenia, leucocytosis, eosinophilia
b) Dermatitis; urticaria; contact dermatitis; photosensitivity
c) Intrahepatic cholestasis with jaundice
d) Acute dystonic reactions, including oculogyric crises (especially from phenothiazines with piperazine side-chains)
e) Galactorrhoea, from increased prolactin release
f) Amenorrhoea.

Dose-related Toxicity
The following are among the manifestations described:

a) Abnormal cutaneous pigmentation
b) Pigmentary retinopathy (from thioridazine, in very high dosage)
c) Epithelial keratopathy, corneal opacities
d) Hypercholesterolaemia
e) Orthostatic hypotension
f) Parkinsonism (from phenothiazines with aliphatic amine or piperidine side-chains)
g) Tardive dyskinesias, which often appear after reduction in dose of phenothiazines with a piperazine type of side-chain; these dyskinesias are thought to be possibly due to denervation hypersensitivity to dopamine (p.133)
h) Akathisia
i) Sedation.

Dysmorphogenicity
There is no clear evidence of phenothiazine dysmorphogenicity.

Butyrophenones

The pharmacology of the butyrophenones is generally similar to that of the phenothiazines. Haloperidol is the most widely used butyrophenone. It is employed particularly in the treatment of psychoses.

Chemistry

Haloperidol (MW 375.88) is a weak base with a pK_a value of 8.25 (Demoen, 1961). Its structural formula is shown in figure 4.13. Haloperidol is practically insoluble in water, but dissolves in organic solvents of moderate polarity.

Pharmacology

Biochemical Pharmacology
The main action of haloperidol, like that of the phenothiazines, is mediated by blockade of dopamine receptors. The drug alters protein structure in the membranes of the synaptic region of neurones (Leterrier et al., 1973) and inhibits acetylcholinesterase (Michalek, 1973).

Pharmacodynamics
The pharmacodynamics of haloperidol are very similar to those of the phenothiazines, particularly those with piperazine side-chains. The peripheral autonomic effects of haloperidol are less developed than those of the phenothiazines.

Pharmacokinetics
Absorption and bioavailability: Haloperidol is absorbed rapidly from the alimentary tract. Peak plasma levels occur 2 to 6 hours after dosage. The bioavailability of the oral preparation in man is 45 % (Forsman and Ohman, 1974).

Distribution: The V_D of haloperidol is 1200 to 2000 litres, suggesting considerable tissue binding (Forsman et al., 1974). The drug is concentrated in the liver and brain of rats. In this species, brain haloperidol levels are 6 to 45 times the simultaneous plasma levels (Marucci et al., 1971). In plasma, 89.6 ± 0.3 % (Hughes et al., 1976) or 92 % (Forsman and Ohman, 1974) of the drug is protein-bound.

Elimination: The terminal half-life of haloperidol is 12.6 to 22.0 hours (Forsman et al., 1974). In man only 1 % of a haloperidol dose is excreted unchanged in urine (Forsman and Ohman, 1974). The biotransformation pathway is thought to be as shown in figure 4.13 (Forsman and Ohman, 1974).

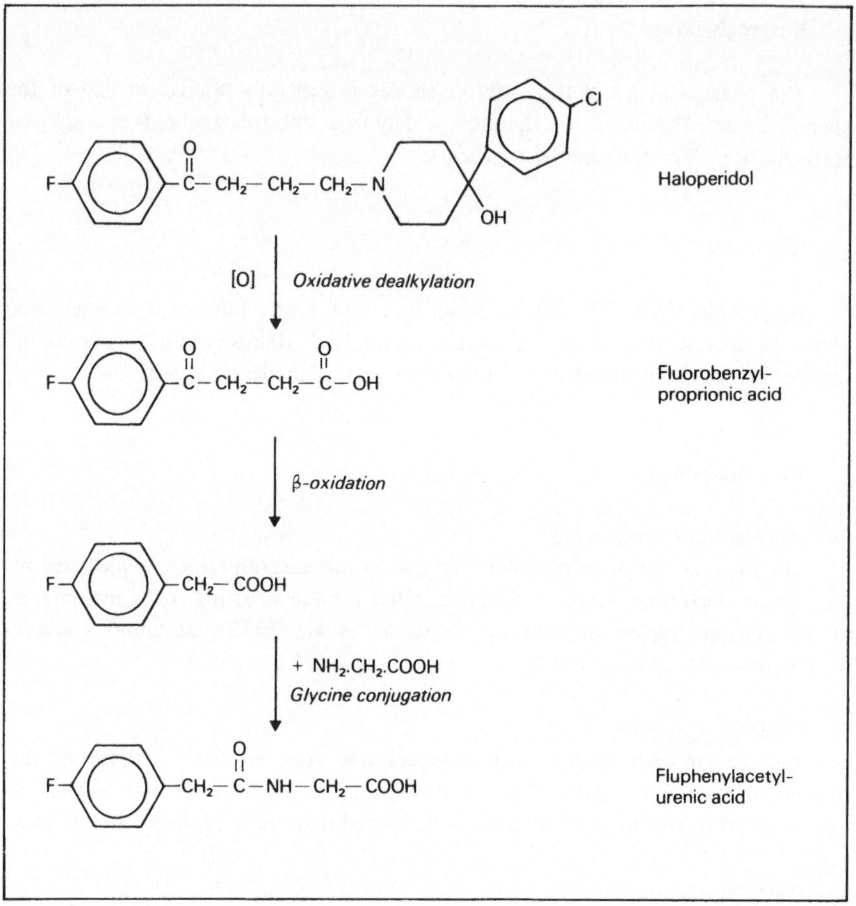

Fig. 4.13. The biotransformation pathway of haloperidol.

Plasma level correlations: In the steady-state, plasma haloperidol levels are proportionate to drug dose, though there is a 5-fold variation in individual level in relation to dose (Forsman et al., 1974).

Interactions
Pharmacodynamic interactions: These are similar to those of the phenothiazines.

Pharmacokinetic interactions: Bishydroxycoumarin is said to compete with haloperidol for plasma protein binding sites (Hughes et al., 1976).

Toxicity

The side effects of haloperidol are similar to those of the piperazine type of phenothiazine. The risk of jaundice is very low. The question of dysmorphogenicity in man is not yet settled.

Metoclopramide

Metoclopramide is used chiefly as an antinauseant and antiemetic, and to enhance motility of the alimentary tract. The drug has been reviewed by Pinder et al. (1976a).

Chemistry

Metoclopramide is a basic drug (fig. 4.14) which is usually used as the hydrochloride.

Pharmacology

Biochemical Pharmacology
Metoclopramide appears to be a highly specific dopamine antagonist.

Pharmacodynamics
Metoclopramide has an antinauseant effect, acting on the medullary chemoreceptor trigger zone. It increases the motility of the alimentary tract.

Pharmacokinetics
Absorption and bioavailability: The action of metoclopramide on alimentary motility begins within 30 minutes of oral intake, suggesting that absorption of the drug is rapid. More exact quantitative data are not available.

Distribution: Data are not available for man. In rabbits glucuronide and sulphonate conjugates of the drug undergo an entero-hepatic circulation though some of the glucuronide may be hydrolysed before resorbption (Arita et al., 1970a).

Elimination: Data are not available for man. In rabbits the biotransformation pathways appear to be as shown in figure 4.14 (Arita et al., 1970b). Cowan et al. (1976) stated that ether cleavage of the methoxy group, di-de-ethylation of the tertiary amine on the side-chain and loss of the whole tertiary amine group also occurred in the rabbit.

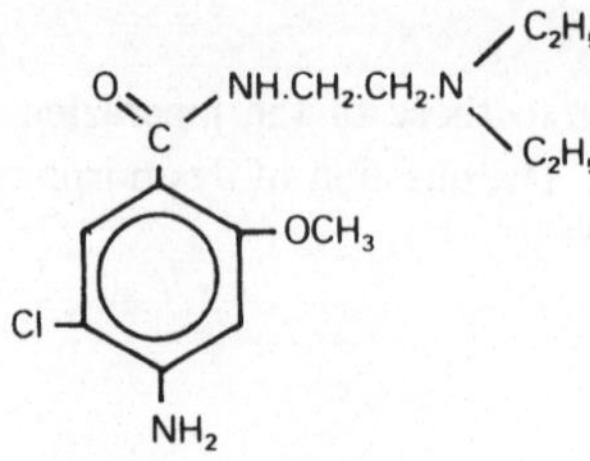

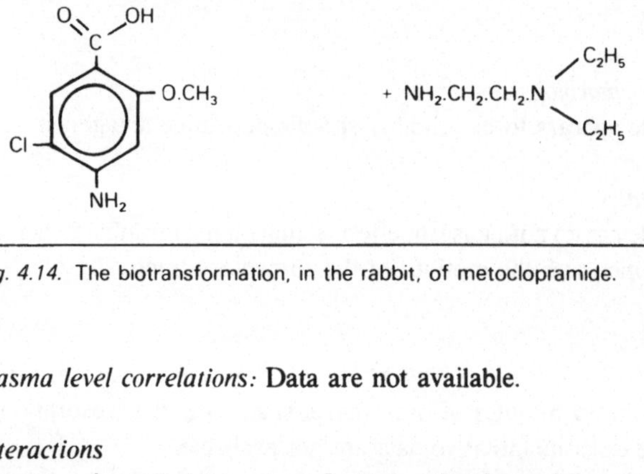

Fig. 4.14. The biotransformation, in the rabbit, of metoclopramide.

The figure shows the metoclopramide structure (MW 299.81) and the following biotransformation pathways:

1) Oxidation of the-NH₂ group on the benzene ring to form a-NO₂ derivative

2) Mono de-ethylation of the tertiary amine group at the end of the side-chain

3) Sulphate conjugation at the-NH₂ group on the benzene ring

4) Glucuronide conjugation at the-NH₂ group on the benzene ring

5) Cleavage at the peptide bond, forming

Plasma level correlations: Data are not available.

Interactions

Pharmacodynamic interactions: In theory the dopamine receptor blocking action of metoclopramide may interfere with the anti-Parkinsonian effects of levodopa and amantadine, should metoclopramide be prescribed for levodopa-induced nausea. However, it has been said that this interaction is not significant in practice (Tarsy et al., 1975).

Pharmacokinetic interactions: The action of metoclopramide in speeding gastric emptying can alter the absorption profiles of other drugs given concurrently. It may, for instance, decrease the overall absorption of a drug with a marginally adequate bioavailability e.g. digoxin (Manninen et al., 1973).

Toxicity

Metoclopramide is said to produce the same type of dyskinetic reaction that may occur with the phenothiazines with a piperazine side-chain.

Treatment of Chorea

The symptomatic treatment of chorea involves the prescription of a sufficient dose of a centrally acting dopamine-blocking agent or dopamine-depleting agent to relieve the involuntary movements and to restore muscle tone to normal. In a sense, treatment is an attempt to produce a sufficient trend towards drug-induced Parkinsonism to cancel out the chorea. At times relatively high doses of dopamine-blocking or dopamine-depleting agents are necessary to achieve the desired therapeutic end. However a satisfactory response can generally be attained without producing an intolerable degree of drowsiness, or of other side effects.

Because chorea is a relatively uncommon disorder, few neurologists are likely to have wide experience of using different dopamine-blocking or dopamine-depleting agents in the disorder. It is likely that many neurologists will have chosen one of the available agents and, if they have obtained satisfactory results, will continue to use this agent only. Among the dopamine-blocking agents thioridazine possesses much less risk of hepatotoxicity than chlorpromazine. As thioridazine dose is increased the drug may produce a Parkinsonian state but has relatively little tendency to cause tardive dyskinesia (unlike the piperazine phenothiazines and haloperidol). Therefore, there may be an argument for regarding thioridazine as the drug of choice in treating chorea. However there is little doubt that other phenothiazines or haloperidol are usually satisfactory. The important point is to use a sufficient dose to relieve the chorea and not to be deterred by knowledge of the conventional smaller dosages employed when the drugs are used as minor tranquillisers. Thus for a choreic patient weighing 50 to 70kg, one might prescribe an initial thioridazine dose of 25mg 2 or 3 times a day. Since this drug has a plasma half-life of 24 hours, it would probably be adequate to prescribe the 50 or 75mg in a single daily dose. With this daily dosage, steady-state conditions might be expected to apply after 5 or 6 days. If by then a sufficient therapeutic response had not occurred an increment of 25 or 50mg may be made in the daily dose. Dosage may be further increased every 5 to 6 days till the chorea is controlled or till side effects preclude any further increase.

If rapid control of chorea is desired (e.g. as when a patient is distressed by severe hemiballismus) a loading dose of twice the proposed initial daily dose may be given over the first 24 hours, followed by the maintenance dose each day. Dosages may be increased every second or third day till the chorea is controlled. Over the next few days the dose is reduced gradually, to find the lowest dose which will maintain control. With dose increments given every other day the chorea tends to be controlled before a steady-state is reached and, if doses are not reduced again, plasma thioridazine levels will rise above the individual's therapeutic threshold for several days before a steady-state is finally achieved.

If tetrabenazine is used, a dose in the range 25 to 200mg per day is likely to be needed. Each patient will require individual dose titration to determine the appropriate dose.

The duration of therapy and the vigour with which therapy is pursued depend to some extent on the type of chorea. Thus in rheumatic chorea, in the absence of active extra-neural rheumatic disease, full pharmacological control of chorea may allow the sufferer to enjoy a reasonably full life and to continue his education or occupation till natural recovery of the condition occurs over weeks or months. During recovery, decreasing phenothiazine dosage may be needed as the patient sometimes begins to become drowsy when taking doses which he previously tolerated comfortably.

Prolonged prophylactic oral penicillin should be given to reduce the possibility of streptococcal reinfection.

In Huntington's disease, if the patient's chorea is a significant problem, vigorous treatment of the dyskinesia is indicated. If, however, the main problem is dementia and behaviour disorder, phenothiazine drugs will be used primarily for their anti-psychotic effect and should be given in dosage sufficient for this purpose.

Hemiballismus usually follows a vascular episode and often settles spontaneously over a few days or weeks. The severity of the involuntary movements makes prompt prescription of sufficient phenothiazine medication desirable. Thereafter it is often possible to reduce the dose over a few weeks and later to withdraw treatment entirely.

It is, of course, not logical to correct levodopa-induced chorea by prescribing drugs with dopamine-blocking or dopamine-depleting actions. The desired anti-Parkinsonian effects of levodopa will be lost together with the undesirable involuntary movements. The same end can be attained more economically by reducing levodopa dosage.

Athetosis

In recent years the term 'athetosis' has become rather uncommon in neurological literature. Sometimes patients have patterns of involuntary movement that are intermediate between classical athetosis and chorea, and for these movements the term 'choreo-athetosis' is often employed. The pathogenesis of these choreo-athetoid movements appears similar to that of chorea, as is the response to drug therapy. Other movements that once might have been called athetoid now probably would be regarded as dyskinetic or dystonic. The therapeutic response of these movement disorders is discussed later in this chapter (p.140).

Thus the old entity of athetosis, as such, seems to be disappearing as knowledge of the pathogenesis of basal ganglia disorder increases.

Tardive Dyskinesia

Disordered Mechanisms

Tardive dyskinesias comprise rather stereotyped choreiform movements which usually occur in the tongue, lips and face, and less often in the limbs and trunk. The movements do not appear until later after months or years of exposure to the causative agent. At the present time the great majority of instances of tardive dyskinesia follow intake of phenothiazine drugs, or butyrophenones. It is generally phenothiazines with piperazine, or less often aliphatic, side-chains which are involved in the genesis of dyskinesia. The onset of the dyskinesia often follows reduction or cessation of drug intake after many months of continuous therapy, often in high dose. Similar dyskinesias occur rarely after phenytoin overdose (Chadwick et al., 1976), as a stage in the evolution of Huntington's disease, and in old people who have not been exposed to neuroleptic agents.

No pathological changes have been found in the brains of persons with drug-induced tardive dyskinesia who have come to autopsy. The dyskinesia usually persists permanently despite cessation of the causative agent unless further treatment is given.

The most effective treatments of the dyskinesia are to increase or resume dosage with the causative agent, to prescribe another phenothiazine or butyrophenone, or to give tetrabenazine. By different means these treatments have the common effect of reducing dopamine actions on striatal neurones. If striatal dopamine concentrations in patients with Parkinsonism are increased too much by giving an overdose of levodopa, movements similar in character to those of tardive dyskinesia may appear. Klawans (1973a,b) interpreted these observations by suggesting that tardive dyskinesia is due to a state of hyper-reactivity to dopamine (akin to denervation hypersensitivity). This state may occur when striatal dopamine receptors are released from a period of prolonged blockade due to various phenothiazine or butyrophenone drugs. It has been found that the use of anticholinergic agents increases tardive dyskinesia (Kiloh et al., 1973; Klawans and Rubovits, 1974). Cyclizine, an antihistamine with anticholinergic actions, can convert localised bucco-linguo-facial dyskinesia into generalised chorea (Klawans and Moskovitz, 1977). The centrally acting anticholinesterase physostigmine relieves tardive dyskinesia (Klawans and Rubovits, 1974). Hence increased central acetylcholine activity also appears to reduce tardive dyskinesia.

Correction of Disordered Mechanisms

As explained above, tardive dyskinesia may be corrected by decreasing dopamine action at striatal receptors. This may be done by:

1) Blockading the receptors with phenothiazines or butyrophenones

2) Decreasing local dopamine concentrations around the receptors by using reserpine or tetrabenazine which increases dopamine release and blocks its re-uptake into axon terminals. Thus a state of local dopamine depletion is produced when all the dopamine released by each nerve impulse is degraded, instead of part being used again via the re-uptake mechanism.

If Klawans' (1973) interpretation is correct, although treatment of drug-induced tardive dyskinesia with phenothiazines or butyrophenones suppresses the abnormal movements, such treatment merely perpetuates the situation which caused the dyskinesia. Once drug dosage is reduced again the dyskinesia will reappear. Treatment with a dopamine-depleting agent (e.g. tetrabenazine) would seem preferable in theory. If this agent is later withdrawn very gradually the dopamine receptors may have recovered from their earlier over-reactivity induced by previous prolonged exposure to receptor-blocking agents. The writers have been unable to find if this expectation has been realised in practice.

Drugs Used in Tardive Dyskinesia

The phenothiazines, haloperidol (the only butyrophenone in common use), and tetrabenazine, have been discussed earlier in this chapter in relation to treating chorea. Reserpine is a drug that is tending to disappear from use and the question of its carcinogenicity has arisen.

Treatment of Tardive Dyskinesia

The incidence of tardive dyskinesia would be reduced if the prolonged intake of phenothiazines and butyrophenones were restricted to persons with severe psychiatric disorders who could not be adequately treated with other drugs. The practice of combining phenothiazines with centrally acting anticholinergics may protect against drug-induced Parkinsonism but appears to facilitate the development of tardive dyskinesia and therefore would be better abandoned. When phenothiazines must be used for long periods there is an argument for employing those with aliphatic or piperidine side-chains (e.g. thioridazine). These derivatives appear to have less tendency to cause tardive dyskinesia than phenothiazine derivatives with piperazine side-chains.

When drug-induced tardive dyskinesia is present it may be relieved by increasing the dose of the causative drug, by adding a different phenothiazine or butyrophenone, or by using tetrabenazine. The dose of the added agent should be increased as necessary, bearing in mind the elimination rate of the drug employed and therefore the time needed to achieve steady-state conditions. If this is done, dose increments are not made so often that finally an excessive dose comes to be used. After some weeks of control of the dyskinesia, dosage may be very gradually reduced in the hope that the dyskinesia will not recur. If it does recur, and the patient wants the dyskinesia treated, dosage will have to be increased again. Since it is difficult to withdraw therapy once tardive dyskinesia has occurred it may be wise to find out if the dyskinesia is really troubling the patient, as distinct from his family and friends, before the initial decision to treat the movement disorder is taken. If the patient is not unduly troubled it may be better to leave the involuntary movements untreated while withdrawing the causative agent, in the hope that the dyskinesia will gradually subside. Unfortunately, this does not always occur.

Dystonias

The dystonias are a group of disorders in which involuntary movements are caused by changes in muscle tone which may be local or more widespread. The involuntary movements themselves tend to be gradual, progressive and repetitive. Several varieties of dystonia exist:

1) Acute dystonic reactions to phenothiazines (mostly those with a piperazine side-chain) and to levodopa overdosage
2) Persisting localised dystonias e.g. spasmodic torticollis
3) Torsion dystonia (dystonia musculorum deformans)
4) Dystonia in Wilson's disease.

Disordered Mechanisms

It is difficult to provide a coherent account of the disordered brain mechanisms which produce dystonia. In Wilson's disease there are severe structural lesions in the basal ganglia and elsewhere in the brain, related to excessive copper retention in the body. In another incapacitating dystonic disorder, dystonia musculorum deformans, which is also usually of genetic origin, no underlying pathological changes have been found in the brain. While dystonic movements can occur in Parkinsonian patients overdosed with levodopa, acute dystonic reactions may also occur in persons without previous neurological disorder, on their first exposure to a phenothiazine drug (taken, for example, to suppress vomiting). Different types of dystonia may sometimes respond to a variety of drugs with different actions, or else show no consistent response to any available drugs. Therefore patterns of pharmacological response throw little light on the mechanisms involved in dystonia. It is difficult to say more than that the basal ganglia appear to be involved and that the disorder may be in some way related to altered dopaminic transmission.

Correction of Disordered Mechanisms

Since one cannot interpret the biochemical mechanisms underlying dystonia it is impossible to propose any logically based, generally applicable, drug therapy for the disorder. All that can be done is to consider the various types of dystonia separately and discuss the treatments that have been found to be useful for them. If there is any therapy that is generally useful in relieving dystonia it is the operative destruction of the ventro-lateral nucleus of the thalamus, but such surgery is relatively nonspecific in that it seems to benefit most of the various dyskinesias, Parkinsonian and non-Parkinsonian.

Drugs Used in Dystonias

With the exception of the agents used to remove copper from the body in Wilson's disease, the drugs used in treating dystonia have already been discussed. The agents used for Wilson's disease are penicillamine and dimercaprol.

Penicillamine

Penicillamine was introduced into therapeutics as an agent for chelating heavy metals and increasing their excretion in urine. The drug is also used in treating cystinuria. Recently it has been found of benefit in the treatment of rheumatoid arthritis and progressive systemic sclerosis (scleroderma).

Chemistry

Chemically, penicillamine is β,β-dimethylcysteine (MW 149.21).

It may be formed by the hydrolysis of penicillin (fig.4.15); the D-isomer is preferred for use in clinical medicine.

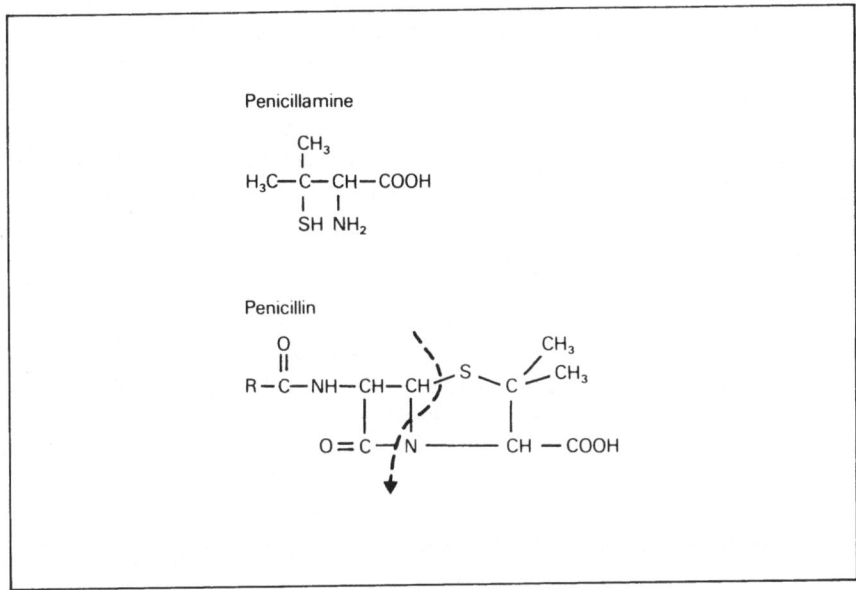

Fig. 4.15. Penicillamine and its formation by hydrolysis from penicillin.

Pharmacology

Biochemical Pharmacology

Penicillamine forms chelates with divalent cations e.g. Cu, Pb, Hg, Zn. It inhibits various enzymes for which pyridoxine is a co-enzyme and it forms penicillamine-cysteine disulphide from cystine (cysteine-cysteine disulphide). The former disulphide is very much more water-soluble than the latter.

Pharmacodynamics

Penicillamine chelates certain heavy metals and enhances their excretion. It increases the solubility of cystine in urine and helps prevent cystine calculus formation. It has an antiarthritic action in rheumatoid disease.

Pharmacokinetics

Absorption and bioavailability: Penicillamine is said to be well absorbed orally.
Distribution: No information is available.

Elimination: The half-life of penicillamine in plasma is about 7 hours. A proportion of the dose is excreted unchanged in urine but some is metabolised in the liver. However penicillamine is less susceptible to the action of certain enzymes (e.g. L-amino acid oxidase, cysteine desulphydrase) than is its desmethyl congener, cysteine.

Plasma level correlations: No data are available.

Interactions

We have been unable to find a record of any interactions involving penicillamine. Since the action of this drug, in a neurological context, does not involve its attachment to 'receptors', it is perhaps not relevant to consider the question of pharmacodynamic interactions.

Toxicity

The situation regarding penicillamine toxicity is somewhat confused because reports in the literature often have not indicated whether the reaction was due to the drug in its relatively non-toxic D-form, or in the DL- or L-forms.

Idiosyncratic Toxicity

Idiosyncratic reactions reported include:

a) Nephrotoxicity
b) Systemic lupus erythematosus-like syndromes
c) Optic neuritis
d) Acute sensitivity reactions such as fever, rashes, leucopenia, eosinophilia, thrombocytopenia (Strickland, 1972)
e) Loss of taste
f) A myasthenia-like syndrome (Bucknall et al., 1975)
g) Polymyositis (Schroeder et al., 1972)

Cross-reactivity exists between penicillin and penicillamine.

Dose-related Toxicity

These reactions include gastrointestinal disturbances e.g. anorexia, nausea and vomiting.

Dysmorphogenicity

No data are available.

Dimercaprol

Dimercaprol was developed as an antidote to the arsenic-containing poisonous gas lewisite. It is now used to treat certain forms of acute or chronic heavy metal poisoning (arsenic, gold, mercury, lead, bismuth, chromium, nickel) and, together with penicillamine, to treat Wilson's disease.

Chemistry

Dimercaprol (2,3-dimercaptopropanol; BAL i.e. British anti-lewisite) is a clear colourless viscous oil with the typical unpleasant odour of a mercaptan. It is soluble in vegetable oils. Its molecular weight is 124.21.

Pharmacology

Biochemical Pharmacology

Dimercaprol, by virtue of its chelating properties, not only binds undesirable cations but also affects certain enzymes which are activated by cations. These enzymes include catalase, carbonic anhydrase and peroxidase, carboxypeptidase (involved in the degradation of bradykinin (p.257) and cytochrome oxidase. *In vitro* dimercaprol will inactivate insulin. Metabolic products of dimercaprol inhibit enzymes containing sulphydryl (-SH) groups.

Pharmacodynamics

The therapeutic action of dimercaprol depends on its ability to chelate polyvalent cations which are then excreted in urine.

Administration of dimercaprol in man may produce a number of unwanted effects:

1) Temporary arterial hypertension and tachycardia lasting up to 2 hours
2) Nausea, vomiting and abdominal pain
3) Headache
4) Burning sensation in the oropharynx and penis
5) A sensation of constriction in the throat, chest and hands
6) Conjunctivitis, rhinorrhoea, salivation, sweating
7) Fever (especially in children)
8) Decreased thyroid function.

Pharmacokinetics

Absorption and bioavailability: Dimercaprol, though to some extent soluble in water, is unstable in aqueous solution. The drug is given by intramuscular injection, since the instability of the drug in an aqueous environment would probably mean that it has a very poor bioavailability if given by mouth.

After intramuscular injection peak plasma levels occur in 30 to 60 minutes, suggesting fairly rapid absorption.

Distribution: Dimercaprol appears to be distributed throughout extracellular fluid.

Elimination: Dimercaprol is eliminated rapidly so that a dose has virtually disappeared from the body within 4 hours of administration.

It seems likely that the sulphydryl groups on dimercaprol are oxidised and that some of the metabolic products are excreted in urine as glucuronides. Elimination is probably mainly by way of biotransformation.

Should dimercaprol form chelates with heavy metals, these chelates are more stable in alkaline than in acid urine. Hence urine pH might have some effect on the elimination of dimercaprol.

Plasma level correlations: Data are not available but in the situations in which dimercaprol is used the aim of therapy is not to achieve any particular tissue level of the drug; rather the intention is to chelate and then excrete heavy metals. Therefore, so long as the patient is not overdosed in the process, a more relevant index of biological effect is provided by serial measurements of urine or plasma content of the particular heavy metal it is desired to chelate.

Interactions

Since the therapeutic action of dimercaprol does not involve receptors it is not relevant to speak of pharmacodynamic interactions. In any event, there is no record available of dimercaprol interactions.

Toxicity

Idiosyncratic Toxicity

There are no reports of definite idiosyncracy.

Dose-related Toxicity

These side effects have been listed under the pharmacodynamics of the drug.

Dysmorphogenicity

No information is available. The circumstances in which the use of the drug is necessary are such that any risk of dysmorphogenicity would usually be acceptable.

Treatment of Dystonia

The medical treatment of the various dystonias is, in many instances, unsatisfactory.

Acute Dystonic Reaction to Drugs

In acute drug-induced dystonia, cessation of the offending substance is often all that is required. If the condition for which the drug was given persists and requires treatment it is preferable to use a non-phenothiazine drug (e.g. cyclizine or meclozine for vomiting; diazepam for acute behavioural disturbance). If a phenothiazine must be used, one with an aliphatic side-chain (e.g. chlorpromazine) or a piperidine side-chain (thioridazine) is less likely to lead to a recurrence of acute dystonia than is a piperazine-like phenothiazine or a butyrophenone such as haloperidol. The latter two classes of drug may have been the likely cause of the drug-induced acute dystonia. Should it be necessary to relieve acute dystonia rapidly because of the patient's distress, an intravenous dose of atropine, benztropine or diazepam will probably be effective. Typical intravenous doses for adults are as follows: atropine 600μg, benztropine 2mg, diazepam 5 to 10mg. Smaller doses should be given to children. Sometimes a second parenteral dose may be necessary several hours later if the dystonia recurs. To obviate the need for this it may be wise to prescribe a few days' oral therapy with an anticholinergic (e.g. orphenadrine 50mg 3 times a day for an adult) after the initial intravenous dose.

Spasmodic Torticollis

No drug therapy is consistently useful in this disorder. Sometimes anticholinergics e.g. orphenadrine 50mg 2 or 3 times a day for an adult, appear of benefit. In other patients a phenothiazine e.g. thioridazine 25 to 50mg twice a day, or amantadine 100mg 2 or 3 times a day seem to lessen the dystonia but after a time many patients seem to abandon the treatment, suggesting a lack of continuing benefit. Gilbert (1972b) reported good results in treating spasmodic torticollis with amantadine, with haloperidol, or with combinations of both. The haloperidol dose was usually in the range 4 to 8mg per day (Gilbert, 1972a). It is difficult to provide any pharmacological interpretation of this benefit derived from apparent antagonists. Couper-Smartt (1973) reported that lithium was of benefit in spasmodic torticollis, and Shaw et al. (1972) found temporary, but rarely lasting, improvement in some cases of spasmodic torticollis given levodopa.

Various surgical procedures have sometimes been used to help relieve the disorder. Affected muscles may be sectioned, or their nerve supply divided. Such peripheral surgery may be followed, after months of benefit, by extension of the disorder to neighbouring, previously unaffected muscles. Ventro-lateral thalamotomy may have more enduring benefit. If medical treatment of spasmodic torticollis fails, and the disorder is severe enough, such surgery might have to be considered.

Torsion Dystonia

Here again no drug therapy is of consistent benefit. As in spasmodic torticollis, the various agents mentioned above which influence basal ganglia function may be tried. Occasionally one will prove of real and continuing benefit. Levodopa produces short term benefit in some patients with the disorder, but the improvement usually does not persist (Eldridge et al., 1973).

In severe cases ventro-lateral thalamotomy may be indicated.

Wilson's Disease

The aim of treatment in Wilson's disease is to reduce the body's copper content thereby preventing manifestations of the disease developing in asymptomatic carriers and reducing the severity of symptoms in patients with the established disorder.

Penicillamine
The treatment of choice is oral penicillamine, for which the usual initial adult dose is 250mg 4 times a day. Later, depending on the patient's tolerance, higher doses up to perhaps 4g/day may be given. What little pharmacokinetic information is available suggests that it may be unnecessary to give the drug more often than 2 or 3 times a day. Penicillamine is best given on an empty stomach so that part of the dose is not wasted by chelating metals of dietary origin. As time passes the penicillamine dose is adjusted, depending on the patient's neurological and hepatic function and on the results of biochemical measurements of indices of copper metabolism. A patient with Wilson's disease is likely to require penicillamine therapy indefinitely.

To reduce absorption of dietary copper, patients with Wilson's disease should take 40mg of potassium sulphide (in a highly flavoured mixture) with meals.

Dimercaprol
It may be necessary to use dimercaprol as an adjunct, or an alternative, to penicillamine in Wilson's disease. Dimercaprol is given by deep intramuscular injection in a dose of 2.5mg/kg body weight. The drug is given at 4-hourly intervals for the first 2 or 3 days of therapy and thereafter the interval is progressively increased to 24 hours, or longer, depending on the therapeutic response and biochemical indices. To avoid breakdown of dimercaprol-metal chelates in an acid environment, patients taking dimercaprol should be given agents to make their urine alkaline, e.g. potassium citrate.

Clearly, penicillamine is a more convenient therapy than dimercaprol and it is now the treatment of choice for Wilson's disease.

Triethylenetetramine (400mg 3 times a day) has been recommended as an alternative to penicillamine in treating Wilson's disease (Walshe, 1973) but little information on the properties of this substance is available.

Myoclonus

Myoclonus is an involuntary movement disorder comprising repetitive brief shock-like contraction of muscles, or groups of muscles.

Disordered Mechanisms

Although myoclonus may arise from basal ganglia disorder, this type of involuntary movement disturbance may also occur with irritative lesions anywhere along the neural pathways which subserve movement. Thus among the varieties of myoclonus are:

Epileptic myoclonus, arising from:
1) the cerebral cortex, in motor Jacksonian epilepsy
2) the cerebral cortex, or possibly the striatum, in epilepsia partialis continuans
3) the upper mid-brain and thalamus, as in the various forms of myoclonic epilepsy (e.g. Lennox-Gastaut syndrome), whether hereditary, related to birth hypoxia or part of progressive degenerations, Lafora body disease (Unverricht-Lundborg syndrome) or Ramsay Hunt's dentato-rubral atrophy.

Non-epileptic myoclonus arising in the cerebrum, for example:
1) the myoclonic jerks of subacute progressive panencephalitis and spongioform encephalopathy
2) a type of post-hypoxic action myoclonus, associated with basal ganglia damage. This disorder responds to therapy with 5-hydroxytryptophan (Growdon et al., 1976) and is worsened by the serotonin blocking agent methysergide (De Lean et al., 1976). Thus 5-hydroxytryptamine deficiency may be involved in its aetiology
3) myoclonus due to levodopa overdosage, in treating Parkinsonism. This type of myoclonus may be improved by methysergide (p.264).

Myoclonus from brain stem disorder, for example:
1) palatal myoclonus, which may respond to 5-hydroxytryptophan (Magnussen et al., 1977)
2) palato-pharyngo-laryngo-oculo-diaphragmatic myoclonus
3) myoclonus of spinal origin, as in rare forms of subacute myelitis
4) myoclonus of peripheral nerve origin, most often facial myoclonus (hemifacial spasm).

The disease processes that cause myoclonus appear to affect axis cylinders as well as cell bodies of neurones. These processes can occur at many different levels of the nervous system. It seems unlikely that there is any single altered chemical mechanism responsible for initiating all instances of myoclonus.

Correction of Disordered Mechanisms

Treatment of myoclonus to some extent depends on its aetiology.

Myoclonus as an epileptic phenomenon is treated with anticonvulsant drugs (see chapter VI). The attempt to treat subacute sclerosing panencephalitis is mentioned in chapter XII (p.347). If myoclonus occurs as an unwanted effect of levodopa therapy, the dose of the causative drug is reduced. Post-anoxic action myoclonus may be treated with 5-hydroxytryptophan (Chadwick et al., 1974; Growdon et al., 1976; van Woert and Sethy, 1974) and there is a report that the anticonvulsant clonazepam is effective (Goldberg and Dorman, 1976). Palatal myoclonus may be treated with 5-hydroxytryptophan (Magnussen et al., 1977). It is not yet known whether palato-pharyngo-laryngo-oculo-diaphragmatic myoclonus responds to this agent. Facial myoclonus may sometimes be treated by surgical correction of any lesion in the cerebello-pontine angle region which irritates the facial nerve (Gardner and Sava, 1962) or by partly paralysing the affected portion of the facial musculature by cutting, crushing or injecting ethyl alcohol into the appropriate portion of the facial nerve.

Drugs Used in Myoclonus

With the exception of 5-hydroxytryptophan, the use of which is still not well established in human therapeutics, the drugs employed in treating myoclonus are discussed in other sections of this book.

Treatment of Myoclonus

The treatment of the different types of myoclonus is discussed above. (Correction of Disordered Mechanisms) or in various other portions of this book.

Tremor

Tremor is a common neurological symptom which sometimes occurs in isolation and sometimes in combination with other neurological manifestations. In some circumstances tremor is simply a normal physiological event. In other instances, though pathological, tremor may not be severe enough to warrant treatment.

Disturbed Mechanisms

The pathogenesis of tremor is not well understood. Experimentally, tremor may be produced by lesions made in a pathway which runs from the dentate nucleus of the cerebellum to the ventro-lateral nucleus of the thalamus, or by appropriate frequencies of electrical stimulation applied to this pathway. The pathway skirts the red nucleus in the mid-brain, and perhaps passes through the inner segment of the globus pallidus. The closer to the dentate nucleus the stimulation is carried out, the more the tremor resembles cerebellar intention tremor, while the closer the stimulation is applied to the thalamus the more the tremor resembles a resting Parkinsonian one. These experimental findings correlate with Holmes' (1904) observations on 'red nuclear' tremor *viz* that lesions near the red nucleus of man produced a tremor with mixed features of cerebellar and Parkinsonian tremor.

Pharmacologically, oxytremorine, a centrally acting cholinergic drug with muscarinic actions, will produce tremor, rigidity and hypokinesis resembling Parkinsonism. Drugs which increase central noradrenergic action e.g. amphetamine, can produce an intention tremor and it is easy to see an analogy between this and the tremor produced by emotion.

The more common forms of tremor are:

1) Physiological tremor, exaggerated by emotion and by thyrotoxicosis
2) Cerebellar type of tremor — an intention tremor due to local disease of the cerebellum or its connections or due to certain toxins which affect cerebellar function (e.g. alcohol)
3) Essential (hereditary) tremor — an intention tremor
4) Parkinsonian tremor — a resting tremor, sometimes mixed with an element of essential tremor.

Correction of Disordered Mechanisms

The possibilities for symptomatic treatment of tremor are limited by our relative ignorance of the biochemical mechanisms and synaptic transmitter substances involved in the production of different types of tremor. However the recent investigations of Shahani and Young (1976) have thrown some light on the situation.

Relief of emotional tension by various forms of psychotherapy, or by the use of tranquillisers e.g. diazepam, may ease physiological tremor which is being made worse by emotional factors. Similarly, relief of other factors which increase physiological tremor e.g. thyrotoxicosis, may be of benefit. The β-adrenergic blocking agent propranolol will reduce emotional and thyrotoxic tremor. It will also relieve tremor due to lithium overdosage (Kirk et al., 1973). Probably central noradrenergic activity is involved in producing these tremors.

No consistently useful drug therapy is known for cerebellar tremor.

A relative overactivity of central noradrenergic transmission may contribute to the production of essential tremor, a disorder which has no known neuropathological basis (Herskovitz and Blackwood, 1969). There are a number of reports that essential tremor is reduced in severity by the β-adrenergic blocking agent propranolol. However, essential tremor is more consistently and more effectively relieved by the intake of small amounts of ethyl alcohol. This beneficial action of alcohol originates centrally, not peripherally (Growdon et al., 1975). Unfortunately, the benefits from alcohol are temporary. It is of interest that haloperidol, a dopamine receptor blocking agent, makes essential tremor worse (Shahani and Young, 1976).

Despite the effect of oxytremorine as a tremorogenic agent, centrally acting anticholinergic drugs provide only limited benefit in Parkinsonian tremor. Ethopropazine is said to be the most effective of these agents (Shahani and Young, 1976). Haloperidol, a dopaminic receptor blocking agent, worsens Parkinsonian tremor but levodopa may relieve it. However, the action of levodopa against tremor takes longer to develop than its action against rigidity and bradykinesis. The response of Parkinsonian tremor to levodopa may be incomplete; thus the genesis of Parkinsonian tremor may involve not only dopaminic pathways. In fact Agnoli et al. (1972) claimed that the antiserotonin antihistamine agent pizotifen did benefit Parkinsonian tremor. Patients with Parkinsonism may have both a resting and an action tremor. The latter is often an expression of essential tremor. If so it may be worsened by levodopa, but relieved by propranolol (Shahani and Young, 1976).

Surgical destruction of the ventro-lateral thalamic nuclei appears capable of relieving all varieties of tremor.

Drugs Used in Treating Tremor

Many of the drugs used in treating tremor are discussed elsewhere in this book in relation to other neurological disorders. Here only β-adrenergic blocking agents will be considered. A number of such agents are already marketed and new agents with various potential therapeutic advantages are being tested. However, the use of β-blockers in neurology is relatively unimportant compared with their use in cardiology. Therefore only two β-blockers, propranolol and pindolol, will be considered here. Propranolol has been the β-blocker most often used in neurology but there are circumstances in which it may be useful to have available a β-blocker with a slightly different pattern of action.

Propranolol and Pindolol

β-Blocking agents have a wide use in cardiology for the treatment of angina pectoris, hypertension and certain supraventricular cardiac arrhythmias. They relieve sympathetic overactivity, as in thyrotoxicosis and anxiety states. In neurology the drugs, particularly propranolol, are useful in essential tremor (Dupont et al., 1973; Tolosa and Loewenson, 1975; Teravainen et al., 1977). The β-blockers are also useful in migraine prophylaxis (Ludgivsson, 1974; Borgesen et al., 1974).

Chemistry

Both propranolol and pindolol bear structural resemblances to the molecule of the β-adrenergic agonist isoproterenol, as do the other β-blockers (fig. 4.16). Propranolol and pindolol are weak bases which are slightly soluble in water. Their corresponding hydrochloride salts are more water soluble.

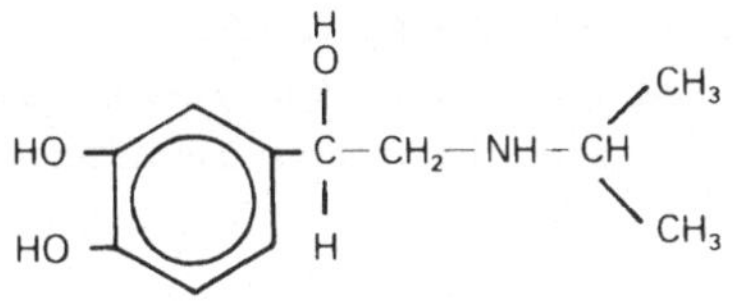
Isoproterenol

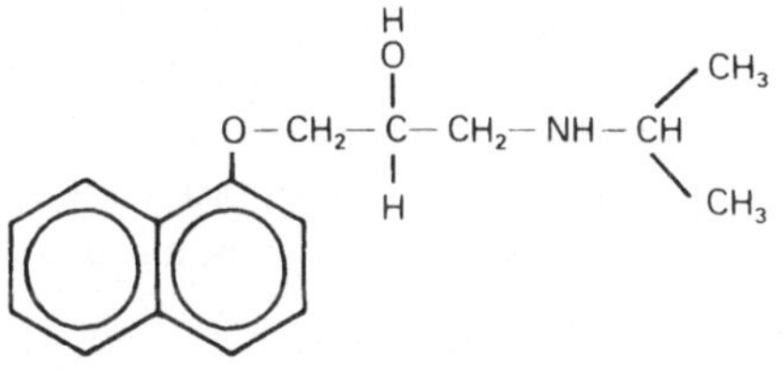
Propranolol MW 259.34

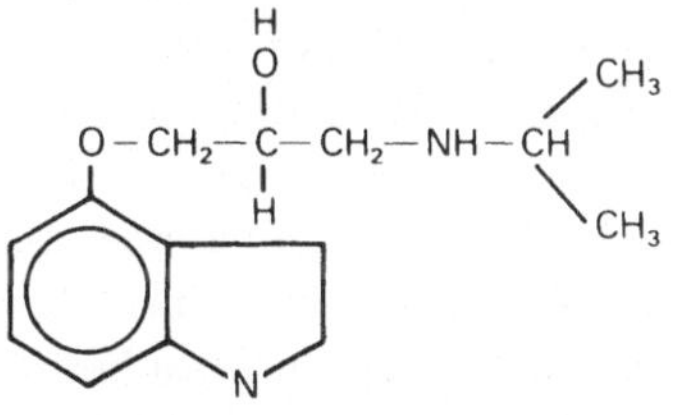
Pindolol MW 248.32

Fig. 4.16. The structural relationship of isoproterenol and the β-blockers propranolol and pindolol.

Pharmacology

Biochemical Pharmacology

The β-blockers act as competitive antagonists at β-adrenergic receptors. These drugs compete with noradrenaline for occupancy of these receptors.

Pharmacodynamics

Propranolol and pindolol are nonspecific β-adrenergic blocking agents (there are relatively specific β-blockers which may, for instance, affect the heart preferentially e.g. practolol, though this drug had to be withdrawn from use because of toxicity). Propranolol lacks intrinsic sympathomimetic activity whereas pindolol possesses such activity. The drugs have the following actions:

1) Heart: propranolol produces bradycardia and decreased cardiac output. These effects are less marked with pindolol. Both produce hypotension, and increase exercise tolerance in patients with angina pectoris. The effects of β-blockade are more obvious in the presence of increased sympathetic tone or circulatory demand (e.g. on exercise). In high doses they have a quinidine-like action
2) Metabolism: β-blockers reduce the hyperglycaemic and lipolytic responses to adrenaline and inhibit glycogenolysis in myocardium, skeletal muscle and liver
3) Respiratory system: β-blockers may produce a degree of bronchospasm
4) Uterus: β-blockers may cause increased contractility
5) Nervous system: β-blockers have local anaesthetic actions. Their mode of action in relieving essential tremor may be central, but may involve a component of direct action on muscle. The site of their preventive action in migraine is uncertain; it might be central, or occur in blood vessel walls.

Pharmacokinetics

Absorption and bioavailability: The pharmacokinetics of these drugs are reviewed by Johnsson and Regardh (1976). The β-blockers are likely to exist predominantly in ionised form at alimentary tract pH, so that they dissolve in gastric and intestinal fluid. The β-blockers are absorbed quickly and completely from the alimentary tract. The absorption half-time for pindolol (assuming first order kinetics) is 25 minutes. However, during the first passage through the liver some β-blockers undergo extensive biotransformation. This applies to propranolol (30 % bioavailable) but not to pindolol (100 % bioavailable). This difference in bioavailability is reflected in the different oral doses of propranolol (e.g. 40mg twice a day) and pindolol (e.g. 5mg twice a day) relative to their 1mg intravenous doses.

Distribution: The apparent volume of distribution of propranolol is 3.6L/kg, and of pindolol 2.0L/kg. These values suggest that both drugs are concentrated in the tissues. In animals β-blockers are concentrated in heart, lungs and liver relative to their levels in plasma. 93% of plasma propranolol is protein-bound and 57% of plasma pindolol. The octanol : water partition ratio of propranolol (5.39 : 1.0) is very much higher than the corresponding ratio for pindolol (0.12 : 1.0); this correlates with the fact that propranolol enters lipid-containing organs (e.g. brain) much more readily than does pindolol.

Elimination: The plasma half-life of propranolol is 2 to 3 hours and of pindolol 3 to 4 hours. The total body clearance of propranolol (1.0L/min) approaches hepatic bloodflow and suggests that extensive hepatic biotransformation occurs. This is in keeping with the known extensive first-pass metabolism of the drug. The lower total body clearance of pindolol (0.4L/min) suggests less active biotransformation and in fact some 40% of a pindolol dose is excreted unchanged in urine. Less than 1% of a propranolol dose is excreted unchanged.

Propranolol is known to undergo a number of possible biotransformation reactions, some of which are shown in figure 4.17. The metabolite 4-hydroxypropranolol is biologically active. Some of the propranolol metabolites shown form glucuronide conjugates, and glucuronide conjugation may also occur at the − OH group on the aliphatic side-chain.

Pindolol undergoes analogous conjugation reactions after aromatic hydroxylation and is also conjugated at the hydroxyl group on the side-chain. In addition,

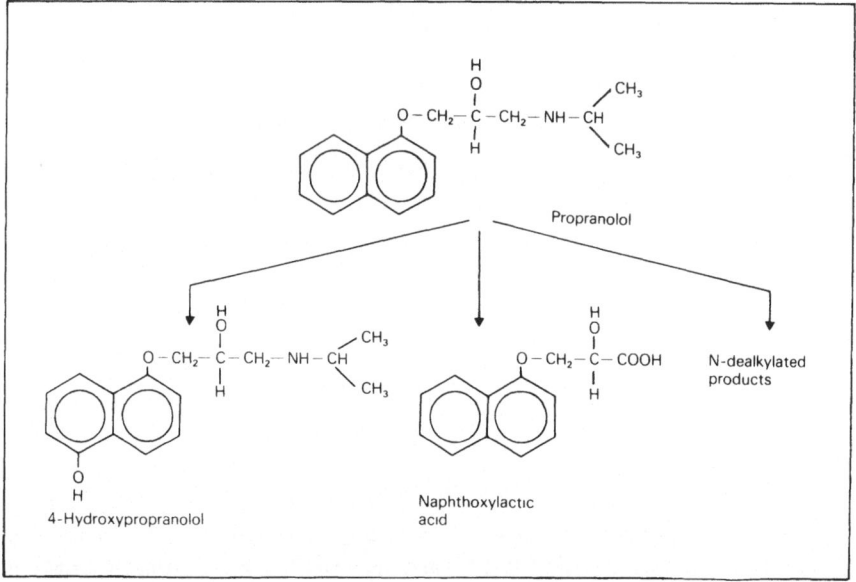

Fig. 4.17. Some biotransformation reactions of propranolol.

ethereal sulphate conjugates may form at the − OH position on the benzene ring, or on the indole ring. The indole ring may open, forming an anthranilic acid derivative.

Plasma level correlations: Data are available correlating levels of β-blocking agents with their cardiovascular effects. Jefferson et al. (1979) found no direct relationship between tremor relief and plasma propranolol level.

Interactions

Pharmacodynamic interactions: β-blocking agents antagonise the effects of sympathomimetic agents at β-receptors. They increase the actions of several antihypertensive agents (e.g. reserpine, α-methyldopa, hydrallazine, guanethidine) and increase the effects of insulin and oral hypoglycaemic agents (and also mask the sympathetic overreactivity which provides a clinical indication of significant hypoglycaemia as well as blocking the sympathetic overactivity in thyrotoxicosis). The β-blockers augment the effects of quinidine on the myocardium and, particularly in the case of propranolol, increase bradycardia due to digoxin.

Bradycardia due to β-adrenergic blockade can be antagonised by anticholinergic agents (e.g. atropine).

Pharmacokinetic interactions: No information is available.

Toxicity

Idiosyncratic Toxicity
Rashes, fever and purpura may occur.

Dose-related Toxicity
The following unwanted effects have been reported:

a) Myocardial failure, particularly in patients with previously impaired myocardial function who receive β-blockers which lack intrinsic sympathomimetic activity e.g. propranolol
b) Increased airways resistance in patients with asthma
c) Hallucinations, nightmares, insomnia and depression.

Dysmorphogenicity
Data on human dysmorphogenicity are not available.

Treatment of Tremor

The use of anti-Parkinsonian agents in treating Parkinsonism, and Parkinsonian tremor, has been discussed (pp.109-117) and the ineffectiveness of drug treatment in the cerebellar type of tremor has been mentioned. There have been suggestions that propranolol is useful in Parkinsonian tremor but the evidence is not very satisfactory. Possibly the distinction has not always been made between true resting Parkinsonian tremor and associated essential tremor.

Essential Tremor

In essential tremor the main problem is often the patient's fear of having Parkinsonism. Once many patients with essential tremor are aware of the diagnosis and prognosis they do not consider their disability severe enough to warrant regular drug therapy. They are often happy to take a minor tranquilliser e.g. 5 to 10mg of diazepam, to minimise any emotionally induced increase in tremor on social occasions, or else use a judiciously timed intake of alcohol to reduce tremor for a few hours on special occasions. Another therapeutic possibility for the patient who simply wants to reduce his tremor on certain occasions is for him to take a single dose of propranolol (e.g. 10 to 40mg) about an hour before the maximum tremor reduction is desired.

Should the patient's essential tremor be severe enough for him to seek regular treatment, propranolol seems the most effective therapy available, though this drug is not a full answer to the problem and does not benefit all cases (Sweet et al., 1974). However, propranolol is certainly a more acceptable alternative to alcohol, for there is danger that patients with essential tremor may become chronic alcoholics if they take alcohol too often while trying to control their tremor. Propranolol therapy is started in low dosage (e.g. 10mg, 3 to 4 times daily). The short elimination half-life of the drug suggests that, with regular intake, steady-state conditions are likely to apply within 24 hours of a dosage change. Therefore the dose can be increased every 1 or 2 days to achieve a degree of tremor relief that satisfies the patient. Doses as large as 240mg per day (Shahani and Young, 1976) or 640mg per day (Jefferson et al., 1979) have been used. Possibly other β-blockers (e.g. pindolol, oxprenolol) could also be used but there is no clear evidence in the literature that these offer greater benefits. In fact there is a recent report that pindolol increases the amplitude of essential tremor (Teravainen et al., 1977).

Shahani and Young (1976) found that the combination of propranolol and diazepam was more effective in essential tremor than propranolol alone.

If medical treatment of essential tremor, or of any other form of tremor fails, the possibility of stereotaxic thalamotomy may be considered.

Asterixis

Asterixis is an involuntary movement disorder which superficially resembles myoclonus. In asterixis there are sudden repetitive temporary losses of postural tone which cause momentary changes in limb position under the influence of gravity.

Asterixis is produced by renal and hepatic insufficiency and by overdosage with various anticonvulsants. It may be treated by correcting the cause.

Tics

Although some tics appear to be emotional disorders of childhood, the syndrome · of Gilles de la Tourette, with its multiple tics and coprolalia, may be organically determined (Sweet et al., 1973). However, no underlying structural neuropathological changes have been described. The disorder often responds to haloperidol.

Restless Legs (Ekbom's Syndrome)

This syndrome, usually of undetermined cause, is said to benefit from phenobarbitone or diazepam (Ekbom, 1966). Similar symptoms (akathisia) may result from chronic phenothiazine intake and may be relieved by cessation of these drugs. Hence it may be undesirable to use phenothiazines for Ekbom's syndrome, though experience suggests that tricyclic antidepressants are sometimes useful. Strang (1967) claimed that propranolol was also useful.

Paroxysmal Choreoathetosis

This uncommon condition produces paroxysms of violent choreo-athetoid movements. In some cases the paroxysms are activated by attempted movement. The pathogenesis of paroxysmal choreoathetosis is uncertain but it has been regarded as a 'striatal epilepsy' because of its paroxysmal nature and response to anticonvulsants. However, it is fair to point out that the anticonvulsant most often used for the condition (phenytoin) has a dopamine blocking action (Mendez et al., 1975). Paroxysmal choreoathetosis also responds to carbamazepine or other anticonvulsants (Kato and Araki, 1969); further the disorder is said to be helped by centrally acting anticholinergics (Rosen, 1964) and by levodopa (Loong and Ong, 1973).

Chapter V

Vertigo, Nausea and Vomiting

Principal Drugs Discussed

Neuroleptic phenothiazines, see also chapter IV

Metoclopramide, see also chapter IV

Antihistamines

The central structures responsible for nausea and vomiting and those mediating vertigo are closely related anatomically and physiologically. Those neurological disorders which cause vertigo often cause nausea and vomiting also. However there are many conditions, neurological (e.g. migraine) and non-neurological (e.g. gastrointestinal disease), which produce nausea and vomiting but do not usually cause vertigo. Nevertheless, it is convenient to discuss vertigo, nausea and vomiting together. The same drugs often provide symptomatic relief for all three symptoms.

Disordered Mechanisms

Vertigo

On the basis of its etymology, the word 'vertigo' should be applied to certain subjective experiences of rotation of the body relative to its surroundings (or vice versa). However, the layman's equivalent of 'vertigo', the words 'giddy' and 'dizzy', take in a broader range of dysequilibratory experience than pure rotational vertigo. Lesions which produce vertigo in some patients may produce non-rotational dysequilibrium in other persons. Therefore it seems reasonable to discuss, under the term 'vertigo', the whole range of hallucinatory experiences of dysequilibrium. The experience we call 'vertigo' or 'giddiness' involves an hallucinatory element, particularly in relation to the head. We do not say we are 'giddy' when we spin ourselves around and are aware of this. However if we feel we still spin after we have actually stopped turning we regard ourselves as 'giddy'.

Vertigo arises when there are inconsistencies in the afferent information which the brain processes to maintain the position of the body in space or when the central processing of this afferent information is faulty. Vertigo or giddiness is not experienced where there are faults purely in the efferent mechanisms which are involved in maintaining balance.

The afferent and central structures involved in maintaining equilibrium include:

Afferent Structures
1) The membranous labyrinths and vestibular fibres of the eighth nerve
2) The proprioceptive system, particularly the pathways from the neck muscles
3) The eyes and optic nerves.

Central Structures
The vestibular nuclear complex, which projects to the spinal cord, cerebellum, and temporal lobes (where equilibratory information probably comes to consciousness).

Lesions in any of these structures may produce hallucinatory experiences of dysequilibrium, with or without accompanying actual dysequilibrium. Disease in the eighth nerve system, and in its central connections, usually produces definite rotational vertigo. Proprioceptive system abnormalities tend to produce vague giddiness and any sense of spinning that is present is located within the patient's own head. Ocular disturbance produces even less well defined giddiness, if it produces any experience of dysequilibrium at all.

The more common disorders which affect these various mechanisms and cause experiences of dysequilibrium are shown in table I.

Nausea and Vomiting

On each side in the floor of the fourth ventricle, beneath the area postrema and in proximity to the vestibular nuclear complex, is the so-called 'chemoreceptor trigger zone.' Just medial to this is the vomiting centre. These regions appear to be interconnected, and the abnormal patterns of activity reaching the vestibular nuclear complex and causing vertigo are also likely to produce nausea and vomiting. Nausea and/or vomiting of neurological origin may also arise from local disease in the brain stem (e.g. tumours) and from various circulating chemicals and drugs which activate the chemoreceptor trigger zone. This zone lies immediately beneath an area in which the blood-brain barrier is defective, so that drugs which cannot enter the brain elsewhere can penetrate into the chemoreceptor trigger zone.

Disease of the alimentary tract can set up afferent impulses via the vagus and sympathetic nerves and these impulses can produce nausea and vomiting if they activate the vomiting centre.

Table I. Disorders affecting afferent and central structures involved in maintaining equilibrium

---

Affections of afferent structures
Affections of membranous labyrinths and vestibular fibres
    bacterial and viral labyrinthitis
    Meniere's disease
    vestibular neuronitis
    paroxysmal positional vertigo of utricular origin
    (post-traumatic, following vestibular neuronitis, and idiopathic)

Affections of proprioceptive system
    posterior neck muscle spasm from various causes

Affections of eyes and optic nerves
    ocular imbalance

Affections of central connections
Vestibular nuclear complex
    ischaemia, as in vertebro-basilar arterial insufficiency
    multiple sclerosis
    tumours
    Wernicke's encephalopathy

Temporal lobe
    epilepsy, and neoplasms (rarely)

Correction of Disordered Mechanisms

Vertigo

Sometimes it may be possible to correct the disorder which causes vertigo (e.g. using antibiotics for bacterial labyrinthitis). On the tenuous hypothesis that Meniere's disease is due to inner ear vasospasm, vasodilating agents (e.g. betahistine) have been used, but their effectiveness is questionable. In the past salt restriction, diuretics and histamine desensitisation were among the treatments that were in vogue for Meniere's disease. None of these treatments has stood the test of time.

On many occasions measures must be used which will suppress the symptom of vertigo, either because the nature of the causal disorder is not understood or because no treatment for the underlying disorder is available. The chemical background to the mechanisms which mediate vertigo is poorly understood. It has been found that phenothiazine drugs (dopamine-blocking agents) and certain antihistamines seem to reduce the severity of vertigo. These antihistamines have anticholinergic effects, as does hyoscine, which has long been found effective in motion sickness. It is therefore possible that overactivity of a cholinergic mechanism and/or of a dopaminic mechanism may be involved in vertigo.

In severe vertigo of peripheral origin, which had failed to respond to medical measures, surgical section of the vestibular fibres of the eighth cranial nerve may be considered (Falconer, 1965). If cochlear function on the affected side is already severely impaired, an alternative possibility is surgical destruction of the end organ. These procedures produce short term severe vertigo, but then relief from the symptom.

Nausea and Vomiting

As with vertigo, it may be possible to treat the cause of nausea and vomiting. If no treatment of the cause is available, nausea and vomiting may be treated symptomatically, using the same drugs that may be helpful in relieving vertigo.

Drugs Used in Treating Vertigo, Nausea and Vomiting

Many of the relevant drugs have been reviewed by Brand and Perry (1966).

Neuroleptic Phenothiazines

The phenothiazines are considered on pages 121-126. However, not all the drugs in this group appear equally useful for treating the symptoms in question. The piperazine derivatives prochlorperazine, trifluoroperazine and thiethylperazine appear useful both as antiemetics and antivertigo agents. Chlorpromazine, a phenothiazine with an aliphatic amine side-chain, appears perhaps less useful in relieving vertigo than in alleviating nausea and vomiting. Phenothiazines diminish the responsiveness of the vestibular system to vertigo-producing stimuli (Johnson and Ireland, 1965).

Metoclopramide

This drug, discussed on pages 129-131, also appears more useful as an antiemetic than in treating vertigo. Its antiemetic effect may be reinforced by its ability to enhance normal peristalsis of the alimentary tract. Phenothiazines appear to lack this latter action.

Antihistamines

Certain antihistamines such as meclozine (Cohen and de Jong, 1972), cyclizine and promethazine are also used in treating vertigo, nausea and vomiting. However the chief use of these drugs, and of other antihistamines, is in treating various allergic disorders in which histamine plays a central role. Some of the antihistamines may also be used as sedatives, particularly in children, and some (with anti-serotonin actions) are used in migraine prophylaxis (p.266).

Chemistry

The structural formulae of the antihistamines cyclizine, meclozine and promethazine are shown in figure 5.1. Promethazine has a pKa value of 9.1. All 3 drugs are basic.

Pharmacology

Biochemical Pharmacology
These antihistamines are competitive inhibitors of histamine at H_1 receptors.

Pharmacodynamics
These drugs have an antiallergic action by inhibiting the effects of histamine (which increases capillary permeability and causes spasm of alimentary and respiratory smooth muscle). The drugs suppress the stimulating effects of histamine on adrenal chromaffin cells but they do not alter the effect of histamine on gastric secretion (an effect which is mediated through histamine H_2 receptors).

The H_1 antagonists under consideration also have anticholinergic actions and local anaesthetic properties. In therapeutic doses in man they tend to depress the central nervous system. Promethazine, in this regard, is more potent than meclozine or cyclizine. Antihistamines may sometimes stimulate the nervous system, producing restlessness, insomnia and convulsions. There is some evidence that the antivertigo and antiemetic effects of the antihistamines correlates with their anticholinergic actions.

Pharmacokinetics
Very little pharmacokinetic information on these drugs is available.

Absorption and bioavailability: The H_1 antagonists are rapidly absorbed after oral and parenteral administration. After oral administration pharmacological effects are detectable in 15 to 30 minutes and reach a peak in about 1 hour.

Distribution: Quantitative data on the distribution and plasma protein binding of these drugs are lacking.

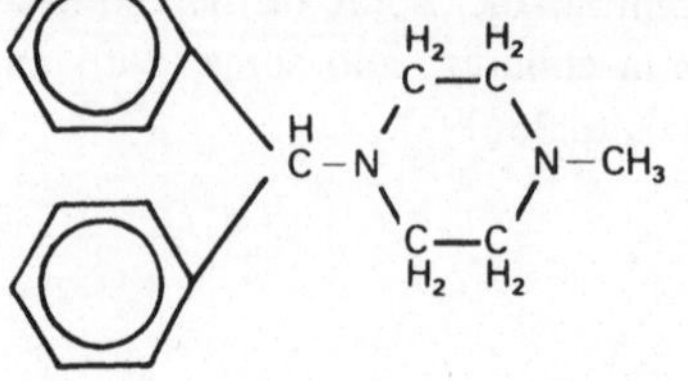

Cyclizine (1-diphenylmethyl-4-methylpiperazine)-MW 266.37

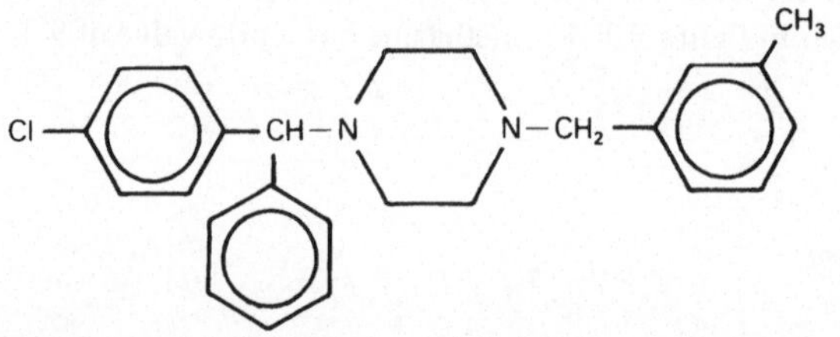

Meclozine (meclizine, 1-(p-chloro-α-phenylbenzyl)-4-(m-methylbenzyl) piperazine — MW 390.96

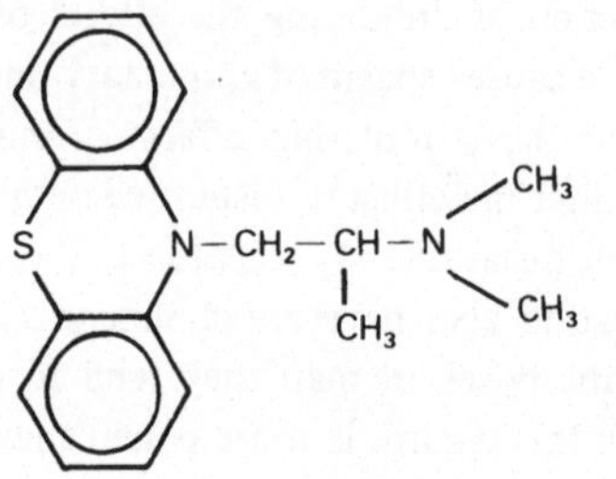

Promethazine — MW 284.41

Fig. 5.1. Antihistamines used in the treatment of vertigo, nausea and vomiting.

Elimination: Plasma half-life data are not available for the drugs under consideration; it is known that cyclizine undergoes extensive metabolism before its excretion in urine.

The durations of action of standard doses of cyclizine, meclozine and promethazine are said to be, respectively, 4 to 6 hours, 12 to 24 hours and 4 to 6 hours.

Plasma level correlations: No data are available.

Interactions

Pharmacodynamic: Antihistamines interact additively with drugs which depress the central nervous system (e.g. alcohol, barbiturates, morphine). They may also interact additively in respect to their anticholinergic action with other agents which have anticholinergic activity (e.g. tricyclic antidepressants). The antineoplastic agent procarbazine may augment the central depressant action of antihistamines. In theory, antihistamines might diminish the action of the drug betahistine, which is metabolised to histamine in the body. Both betahistine and antihistamines might be used simultaneously to treat vertigo.

Pharmacokinetic: Chronic antihistamine administration can induce the hepatic microsomal enzyme system though whether this significantly alters the actions of other drugs given to man is open to question.

Toxicity

Idiosyncratic Toxicity

Cutaneous allergies may arise from the topical use of antihistamines but are rare with systemic use, as are blood dyscrasias.

Dose-related Toxicity
Reported effects include:

a) Sedation, lassitude, incoordination, diplopia, euphoria, nervousness, dizziness, tremor, hallucinations, headache
b) Dry mouth, anorexia, nausea, constipation or diarrhoea
c) Urinary frequency
d) Hypotension
e) Photosensitivity (with promethazine).

Dysmorphogenicity

In laboratory animals cyclizine and meclozine cause fetal abnormalities, but evidence of significant human dysmorphogenicity is lacking.

Hyoscine

This drug is considered on pages 104-109.

Betahistine

Betahistine, a vasodilator, has been claimed to be useful in treating Meniere's disease. The evidence that betahistine is effective in this disorder is so weak that further discussion here of the drug does not seem justified.

Treatment of Vertigo, Nausea and Vomiting

Vertigo

Treatment of the Causative Disorder or Provoking Factors
The conditions will be considered in the order in which they are listed in table I.

Labyrinthitis: Bacterial infection of the labyrinth is treated with the appropriate antibiotic or antibiotics. Sometimes mastoid surgery may be necessary. No treatment is available for the causal organisms in so-called viral labyrinthitis.

Meniere's disease: Over the years a number of theories as to the aetiology of Meniere's disease have been in vogue, but the cause of the condition remains obscure. As indicated above, various treatments based on these theories have been employed, without conspicuous success.

Vestibular neuronitis: The aetiology is uncertain and no treatment of the cause is possible.

Utricular positional vertigo: The various causes of this syndrome are untreatable. However, if the movement which provokes the patient's vertigo can be identified, and the patient is taught to avoid this movement, the vertigo often seems to subside. Occasionally restricting neck movement by a collar may be necessary to prevent the patient provoking the vertigo.

Neck muscle spasm: This can be treated by local application of heat, by massage and physiotherapy, by the use of muscle-relaxing drugs (e.g. diazepam), analgesics (e.g. aspirin) and occasionally by infiltration of dilute local anaesthetic agent around the motor points of the affected neck muscles. A supporting collar may be helpful.

Ocular imbalance: The correction of this is a matter for an ophthalmologist and may involve the patient in orthoptic exercises or in wearing spectacles with prismatic lenses.

Disorders of the vestibular nuclear complex: The various diseases which involve this region are discussed in other sections of this book.

Temporal lobe epilepsy: This is discussed in chapter VI.

Symptomatic Treatment
Where no treatment of the cause of vertigo is available, or when vertigo requires relief while its cause is being treated, phenothiazine or antihistamine antivertigo drugs may be used. Possibly the phenothiazines are more effective than the anti-

histamines, but phenothiazines have the disadvantage that they may trigger acute dystonic reactions which cause interruption of the therapy. Sometimes these reactions have to be corrected by further drug treatment (p.141).

Phenothiazines: The initial phenothiazine dose, given orally, ranges between 5mg prochlorperazine twice daily for a child and 10mg 2 or 3 times a day for an adult, or 1 to 2mg trifluoroperazine 2 or 3 times a day or 6.5mg thiethylperazine 3 times daily. Should the patient be unable to take the drugs orally (usually because of vomiting) 25mg of prochlorperazine may be given to an adult once or twice daily (or 6.5mg thiethylperazine twice daily) as a rectal suppository. Alternatively 12.5mg prochlorperazine or 1 or 2mg trifluoroperazine may be injected intramuscularly or intravenously in an adult, with a smaller dose for a child. Subsequent dosage will depend on the therapeutic response and the patient's tolerance of the treatment.

Vertigo usually subsides over a few days so that continued phenothiazine medication is rarely necessary. If continued treatment is needed, as in frequently recurring attacks of Meniere's disease or paroxysmal positional vertigo, the lowest effective oral maintenance dose should be used because of the risk of producing tardive dyskinesias. In these circumstances continued use of antihistamines may be preferable to long term use of phenothiazines, so long as the antihistamines prove effective. If long term phenothiazines are used, pharmacokinetic considerations suggest that only one dose a day should be necessary to maintain reasonable plasma drug concentrations over the dosage interval.

Antihistamines: The antihistamines that are used to treat vertigo probably are not as effective for the purpose as are the phenothiazines, but their side effects rarely make it necessary to abandon therapy. The apparent durations of action of cyclizine and promethazine are relatively short (4 to 6 hours) so that these drugs probably need to be given several times a day. In the more acute situation this could be an advantage while the effective dose is being found for the patient. In longer term use the more prolonged action of meclozine should permit the convenience of once or twice daily dosage. Initially in an adult, cyclizine could be given in a 50mg oral or intramuscular dose and repeated 4 or more times a day. A promethazine dose of 25mg, orally or by injection, is given 3 times a day. If sedation were an advantage in managing a patient with vertigo, promethazine might be preferred to cyclizine. Many adults will tolerate a meclozine dose of 25mg twice daily without side effects and can take this amount of drug for months, if necessary.

Nausea and Vomiting

Treatment of the Cause
The causes of neurogenic nausea and vomiting, including the causes of vertigo which may be associated with nausea and vomiting, should be treated, where possible. The treatment of individual causes is too extensive a matter to consider here.

Symptomatic Treatment

The various drugs used in treating vertigo can be used, in similar dosage, to treat nausea or vomiting. Often the drugs must be given rectally or parenterally till nausea and vomiting are sufficiently controlled to permit oral therapy.

Phenothiazines with aliphatic side-chains (e.g. chlorpromazine) though seemingly of little use in treating vertigo, are reasonably effective antiemetics e.g. in a dose of 25 or 50mg 3 times a day for an adult. Acute dystonic reactions are far less likely with chlorpromazine than with the short term use of phenothiazines with piperazine side-chains.

Metoclopramide 10mg 3 times a day orally or intramuscularly is an effective antiemetic which may have the additional benefit of increasing the normal peristalsis of the alimentary tract.

Chapter VI

Paroxysmal Disorders

Principal Disorders and Drugs Discussed

Epilepsy
   Phenytoin
   Carbamazepine
   Barbiturates
   Ethosuximide
   Troxidone, Benzodiazepines
   Valproic acid
   Sulthiame
   Chlormethiazole

Syncope
   Ephedrine
   Fludrocortisone, (See also chapter II).

Epilepsy

A great deal more is known of the clinical pharmacology of epilepsy than of the clinical pharmacology of any other neurological disorder. The problem in writing the present account has been to decide what to omit in order to prevent this chapter from occupying too much of the book.

Disordered Mechanisms in Epilepsy

Hughlings Jackson's (1870) statement that 'a convulsion is but a symptom and implies only that there is an occasional, an excessive and a disorderly discharge of nerve tissue . . .' summarises the situation regarding the mechanisms of epilepsy.

Clinical epilepsy appears to arise in neuronal collections in the cerebral cortex or in the deep grey nuclei of the basal ganglia, thalamus and mid-brain. Within these structures groups of neurones are brought into a state of heightened excitability which may reach a stage at which spontaneous electrical discharging occurs. If this discharging involves a sufficient number of neurones, a clinically apparent epileptic seizure occurs. The manifestations of this seizure are determined by the normal function of that portion of brain in which the discharge arises and by the functions of those portions of brain which the discharge activates during its spread.

The factors which bring local collections of neurones to the point of occasional and excessive discharge appear to be either hereditary influences or acquired brain disorder.

Apart from hereditary brain lesions affecting grey matter (e.g. tuberose sclerosis), it appears that an instability of function of certain neurones in parts of the thalamus and in the mid-brain reticular formation (the mesodiencephalic reticular formation) can be inherited. It is not yet known if the inheritance is of a primary state of chronic partial depolarisation of these neurones or a diminished inhibition of these due to abnormality elsewhere. Acquired lesions of grey matter, irrespective of cause, appear capable of producing hyperexcitability in neurones adjacent to the lesions. This hyperexcitability appears due to loss of inhibition from damage to neighbouring (inhibitory) neurones.

As well as this local hereditary or acquired hyperexcitability in groups of neurones, due to locally acting factors, epilepsy may be due to factors which increase the excitability of the brain generally. Such factors include fever, hypoxia, hyponatraemia, hypocalcaemia, alkalosis, hypoglycaemia, and sudden withdrawal of chronic sedation. In normal brain such diffusely acting factors appear to bring the mesodiencephalic reticular formation to its point of spontaneous discharge before the remaining grey matter reaches its epileptic threshold, though probably the discharges so initiated are facilitated in their spread by the general state of brain hyperexcitability. However, should there already be an area of local hyperexcitability in the grey matter, the diffusely acting excitatory factors are likely to bring the locally abnormal area to the point of producing epileptic discharges before the remainder of the cortical or deep central grey matter reaches this state. Thus, diffusely acting factors can initiate epilepsy arising from pre-existing local abnormalities in the grey matter or, in the absence of such abnormalities, they may produce epilepsy originating in the general region of the mesodiencephalic reticular formation.

While the clinical patterns of epilepsy are determined both by the site of origin of epileptic discharges and the patterns of their spread, it seems likely that pattern of discharge spread may depend to some extent on the presence of local brain abnormalities. Thus in hereditary instability of the mesodiencephalic reticular formation the typical pattern of epilepsy is that of petit mal absence seizures, with associated 3 Hz generalised spike and wave discharges in the surface EEG. However when the mesodiencephalic reticular formation or neighbouring brain regions are made unstable by acquired disease, any epileptic activity which begins in this general area has a pattern of spread which is rather different from that of hereditary petit mal. There are more bilateral myoclonic manifestations and the surface EEG shows a generalised polyspike and wave or 2 to 2.5 Hz spike and wave discharge pattern.

The classification of epilepsy that is increasingly used today, and that which will be employed here, is that produced by the International League against Epilepsy (Gastaut, 1969). This classification is based primarily on the site of origin of the seizures.

Generalised Epilepsy

Seizures originating in, or involving very rapidly, the mesodiencephalic reticular formation are called *generalised* seizures. If of hereditary origin they typically produce petit mal absence attacks; if of acquired origin there is usually some associated bilateral and symmetrical muscle jerking (myoclonic epilepsy). There is some evidence that the latter type of generalised epilepsy may originate outside the mesodiencephalic reticular formation (e.g. in the inferior surface of the frontal lobe) and may generalise very rapidly through cortico-cortical pathways without necessarily activating the mesodiencephalic reticular formation. Nevertheless the surface EEG shows apparently bilaterally symmetrical and synchronous diffuse cortical activation. In association with either type of generalised seizure, or sometimes occurring alone, there may be sufficient activation of descending motor pathways from the cortex to produce a bilateral tonic, clonic, or tonic-clonic epileptic fit. These are the principal manifestations of generalised epilepsy.

Partial Epilepsy

Epilepsy arising in grey matter outside the mesodiencephalic reticular formation (in practice nearly always in the cerebral cortex) is called partial (formerly 'focal') epilepsy. Such partial epilepsy is nearly always due to acquired pathology. Its clinical manifestations are protean. If discharges from a focus anywhere in the cortex activate the cortex diffusely, perhaps via the mesodiencephalic reticular formation, there may be superimposed on the features of the partial seizure manifestations of generalised epilepsy (e.g. loss of consciousness, with or without bilateral tonic, clonic or tonic-clonic fitting). Thus there may be a secondary generalisation of the partial epilepsy. It should be noted that the term 'secondary generalised epilepsy' is sometimes used in different senses by different writers. Used as above, the term refers to the secondary generalisation of a partial seizure. However the term may also be used to refer to those generalised epilepsies which appear to arise in or near the mesodiencephalic reticular formation but which are secondary to acquired lesions in this region. Thus the word 'secondary' may refer either to the aetiology of the epilepsy, or to the pattern of its spread in the brain.

Thus far epilepsy has been considered predominantly from an electro-physiological point of view, but it is also necessary to consider the relevant biochemical mechanisms. The biochemical mechanisms involved in the initiation of mesodiencephalic discharge of hereditary origin are unknown. In all types of acquired epilepsy of cerebral origin it is unnecessary to posit any primary biochemical disturbance. Simple loss of inhibition from damage to, or destruction of, other neurones seems a sufficient explanation. When diffusely acting factors (e.g. fever, hypoxia, hypoglycaemia, hypocalcaemia etc.) produce epilepsy they probably do so by virtue of altering ionic concentration gradients (and therefore potential differences) across neuronal cell membranes so that a degree of depolarisation occurs. Fever, hypoxia and hypoglycaemia may have their epileptogenic effects by disturbing neuronal energy production so that less ATP is formed to meet the needs of the sodium pump which, by active extrusion of Na^+, maintains the normal resting membrane potential. Low extracellular Ca^{++} and H^+ concentrations may act at cell membrane level to decrease the potential difference across the neuronal cell membrane. Thus those biochemical factors which favour the initiation of epileptic discharges, and the spread of these discharges, may act at least in part by a common final mechanism *viz* alteration of ionic concentration gradients across neuronal cell membranes leading to depolarisation of these membranes.

Factors thought to influence the initiation and spread of epileptic discharges have been discussed above but there remains to be answered the question as to why a discharge, once initiated, ever terminates. The old explanation that the discharge continues till the neurones involved have exhausted their available energy supply is no longer tenable. It would appear likely that excessive neuronal discharges activate inhibitory feedback mechanisms which after a time usually suppress further epileptic discharges.

Correction of Disordered Mechanisms

Epilepsy is a symptom and in general the treatment of a symptom should be directed at correcting its cause. When the diffusely acting biochemical factors discussed above are present they can usually be corrected. When epilepsy is due to acquired disease in the cerebral cortex or deep grey matter it may occasionally be possible to correct the underlying causative lesion (e.g. cerebral syphilis). Very much more often the causative lesion has become inactive before the epilepsy begins. Death or loss of function of neurones may disinhibit other neurones, thus producing epilepsy. Here the causative lesion cannot be treated. In the hereditary generalised epilepsies it is also not possible to treat the cause.

Where the cause of epilepsy cannot be treated therapy should be directed at:

1) Correcting the state of partial depolarisation that exists at the site of initiation of the epilepsy, and/or
2) Limiting the spread of epileptic discharges.

Correcting the Abnormality of Neuronal Polarisation in the Epileptic Focus

Correction of the state of partial depolarisation that exists in a focus of epileptogenesis would appear to require an agent that acts selectively in the focus itself and does not affect the brain generally. This agent should produce a relative hyperpolarisation in neurones in the focus. There is some evidence that the anticonvulsant phenytoin may have a selective action in damaged, epileptogenic neurones, in which it activates the enzyme Na^+, K^+-linked adenosine triphosphatase (Esceta and Appel, 1971). In epileptogenic neurones phenytoin may produce increased Na^+ extrusion across the cell membrane, and this tends to correct the partial depolarisation of the membrane. Whether other anticonvulsants have such a selective action is unknown.

The other, cruder, possibility is to remove or destroy surgically the neurones in the epileptic focus, if this portion of brain is considered expendable. Even if the area to be removed or destroyed appeared expendable in relation to overall requirements for brain function, in our present imperfect state of knowledge of cerebral physiology it would be exceedingly difficult to be sure that removal or destruction of neurones in one area did not disinhibit other neurones and set up a new epileptic focus.

Limiting the Spread of Epileptic Discharges

Since clinically apparent epilepsy is most unlikely to occur till epileptic activity has spread from its site of origin to involve other neurones, limiting the spread of epileptic activity will usually have the effect of preventing clinical epileptic seizures. Here there are two main biochemical therapeutic possibilities:

1) To decrease the overall excitability of neurones. This can be achieved by the use of certain drugs, including many of the anticonvulsants. However, neurones not involved in the epileptic process may be affected as well as the neurones it is desired to influence (except possibly in the case of phenytoin, which may have a more selective action in this regard than the other anticonvulsants).

2) To impede synaptic transmission between the relevant neurones. The synapse is the vulnerable point for chemical modulation of neuronal function. Impeding synaptic transmission offers the possibility for selectivity of anticonvulsant action, since different neural pathways involve different, and specific, synaptic transmitter chemi-

cals. Certain anticonvulsants do alter concentrations of synaptic transmitter molecules in brain. This may explain, or contribute to, their anticonvulsant effects. However, present knowledge is incomplete regarding the patterns of selective propagation of epileptic discharges within the brain, and the nature of molecules mediating synaptic transmission in the various pathways involved in epileptogenesis. Thus it is impossible to equate the effects of anticonvulsants on synaptic transmitters with specific blocking of particular pathways involved in epileptogenesis.

The other possibility that exists for preventing the spread of epileptogenic activity is to interrupt the pathway through which the activity spreads, surgically. For this possibility to be practicable the relevant pathways must be expendable and one should know that, once one pathway has been interrupted, epileptic activity will not then spread through other pathways.

In practice, in the great majority of instances, the treatment of epilepsy resolves itself into the prescription of anticonvulsant drugs whose modes of action are not fully known.

Drugs Used in the Treatment of Epilepsy

The clinical pharmacology of the anticonvulsants has been the subject of several reviews e.g. Woodbury et al. (1972), Richens (1976), Eadie and Tyrer (1980). The following groups of drugs will be considered: hydantoins, carbamazepine, barbiturates, succinimides, oxazolidinediones, benzodiazepines, valproic acid, sulthiame and chlormethiazole.

Phenytoin

Phenytoin (diphenylhydantoin) has been widely used as an anticonvulsant since its introduction by Merritt and Putnam, (1938). The drug is useful in preventing generalised tonic-clonic seizures and in all varieties of partial epilepsy. It is also employed as a cardiac antiarrhythmic agent, in the prophylaxis of certain varieties of migraine and, occasionally, in treating myotonia and tic douloureux.

Chemistry

Phenytoin (till recently officially known as diphenylhydantoin in the USA) is 5,5'-diphenylhydantoin (MW 252.26). The drug is a white crystalline material. It is a weak acid with a pKa of 8.2 (Agarwal and Blake, 1968), though formerly the pKa was said to be 9.2 (Dill et al., 1956). Phenytoin dissolves in organic solvents, but is very poorly soluble in water. The drug is often given by mouth as its sodium salt. This may sometimes cause confusion when commercial preparations of phenytoin and sodium phenytoin are compared as, on a molar basis, 92mg of phenytoin base is very nearly equivalent to 100mg of sodium phenytoin. The structural formula of phenytoin is seen in figure 6.1. Tautomerisation to an enol form at the C atom in the 2 position permits formation of the sodium salt.

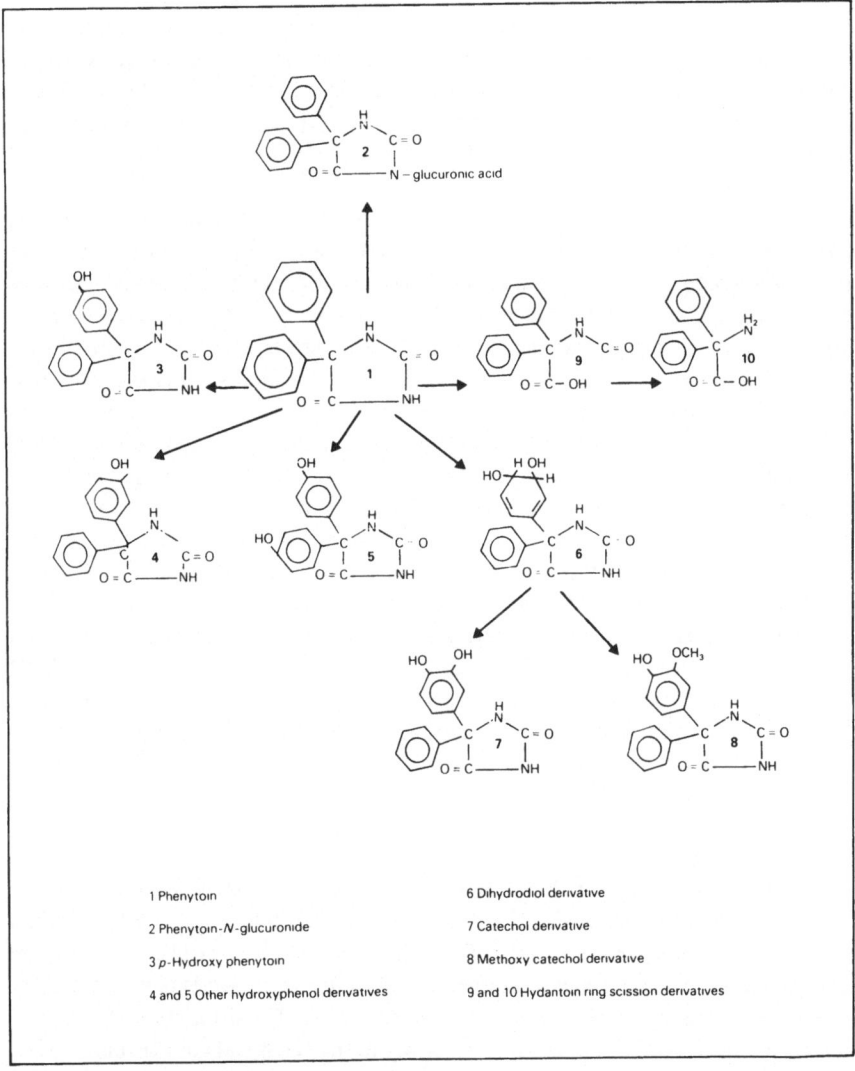

Fig. 6.1. Phenytoin and its metabolic pathways.

Pharmacology

Biochemical Pharmacology

Although there have been conflicting findings in relation to the effects of phenytoin on Na^+ flux across neuronal cell membranes (e.g. Pincus, 1972), it does appear that in neurones from experimental epileptogenic foci phenytoin activates the enzyme Na^+, K^+-linked adenosine triphosphatase (Schwartz et al., 1975). This enzyme is a major component of the membrane sodium pump mechanism and its activation would have the effect of increasing Na^+ extrusion from epileptogenic neurones and increasing K^+ entry into these neurones. This ion movement would increase the potential difference across the cell membranes of epileptogenic neurones, thus tending to correct the state of chronic partial depolarisation which renders the neurones potentially epileptogenic. This activation of the sodium pump may well be the essential anticonvulsant action of phenytoin.

Phenytoin has other actions which may bear on its anticonvulsant effect. It blocks neuronal responses to dopamine (Mendez et al., 1975). It produces dose-dependent alterations in the release of acetylcholine (Woodbury, 1969) and increases brain levels of both GABA (Saad et al., 1972) and 5-hydroxytryptamine (Chase et al., 1969). Phenytoin is a monoamine oxidase inhibitor (Azzard et al., 1973) and causes a decrease in the activities of brain γ-amino butyrate transaminase and succinic semialdehyde dehydrogenase (Nakamura and Bernheim, 1961). It may cause folate deficiency (Davis and Woodliff, 1971) possibly by diminishing folate absorption from the alimentary tract (Hoffbrand and Necheles, 1968) or by increasing the hepatic usage of folate, by causing induction of the hepatic mixed-oxidase systems for which folate is a co-factor (Maxwell et al., 1972). Certain folate derivatives (e.g. pteroyl monoglutamate, formyltetrahydrofolate) are cerebral excitants (Spector, 1972) so that phenytoin-induced folate deficiency might itself produce an anti-epileptic state.

Phenytoin at therapeutic concentrations can impair oxidative metabolism in rat neural tissue (Spector, 1972). The drug can inhibit certain types of brain NADH dehydrogenase (Giuditta, 1962) but can also divert glutamic acid into the Krebs cycle, possibly thereby providing increased amounts of ATP for the sodium pump (Woodbury, 1969). If and how these various metabolic actions have any significant anticonvulsant effect remains obscure.

Pharmacodynamics

Phenytoin abolishes the tonic phase of maximal electroshock seizures in experimental animals (Toman et al., 1946). It minimises after-discharges in the cerebral cortex and thalamus (Boyer, 1966). The anticonvulsant effect of phenytoin may be due at least in part to its effects on cerebellar Purkinje cells, and is diminished if the cerebellum is removed experimentally (Julien, 1972). The drug reduces the post-tetanic potentiation that can occur at synapses in the cat spinal cord (Esplin, 1957). Phenytoin stabilises the membrane of peripheral nerves (Morrell et al., 1958).

Pharmacokinetics

Absorption and bioavailability: Phenytoin is poorly soluble in water at physiological pH. With the exception of an excipient interaction (with calcium sulphate) which substantially reduced the lipid-solubility of phenytoin and prevented absorption of perhaps 25 % of the dose (Tyrer et al., 1970; Bochner et al., 1972a) there has been little clearcut evidence of incomplete absorption of the drug if given by mouth. However a number of studies have shown that the rate of phenytoin absorption varies from preparation to preparation, peak plasma levels occurring 3 to 12 hours from dosage. Dill et al. (1956) showed that the drug was absorbed faster when given as the free acid rather than as its sodium salt, but this difference was thought to be an effect of particle size. While in normal subjects only 5 % of a therapeutic dose of phenytoin may be excreted unchanged in faeces (Eadie and Tyrer, 1980) the solubility characteristics of phenytoin raise the possibility that, in states of gastrointestinal hurry, absorption of the drug after oral administration may be incomplete and variable.

Absorption of phenytoin from intramuscular injection sites is very slow, and rather unpredictable (Wallis et al., 1968). The diluent for the injections is strongly basic (pH around 12) and intramuscular injections may produce local muscle damage. Phenytoin is not very suitable for intramuscular injection owing to the relatively large volume of alkaline fluid that must be injected to provide an adequate dose of the drug. The low solubility of the drug at tissue pH leads to its precipitating out at injection sites and then dissolving again slowly before being absorbed. A 50 % increase in daily phenytoin dose is required to maintain plasma phenytoin levels when intramuscular injection is substituted for oral intake (Wilder and Ramsay, 1976). Intramuscular administration of phenytoin is too inefficient for reliable therapy.

Phenytoin may precipitate out in intravenous solutions with a neutral or acid pH if it is injected into these so that it can be given intravenously. The phenytoin in solution can be injected slowly into the tubing of a running intravenous drip; however, if too much is given too rapidly, the solvent, which contains propylene glycol, can cause hypotension.

Distribution: Phenytoin has an apparent volume of distribution in man of 0.6 L/kg, consistent with a widespread distribution in body water. In the rat, Noach et al. (1958) showed brain phenytoin levels were a little higher than the plasma levels and that levels in liver, salivary glands and kidneys were higher than those in brain.

In man some 90 % of the drug in plasma is protein-bound (Lund et al., 1971; Conard et al., 1971; Lund et al., 1972; Hooper et al., 1974a). Binding is less in the neonate (Ehrenbo et al., 1971) and decreases with age after puberty (Hooper et al., 1974a). Phenytoin binding to plasma protein falls in the presence of low albumin and high bilirubin levels (Rane et al., 1971; Hooper et al., 1974a; Olsen et al., 1975). Binding is reduced in patients with uraemia (Blum et al., 1972; Shoeman and Azarnoff, 1972; Odar-Cederlof and Borga, 1974) and in persons with liver failure (Hooper et al., 1974a). Phenytoin may be displaced from plasma protein binding sites by free fatty acids (Rudman et al., 1971), salicylic acid and phenylbutazone (Lunde et al., 1970) and possibly sulthiame (Hooper et al., 1973).

Phenytoin enters CSF and saliva. In both fluids drug concentrations are similar to those in plasma water (Triedman et al., 1960; Firemark et al., 1963; Lund et al., 1972; Bochner et al., 1974).

Phenytoin crosses the placenta; concentrations are similar in maternal and in umbilical cord plasma. It appears in human milk, where concentrations are 25 to 50% of those of whole plasma (Mirkin, 1971).

Elimination: Phenytoin is eliminated chiefly by biotransformation, only about 5% of a dose being excreted unchanged in the urine (Glazko et al., 1969). Since up to 5% of an oral dose may be lost in faeces, it appears that about 90% of a dose is eliminated by biotransformation. The major phenytoin metabolite in man is 5-*p*-hydroxyphenyl-5-phenylhydantoin, *p*-hydroxyphenytoin) which is pharmacologically inert. Some 60 to 80% of a phenytoin dose is excreted as this metabolite but the proportion of the dose thus converted decreases as larger doses of phenytoin are given (Eadie et al., 1976). Some patients may still remain in the steady-state as regards drug intake and output while the proportion of the dose converted to 5-*p*-hydroxyphenytoin falls, as phenytoin dose is increased. Therefore it seems possible that biotransformation of phenytoin to other metabolites increases as phenytoin dose increases. The known metabolic pathways of phenytoin are shown in figure 6.1.

It has been shown that, in man, biotransformation of phenytoin becomes saturated at plasma and tissue phenytoin concentrations which are encountered therapeutically (Bochner et al., 1972a). The elimination of the drug tends to follow Michaelis-Menten rather than first order kinetics and a number of authors have calculated apparent K_m and V_{max} values for the overall process. Their mean figures are shown in table I.

Although the kinetics of phenytoin elimination make it inappropriate to speak of the half-life of the drug (a parameter which depends on a drug being eliminated by first order kinetics) a number of authors had calculated a half-life for the drug before the true kinetics of its elimination were appreciated. One of the values calculated was that of Arnold and Gerber (1970) — 22.0 ± 9.0 hours, but the calculated half-lives would have varied, depending on the ranges of plasma phenytoin levels on which the calculations were based.

The renal excretion of phenytoin appears to be by glomerular filtration, with passive resorption of the drug during its passage down the renal tubules. The metabolite *p*-hydroxyphenytoin is present in plasma mainly as its glucuronide, of which 44% is bound to plasma protein (Bochner et al., 1973). The unbound glucuronide appears to be filtered through the renal glomeruli and in addition may be actively secreted into urine (Bochner et al., 1973).

Table I. Values found for the elimination of phenytoin in man

Km		V_{max}		Reference
adults	children	adults	children	
6.77µg/ml		6.1mg/kg/day		Gerber and Wagner (1972)
16.3µg/ml		14.4mg/L/day		Atkinson and Shaw (1973)
3.0-5.8µg/ml				Richens and Dunlop (1975)
5.8µg/ml	5.3µg/ml	8.1mg/kg/day	12.5mg/kg/day	Eadie et al. (1976)

Plasma level correlations: The correlation between steady-state plasma phenytion concentrations and therapeutic and toxic effects has been much studied. It is fairly generally accepted that the therapeutic range of plasma phenytoin concentration is 10 to 20µg/ml (Kutt et al., 1964) and that the incidence of toxic manifestations increases as phenytoin levels rise above 20µg/ml, although occasional patients tolerate much higher plasma drug levels without apparent adverse effect. Conversely, occasional patients may achieve a clinically adequate anticonvulsant effect at plasma phenytoin concentrations below 10µg/ml. Paradoxically, at phenytoin plasma levels well above 20µg/ml some, but not all, patients may show a loss of anticonvulsant effect (Lascelles et al., 1970). The therapeutic range of plasma phenytoin levels for control of cardiac arrhythmia appears similar to that for anticonvulsant effect (Bigger et al., 1968).

Peak plasma phenytoin levels occur 2 to 8 hours after oral dosage (Triedman et al., 1960). With regular dosage steady-state conditions occur after 4 to 8 days (Triedman et al., 1960) or 7 to 8 days (Buchanan et al., 1972). The higher the dose the longer it takes for the steady-state to be achieved (Buchthal and Svensmark, 1959), possibly because of the increasingly apparent effects of the non-linear elimination kinetics of the drug at higher plasma phenytoin levels. In the steady-state, plasma phenytoin levels remain virtually constant over the dosage interval with once daily administration of the drug (Haerer and Buchanan, 1972; Strandjord and Johanessen, 1972; Vajda et al., 1975). This probably reflects the relatively slow absorption of the drug after oral administration and the significant influence of Michaelis-Menten rather than first order elimination kinetics when plasma phenytoin levels are in the therapeutic range.

In treated populations there is a linear relation between plasma phenytoin level and drug dose but there is a wide scatter of individual points about the regression line. The relation between plasma phenytoin level and dose (on a body weight basis) differs between adults and children (Svensmark and Buchthal, 1964; Jalling et al., 1970; Borofsky et al., 1972; Eadie et al., 1973). The latter authors' data suggested that the relation between plasma drug level and dose changed around the time of puberty. This correlates with the different V_{max} for the elimination of phenytoin in children and in adults found by Eadie et al. (1976). Children on the average required higher doses than adults to achieve plasma phenytoin levels in the therapeutic range. The data of Eadie et al. (1973) suggested that the average Australian adult would achieve a plasma phenytoin level of 15µg/ml with a dose of a little over 6mg/kg/day, whereas the average child under 10 years required a phenytoin dose of about 11.5mg/kg/day to achieve this plasma phenytoin level. Sex does not appear to have a significant effect on the relation between plasma phenytoin levels and drug dose (Eadie et al., 1973; Houghton et al., 1975). Phenytoin requirement increases during pregnancy (Lander et al., 1977).

In treated individuals the relation between steady-state plasma phenytoin level and dose is not linear. This is a consequence of the drug's dominantly Michaelis-Menten type of elimination kinetics. As larger doses are given to a patient, he can biotransform proportionately less of the dose (and biotransformation of phenytoin is its main route of elimination). Consequently proportionately more of each dose increment accumulates in the body and steady-state plasma phenytoin levels increase to a disproportionately great extent with each dose increment (Bochner et al., 1972; Richens, 1976). The practical consequences of this non-linearity are of great importance when patients' phenytoin doses are changed. It is very easy to overdose or underdose patients with what appear to be relatively minor dosage alterations.

Interactions

Pharmacodynamic interactions: Clinical observation suggests that phenytoin interacts additively with certain other anticonvulsants to produce an enhanced antiepileptic effect. It seems probable that this is more than a matter of pharmacokinetic interaction, but there is no clear evidence that any synergism is involved.

In the striatum phenytoin acts as a dopamine antagonist. Its use can cause deterioration in Parkinsonism which is being treated with levodopa, and can make Huntington's chorea worse (Mendez et al., 1975).

Pharmacokinetic interactions: Many pharmacokinetic interactions of phenytoin are known:

1) Interactions altering plasma concentrations of other substances. These interactions involve two principal mechanisms: in the first, phenytoin may displace other substances from plasma protein binding sites. Displaced substances include thyroxine (Larsen et al., 1970; Schussler, 1971; Finucane and Griffiths, 1976), methotrexate (Hartshorn, 1970) and tricyclic antidepressants (Borga et al., 1969). In the second interaction mechanism phenytoin may induce the hepatic microsomal mixed-oxidase system in man (Petruch et al., 1974) and thereby enhance the biotransformation and reduce plasma levels of the following:

Folate (Jensen and Olesen, 1970). This is discussed further on pages 170 and
398; rarely the folate deficiency leads to megaloblastic anaemia
Cortisol (Choi et al., 1971)
Dexamethasone (Jubiz et al., 1970)
Metapyrone (Miekle et al., 1969)
Digitoxin (Solomon et al., 1971)
Dicoumarol (Hansen et al., 1971a)
Phenobarbitone (Morselli et al., 1971)
25-Hydroxycholecalciferol (Hahn et al., 1972) — as discussed later in relation to
phenytoin-induced osteomalacia
Carbamazepine (Christiansen and Dam, 1973; Hooper et al., 1974b)
Dicophane (Davies et al., 1969)

Phenytoin may cause a rise in plasma caeruloplasmin levels (Cantu and Schwab,
1966) may reduce plasma levels of immunoglobulins A, G and M in some
patients (Aarli, 1976) and may inhibit antidiuretic hormone release (Fichmann
et al., 1970).

2) Interactions altering plasma phenytoin levels. Plasma phenytoin levels were
reduced by an interaction in which calcium sulphate dihydrate, present as an excipient
in some sodium phenytoin capsules, altered the properties of the phenytoin so that
about 25% of the dose failed to be absorbed (Bochner et al., 1972b). Other interactions which might reduce plasma phenytoin levels are those in which the drug is displaced from plasma protein by salicylic acid and phenylbutazone (Lunde et al., 1970)
and possibly by sulthiame (Hooper et al., 1973). Further, phenytoin biotransformation may be increased by the actions of other drugs which induce the hepatic microsomal drug metabolising enzymes. Drugs which have been thought to decrease
plasma phenytoin levels in the latter manner include:

Phenobarbitone (Cucinell et al., 1965; Kristensen et al., 1969)
Folic acid (Olesen and Jensen, 1970; Baylis et al., 1971)
Ethyl alcohol (Kater et al., 1969)
Carbamazepine (Hansen et al., 1971b,c; Cereghino et al., 1973)
Clonazepam (Edwards and Eadie, 1973)

It should be noted that, with the possible exception of folic acid, the effect of
these substances in reducing plasma phenytoin levels is not consistent. Kutt et al.
(1969) suggested that not only does phenobarbitone induce liver microsomal mixed-
oxidase enzymes but that this drug may also compete for the metabolic pathway that
it induces. Thus the net effect of adding phenobarbitone to phenytoin therapy may be
to decrease, leave unaltered or increase plasma phenytoin levels. In practice this
variability of response seems to occur. Similar considerations appear to apply for
ethyl alcohol (Kutt and Louis, 1972) and personal experience suggests that they may
well apply for carbamazepine and clonazepam.

Many interactions which raise plasma phenytoin levels are known. These interactions are easy to detect clinically and biochemically since, with plasma phenytoin levels in the therapeutic range, the body's biotransformation capacity for the drug is nearly saturated. Therefore any further drug-induced slowing of metabolism can produce a major rise in plasma phenytoin level. Drugs which have been recorded as producing such interactions include:

Chloramphenicol (Christensen and Skovsted, 1969; Ballek et al., 1973)
Chlordiazepoxide (Kutt and McDowell, 1968; Vajda et al., 1971)
Chlorpromazine (Kutt and McDowell, 1968)
Diazepam (Vajda et al., 1971), though Houghton and Richens (1974) reported a contrary finding
Dicoumarol (Hansen et al., 1966)
Disulfiram (Olesen, 1966; Svendsen et al., 1976)
Ethosuximide (Frantzen et al., 1967)
Frusemide (Eadie and Tyrer, 1980)
Halothane (Karlin and Kutt, 1970)
Isoniazid (Kutt et al., 1966)
Mephenytoin (Roseman, 1961)
Methylphenidate (Kutt and Louis, 1972)
Phenylacetyl urea (Huisman et al., 1970) and pheneturide (Houghton and Richens, 1974)
Phenylbutazone (Hansen et al., 1966)
Phenyramidol (Solomon and Schrogie, 1967)
Prochlorperazine (Kutt and McDowell, 1968)
Propranolol (Eadie and Tyrer, 1980)
Propoxyphene (Kutt, 1971)
Sulphaphenazole (Hansen et al., 1966)
Sulthiame (Hansen et al., 1968; Olesen and Jensen, 1969; Richens and Houghton, 1973)
Troxidone (Roseman, 1961)
Valproic acid (Vajda et al., 1976)
Warfarin (Rothermich, 1966)

Toxicity

Idiosyncratic Toxicity

Phenytoin occasionally produces idiosyncratic reactions. These include skin rashes, usually morbilliform but, rarely, more severe e.g. erythema multiforme (Watts 1962) or exfoliative dermatitis (Stein and Pembrook, 1965). A syndrome of lymphadenopathy, fever and eosinophilia may be associated with the skin rash on rare occasions and in these circumstances hepatitis may occur (Weedon, 1975).

Lupus erythematosus has occurred occasionally in patients taking phenytoin (Rallison et al., 1961). Hypoplasia of the various formed elements of the blood is a rare accompaniment of phenytoin therapy, as is thyroiditis. Occasionally a lymphoma-like syndrome complicates phenytoin treatment (Saltzstein and Ackerman, 1959). The lymph gland enlargement usually subsides in a few weeks after phenytoin intake ceases. There have been some suggestions that phenytoin therapy may lead to malignant lymphoma (Hyman and Sommers, 1966; Anthony, 1970; Rausing and Trell, 1971).

Dose-related Toxicity

Orally administered phenytoin may cause nausea and vomiting, especially if large single doses are taken. At intramuscular injection sites phenytoin may cause muscle damage and the solvent in phenytoin preparations for intravenous injection (propylene glycol) can cause hypotension (Wallis et al., 1968).

Phenytoin overdosage typically produces nystagmus (often appearing when plasma phenytoin levels are 20 to 25µg/ml). At higher plasma phenytoin levels ataxia of gait, diplopia, nausea and vomiting may occur (Kutt et al., 1964). Sometimes phenytoin overdosage does not produce this typical picture; instead there may be mental changes, depression, sphincter incontinence, choreo-athetoid movements and worsening of epilepsy. Phenytoin overdosage may slow conduction velocities in peripheral motor nerves (Birket-Smith and Krogh, 1973). It is uncertain whether phenytoin can cause loss of cerebellar Purkinje cells, or whether loss of these cells is due to anoxia accompanying epileptic seizures for which phenytoin has been given (Dam, 1972).

Gum hypertrophy (Kimball, 1939) is a characteristic side effect of chronic phenytoin therapy, particularly in the young. There is some argument as to the extent to which gum hypertrophy is dose-related (Kutt and McDowell, 1968) and as to the role of dental hygiene. In children, particularly those with dark hair, phenytoin therapy may lead to overgrowth of body hair (Livingstone, 1972).

Chronic phenytoin therapy may cause hypocalcaemia with raised serum alkaline phosphatase levels (Richens and Rowe, 1970; Hunter et al., 1971). The possibility of hypocalcaemia is increased as phenytoin dose rises. The hypocalcaemia is sometimes associated with significant osteomalacia (Dent et al., 1972). The mechanism responsible for hypocalcaemia and osteomalacia appears to be induction of liver enzymes by the phenytoin, with resultant metabolism of cholecalciferol to products other than 25-hydroxycholecalciferol, the precursor of the biologically active 1,25-dihydroxycholecalciferol (Hunter, 1976).

Phenytoin intake is associated with the frequent occurrence of immunological abnormalities e.g. low levels of IgA, depression of phytohaemagglutinin-induced lymphocyte transformation *in vitro* and absence of delayed skin hypersensitivity to certain common skin test allergens (Sorrell et al., 1971).

Long term phenytoin intake can be associated with mild peripheral neuropathy (Lovelace and Horwitz, 1968).

If phenytoin is taken during pregnancy the offspring may have evidence of vitamin K deficiency, with coagulation defects (Mountain et al., 1970)

Dysmorphogenicity

For several years increasing evidence has accumulated that phenytoin may be a teratogen in man. It is known to be a teratogen in rats and mice (Harbison and Becker, 1969; 1972). The drug taken during human pregnancy may be associated with hypoplasia of the terminal phalanges in the offspring (Danks et al., 1974). There is reasonably strong evidence that phenytoin given to pregnant women doubles or trebles the risk of more serious malformations including cleft-palate, hare-lip, congenital heart lesions and diaphragmatic herniae (Annegers et al., 1974). The matter is not settled beyond doubt, for often more than one anticonvulsant has been taken, the data have been obtained from retrospective surveys with their attendant limitations, and the possibility of the malformations being associated with epilepsy rather than the treatment of epilepsy remains, as the large survey of Shapiro et al. (1976) suggested.

Other Hydantoins

The only other hydantoin anticonvulsants which enjoy appreciable use are methoin (mephenytoin) and ethotoin, though albutoin has been used on occasions in the USA (Cereghino et al., 1974).

Methoin

Methoin (5-ethyl-3-methyl-5-phenylhydantoin) appears to be as potent an anticonvulsant as phenytoin and in some circumstances is more effective. It does not cause gum hyperplasia but its use carries an appreciable risk of aplastic anaemia. Because of this it would seem that its use can rarely be justified till all other suitable anticonvulsants have failed. Its use is discussed, and some scanty pharmacokinetic information provided, by Troupin et al. (1976). Its *N*-desmethyl metabolite, formed in man, is 5-ethyl-5-phenylhydantoin ('Nirvanol'). This substance is known to be toxic to bone marrow but it is also an anticonvulsant (Kupferberg and Yonekawa, 1975).

Ethotoin

Ethotoin (3-ethyl-5-phenylhydantoin) is not a very effective anticonvulsant and is relatively little used. It might find a place in patients who cannot tolerate phenytoin because of idiosyncratic toxicity and in whom alternative anticonvulsants fail or are not tolerated.

Few pharmacokinetic data for the drug are available, but Yonekawa et al. (1975) found a half-life of 8.5 hours in one patient, while Lund et al. (1975) suggested that the elimination of the drug may not follow first order kinetics. Its pattern of biotransformation is described by Dudley et al. (1970).

Carbamazepine

Carbamazepine rather closely resembles phenytoin in its clinical effects. The drug is used chiefly as an anticonvulsant for all types of partial epilepsy, for tonic-clonic fits, and sometimes for myoclonic seizures. It is not effective in petit mal absence epilepsy. Carbamazepine is also the drug of choice in treating tic douloureux and it may be of benefit in certain other neuralgias and in diabetes insipidus.

Chemistry

Carbamazepine (MW 236.3) is a white powder which is soluble in polar organic solvents but almost insoluble in water. The molecule is essentially neutral and the structural formula is shown in figure 6.2. Carbamazepine has a general similarity of configuration to the tricyclic antidepressants. All are iminostilbene derivatives.

Pharmacology

Biochemical Pharmacology
Little information is available relating to the anti-epileptic action of carbamazepine. Sawaya et al. (1975) showed that therapeutic concentrations of the drug inhibited succinic semialdehyde dehydrogenase in mouse brain homogenate.

Pharmacodynamics
Carbamazepine raises the threshold for electro-shock induced seizures in rats and for strychnine induced convulsions in mice. It alters the thresholds for monosynaptic and polysynaptic spinal reflexes in mice (Theobald and Kunz, 1963). The drug does not antagonise the effects of pentylenetetrazole. It abolishes after-discharges in the amygdala and hippocampus of the cat and decreases the propagation of activity from these regions to the thalamus (Hernandez-Peon, 1962). Carbamazepine raises the cortico-thalamic threshold for after-discharge in the cat (Kobayashi et al.,

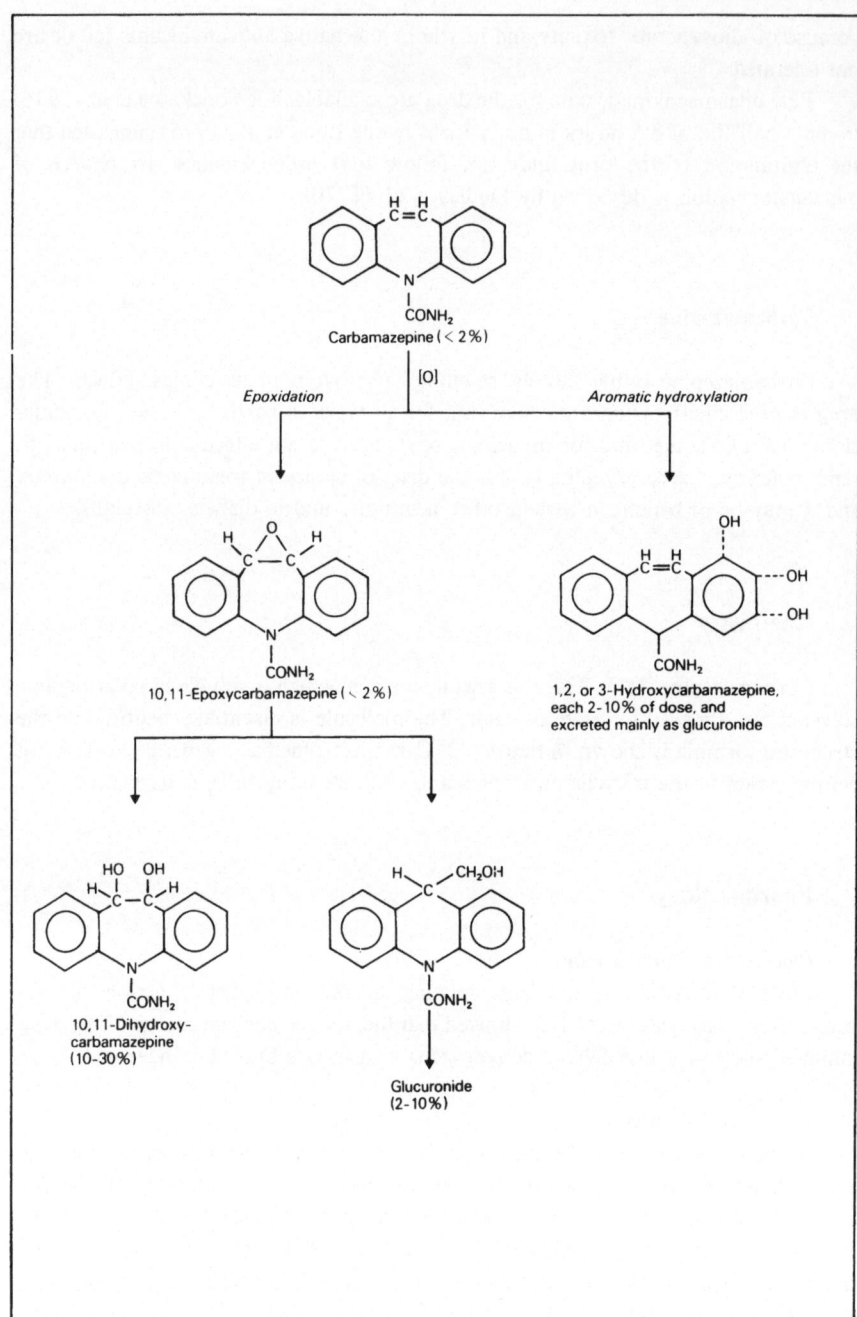

Fig. 6.2. The biotransformation pathways for carbamazepine.

1967). It decreases pain responses in rabbits and guinea pigs (Theobald et al., 1968) and diminishes synaptic transmission in the spinal trigeminal nucleus of cats (Fromm and Killian, 1966). Post-tetanic potentiation is decreased in the rabbit spinal cord and the drug lowers the amplitude and increases the duration and latency of evoked afferent potentials in the sciatic nerve (Krupp, 1969).

Pharmacokinetics

Absorption and bioavailability: Carbamazepine is given to man only by the oral route. The drug is very poorly soluble in aqueous fluids and its bioavailability is unreliable (Kauto and Tammisto, 1974; Cotter et al., 1977). The latter authors showed that peak plasma drug levels took as long as 18 to 22 hours to be achieved when tablets were used but took less than 5 hours when carbamazepine was taken in a specially prepared solution. Assuming first order absorption kinetics, the mean absorption half-time of carbamazepine from tablets was calculated to be 7.4 hours and the absorption rate appeared to slow as the dose was increased.

It seems possible that on some occasions the amount of carbamazepine absorbed from a dose of the drug may be substantially less than the dose given.

Distribution: Values of around 1 L/kg are quoted for the apparent volume of distribution of carbamazepine in man. These values may be an overestimate as they are usually based on the premise that the whole of an orally administered dose of the drug in tablet form has been absorbed. Representative published values for the V_D are 0.82 to 1.04L/kg (Morselli et al., 1975), 1.07 ± 0.22L/kg (Rawlins et al., 1975) and 1.20 ± 0.45L/kg (Eichelbaum et al., 1975). When carbamazepine was given in solution the V_D was 0.83 ± 1.0L/kg (Cotter et al., 1977). It seems likely that carbamazepine is distributed throughout total body water and that some is bound to tissues. Carbamazepine is fairly uniformly distributed through the bodies of experimental animals (Morselli et al., 1971). Brain to plasma ratios of carbamazepine in man range from 2.25:1 to 1.1:1 (Morselli et al., 1975).

An average of 73% (Hooper et al., 1975) or 76% (Di Salle et al., 1974) of the drug in plasma is protein-bound. The percentage binding is relatively constant over the plasma carbamazepine concentration range 5 to 50µg/ml. Anticonvulsants in common use do not appear to compete with carbamazepine for plasma protein binding sites. The binding of carbamazepine is decreased in the plasma of patients with hepatic insufficiency but not in plasma from patients with renal insufficiency. Figures for CSF carbamazepine levels expressed as a percentage of the drug's plasma levels are 15% (Meinardi, 1972), $21 \pm 5\%$ (Johannessen and Strandjord) or 19 to 30% (Johannessen et al., 1976). Thus carbamazepine levels in CSF roughly correspond with levels in plasma water. Salivary carbamazepine concentrations are also similar to those in plasma water (Troupin and Friel, 1975). Carbamazepine crosses the human placenta (Rane et al., 1975). Carbamazepine concentrations in milk average 60 % of those in maternal plasma (Pynnonen and Sillanpaa, 1975).

Elimination: Carbamazepine elimination appears to follow first order kinetics. The half-life is 1.46 to 1.54 days (Palmer et al., 1973), 37.5 ± 13.1 hours (Cotter et al., 1977) or $37.5 \pm$ (95 % confidence limits) 5.5 hours (Gerardin and Hirtz, 1975). It should be noted that these figures apply to subjects taking a first dose of carbamazepine alone; elimination appears appreciably faster if patients are taking phenytoin simultaneously. Elimination may also increase after repeated dosage with carbamazepine (Eichelbaum et al., 1975). Pitlick et al. (1976) showed in 6 subjects that the half-life fell from 33.9 ± 3.5 hours after a first dose of carbamazepine to 19.8 ± 4.0 hours after 3 weeks of therapy. Gerardin et al. (1976) noted that the half-life shortened as the dose was increased. This effect was also noted by Cotter et al. (1977).

Elimination of the drug is almost entirely by biotransformation, less than 2 % unchanged carbamazepine appearing in urine. The principal metabolic product found in plasma (10,11-epoxycarbamazepine) is an active anticonvulsant with a half-life of 6 to 14 hours (Morselli et al., 1975). The known pathways of biotransformation are as shown in figure 6.2 (Faigle et al., 1975).

Plasma level correlations: The therapeutic range of plasma carbamazepine levels is not yet defined. The drug has often been used in conjunction with other anticonvulsants after the latter have failed to control epilepsy, and in these circumstances it is difficult to define a therapeutic range. On the basis of the therapeutic response in tic douloureux it was suggested that the lower therapeutic limit is 6µg/ml (Eadie and Tyrer, 1974). A rather flexible upper limit of 12 to 15µg/ml appears reasonable.

This is in general accord with the observation of Morselli et al. (1975) that plasma carbamazepine levels of 7 to 12µg/ml are associated with a 'better therapeutic response' and with the range of 6 to 10µg/ml suggested by Simonsen et al. (1975). These provisional therapeutic ranges are higher than those suggested a few years ago, when the suggested upper limit was 6µg/ml (Meinardi, 1972).

In treated populations most authors have found either no statistically significant correlation between plasma carbamazepine level and drug dose (Reynolds, 1973; Morselli et al., 1975) or else a poor correlation (Cotter et al., 1975; Rane et al., 1976). The reasons for this lack of correlation include the uncertain bioavailability of the drug, referred to above, and the fact that many subjects have also been taking phenytoin or phenobarbitone, both drugs now known to alter the elimination of carbamazepine and hence its plasma level (Christiansen and Dam, 1973). However the correlation between steady-state plasma carbamazepine level and drug dose is still very poor in patients taking carbamazepine alone (Lander et al., 1977). Age and sex do not appear to alter the relation between steady-state plasma carbamazepine levels and drug dose in epileptic patients (Hooper et al., 1974).

In individual patients taking carbamazepine alone the few published data suggest that steady-state plasma drug levels rise less in proportion to dose increment as the dose is increased (Cotter et al., 1975). It is uncertain to what extent the poor bio-availability of the drug contributes to this effect. The increase in the carbamazepine elimination rate constant with increasing drug dose (as mentioned above) may also contribute to this effect. In persons taking carbamazepine with phenytoin, steady-state plasma carbamazepine level shows a tendency to an increasing rise with each dosage increment (Hooper et al., 1974b). It is possible that in the presence of pheny-toin, the elimination of carbamazepine becomes rate-limited under conditions of drug concentration that occur therapeutically i.e. that the biotransformation of car-bamazepine is saturable in these circumstances.

Interactions
Pharmacodynamic interactions: Carbamazepine, added to other anticonvulsant medication, can increase overall anti-epileptic activity but it is not known whether this represents more than an additive effect.

Pharmacokinetic interactions: Although carbamazepine binds to plasma proteins it has not been shown to displace other drugs from protein binding sites, nor is it dis-placed by salicylic acid or by other anticonvulsants in common use (Hooper et al., 1975).

Carbamazepine may induce hepatic microsomal drug metabolising enzymes (Morselli et al., 1972). This may allow the drug to increase its own elimination rate if taken chronically (Gerardin and Hirtz, 1975). It is known that carbamazepine in-creases the metabolism of warfarin (Hansen et al., 1971c). Carbamazepine therapy causes a fall in plasma phenytoin level in some, but not all, patients (Hansen et al., 1971b,c; Cereghino et al., 1973; Hooper et al., 1974b). However, in a population study Lander et al. (1975) could not confirm this interaction. Cereghino et al. (1973) obtained some evidence that carbamazepine therapy raised plasma phenobarbitone and primidone levels. Eadie et al. (1977), in another population study failed to detect these effects but noted that carbamazepine appeared to increase the conversion of pri-midone to phenobarbitone.

Christiansen and Dam (1973) showed that phenobarbitone or phenytoin ad-ministration caused a fall in plasma carbamazepine levels. This effect of phenytoin was confirmed by Hooper et al. (1974). Increased formation of 10,11-epoxycar-bamazepine occurs (Christiansen and Dam, 1975) in these circumstances.

Toxicity

Idiosyncratic Toxicity
Carbamazepine occasionally causes rashes of various kinds (e.g. erythema, pur-pura, erythema multiforme or exfoliative dermatitis). One instance of a lupus-like

syndrome has been noted (Simpson, 1966). Rarely aplastic anaemia and jaundice have occurred.

Dose-related Toxicity
In overdosage carbamazepine usually causes nystagmus, diplopia, drowsiness, fatigue, ataxia and feelings of dysequilibrium (Livingstone et al., 1967). Occasionally the drug causes nausea and vomiting. Effects on folic acid and vitamin D metabolism do not appear to have been recorded.

Dysmorphogenicity
Although carbamazepine causes fetal abnormalities in experimental animals there is one report that given to pregnant women it may reduce the risk of dysmorphogenesis from other anticonvulsants given in combination with it (Starreveld-Zimmerman et al., 1973).

Barbiturate Anticonvulsants

There are three barbiturates which are in reasonably common use in long term anticonvulsant therapy (if primidone is regarded as a barbiturate, though strictly it is a desoxy-barbiturate): phenobarbitone, methylphenobarbitone and primidone. Methylphenobarbitone and primidone are partly biotransformed to phenobarbitone within the body and it is likely that much of the anticonvulsant effect of methylphenobarbitone and primidone is mediated through phenobarbitone. Therefore it is convenient to discuss all 3 drugs together. Amylobarbitone, of occasional use in status epilepticus, will then be discussed.

Phenobarbitone: Methylphenobarbitone: Primidone

Though phenobarbitone was widely used as a sedative until comparatively recent times, all 3 drugs are now used mainly as anticonvulsants. They are useful in all varieties of partial epilepsy, in the prevention of tonic, clonic or tonic-clonic fits, and in myoclonic epilepsy, particularly in those varieties which occur in adolescents and adults. The barbiturate anticonvulsants are of little use in petit mal absence seizures.

Chemistry

The structural formulae of phenobarbitone (MW 232.23), N-methylphenobarbitone (MW 246.26) and primidone (desoxyphenobarbitone) [MW 218.25] are shown in figure 6.3. All 3 substances are white powders which are poorly soluble in

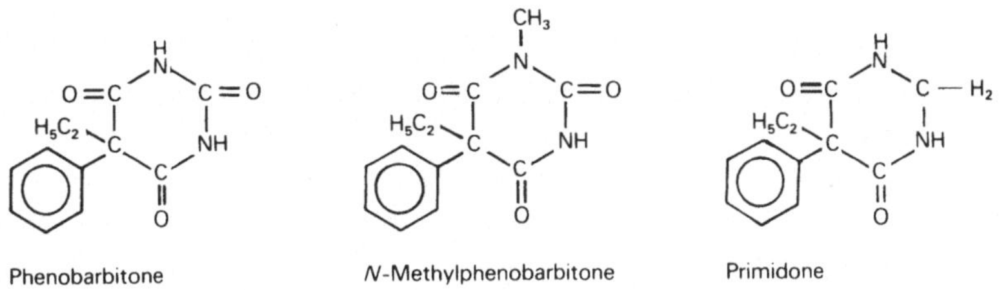

Fig. 6.3. The structural formulae of the barbiturate anticonvulsants.

water. Phenobarbitone and methylphenobarbitone are moderately soluble in the more polar organic solvents, while primidone is less soluble. They are all weak acids (phenobarbitone pKa 7.2; methyl phenobarbitone pKa 7.6; primidone is virtually neutral in aqueous solution). Phenobarbitone is sometimes prescribed as its more water-soluble sodium salt.

Pharmacology

Biochemical Pharmacology

Phenobarbitone impedes Na^+ and K^+ fluxes across cell membranes (Bunker and Vandam, 1965) and may decrease intraneuronal Na^+ concentration (Pincus et al., 1970). Phenobarbitone thus increases the polarisation of neurones, making them less excitable. In such neurones phenobarbitone selectively increases membrane permeability to the passage of K^+ (Prichard, 1972). The drug does not activate the sodium pump (Formby, 1970).

Phenobarbitone increases γ-aminobutyrate levels in mouse brain (Saad et al., 1972) but its action in depressing terminal mitochondrial oxidation occurs to a significant extent only at supratherapeutic concentrations (Cowger and Labbe, 1967). However, at therapeutic concentrations, in rat microsomes and synaptosomes, phenobarbitone reduces oxygen consumption; this effect is reversed by noradrenaline or tetrahydrofolate (Spector, 1972). In chronic phenobarbitone treatment folate deficiency may ensue. Presumably folate depletion could allow phenobarbitone to exert a generally depressant effect on neuronal metabolism. This latter effect of phenobarbitone also occurs with primidone (Spector, 1972). Otherwise no information is available regarding any special biochemical effects of methylphenobarbitone or primidone, as distinct from the effects of the phenobarbitone produced from metabolism of these drugs.

Pharmacodynamics

Phenobarbitone is a general depressant of neuronal excitability. It reduces postsynaptic excitatory potentials (Schmidt and Wilder, 1968) and may enhance presynaptic inhibition (Eccles, 1964) but has little effect on post-tetanic potentiation (Fromm and Landgren, 1963). In experimental animals it increases the threshold for minimal electro-shock seizures, reduces the tonic phase of maximal electro-shock seizures and protects against seizures induced by pentylenetetrazole (Woodbury and Kemp, 1970). It elevates the after-discharge threshold in both cerebral cortex and thalamus (Boyer, 1966).

Studies in the rat indicate that methylphenobarbitone is an anticonvulsant in its own right (Craig and Shiedman, 1971). The anticonvulsant effect of primidone itself is uncertain. It is rapidly biotransformed to phenylethylmalonamide, which protects against hexafluorodiethyl ether-induced convulsions in the rat (Gallagher et al., 1970) and this metabolite may account for the apparent anticonvulsant effect of primidone. Frey and Hahn (1960) showed that primidone offered little protection against experimental epilepsy in the guinea pig, an animal which forms little phenobarbitone from primidone.

Pharmacokinetics

Absorption and bioavailability: After oral administration the absorption of *phenobarbitone* is thought to be complete (Maynert, 1972) but relatively slow. Maximum plasma concentrations may not occur till 6 to 18 hours after dosage (Lous, 1954). The rate of absorption of phenobarbitone from injection sites is unknown.

Indirect evidence suggests that *methylphenobarbitone* is incompletely absorbed after oral dosage (Maynert, 1972). However, personal unpublished studies suggested comparative rapid absorption of the drug (T_{max} within 7 hours of dosage in 7 of 8 subjects), which makes poor bioavailability of the drug unlikely. The argument that the bioavailability of methylphenobarbitone is poor has been based on the approximately 2:1 ratio of its dose to that of phenobarbitone to produce similar biological effects. The T_{max} data cited above make it more likely that the pattern of elimination of methylphenobarbitone accounts for the dosage discrepancy between it and phenobarbitone.

Absorption of orally administered *primidone* is said to be fairly rapid, with peak plasma levels an average of 3 hours from dosage (Booker et al., 1970; Gallagher and Baumel, 1972).

Distribution: The apparent volume of distribution of *phenobarbitone* is 0.7L/kg (Van der Kleijn et al., 1975). The drug is fairly evenly distributed throughout the body tissues and fluids (Goldbaum and Smith, 1954). There is no selective accumulation of phenobarbitone in any brain region (Domek et al., 1960). Brain and serum phenobarbitone levels are similar (Buchthal and Svensmark, 1959). Maternal and fetal plasma levels of phenobarbitone are similar (Melchior et al., 1967). Some 50 % of the drug in plasma is protein-bound and CSF levels are 40 % of plasma levels

(Baumel et al., 1972). There is no close relationship between salivary and plasma phenobarbitone levels (Troupin and Friel, 1975).

Little has been published on the distribution of *methylphenobarbitone*. Personal unpublished data suggest that its apparent volume of distribution may be about 4 to 5 times that of phenobarbitone in the same subject, suggesting more extensive tissue binding of methylphenobarbitone. In 4 subjects the average V_D was 1.9L/kg. Data on the plasma protein binding of methylphenobarbitone are lacking.

Primidone has an apparent volume of distribution of 0.6L/kg and there is no special regional distribution (Van der Kleijn et al., 1975). Primidone is not bound to plasma proteins (Gallagher and Baumel, 1972). Its levels in CSF are at least equal to those in plasma (Sherwin, 1975). It crosses the placenta (Martinez and Synder, 1973). The primidone metabolite, phenylethylmalonamide, also appears not to be protein-bound (Schafer, 1975).

Elimination: The half-life of *phenobarbitone* has a mean value of 3 to 4 days (Mark, 1963), a mean of 4 days (Buchthal and Lennox-Buchthal, 1972) or 4.3 to 6.7 days (Lous, 1954). In children the half-life is shorter, being 1.5 to 3.1 days (Garrett-

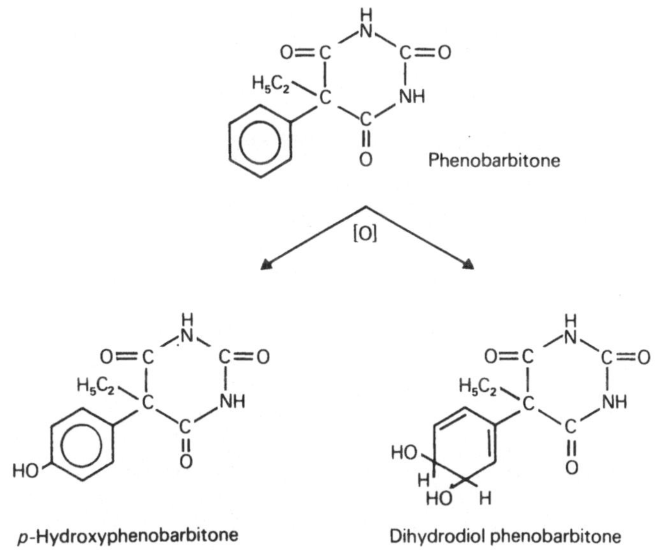

Fig. 6.4. Phenobarbitone and its metabolites.

son and Dayton, 1970). A mean of 21 % of the dose is excreted unchanged in urine (Lous, 1954). The renal excretion of phenobarbitone is pH dependent. The major metabolite is *p*-hydroxy-phenobarbitone (Butler, 1956) 50 % of which is excreted in urine in conjugated form (as a glucuronide and possibly as a sulphate). A dihydrodiol metabolite has also been identified (Harvey et al., 1972). The hydroxy metabolite of phenobarbitone (fig. 6.4) does not appear to be an effective anticonvulsant.

No published elimination data for *methylphenobarbitone* can be traced. Personal unpublished data suggest its half-life has a mean value of 32 hours (range 17 to 76 hours in 8 adults). Less than 5 % of a dose appears in urine as unchanged methylphenobarbitone. The drug is believed to be biotransformed to phenobarbitone, which is then further metabolised. Since, to achieve the same biological effect, the dose of methylphenobarbitone is approximately twice that of phenobarbitone, it appears likely that no more than 50 % of a methylphenobarbitone dose is converted to phenobarbitone. Direct measurement in one patient suggests that this is the case. If so, methylphenobarbitone must have an as yet unknown pattern of biotransformation apart from oxidative *N*-desmethylation to phenobarbitone.

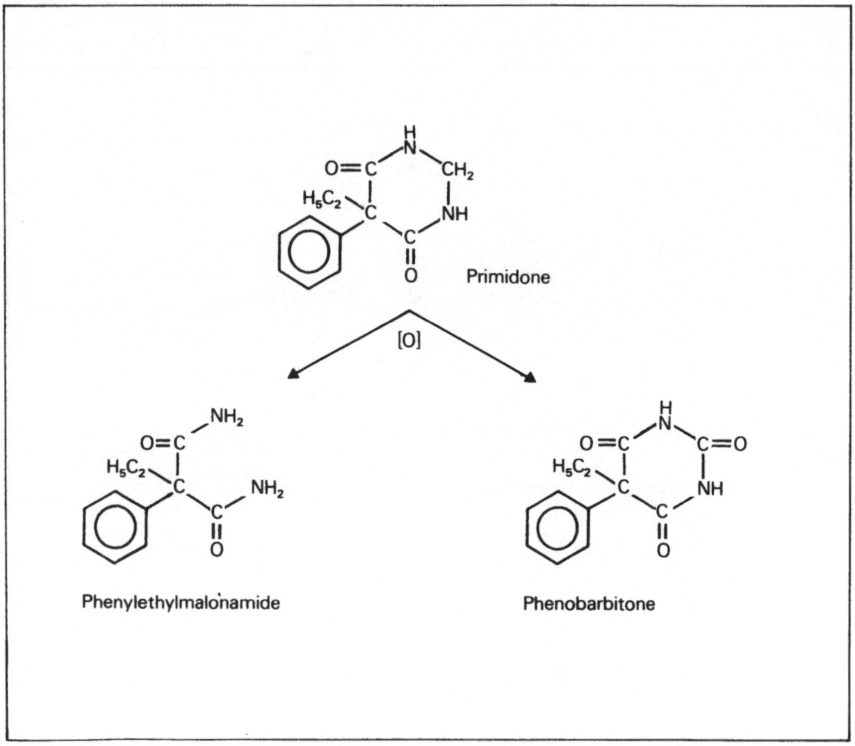

Fig. 6.5. The biotransformation of primidone.

Primidone has a half-life of 10 to 12 hours (Booker et al., 1970) or 6.5 ± 1.0 hrs (Gallagher and Baumel, 1972). The extent of urinary excretion of unchanged primidone is unknown. In the steady-state 15% (Butler and Waddell, 1956) or 24.5% (Olesen and Dam, 1967) of a primidone dose is oxidised to phenobarbitone. Gallagher and Baumel (1972) found some evidence that this biotransformation of primidone to phenobarbitone could become saturated under therapeutic conditions. The known biotransformation pathways for primidone are shown in figure 6.5.

Plasma level correlations; The lower therapeutic limit of plasma *phenobarbitone* level appears to be either 10µg/ml (Buchthal et al., 1968) or 15µg/ml, for febrile convulsions (Faero et al., 1972). The upper therapeutic limit is more difficult to define as the plasma drug level at which side effects from overdosage appear is variable. Some would set the upper limit at 40µg/ml (Van Meter et al., 1970). At the present time the therapeutic range of 10 to 25µg/ml, suggested by Buchthal and Lennox-Buchthal (1972), may be a reasonable one to accept.

Because of its relatively long half-life, there is a period of 2 to 4 weeks after phenobarbitone dose is changed before steady-state conditions will apply. In the steady-state, the plasma phenobarbitone level is linearly related to drug dose in a treated population, though there is considerable inter-individual variation of plasma drug levels at any one dosage. Excluding neonates, the relation between plasma phenobarbitone level and drug dose becomes steeper as the population ages; males tend to require higher doses than females to achieve the same plasma drug levels (Eadie et al., 1976). Contrary to what was said earlier (Richens, 1974), the relationship between plasma phenobarbitone level and drug dose does not appear to be linear. As dose is increased in the individual, steady-state plasma phenobarbitone levels rise by increasing amounts with each dose increment (Eadie et al., 1977). The reason for this non-linearity is not yet known.

When *methylphenobarbitone* is given, there is a delay of several weeks before steady-state conditions appear to apply. When therapy is begun phenobarbitone begins to appear in plasma within 8 hours in some subjects, but in others only after 1 to 2 days (personal unpublished data). Steady-state plasma phenobarbitone levels are some 7 to 10 times greater than those of methylphenobarbitone when plasma levels of the former are in the range 10 to 20µg/ml (personal unpublished data). Consequently plasma phenobarbitone levels rather than plasma levels of methylphenobarbitone may be used as a guide to therapy. Plasma phenobarbitone levels in the steady-state correlate better with methylphenobarbitone dose than do plasma methylphenobarbitone levels themselves. There is considerable inter-individual variation between plasma phenobarbitone levels and methylphenobarbitone dose in a treated population. Older subjects tend to have higher plasma phenobarbitone levels in relation to methylphenobarbitone dose (on a body weight basis) than do younger subjects, and adult males tend to have higher levels than adult females in relation to drug dose (Eadie et al., 1977). In individual patients the relation between plasma phenobarbitone level and methylphenobarbitone dose is linear. This makes it easier to manipulate plasma phenobarbitone levels when methylphenobarbitone is used than when phenobarbitone itself is used.

Phenobarbitone begins to appear in plasma 2 days after *primidone* intake begins (Huisman, 1969; Booker et al., 1970). Because of the relatively long half-life of phenobarbitone, steady-state conditions are likely to require 2 to 4 weeks to develop. In the steady-state, plasma levels of primidone and its metabolites phenobarbitone and phenylethylmalonamide, are all related to primidone dose. Gallagher and Baumel (1972) found plasma phenobarbitone levels were about 2.5 times plasma primidone levels and that phenylethylmalonamide levels were about 10% greater than primidone levels. Since the anticonvulsant role of unmetabolised primidone is uncertain there is little point in attempting to define therapeutic ranges of plasma primidone levels. It would be difficult to establish therapeutic correlations for phenylethylmalonamide levels in the presence of phenobarbitone. Plasma phenobarbitone levels are usually taken as an index of the anticonvulsant activity of primidone, as they are for methylphenobarbitone. Age and sex do not appear to influence the relationship between plasma phenobarbitone level and primidone dose (Eadie et al., 1977).

Interactions

Pharmacodynamic interactions: The barbiturate anticonvulsants may have an increased anti-epileptic effect when combined with other anticonvulsants (e.g. phenytoin). Whether this is more than an additive interaction is uncertain. These barbiturates may also interact additively with other sedatives (e.g. alcohol, tricyclic antidepressants).

Pharmacokinetic interactions: Phenobarbitone is a wellknown inducer of the hepatic microsomal mixed-oxidase system (Conney, 1967). Its administration leads to increased metabolism, more rapid elimination and hence lowered plasma levels of:

    Cortisol (Burstein and Klaiber, 1965)
    Bilirubin (Thompson et al. 1969)
    Bishydroxycoumarin, warfarin (Cucinell et al., 1965)
    Phenylbutazone (Levi et al., 1968)
    Digitoxin (Conney, 1967)
    Aminopyrine (Vesell and Page, 1969)
    Dicophane (Davies et al., 1969)
    Tricyclic antidepressants (Sjoqvist et al., 1971)
    Oestrogens (in experimental animals, but not confirmed in man)
    Doxycycline (Neuvonen and Penttila, 1974).

Phenobarbitone administration was thought to enhance the biotransformation of griseofulvin, but more recent evidence (Riegelman et al., 1970) suggests that the effect of phenobarbitone is to impair the absorption of griseofulvin from the alimentary tract.

The following substances have been reported to cause a fall in plasma phenobarbitone levels:

Dicoumarol (Cucinell et al., 1965)
Phenylbutazone (Conney, 1967)
Phenytoin (Morselli et al., 1971)

Plasma phenobarbitone levels may be increased by administration of the following:

Phenylacetylurea (Huisman et al., 1970)
Carbamazepine (Cereghino et al., 1973)
Valproic acid (Vakil et al., 1976)
Ketogenic diet (Livingstone, 1972)

No specific interactions appear to have been recorded for methylphenobarbitone.

Phenytoin is known to increase the formation of phenobarbitone from primidone (Reynolds et al., 1975). Carbamazepine appears to have a similar effect (Eadie et al., 1977). Carbamazepine administration may raise plasma primidone levels (Cereghino et al., 1973).

Toxicity

Idiosyncratic Toxicity

The barbiturate anticonvulsants occasionally cause skin rashes, usually erythematous, rarely progressing to exfoliation (McGeachy and Bloomer, 1953). Agranulocytosis and aplastic anaemia are very rare complications, as are jaundice and hepatitis (Welton, 1950). It has been claimed that primidone occasionally causes impotence (Livingstone, 1972) but the evidence for this is not very convincing.

Dose-related Toxicity

The barbiturate anticonvulsants all produce drowsiness. In some patients this is particularly troublesome with the first doses of primidone; a degree of tolerance to the sedative effects of the drugs appears to develop. These drugs also produce irritability and hyperactivity in some children and may cause confusion in the aged. During therapy the drugs may cause personality alterations and an insidious decline in intellectual performance. In overdosage, barbiturate anticonvulsants cause dizziness, ataxia, nystagmus and diplopia.

Phenobarbitone therapy may cause folate deficiency, with or without overt macrocytic anaemia (Chanarin et al., 1958; Davis and Woodliff, 1971). Chronic phenobarbitone intake may be associated with hypocalcaemia. The mechanisms involved appear similar to those which apply for phenytoin (p.170, 177).

Dysmorphogenicity

Evidence has accumulated that phenobarbitone (and consequently methyl-phenobarbitone and primidone) causes fetal abnormalities in man (Staples, 1972). The evidence is epidemiological and to some extent confused by the fact that multiple anticonvulsants are often involved in the possible dysmorphogenicity. However, most of the evidence seemed to indicate that phenobarbitone was a dysmorphogen, though a less potent one than phenytoin (Fedrick, 1973). On the other hand the more recent major study of Shapiro et al. (1976) appears to exculpate phenobarbitone.

There is some evidence that phenobarbitone therapy in the pregnant woman may be associated with coagulation defects in the newborn and sometimes with a clinical bleeding tendency, which can be reversed by vitamin K_1 administration (Mountain et al., 1970).

Amylobarbitone

Amylobarbitone has been widely used as a sedative and hypnotic though in recent years it has been replaced to some extent by various benzodiazepine derivatives. Given intravenously it is a very useful anticonvulsant for status epilepticus. It is unsuitable for use in long term anticonvulsant medication because of the amount of drowsiness it produces.

Chemistry

Amylobarbitone (amobarbitol; 5-ethyl-5-isopentylbarbituric acid: MW 226.27) is a crystalline material which is poorly soluble in water at neutral pH. the drug is sometimes given as its more water-soluble sodium salt.

Pharmacology

Biochemical Pharmacology

Amylobarbitone is a classical inhibitor of the terminal mitochondrial oxidation pathway. The net effect of its use is to diminish the amount of energy potentially available to the cell and which can be stored as adenosine triphosphate.

Pharmacodynamics

Because of its effects on the energy available in neurones, amylobarbitone is a general depressant of neuronal function. The activity of higher centres is suppressed first, but given in sufficient dose amylobarbitone can depress all levels of the nervous system, including vegetative functions.

Pharmacokinetics

Inaba et al. (1976) have provided some pharmacokinetic data for the drug. It has a 99% bioavailability if given by mouth, a V_D of 0.5 to 1.1 L/kg, and is eliminated by first order processes with a $T_{1/2}$ of 23.8 ± 6.7 hours, and a clearance of 36.7 ± 10.0 mls min. Less than 1% of a dose is excreted unchanged in urine (Balasubramaniam et al., 1970), 36% appearing as 3-hydroxyamylobarbitone.

Plasma level correlations: When given intravenously for status epilepticus, the anticonvulsant action of amylobarbitone occurs while the drug is still in a distributional phase so that definitive equilibria may not have been established between plasma and receptor concentrations of the drug.

Interactions

Amylobarbitone is likely to interact additively with other sedatives and with ethyl alcohol. Given chronically it may induce the hepatic mixed-oxidase system, thus enhancing the biotransformation of certain other drugs given simultaneously.

Toxicity

There may be occasional allergic rashes, but the main toxic effect of amylobarbitone is excessive sedation, which in more severe overdosage can go on to un-

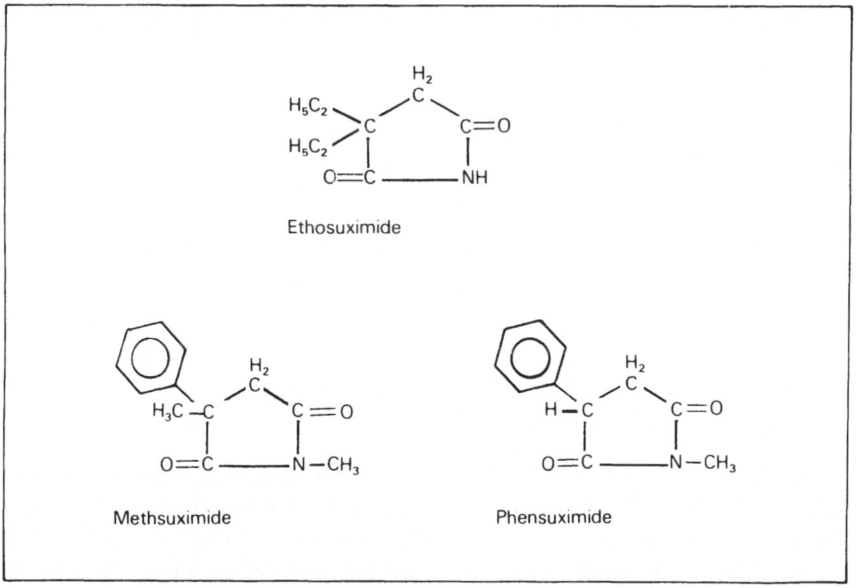

Fig. 6.6. The succinimide anticonvulsants.

consciousness, coma, cardio-respiratory depression and death. Sudden cessation of continued high dose amylobarbitone intake can cause drug-withdrawal fitting.

Succinimides

Of the three succinimide derivatives which are available — ethosuximide, methsuximide and phensuximide (fig. 6.6) — only the first is now in frequent use. It will therefore be considered in some detail, but only an outline of its congeners will be given.

Ethosuximide

The sole medical use of ethosuximide is as an anticonvulsant for absence epilepsy (petit mal) and sometimes for myoclonic seizures (particularly those of hereditary origin).

Chemistry

Ethosuximide (2-ethyl-2-methylsuccinimide) is a white crystalline powder (MW 204.22) which is sparingly soluble in water but soluble in the more polar organic solvents. It is a weak acid with a pK_a of 9.3.

Pharmacology

Biochemical Pharmacology
The chemical mode of action of ethosuximide is uncertain. The drug may enhance the transport of glucose from blood to brain cells (Nahorski, 1972) but this observation hardly provides a sufficient basis for the anti-epileptic action of the drug. In mouse brain homogenate therapeutic concentrations of the drug inhibit gamma aminobutyrate transaminase (Sawaya et al., 1975).

Pharmacodynamics
In the rat ethosuximide protects against epileptic attacks in the best available animal model for petit mal absence epilepsy, *viz* pentylenetetrazole-induced seizures (Chen et al., 1963). The drug elevates the threshold for minimal electro-shock seizures but has relatively little effect on maximal electro-shock seizures. It diminishes spike production in cobalt-induced epileptogenic foci in the rat.

Pharmacokinetics

Absorption and bioavailability: Ethosuximide is almost always given by mouth. The drug is well absorbed, with peak plasma levels 1 to 4 hours (Hansen and Felberg, 1964; Dill et al., 1965) or 3 to 7 hours after dosage (Hvidberg and Dam, 1976). The absorption of ethosuximide is faster from syrup than from capsules (Buchanan et al., 1969).

Distribution: The apparent volume of distribution in children and adults is about 0.7L/kg, i.e. approximately the volume of body water (Hvidberg and Dam, 1976). Plasma and brain concentrations of the drug are similar (Dill et al., 1965). There is little or no binding of the drug to plasma protein. CSF levels (Sherwin and Robb, 1972) and salivary levels (Eadie et al., 1977) are similar to whole plasma levels of ethosuximide.

Elimination: The plasma half-life of the drug is about 30 hours in children, and over 60 hours in adults (Buchanan et al., 1969) with a mean value for adults of 2.33 days (Buchanan et al., 1973). Some 19% of a dose (Buchanan et al., 1973) or 30% (range 17 to 38%), [Glazko, 1975] is excreted unchanged in urine. The known metabolic pathways are shown in figure 6.7.

Plasma level correlations: Experience has shown that plasma ethosuximide levels of 40 to 80µg/ml offer the best chance of controlling absence seizures (Sherwin and Robb, 1972; Penry et al., 1972), though the upper limit of the therapeutic range has been set higher, at 100µg/ml (Brown et al., 1975). Personal experience has shown that some patients tolerate plasma ethosuximide levels up to 150µg/ml with improved control of seizures.

While there is considerable interindividual variation in the relation between plasma ethosuximide levels and drug dose, in treated populations plasma ethosuximide levels tend to be proportionate to dose. Sherwin and Robb (1972) showed that, on the average, children required higher ethosuximide doses on a body weight basis than adults to achieve the same plasma ethosuximide levels. Little has been published on the relationship between ethosuximide dose and steady-state plasma levels in the individual, but the findings of Eadie (1976) raised the possibility that the relation is not linear, with increasing rises in plasma drug level in proportion to increases in drug dose.

The long half-life of ethosuximide indicates that its steady-state plasma levels will show little fluctuation over a dosage interval of 12 to 24 hours.

Interactions

Pharmacodynamic interactions: Recent experience suggests that ethosuximide has at least an additive effect against absence epilepsy, if given together with clonazepam.

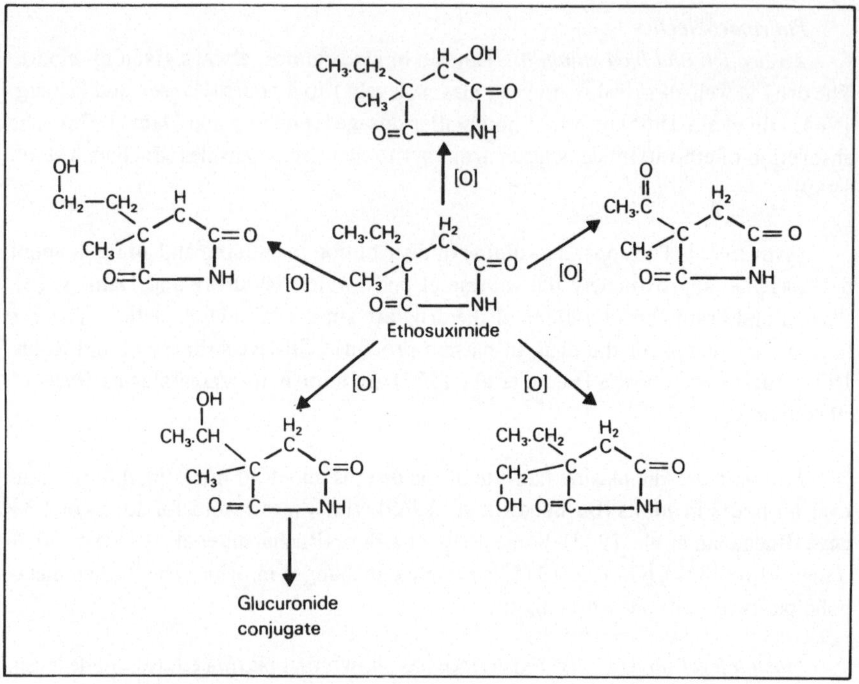

Fig. 6.7. The metabolic pathways of ethosuximide.

Pharmacokinetic interactions: Ethosuximide causes plasma phenytoin levels to rise (Frantzen et al., 1967). In rats the drug can induce the hepatic mixed-oxidase system (Orton and Nicholls, 1972). Should this effect occur in man it could alter the metabolism of many concurrently administered drugs. However Gilbert et al. (1974) failed to find evidence supporting the existence of such an effect in man.

Toxicity

Idiosyncratic Toxicity
Skin rashes are rare, but erythema multiforme and a lupus-like syndrome have been reported (Buchanan, 1972). Rare instances of leucopenia and pancytopenia are known (Kiorboe et al., 1964; Cohn, 1968).

Dose-related Toxicity
High local concentration of the drug in the upper alimentary tract may cause anorexia, nausea, vomiting and upper abdominal distress. At higher plasma drug

levels (over 100µg/ml) there may be tiredness, headache and sensations of dysequilibrium.

Dysmorphogenicity

The types of epilepsy for which ethosuximide is used have often become inactive before the age at which reproduction usually occurs. Hence the question of dysmorphogenicity of the drug is not of great practical importance and adequate data are lacking.

Methsuximide

Although methsuximide (MW 203.23) is less effective than ethosuximide against absence epilepsy it is reputed to have some action against partial epilepsy arising in the temporal lobe. The drug has a short half-life (2.6 hours — Glazko and Dill, 1972; 1.4 hours — Porter et al., 1977). It is substantially biotransformed to its N-desmethyl derivative. This substance is also an anticonvulsant and has a half-life of 36 to 48 hours (Barrow et al., 1974) or 36 hours (Porter et al., 1977). Therefore with continued methsuximide intake the dominant antiepileptic effect comes to be exerted through the metabolite, for which a therapeutic range of plasma levels of 10 to 40µg/ml has been proposed (Barrow et al., 1974). It is believed that hydroxylated metabolites also occur (Horning et al., 1973; Dudley et al., 1974).

Phensuximide

Phensuximide (MW 189.21) is said to be of some benefit in petit mal absence epilepsy. Structurally it resembles methsuximide (fig. 6.6). The drug is said to be absorbed rapidly after oral administration. It has a plasma half-life of 4 hours (Kinkel, 1972) of 7.8 hours (Porter et al., 1977). It undergoes N-demethylation and benzene ring hydroxylation to form phenolic, dihydrodiol and catechol derivatives (Horning et al., 1974). The succinimide ring may also undergo cleavage. Plasma levels and clinical correlations for the drug do not appear to have been studied in man.

Oxazolidinediones

Although a number of oxazolidinediones have been marketed, most are not now in common use, as more effective drugs have been developed for absence epilepsy (e.g. ethosuximide, clonazepam, valproic acid). Troxidone (trimethadione) is the only survivor of the oxazolidinedione group of drugs that appears worthy of discussion, though troxidone too is a drug which is disappearing from use.

Troxidone

This drug is sometimes used to treat absence epilepsy.

Chemistry

Troxidone (MW 143.14) is a water-soluble white powder. The molecule is essentially neutral. Much of the apparent anticonvulsant activity of troxidone is mediated through its N-desmethyl derivative (dimethadione) which is a weak acid with a pKa of 6.13.

Pharmacology

Biochemical Pharmacology

Troxidone can decrease intracellular Na^+ concentration (Pincus et al., 1970). Troxidone and dimethadione activate the sodium pump (Brink and Freeman, 1972), while dimethadione produces an extracellular acidosis (Butler et al., 1966) which might also alter the polarisation of neuronal cell membranes. Troxidone increases serotonin synthesis in rat brain (Diaz, 1974).

Pharmacodynamics

Troxidone prevents pentylenetetrazole-induced seizures in experimental animals. It elevates thalamic seizure thresholds and thresholds for after-discharges (Schallek and Kuehn, 1963), yet it has no effect on cortical or hippocampal after-discharges. Troxidone does not alter post-tetanic potentiation, or presynaptic or postsynaptic inhibition (Woodbury, 1969). In man, the drug does not modify the clinical pattern of maximum electro-shock seizures produced during the course of psychiatric therapy (Toman et al., 1946).

Pharmacokinetics

Absorption and bioavailability: In practice troxidone is given only by mouth. It appears to be absorbed rapidly, with peak plasma levels 30 minutes after dosing (Booker, 1972). Data on the extent of its absorption are lacking.

Distribution: In dogs troxidone appears to be distributed through body water, but the volume of distribution of dimethadione is smaller (Frey and Schulz, 1970). The drug undergoes little or no binding to plasma protein (Booker, 1972). There is no selective regional concentration of troxidone in brain (Ferngren and Paalzow, 1969), nor is there selective concentration of dimethadione (Roos, 1965).

Elimination: The half-life of troxidone is about 16 hours (Booker, 1972) but the half-life of dimethadione is about 240 hours (Butler, 1955). While troxidone is eliminated chiefly by biotransformation to dimethadione, the latter is eliminated unchanged in urine, in which about 6% of the dose is excreted daily (Butler and Waddell, 1958). The urine excretion of dimethadione is pH dependent, decreasing in acid urine.

Plasma level correlations: In treated populations plasma troxidone and dimethadione level are both related to drug dose. Because of its much slower elimination, plasma levels of dimethadione come to be much higher than levels of troxidone by the time the steady-state is reached. In the steady-state the average ratio of dimethadione to troxidone in plasma is 12 : 1 (Booker, 1972). It has been observed that plasma dimethadione levels somewhat in excess of 700µg/ml offer the best chance of controlling absence seizures (Jensen, 1962; Chamberlin et al., 1965; Booker, 1972).

The relation between plasma levels and troxidone dose in the individual is not known.

Interactions

Pharmacodynamic interactions: Troxidone probably interacts additively with ethosuximide in the control of absence seizures.

Pharmacokinetic interactions: Roseman (1961) claimed that troxidone caused raised plasma phenytoin levels. *In vitro* troxidone can inhibit the demethylation of *N*-methylbarbitone (Butler et al., 1965), but whether it inhibits this and other dealkylations *in vivo* is unknown.

Toxicity

Idiosyncratic Toxicity

Troxidone may cause skin rashes of varying pattern. At times exfoliative dermatitis has occurred. Instances of a nephrotic syndrome following troxidone usage have been reported (Barnett et al., 1948; Heymann, 1967) and also myasthenia (Peterson, 1966; Booker et al., 1970). Pancytopenia and aplastic anaemia occur occasionally (Wells, 1957); mild to moderate neutropenia is more common, occurring in 20% of persons taking the drug (Davis and Lennox, 1949).

Dose-related Toxicity

Local alimentary irritative effects of the drug are rare. It may cause sedation and troublesome glare phenomena are frequent (Sloan and Gilger, 1947).

Dysmorphogenicity

German et al. (1970) found an increased incidence of malformed babies in mothers taking oxazolidinediones. However, the types of epilepsy for which troxidone is useful would rarely persist to an age at which pregnancy was likely and troxidone is a drug which is disappearing from use. Therefore the question of fetal abnormality from troxidone is of little practical importance.

Benzodiazepines

The benzodiazepines are an important group of drugs with very widespread use. A number of the benzodiazepines yield the common metabolite *N*-desmethyl diazepam (i.e. nordiazepam), which is an anticonvulsant. Hence many of the group have anticonvulsant effects. Here only three will be discussed, *viz* diazepam, nitrazepam and clonazepam.

Diazepam: Nitrazepam: Clonazepam

Diazepam has achieved extensive use as a tranquilliser and sedative, and nitrazepam as a hypnotic. Orally, both drugs are used as anticonvulsants, principally in myoclonic epilepsy, though sometimes in other forms of seizure. For some years parenteral diazepam has been the treatment of choice for status epilepticus. Clonazepam, a more recently introduced benzodiazepine, is probably a more effective oral and parenteral anticonvulsant than its congeners. It is also useful in tic douloureux. Pinder et al. (1976) have provided a major review of the properties and use of clonazepam.

Chemistry

The three benzodiazepines under consideration are relatively water insoluble bases which dissolve in organic solvents of moderate polarity. The respective pKa values are diazepam 3.3; nitrazepam 3.4, 10.8; clonazepam 1.5, 10.5. Their structural formulae are shown in figure 6.8.

Pharmacology

Biochemical Pharmacology

The benzodiazepines affect brain transmitter amine levels and therefore may exert an anticonvulsant effect by altering synaptic transmission in certain neural path-

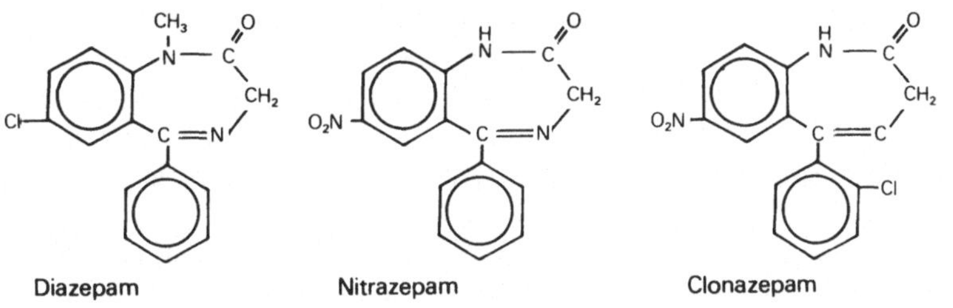

Fig. 6.8. The benzodiazepine anticonvulsants.

ways. Thus all three benzodiazepines here considered increase brain noradrenaline levels (Fennessy and Lee, 1972). Diazepam exerts this effect by decreasing turnover of this amine in the thalamus, mid-brain, cerebral cortex and cerebellum (Taylor and Laverty, 1969). Brain dopamine levels are increased by nitrazepam and clonazepam, and brain serotonin levels by clonazepam (Fennessy and Lee, 1972). Diazepam, in a dose of 5mg/kg, increases acetylcholine levels in the mouse cerebral hemispheres and diencephalon but not in the brain stem (Consolo et al., 1974). The drug inhibits cyclic AMP phosphodiesterase in cat brain (Dalton et al., 1974). Young et al. (1974) suggested that benzodiazepines may bind to glycine receptors in the nervous system and mimic the effects of glycine. More recent evidence favours an action in relation to GABA receptors (Costa and Guidotti, 1979).

Pharmacodynamics

Benzodiazepines have effects against both electrically and pentylenetetrazole-induced seizures in several animal species (Randall and Schallek, 1968). These drugs inhibit the photic epileptic responses which occur in the baboon *Papio papio,* but do not affect post-tetanic potentiation. Diazepam and nitrazepam elevate after-discharge thresholds in the hippocampus, amygdala and thalamus, but not in the neocortex. Clonazepam and diazepam have an anticonvulsant effect against cocaine-induced limbic seizures in the rat (Eidelberg et al., 1965), while clonazepam inhibits cortical experimental epileptic foci produced by alumina application (Mutani and Fariello, 1971). At spinal cord level diazepam suppresses excess activity in lower motor neurones, either by blocking polysynaptic pathways or by increasing presynaptic inhibition (Nathan, 1970).

Pharmacokinetics

Absorption and bioavailability: Orally administered *diazepam* is absorbed rapidly with T_{max} values of about 1 hour (De Silva et al., 1966). Absorption is reasonably complete, with only about 10% of an oral dose appearing in the faeces (Schwartz et al., 1965). Diazepam is better absorbed from tablets than from a suspension (Berlin et al., 1972). After intramuscular injection diazepam is absorbed less rapidly than after oral administration (Gamble et al., 1973; Hillestad et al., 1974). The drug is absorbed relatively quickly after rectal administration as a solution (T_{max} 10 to 20 mins) but less rapidly if given in a suppository (T_{max} 60 mins) according to Agurell et al. (1975).

Orally administered *nitrazepam* is fairly rapidly absorbed with a T_{max} of 2 hours (Rieder and Wendt, 1971) and an absorption rate constant of 2.16/hour (Rieder, 1973). Some 14 to 20% of an oral dose appears in the faeces.

Oral *clonazepam* is fairly rapidly absorbed with a T_{max} of 2 to 4 hours (Berlin and Dahlstrom, 1975). About 10% of an oral dose fails to be absorbed. The absorption of the drug from intramuscular injection sites does not appear to have been studied.

Distribution: The apparent volumes of distribution of the benzodiazepines are relatively high, suggesting substantial tissue binding of the drugs. The V_D of diazepam is 0.7 to 2.6L/kg; that of nitrazepam is 2.1L/kg; that of clonazepam is 2.6L/kg (Sjo et al., 1975; Berlin and Dahlstrom, 1975).

Figures for plasma protein binding are: diazepam 90%, nitrazepam 55%, clonazepam 47% (Muller and Wollert, 1973) and desmethyldiazepam 96.6% (Klotz et al., 1976). Diazepam binding is reduced in uraemic serum (Sjoholm et al., 1976). After injection diazepam is rather selectively taken up by adipose tissue and, in the nervous system, by the spinal cord, thalamus and cerebral cortex. Post-distributional levels are higher in the cerebral white matter, dentate nucleus, pons and medulla than in the cerebral grey matter, hypothalamus and caudate nucleus. Total brain levels of diazepam are much higher than blood levels of the drug (van der Kleijn, 1969).

In man diazepam does not undergo an enterohepatic circulation (Mahon et al., 1976). CSF diazepam levels are about 3% of simultaneous plasma levels (Kanto et al., 1975).

Diazepam and nitrazepam are found in human milk at 10% (Erkkola and Kanto, 1972) and 50% (Rieder and Wendt, 1971) of their respective plasma concentrations. Diazepam and also desmethyldiazepam levels are similar in maternal and umbilical cord plasma (Mandelli et al., 1975).

Elimination: Representative values for the half-life of diazepam are 2.25 days (Hillestad et al., 1974), 0.88 to 1.54 days (Kaplan et al., 1973) and 0.83 to 1.75 days (van der Kleijn et al., 1971). Less than 1% of a dose of the drug appears unchanged in urine (Kaplan et al., 1973). Elimination of diazepam takes place almost entirely by

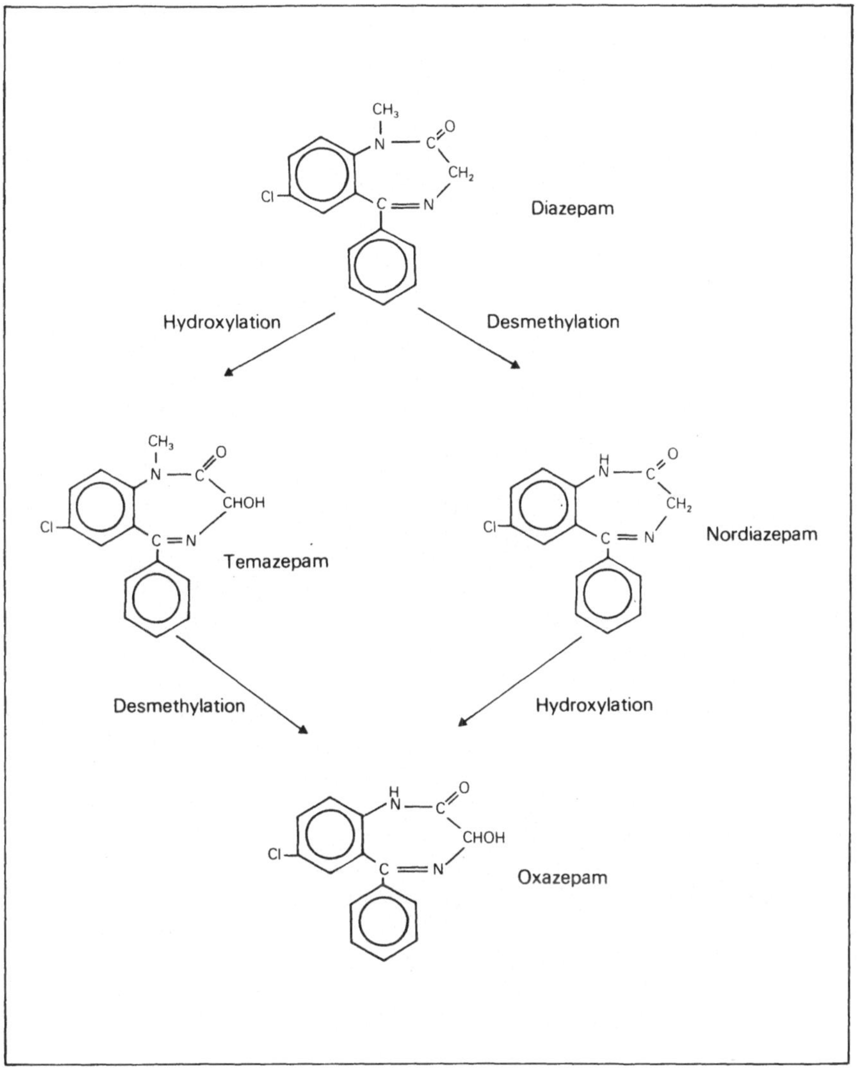

Fig. 6.9. The biotransformation of diazepam.

biotransformation. The known pathways are shown in figure 6.9. The hydroxylated derivatives form glucuronide conjugates which are excreted as such in urine.

Nordiazepam (desmethyldiazepam) is both an anticonvulsant and tranquilliser, with a half-life of 60 to 95 hours (van der Kleijn et al., 1971). Oxazepam also is a tranquilliser and an anticonvulsant (Lou, 1968) with a half-life of 9 to 21 hours (Vessman et al., 1973).

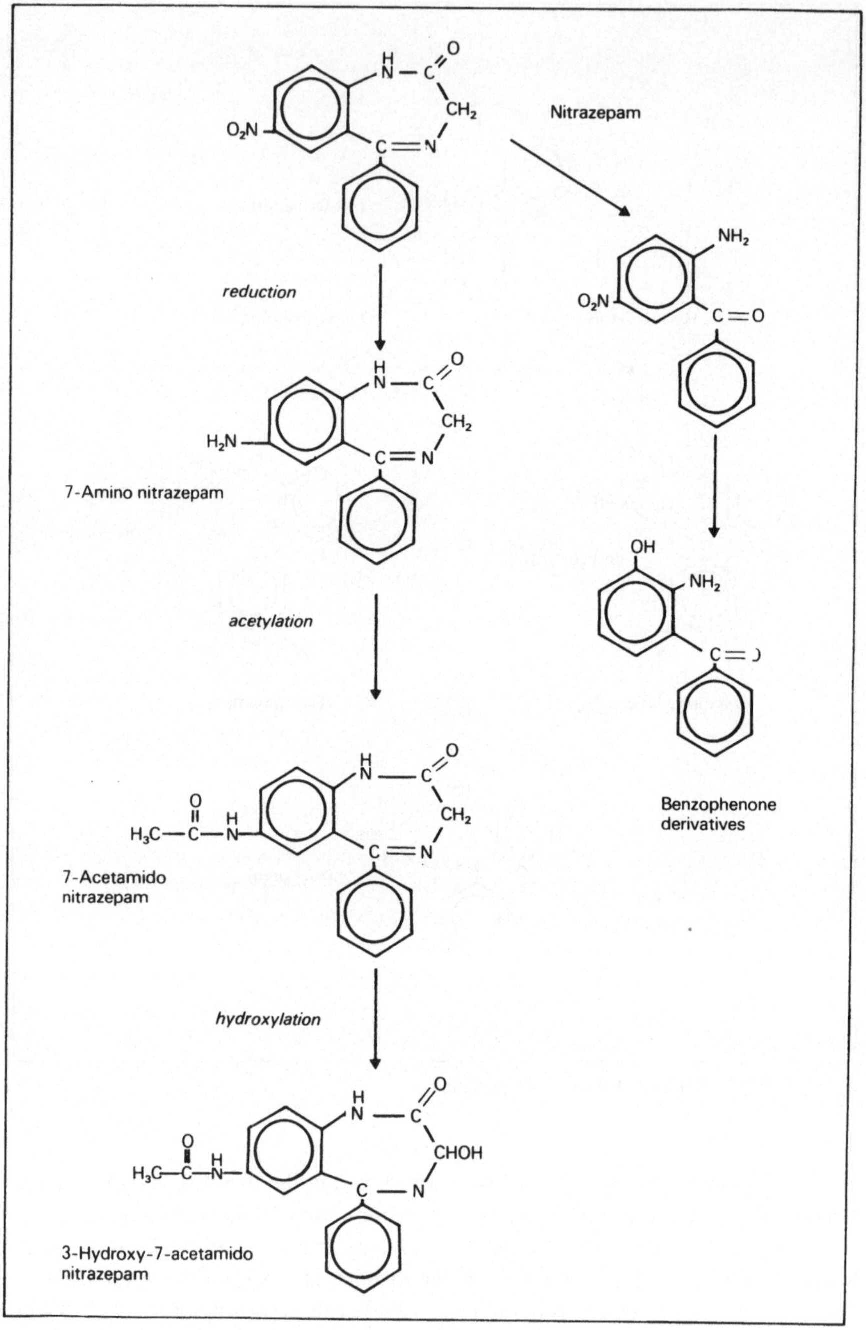

Fig. 6.10. The biotransformation of nitrazepam.

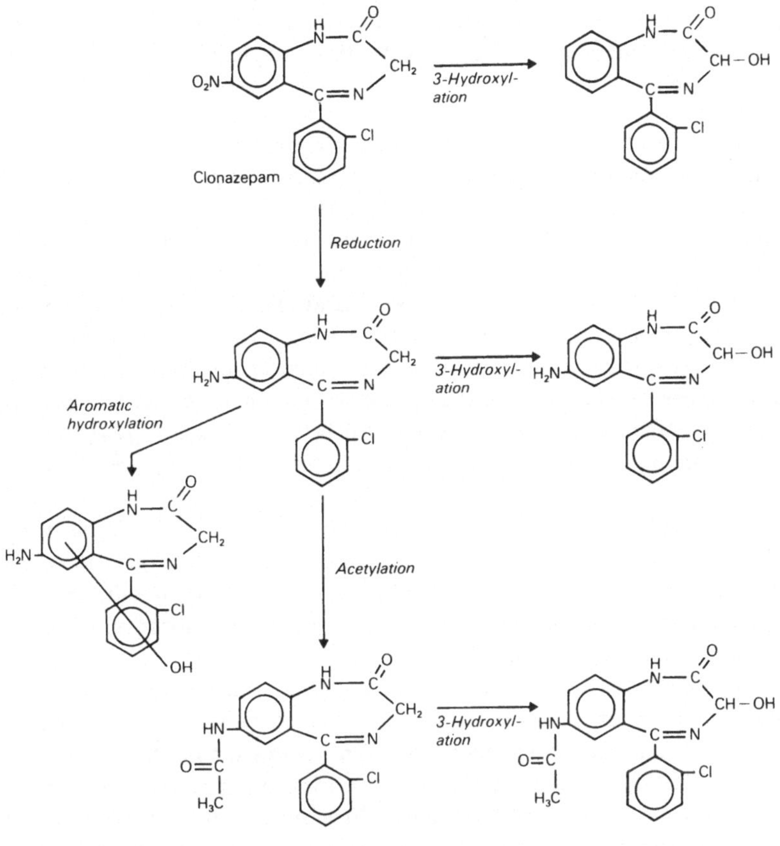

Fig. 6.11. The biotransformation of clonazepam.

Nitrazepam has a half-life of 21 to 25 hours (Rieder and Wendt, 1971) or a β-phase half-life of 25.1 hours (Rieder, 1973). Very little unchanged nitrazepam appears in urine. The known biotransformation pathways for the drug are as set out in figure 6.10. The chief metabolites found in urine are the 7-amino and 7-acetamido derivatives.

Clonazepam has a plasma half-life of 1 to 2 days (Naestoft et al., 1973), 26.4 hours (Kaplan et al., 1974) or 22 hours (Knop et al., 1975). About 2% of the dose is excreted unchanged in urine, but the drug has a total plasma clearance of about 0.05L/kg/h (van der Kleijn et al., 1975). Elimination is chiefly by biotransformation, and the known pathways involved are shown in figure 6.11. The 7-amino and 7-acetamido derivatives are the chief metabolites found in plasma. Clonazepam metabolites are also found in faeces, suggesting that these metabolites may have undergone biliary excretion.

Plasma level correlations: After the initial administration of *diazepam* about 24 to 36 hours are required for nordiazepam to appear in plasma (de Silva et al., 1966; Foster and Frings, 1970). Oxazepam plasma levels are so low as to be virtually unmeasurable in these circumstances. With regular diazepam dosage, by the time the steady-state is reached, plasma nordiazepam levels are a little higher than plasma diazepam levels. There are relatively few data available on the relation between plasma diazepam level and drug dose in a treated population or in individuals. It has been suggested that plasma diazepam levels in excess of 600ng/ml are required to control epilepsy (Booker and Celesia, 1973). A minimum plasma diazepam concentration of 400ng/ml is needed to relieve anxiety (Dasberg et al., 1974). In practice such levels are unlikely to be achieved with conventional oral therapeutic doses of diazepam.

Little information is available on plasma *nitrazepam* levels in treated patients, though it is known that, in the steady-state, plasma levels of nitrazepam and of its 7-amino and 7-acetamido derivatives are all similar (Rieder and Wendt, 1971). The therapeutic range of plasma nitrazepam levels to achieve an anticonvulsant effect is not known.

Steady-state plasma *clonazepam* levels are directly related to drug dose in treated populations (Huang et al., 1973) and in treated individuals (Eadie, 1976). Sufficient experience has not yet accumulated to set firm figures for the therapeutic range. Huang et al. (1973) suggested that levels above 15ng/ml correlated with protection against myoclonic seizures and levels above 30ng/ml with protection against other varieties of seizure. Hvidberg and Dam (1976) suggested a therapeutic range of 20 to 70ng/ml.

Interactions

Pharmacodynamic interactions: Diazepam increases the action of certain sedative and hypnotic substances (e.g. alcohol, barbiturates), possibly through pharmacodynamic interactions.

Pharmacokinetic interactions: Diazepam displaces tri-iodothyronine from thyroxine-binding globulin (Schussler, 1971) and causes an increase in plasma testosterone levels (Arguelles and Rosner, 1975) and in plasma phenytoin levels (Vajda et al., 1971). Although clonazepam therapy usually causes a decrease in plasma phenytoin levels (Edwards and Eadie, 1973), in some patients phenytoin levels rise.

Benzodiazepine therapy does not alter plasma levels of tricyclic antidepressants (Silverman and Braithwaite, 1973).

Toxicity

Idiosyncratic Toxicity
Occasional drug rashes occur.

Dose-related Toxicity
High doses of the benzodiazepines produce sedation and confusion, with disturbances of equilibrium. Nitrazepam may produce increased salivary and bronchial secretion (Millichap and Ortiz, 1966). Clonazepam causes aggressiveness in some patients. In epilepsy abrupt cessation of clonazepam therapy may cause status epilepticus (Edwards, 1974).

Dysmorphogenicity
There is as yet no evidence that nitrazepam and clonazepam cause fetal abnormalities in man but there are reports that diazepam therapy has been associated with an increased incidence of oral clefts (Aarskog, 1975).

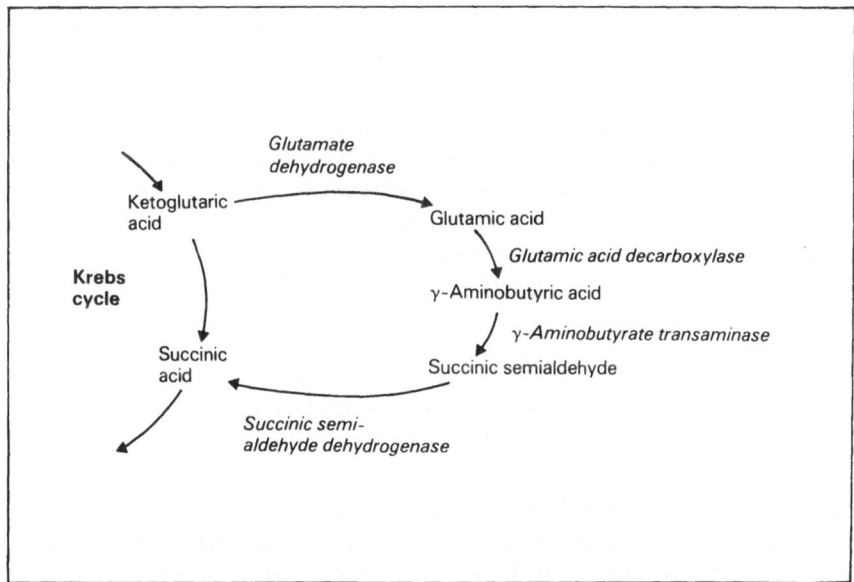

Fig. 6.12. The GABA shunt.

Valproic acid

This drug is used almost solely as an anticonvulsant. Simon and Penry (1975) and Pinder et al. (1977b) have provided detailed reviews of its properties and use.

Chemistry

Valproic acid (di-n-propyl-acetic acid; MW 166.20) is a white hygroscopic powder with a pKa of 4.95; the structural formula is shown in figure 6.13. The drug is usually administered orally as its sodium salt. Attempts have been made to alter the pharmacokinetic profile of the drug by administering it as its dipropylacetamide derivative.

Pharmacology

Biochemical Pharmacology
Valproic acid inhibits the enzymes glutamic acid decarboxylase and γ-aminobutyrate transaminase, the latter more markedly than the former. Harvey (1976) suggested that valproic acid inhibited succinic semialdehyde dehydrogenase rather than γ-aminobutyrate transaminase. The net effect of these inhibitions is to raise brain γ-aminobutyrate levels (Godin et al., 1969). Ciesielski et al. (1975) also showed that valproate will support brain respiration, suggesting that it might be able to substitute for γ-aminobutyrate on the γ-aminobutyrate transaminase receptor. Valproate is partly converted into triglycerides and phospholipids in the rat liver, but also into fatty acids such as 2-n-propylglutaric acid and 2-n-propylhydroxypentanoic acid (Kuhara and Matsumoto, 1974). Short chain fatty acids, supplied by means of a ketogenic diet, have a similar spectrum of anti-epileptic action to valproate. It has been argued that anticonvulsant effects of valproate may not be mediated through altered γ-aminobutyrate levels, since brain levels of this amino acid transmitter are not sufficiently raised by therapeutic concentrations of valproate (Harvey, 1976). However whole brain levels of γ-aminobutyrate may not necessarily reflect γ-aminobutyrate levels in axon terminals and these are more relevant levels for the anti-convulsant effect of valproate. The greater part of brain γ-aminobutyrate is involved in the GABA shunt as a metabolic intermediate (figure 6.12).

Pharmacodynamics
In several animal species valproate protects against seizures induced by max-imum electro-shock and pentylenetetrazole and raises the threshold for minimal seizures induced by these agents. It protects against audiogenic seizures in mice and rats, seizures produced from a hippocampal cobalt focus in cats and photomyoclonic

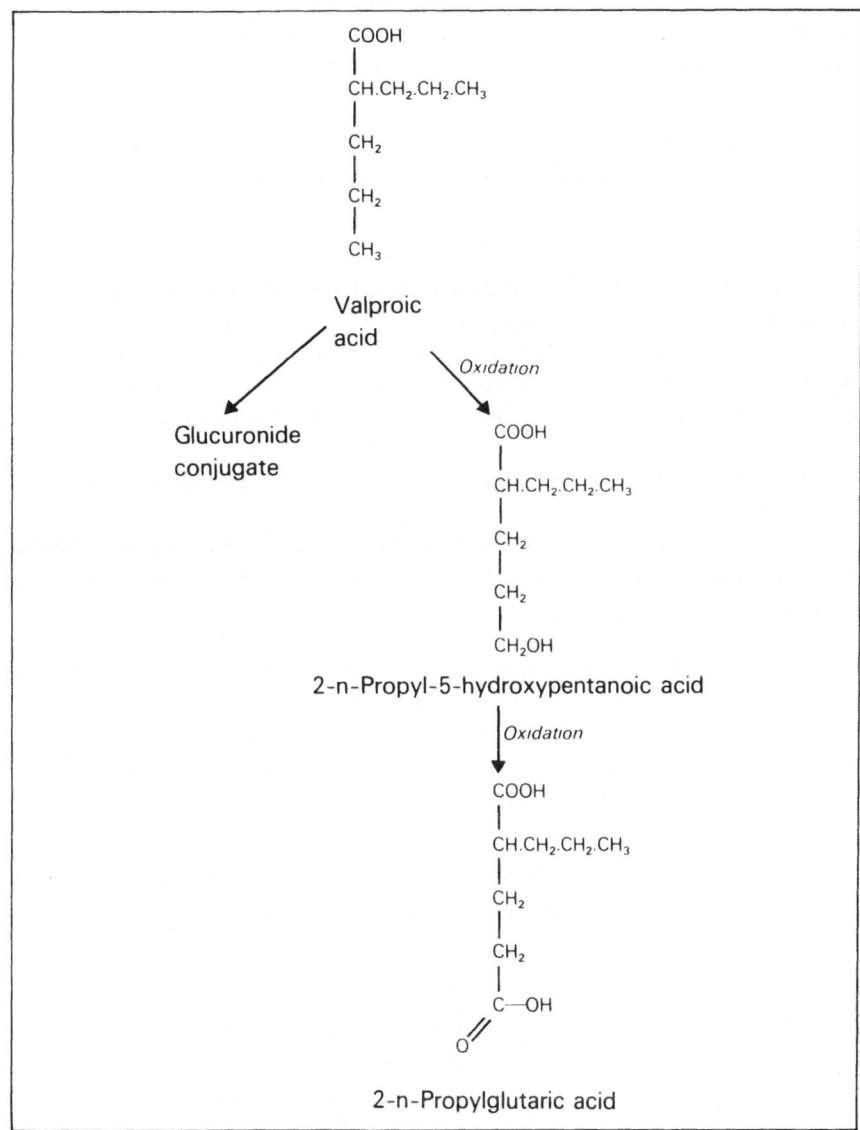

Fig. 6.13. The biotransformation of valproic acid.

seizures in the baboon *Papio papio.* Valproate has no action on seizures induced by strychnine, picrotoxin and cocaine.

In man the drug appears most effective in myoclonic and petit mal absence epilepsy (Simon and Penry, 1975). Its apparent effectiveness in other types of epilepsy may be due to effects on other anticonvulsants (Volzke and Doose, 1973) because of pharmacokinetic interactions.

Pharmacokinetics

Absorption and bioavailability: After oral administration valproate is absorbed rapidly, with a T_{max} of less than 1 hour (Schobben et al., 1975).

Distribution: The V_D of valproate is 0.15 to 0.40L/kg (Schobben et al., 1975). However Richens et al. (1976) found a V_D of 0.198 ± 0.029L/kg in 8 epileptic adults and a V_D of 0.127 ± 0.040L/kg in 10 normal adult volunteers. Limited personal experience suggests the drug has a greater V_D in epileptic children than in adults; in the latter the distribution appears to correspond roughly with extracellular water (Eadie et al., 1977).

The plasma protein binding of valproate is 84% (Meinardi et al., 1975), or 90% (Jordan et al., 1976).

Eymard et al. (1971) showed, in rats and mice, that at the time of peak plasma valproate levels brain valproate levels were only about 2 to 3% of the levels in muscle, and below 2% of those in the liver.

Elimination: The half-life of valproate has been measured at 10.3 ± 2.6h (Schobben et al., 1975), or 5.88 ± 0.47h in epileptic adults, and 9.00 ± 1.01h in normal adults (Richens et al., 1976). Some 7% of the dose is excreted unchanged in urine (Schobben et al., 1975) so that elimination is mainly by omega oxidation to various fatty acid derivatives as indicated earlier (figure 6.13).

Plasma level correlations: Because of the rapidity of its elimination relative to those of the other anticonvulsants, steady-state plasma valproate levels are likely to show more fluctuation over a dosage interval. Steady-state plasma valproate levels are proportionate to dose though there is substantial interindividual variation (Hassan et al., 1976). The relation of plasma level to dose in the individual does not appear to have been studied in detail. A tentative lower therapeutic limit of 50µg/ml has been suggested (Vajda et al., 1976). Van der Kleijn et al. (1975) suggested a range of 60 to 80µg/ml. Meinardi (1976) noted that muscular weakness and tremor usually appeared when valproate levels exceeded 110µg/ml.

Interactions

Pharmacodynamic interactions: There are some intimations that valproate may have additional anticonvulsant effects when combined with other antiepileptic agents, though the possibility of pharmacokinetic interactions causing increased anticonvulsant activity in these circumstances has not yet been thoroughly studied.

Pharmacokinetic interactions: Valproate *in vitro* produces a minor degree of displacement of phenytoin and phenobarbitone from plasma protein binding sites (Jordan et al., 1976). There are several reports that valproate therapy causes a substantial rise in plasma phenobarbitone levels (Schobben et al., 1975; Harvey, 1976; Vakil et al., 1976). In rat liver microsomes, valproate inhibits the hydroxylation of phenytoin (Sapeika and Kaplan, 1974) and in this species valproate therapy causes a rise in brain phenytoin levels (Lascelles, 1976). In man, Vajda et al. (1976) noted a rise in serum phenytoin levels when valproate was given, though our experience suggests that this pattern of interaction does not always occur. Loiseau et al. (1975) suspected that ethosuximide, clomipramine and diazepam all raised plasma valproate levels.

Toxicity

The side effects of valproate were reviewed by Noronha and Bevan (1976).

Idiosyncratic Toxicity
The writers know of one instance of severe hepatotoxicity associated with the use of valproate.

Dose-related Toxicity
Nausea, abdominal cramps and occasional vomiting may develop early in the course of therapy but usually subside with time. Drowsiness may occur, and alterations in appetite. A mild degree of hair loss has occurred in some cases and the behaviour of children may deteriorate. Valproate inhibits secondary platelet aggregation in some patients but there is as yet no evidence that this effect is clinically significant (Richardson et al., 1976). The Australian Pharmaceutical Benefits List carries a warning that the drug is suspected of causing testicular damage (at least in animals).

Dysmorphogenicity
Adequate data are not yet available on the human dysmorphogenicity of valproate. The experimental data are reviewed by Whittle (1976). In rats spinal and renal defects may occur and in mice encephaloceles, ablepharia and rib fusions.

Sulthiame

Although sulthiame has been in use as an anticonvulsant for partial epilepsy over a number of years, its efficacy as a major anti-epileptic drug in its own right appears dubious (Green et al., 1974).

Chemistry

Sulthiame (MW 290.37) is a white crystalline acidic sulphonamide derivative which is poorly soluble in water and ethanol.

Pharmacology

Biochemical Pharmacology

Sulthiame inhibits the enzyme carbonic anhydrase. The drug may thus possibly produce an intracellular acidosis which will reduce Na^+ entry into cells and increase the polarisation of the cell membrane. The therapeutic effect of sulthiame correlates with a lowering of plasma pH (Geets and Pinon, 1971). Sulthiame, at therapeutic concentrations, reduced oxygen consumption in a rat brain microsome-synaptosome preparation (Spector, 1972). This action was antagonised by noradrenaline or formyltetrahydrofolate.

Pharmacodynamics

Sulthiame reduces the clonic component of electro-shock induced seizures in experimental animals but does not protect against pentylenetetrazole-induced seizures (Wirth et al., 1961).

In man the drug was considered relatively specific for partial epilepsy, though there have been reports that it is of benefit in myoclonic epilepsy. However, the study of Green et al. (1974) showed that sulthiame, if used alone, was so much inferior to phenytoin that its continued use as a primary anticonvulsant seems hard to justify. However the drug may have anti-epileptic effects by virtue of pharmacodynamic interactions with other anticonvulsants. These effects could be attained more simply by adjusting the dose of the primary anticonvulsants.

Pharmacokinetics

Absorption and bioavailability: In rats the isotopically labelled drug is well absorbed (Duhm et al., 1963). Data for man are lacking.

Distribution: Distribution data in man are lacking. In rats Duhm et al. (1963) found sulthiame levels in brain and blood were similar, but the drug was more concentrated in red cells than in serum.

Elimination: Some 60 to 70% of a sulthiame dose is excreted unchanged in urine in man (Diamond and Levy, 1963). Within 24 hours of dosage, 32% of the dose is present in urine (Olesen, 1968). More exact elimination data are lacking. In the rat the drug was found to form an inactive hydroxylated metabolite (Duhm et al., 1963).

Plasma level correlations: Practically no information is available. Olesen (1968) showed that sulthiame doses of 200 to 1000mg per day produced plasma drug levels in the range 0.5 to 12.5µg/ml. No therapeutic range is known for the drug.

Interactions

Pharmacodynamic interactions: None are known.

Pharmacokinetic interactions: There is some evidence raising the possibility that sulthiame may displace phenytoin from plasma protein binding sites (Hooper et al., 1973). In rats already receiving phenytoin, the addition of sulthiame raised brain but not plasma phenytoin levels (Morselli et al., 1970). In man sulthiame therapy raised plasma phenytoin concentrations (Hansen et al., 1969; Olesen and Jensen, 1969; Richens and Houghton, 1973).

Toxicity

Idiosyncratic Toxicity
The drug occasionally produces headaches and mental changes (e.g. hallucinations). Rarely there is increased salivation. An instance of renal tubular necrosis has been recorded (Aviram et al., 1965).

Dose-related Toxicity
Sulthiame sometimes causes a degree of gastric irritation. In higher doses it may cause drowsiness, ataxia and anorexia. Hyperpnoea with breathlessness and peripheral paraesthesiae are regularly encountered with higher doses of the drug.

Dysmorphogenicity
No human data are available bearing on this question.

Chlormethiazole

Chlormethiazole is used to control delerium tremens and various agitated and hallucinatory states. The drug has been advocated as a sedative and hypnotic in the elderly. Given intravenously it may be very useful in controlling status epilepticus. The pharmacokinetic properties of the drug, and its potential for causing dependence, make it unsuitable for long term use as an anticonvulsant.

Chemistry

Chlormethiazole (MW 161.66) is a base with a pKa of 3.2. Its structural formula is shown in figure 6.14. It is a viscous oily liquid which is sometimes given as its highly water-soluble ethane disulphonate derivative.

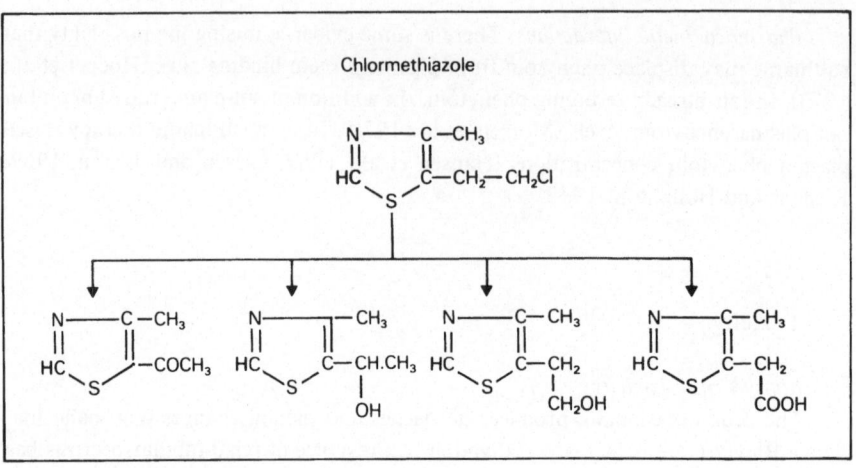

Fig. 6.14. The metabolic pathways suggested for chlormethiazole.

Pharmacology

Biochemical Pharmacology

The biochemical actions of the drug are not well understood. It may inhibit Na^+ uptake into cerebral tissue after electrical stimulation *in vivo* (Wallgren et al., 1947).

Pharmacodynamics

These have been reviewed by Lechat (1966). Chlormethiazole is an anticonvulsant, antagonising experimental seizures induced by pentylenetetrazole, bemegride, isoniazid and electro-shock. It does not antagonise strychnine seizures. It is also a sedative and hypnotic. The drug inhibits the medullary vegetative centres and blocks polysynaptic reflexes in the spinal cord.

Pharmacokinetics

Absorption and bioavailability: Chlormethiazole is said to be rapidly and completely absorbed from the alimentary tract in experimental animals. The calculations of Moore et al. (1975a) suggest that because of first-pass metabolism the drug has a 15% systemic availability after oral administration.

Distribution: The apparent volume of distribution of chlormethiazole in man averages 5.4L/kg, suggesting considerable tissue binding (Moore et al., 1975a). Some 63% of the drug in plasma is protein bound.

Elimination: After intravenous injection the terminal half-life (β phase) of chlormethiazole is 4.05 ± 0.60h. Less than 5% of the dose is excreted unchanged in urine

(Moore et al., 1975a). The plasma clearance of the drug is relatively high, being 22.97 ± 4.07ml/min/kg (Moore et al., 1975a). This suggests rapid and extensive hepatic metabolism of the drug (hepatic blood flow averages 24.3mls/min/kg). The suggested metabolic pathways for the drug are shown in figure 6.14 (Moore et al., 1975b). In addition, 4-methyl-5-thiazoleacetaldehyde may be a metabolite. However, even when these metabolites were measured in urine the fate of over 80% of a chlormethiazole dose was not accounted for.

Plasma level correlations: Few data are available. When the drug is used intravenously to treat status epilepticus, the therapeutic effect probably occurs while the distributional phase is still going on.

Interactions

Chlormethiazole might be expected to enhance the effects of other sedatives taken concurrently. Little is recorded about interactions of the drug.

Toxicity

Idiosyncratic Toxicity

Urticaria and erythema occur rarely (Sattes, 1966).

Dose-related Toxicity

Side effects are reviewed by Svedin (1966). Tingling in the nose and sneezing occur frequently and may start very soon after intravenous administration begins. Conjunctival injection and bronchorrhoea may occur. The drug is a hypnotic and produces drowsiness, dysarthria, nystagmus and hiccup. Given intravenously, the drug is said to produce tachycardia without blood pressure or cardiac output change. With intravenous use of solutions more concentrated than 0.8% there is some risk of haemolysis. Despite its structural resemblances to part of the molecule of thiamine, chlormethiazole will not correct manifestations of thiamine deficiency.

The drug has a potential for producing dependence (Lundquist, 1966).

Dysmorphogenicity

Chlormethiazole does not appear to cause fetal abnormalities in experimental animals (Lechat, 1966).

The Treatment of Epilepsy

Some General Principles

Patients with epilepsy usually present to the neurologist after they have had one or more episodes of disturbed cerebral function. The neurologist should first decide

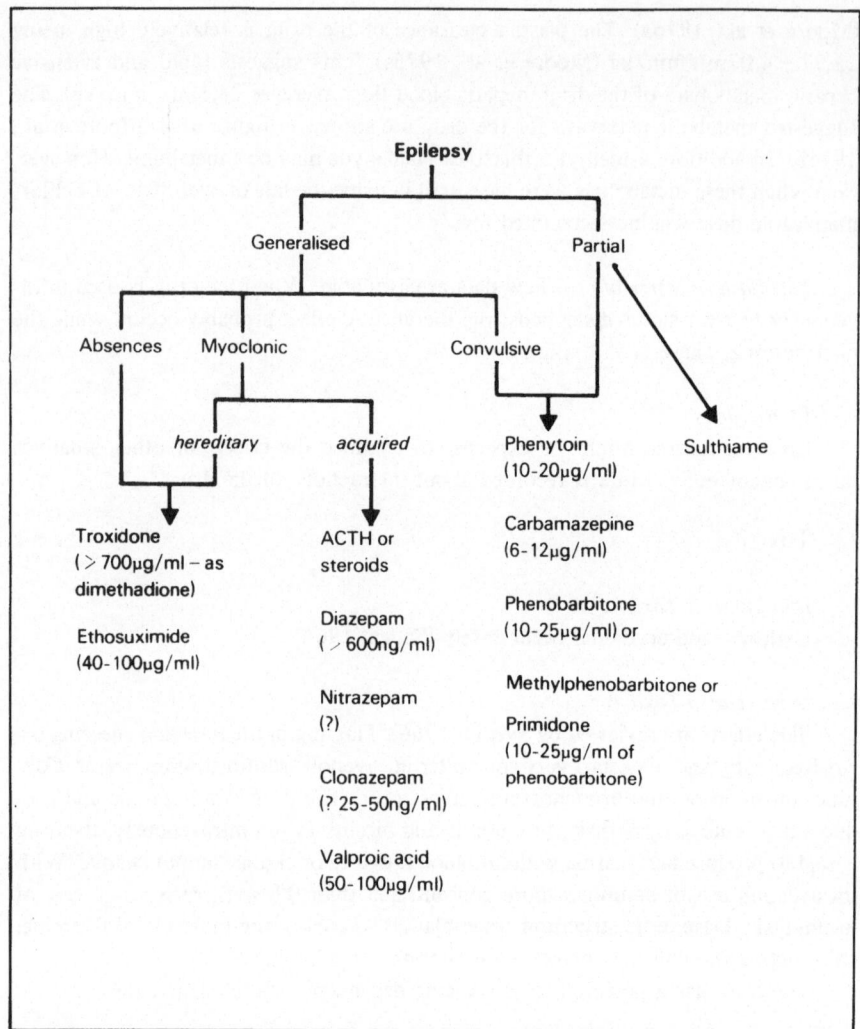

Fig. 6.15. Therapeutic plasma drug level ranges for the principal anticonvulsants used in the various types of epilepsy.

whether these episodes are epileptic. If the episodes are epileptic, he should then try to determine their cause, as they may be due to some disorder requiring treatment in its own right e.g. cerebral tumour, hypocalcaemia, hypoglycaemia. If there is no causative factor which, if corrected, will remove the risk of further epileptic attacks, the neurologist should then consider the question of prevention. Occasionally he may assess the risk of further seizures as too low to warrant preventative treatment. Very much more often he is likely to consider that prevention is indicated. The aim of therapy is to prevent all further seizures, however minor, for so long a time that the affected neurones lose their potential for producing epileptic discharges. Generally this seems to require 3 to 4 years of complete freedom from all traces of epilepsy. Where possible, the clinical evidence of this complete suppression of epilepsy should be confirmed by the clearing of epileptiform activity from the patient's EEG. The drugs used in preventing a patient's epilepsy are determined by his type (or types) of seizure. The appropriate drug (or drugs) should be prescribed in sufficient dose to suppress all traces of epilepsy, if such dosage can be tolerated. If maximum tolerated doses of an anticonvulsant drug have not completely suppressed the epilepsy a second appropriate anticonvulsant (or even a third) should be added. The neurologist should seek the best compromise he can find between reduction of epilepsy and disability from drug side effects. In these circumstances there is little prospect that the patient's epilepsy will be cured and the aim of treatment has become minimisation of disability.

When a patient has frequent seizures it is relatively easy to know when drug therapy has suppressed these seizures. However, many patients have seizures only at long and irregular intervals. In such cases it may take many months, or years, to find the correct drug dose which achieves complete suppression of epilepsy, if dosage adjustments are made purely on a basis of failure of clinical response. In these circumstances, adjustment of drug dosages to achieve plasma drug concentrations in the therapeutic ranges for the drugs can save considerable time and disappointment. The therapeutic ranges for the various anticonvulsants in common use, correlated with the types of epilepsy for which particular drugs usually are of greatest value, are set out in figure 6.15. In this figure the individual drugs and their therapeutic ranges are placed in columns underneath the types of epilepsy for which the drugs are most useful. As one moves down the columns the anticonvulsants come to have an increasingly broad spectrum of action (though they do not necessarily increase in efficacy). Thus ethosuximide is sometimes useful in myoclonic epilepsy, as are phenobarbitone and its congeners, while clonazepam and valproate appear fairly broad spectrum anticonvulsants.

Prevention of Specific Types of Epilepsy

Absences (Petit Mal)

Absences are nearly always frequent, usually occurring several or more times daily. It is easy thus to assess the response to therapy clinically. In recent times the drug of choice has been ethosuximide. The anticonvulsant effect correlates with the plasma level of the drug (therapeutic range 40 to 100µg/ml). The relatively long half-life of ethosuximide (30 hours in children) suggests the drug could be given once daily to maintain therapeutic plasma levels within reasonable limits across the dosage interval.

However the usual daily dose is large (often 3 to 6 capsules, each of 250mg) therefore the drug may be more conveniently given twice daily. There will then be less fluctuation in plasma drug level. Initial ethosuximide dosage for small children is about 250mg twice daily, and for older children 750mg daily. Steady-state conditions (and maximum pharmacological effects from the dose) might be expected to apply in children about 1 week from the last dosage change. Therefore dosages may be changed as often as weekly in children (possibly about fortnightly in adults, in whom ethosuximide elimination is slower), if a satisfactory therapeutic response has not been achieved. The dose may be increased as necessary till absences cease, or until troublesome side effects supervene. In absence epilepsy, plasma ethosuximide measurements often serve simply as an indication of the drug concentration in the individual at which suppression of epilepsy occurs. This knowledge can be useful if the epilepsy subsequently escapes from control. Patients may tolerate plasma ethosuximide levels well above 100µg/ml and obtain improved control of epilepsy. Available data suggest that plasma ethosuximide levels rise with disproportionate rapidity as the dose increases, at least in patients taking ethosuximide with phenytoin (Eadie, 1976). This should be borne in mind if ethosuximide doses are adjusted on a basis of plasma level measurements.

There is a significant risk that children with absence seizures will develop tonic-clonic fits as time passes. Some believe that this risk is increased by treating with ethosuximide (or troxidone) alone, and that an anticonvulsant for major seizures should be given concurrently with ethosuximide from the outset. This is the authors' practice. Phenytoin, phenobarbitone or a congener, or carbamazepine may be used and prescribed for a few days before ethosuximide therapy is begun. Appropriate dosage of these major anticonvulsants is considered later. Increase in phenytoin dose appears to increase plasma ethosuximide levels, and *vice versa*.

Serious side effects from ethosuximide are uncommon. In the past these might have made its replacement with troxidone necessary, though in general troxidone is a more toxic drug than ethosuximide. Now clonazepam, or valproate, should be used if ethosuximide fails, or cannot be tolerated. The use of these drugs is considered in relation to myoclonic epilepsy (p.219). As clonazepam and valproate seem to protect against major fits, it may not be necessary to use a second anticonvulsant to prevent major epilepsy if clonazepam or valproate is used for absences.

Ethosuximide therapy is ordinarily continued till the patient has had no attacks for 4 years, or till he or she is about 14 years of age, whichever is the later. By this time many patients lose their tendency to have absences. However, the anticonvulsant for major seizures might need to be continued for several years after ethosuximide is withdrawn.

Myoclonic Epilepsy

Infancy: In infancy myoclonic seizures are associated with the EEG appearance of hypsarrhythmia (West's syndrome). In rare instances this is due to pyridoxine deficiency and it may be wise to prescribe oral pyridoxine (e.g. 25 to 50mg 3 times a day) in all cases without waiting for formal confirmation of the aetiological diagnosis. Hypsarrhythmia is associated with progressive mental retardation. The associated myoclonic seizures may be prevented in some cases by clonazepam, or valproate, but these drugs are said not to influence the mental retardation. However in about 50 % of cases corticotrophin or a corticosteroid stops the seizures and also prevents the mental retardation. Therefore these agents are the drugs of choice in hypsarrhythmia and the benzodiazepines or valproate are used for symptomatic relief of the epilepsy if the corticosteroids fail. The doses used are 20 to 40 units of ACTH gel (or 0.5 to 1.0mg tetracosactrin) by injection once daily, or 20 to 40mg prednisone orally in divided doses each day. De Negri and Lamedica (1973) have stated that enough corticotrophin or tetracosactrin should be given in the treatment of hypsarrhythmia to raise plasma cortisol levels above 40µg/100mls. Treatment should continue till 1 week or so after all seizures stop and after the EEG reverts to normal. Higher doses may be used if benefit does not occur after 2 weeks of therapy with the doses suggested above. If steroid therapy fails after 6 weeks of use in high dosage the prognosis is very poor indeed. Even if the hypsarrhythmia ceases with treatment there is still a risk that other patterns of epilepsy will appear later in life.

Childhood: Myoclonic epilepsy in childhood is often a severe disorder with recurrent, sometimes violent, myoclonic jerks which become a major handicap to the sufferer (Lennox-Gastaut syndrome). It often does not respond well to therapy. The most effective agents are clonazepam and valproic acid. Clonazepam, with a half-life of about 24 hours, should need to be taken only twice a day to maintain reasonably constant plasma levels. Its therapeutic range is not well established and, if doses are increased gradually, patients may tolerate plasma clonazepam levels well above the upper limit of the proposed therapeutic range of 25 to 50µg/ml. If the drug is introduced gradually, with dose increments at weekly intervals (to allow time for a steady-state and maximum potential benefit to be attained between increments) the incidence and severity of side effects such as drowsiness and unsteadiness appear to be lessened. The suggested initial clonazepam dose in a child is 1mg orally twice daily, with 1mg dose increments each week till side effects supervene, or the seizures stop. The upper limit for the therapeutic dose is not known and plasma drug levels seem to increase in direct proportion to the dose.

Overall, valproic acid is probably as useful as clonazepam in childhood myoclonic epilepsy; side effects are usually not severe. The drug has a relatively short half-life (8 to 10 hours) so that steady-state conditions should prevail after 2 or 3 days, and doses may be increased twice weekly. To avoid excessive fluctuations in plasma levels over a dosage interval, valproate needs to be given 3 times a day. There may be an advantage in taking valproate after meals; in this circumstance slowed gastric emptying would prolong the absorption phase, which could allow steady-state valproate levels to vary less widely across the 8 to 10 hour dosage interval. The initial valproate dose for the average child is 100 to 200mg 3 times a day, with twice weekly dose increments as necessary to control seizures. Once plasma valproate levels exceed 100μg/ml side effects may become troublesome and there is a possibility of clinically significant disturbance of platelet function. Valproate interacts with phenobarbitone to raise plasma levels of the latter.

If clonazepam and valproate are unavailable, or unsuitable, an alternative is nitrazepam, beginning with 2.5mg twice daily. Dose increments of this drug are made at the same intervals as for the other benzodiazepine, clonazepam, and the dose is increased till epilepsy is controlled or till side effects preclude any further increase. Other therapeutic possibilities are to use one of the barbiturate anticonvulsants, or carbamazepine, and there have been occasional reports that sulthiame is useful in myoclonic epilepsy (Lerman and Nussbaum, 1975). It may also be worth using ethosuximide, if necessary in maximum tolerated doses. If the Lennox-Gastaut syndrome can be fully controlled, therapy should be continued for at least 4 years before a reduction in dosage is contemplated.

Adolescence and adult life: Myoclonic epilepsy in adolescents and adults, unless due to a progressive cerebral degeneration (e.g. Lafora body disease), is often a more benign condition than myoclonic epilepsy in earlier life. It usually responds well to barbiturate anticonvulsants (dosage of which is discussed later) and may generally be cured by several years' full suppression of seizures. The various benzodiazepines, or valproate, are likely to be effective if the barbiturates fail, or cannot be tolerated.

All Other Types of Epilepsy

This section includes generalised epilepsy producing convulsive fits (tonic, clonic or tonic-clonic) and all varieties of partial epilepsy, with or without subsequent generalisation.

All these types of epilepsy are best treated with phenytoin, or carbamazepine, or the barbiturate anticonvulsants (phenobarbitone, methylphenobarbitone or primidone), alone or in combination. Sulthiame may be of use for partial seizures and clonazepam and valproate appear useful for all these types of epilepsy though neither drug has yet been available long enough to find its definitive place. In the types of epilepsy being discussed here, seizures often occur at infrequent and irregular intervals and it is in these circumstances that measurement of plasma anticonvulsant levels has its greatest advantage in managing patients.

Phenytoin: The average oral phenytoin dose required to achieve the therapeutic range of plasma drug levels (10 to 20μg/ml) is 5mg/kg/day for adults and about twice this amount for children. To avoid overdosing a minority of patients it is wise to use rather lower doses initially and to increase the dose as necessary, guided by plasma phenytoin level estimation after the steady-state has been reached. A new steady-state takes about 4 or 5 days to develop after a phenytoin dose change. The relatively slow absorption of phenytoin after oral administration, and its relatively slow elimination, mean that the drug needs to be given only once daily to maintain virtually constant plasma drug levels. However, the drug is often given twice daily. If dose increments are necessary, the non-linear relation between plasma phenytoin level and phenytoin dose in the individual should be borne in mind to reduce the risk of overdosage. A family of curves (Eadie and Tyrer, 1980) and a nomogram (Richens, 1975 — corrected version) are available to assist in dosage adjustment. If plasma phenytoin levels in the therapeutic range fail to control a patient's epilepsy, drug dosage may be increased slightly to increase the plasma phenytoin level in the hope that this will control the epilepsy. In doing this one should realise that phenytoin toxicity does not always produce a typical picture of ataxia, nystagmus, double vision, nausea and vomiting, and that many manifestations of physical or mental ill-health may be due to the drug. Hence vague symptoms occurring at plasma phenytoin levels above 20µg/ml may be due to the drug and the presence of such symptoms suggests the need for assessing the effect of dose reduction.

Carbamazepine: There is relatively little correlation between plasma carbamazepine levels and drug dose in the treated population. In practice, in patients not receiving other anticonvulsants, oral carbamazepine doses of 100mg twice daily for young children, 100 to 200mg twice daily for older children and 200 or 300mg twice daily for adults are likely to produce plasma carbamazepine levels in the therapeutic range of 6 to 12µg/ml. Plasma drug levels should remain fairly constant if the drug is given twice daily as it is slowly absorbed and its half-life is over 24 hours. After dosage change the new steady-state is likely to take about a week to develop. Therefore it is preferable not to change carbamazepine dosage more frequently than once a week. If carbamazepine doses are built up at weekly intervals the major side effect of the drug, drowsiness, is not likely to be troublesome. Patients can often tolerate plasma carbamazepine levels well above 12µg/ml if the drug dose has been increased gradually.

Barbiturates: Of the three barbiturate anticonvulsants, the authors' preference is for methylphenobarbitone. It could be argued that phenobarbitone itself would be the simplest of these three drugs to use, because with methylphenobarbitone one has to consider an active metabolite (phenobarbitone) as well, and with primidone two active metabolites. In the authors' view the disadvantage of the more complex pharmacokinetic situation in the case of methylphenobarbitone is more than counterbalanced by the greater ease in manipulating plasma levels of the derived phenobarbitone, as compared with the situation when phenobarbitone itself is prescribed (p.190). However, choice between the three drugs in many instances is probably determined by personal preference. The three drugs are probably fairly nearly equivalent in effect if given in doses which produce the same plasma phenobarbitone level. Since phenobarbitone is eliminated slowly (half-life 4 days in adults and about 2 days in children) a once daily dosage regimen would suffice for all three drugs if plasma phenobarbitone levels were the only consideration. However for primidone (half-life less than 12 hours), though not for methylphenobarbitone (half-life about 30 hours), elimination of the parent drug is fast enough to permit appreciable change in plasma drug levels and the occurrence of a temporary soporific effect during each dosage interval. Therefore twice daily dosage, with reduced peak levels of unmetabolised drug, may be desirable for primidone and no disadvantage for its congeners. The average oral phenobarbitone dose to produce a steady-state 'therapeutic' plasma level of 15μg/ml is 1.75mg/kg/day, for methylphenobarbitone 2.75mg/kg/day and for primidone 7.75mg/kg/day. The required dose is higher in young children and lower in the aged, at least for phenobarbitone and methylphenobarbitone. Bearing these relationships in mind one aims to give a 70kg adult 90 or 100mg of phenobarbitone daily, or 180mg of methylphenobarbitone or 500mg of primidone. Because full doses of barbiturate anticonvulsants often make patients drowsy at first, unless one is in a hurry to obtain a full therapeutic effect it may be better to prescribe half the calculated dose for a week, three quarters of the dose in the second week, and the full dose thereafter. Since it takes about 5 times the half-life of a drug for a steady-state to be reached (i.e. $4 \times 5 = 20$ days in the case of phenobarbitone) it will require some 3 weeks from the beginning of therapy before meaningful steady-state plasma phenobarbitone levels can be obtained, whichever barbiturate anticonvulsant is given. If these levels are not satisfactory i.e. not in the therapeutic range, or if epilepsy continues, dosage should be increased unless side effects preclude this. In increasing the dose it should be remembered that plasma phenobarbitone levels (at least up to 40μg/ml) will rise in direct proportion to the dose if methylphenobarbitone is used, but will rise more rapidly than this if phenobarbitone itself is used. The effect on plasma phenobarbitone level of changing the drug dose should be checked no sooner than 3 weeks after the dosage change.

Sulthiame: Little pharmacokinetic information is available regarding sulthiame. If it is decided to use this drug an adult may be given 200mg twice daily and, if there are no unacceptable side effects (mostly paraesthesiae and hyperventilation) doses may be increased every few weeks as necessary to control epilepsy. Children should be given lower initial doses e.g. 50mg twice daily for a 1 or 2 year old and 100mg twice daily for an older child.

The use of clonazepam and valproic acid has been discussed earlier.

If the forms of epilepsy under discussion can be completely controlled by treatment, full doses of therapy are continued for 3 or 4 years. A decision about discontinuing treatment is then taken. If the epilepsy cannot be controlled by maximum tolerated doses of appropriate drugs (or drug combinations) all that can be done is to control the epilepsy as well as possible with drug doses that do not distress the patient more than his epilepsy does.

Anticonvulsant Combinations

Combinations of anticonvulsants are used:

1) When the patient has more than one type of epilepsy and each type of epilepsy is best treated by a different drug. Thus the combination of petit mal absences and major tonic-clonic fits is often treated with ethosuximide and phenytoin.

2) When maximum tolerated doses of one anticonvulsant have partly suppressed, but not completely controlled, a patient's epilepsy. Here a second appropriate anticonvulsant should be added to the first.

In combining anticonvulsants it is irrational to combine phenobarbitone, methylphenobarbitone or primidone. In the body the latter two drugs yield phenobarbitone and maximum tolerated concentrations of this should have already been achieved from the first drug used. When two drugs are combined there is the possibility of pharmacokinetic interactions between the drugs. The better known of these have been listed when the individual drugs were considered earlier in this chapter, and such interactions should be anticipated when the relevant drugs are combined. Whenever one anticonvulsant is added to another the plasma levels of both drugs should be measured once enough time has passed for new steady-state conditions to apply. It may be necessary to adjust the doses of one or both drugs in order to obtain the maximum benefit from the combination.

Sometimes it becomes necessary to combine three or more anticonvulsants.

Problems of Long Term Anticonvulsant Therapy

Many anticonvulsant side effects, particularly the idiosyncratic ones, arise soon after the drugs are introduced in a patient. However, there may be delayed toxic effects. These include evidence of folate deficiency (p.395), including megaloblastic anaemia, vitamin D deficiency with hypocalcaemia, intellectual dulling and, in the case of phenytoin, immunological abnormalities and possibly pseudolymphomatous change. For reasons which are not always clear, anticonvulsant dosage requirements (as indicated by plasma drug levels) may change over months or years and necessitate dosage change.

Loading Doses of Anticonvulsants

Several anticonvulsants (e.g. phenytoin, diazepam) are absorbed slowly and inefficiently if given by intramuscular injection and others are not available as parenteral preparations (e.g. carbamazepine, primidone, ethosuximide). If a therapeutic anticonvulsant level is desired within 24 hours of beginning therapy, and intravenous administration of drugs is not judged necessary, an oral loading dose of twice the expected daily maintenance dose may be given for many of the anticonvulsants. This loading dose may with advantage be divided into 2 to 4 parts given at half-hourly to hourly intervals. This reduces the chance of too large a single dose irritating the stomach and causing vomiting, which would make the amount of drug absorbed uncertain. After the loading dose, the ordinary twice daily maintenance doses of the

drug are given regularly. Such a regimen offers a good chance of producing therapeutic plasma levels within the second 24 hours of dosage and the risks of later overdosage are low.

Inability to Take Anticonvulsants Orally

If a patient becomes unable to swallow, his anticonvulsants must be given parenterally, or by duodenal tube. As pointed out above, parenteral preparations of some
drugs are not available and these must then be given by duodenal tube. For other anticonvulsants, such as phenytoin, the drug is absorbed so poorly from intramuscular
injection sites that it is necessary to increase the daily dose by 50 % to maintain
plasma levels. Phenobarbitone appears to be more efficiently absorbed from intramuscular injection sites. Diazepam (in solution) is the only anticonvulsant known to
be well absorbed from the rectum (Agurell et al., 1975).

Methods of coping with the problems produced by the inability to swallow anticonvulsants have not yet been well worked out but the comments above may serve as
some guide to dosage requirement till better information becomes available.

Epilepsy in the Neonate

As well as sometimes being due to intracranial haemorrhage and cerebral birth
trauma, epilepsy in the neonate is often produced by disorders which are uncommon
causes for epilepsy later in life. Such causes include meningitis, hypocalcaemia and
other electrolyte disturbances, and hypoglycaemia. After the possible occurrence of
these disorders is investigated in neonates with epilepsy and, if present, treated, it may
be necessary to give anticonvulsants. Not a great deal of work has been done on anticonvulsant dosage in relation to plasma levels of the drugs in neonates. However neonates eliminate many drugs more slowly than older children and proportionately
lower doses of phenytoin or phenobarbitone than in infants, even on a body weight
basis, may be needed. The treatment of neonatal seizures is discussed by Holden and
Freeman (1975).

Benign Febrile Convulsions of Infancy

Some 5 % of infants get febrile convulsions. The majority of these infants do not
suffer from epilepsy in later life. Therefore it can be argued that febrile convulsions
do not require treatment. However, it seems to be increasingly recognised that one
often cannot predict which infant with febrile convulsions will go on to subsequent
epilepsy till the event (usually a prolonged convulsion with consequent cerebral hy-

poxia) has occurred which may cause an enduring epileptic tendency. Therefore there is a growing body of opinion that anticonvulsant prophylaxis should be given against febrile convulsions once the first attack has occurred in a child, and that that therapy should continue till the child is about 4 years of age.

Phenytoin has been shown to be ineffective in preventing febrile convulsions, even when therapeutic plasma levels of the drug have been attained (Melchior et al., 1971). Phenobarbitone, in plasma levels above 15μg/ml, was effective in the studies of Faero et al. (1972) but was not statistically significantly better than placebo in the study of Heckmatt et al. (1976), though fewer patients receiving phenobarbitone had febrile convulsions than did the control group. However, Wolf (1977) showed that continuous phenobarbitone prophylaxis did provide significant protection against febrile seizures. Phenobarbitone, in regular daily doses producing plasma phenobarbitone levels above 15μg/ml appears the therapy of choice for preventing febrile convulsions. However there is little doubt that phenobarbitone can make some children extremely irritable or drowsy and inattentive. In such children it may be necessary to try carbamazepine, though this drug has not been shown to be efficacious in febrile convulsions. There is one report that valproate is effective in preventing febrile convulsions (Cavazzuti, 1975). The effectiveness of clonazepam in this disorder is not known.

Because febrile convulsions usually occur soon after the onset of fever there is no simple, safe and reliable method of achieving adequate plasma anticonvulsant concentrations quickly enough if the drugs are given only when fever occurs. Hence continuous anticonvulsant therapy is necessary to provide protection.

Epilepsy in Pregnancy

In Western society epilepsy during the child-bearing years is nearly always of a variety which requires phenytoin, carbamazepine or the barbiturate anticonvulsants for its treatment. Plasma levels of phenytoin and phenobarbitone tend to fall as pregnancy progresses (Lander et al., 1977), hence it is desirable to monitor plasma anticonvulsant levels frequently during the pregnancy and the puerperium. It is likely that anticonvulsant doses will have to be increased during pregnancy to maintain protection against epilepsy and then reduced again during the puerperium to avoid overdosage manifestations.

Whether the taking of anticonvulsants, or the presence of epilepsy, is dysmorphogenic may be argued (see p.178) but it seems generally agreed that the overall disadvantages of discontinuing anticonvulsants during pregnancy are greater than the consequences of possible fetal malformations.

Anticonvulsants given during pregnancy may cause a bleeding tendency in the neonate. This can be overcome by giving the mother vitamin K while she is in labour.

In general anticonvulsant concentrations in breast milk are such that unless the mother is substantially overdosed, drug intake from breast feeding is unlikely to significantly affect the baby's clinical condition.

Status Epilepticus

Generalised convulsive status epilepticus requires prompt treatment to maintain the patient's vital functions and to stop his seizures. While this treatment is being given the factors which caused the status epilepticus should be determined, in case some treatable primary cause is operating (e.g. hypoglycaemia, meningitis, cerebral tumour).

The care of the patient with status epilepticus involves maintenance of the airway and state of arterial oxygenation, provision of parenteral fluids, care of the bladder, protection against injury, and the treatment of any secondary infection (e.g. pneumonia).

For some years diazepam has been the drug of choice in treating status epilepticus. Diazepam is given intravenously, at the rate of 1 to 2mg per minute in an adult, up to a dose of perhaps 10mg. If the convulsing does not cease in 2 or 3 minutes, further diazepam is given till convulsing does stop, or until significant hypotension or respiratory depression occurs. Clonazepam, in initial doses about one-tenth to one-fifth of those used for diazepam, may also be used in treating status epilepticus. The effective dose in the individual has to be found by trial.

The most effective alternatives to these benzodiazepines appear to be chlormethiazole and amylobarbitone. Chlormethiazole is given in a 0.8% intravenous solution (in a drip) at the rate of 4ml per minute till convulsing stops or unwanted effects necessitate a reduced rate of administration. Amylobarbitone sodium in freshly prepared aqueous solution, is injected intravenously at the rate of 50mg per minute to an adult till convulsing stops, or respiration is depressed, or until 500mg has been given. Should the above measures fail, thiopentone anaesthesia may become necessary to stop the status epilepticus.

Once status epilepticus is controlled it is necessary to institute continued anticonvulsant therapy to prevent relapse. Of the above drugs used to treat status epilepticus, only clonazepam is regularly used as a maintenance anticonvulsant. For the adult patient further 1mg or 2mg intravenous doses of clonazepam 6-hourly may be required till the patient can swallow when oral clonazepam 2mg 3 or 4 times a day may be given. Clonazepam is a relatively untried maintenance anticonvulsant in these circumstances. Once status epilepticus is stopped one may prefer to give intravenous phenytoin in a dose of 10mg/kg over a few hours into the tubing of a drip. Thereafter the patient's therapy may be changed to oral phenytoin 5 to 6mg/kg/day once he can swallow (and so long as he is not already receiving phenytoin, when a lower dose will be required). Further anticonvulsant dosages should be determined by plasma drug levels and the patient's clinical state.

Syncope

Syncope is perhaps more the province of the cardiologist than of the neurologist. However the neurologist is so often called in to differentiate between syncope and epilepsy that he finds it necessary to have some knowledge of the management of syncope.

Disordered Mechanisms

Syncope occurs when there is insufficient perfusion of the brain with blood. This may occur because of:

1) Reduction in total blood volume, due to haemorrhage, dehydration etc.

2) Failure of a diseased heart to deliver sufficient blood to the brain, as in acute myocardial infarction, cardiac arrhythmia, aortic or pulmonary valve stenosis

3) Failure of a healthy heart to deliver sufficient blood to the brain because of defective reflex mechanisms governing arterial and venous blood pressures. The reflex mechanisms may be defective because of:

a) neurological lesions which interrupt central or peripheral sympathetic pathways e.g. severe spinal cord lesions, extensive peripheral neuritis, hereditary degeneration of autonomic pathways as in the Shy-Drager syndrome and olivo-ponto-cerebellar atrophy

b) functional disorders (e.g. postural, emotional, micturition, cough and carotid sinus syncope, and the use of antihypertensive drug therapy).

In particular patients, the various factors which can cause syncope may sometimes act in combination (e.g. patients taking too large a dose of antihypertensive drugs are more likely to faint when standing than when lying down).

Correction of Disordered Mechanisms

The management of syncope depends on correct diagnosis of the nature and cause of the symptom. The main differential diagnosis is from epilepsy. In this connection it should be realised that bilateral myoclonic jerking, and even fitting, may occur if the syncope leads to a sufficient degree of brain ischaemia. The risk of secondary ischaemic fitting is increased if the patient faints and remains in the upright position or is propped up before he recovers from his faint. Syncope may also have to be differentiated from drop attacks (due to myoclonic epilepsy, to vertebro-basilar artery insufficiency, to a loose odontoid peg or to cataplexy).

Diagnosis of the cause of syncope is important, as many of the causes are treatable. Thus in hypovolaemia plasma volume may be expanded by the administration of blood or fluid. Drugs and, in some circumstances surgery, may be used to correct cardiac disorders. In general there is no direct treatment available for those neurological lesions which interrupt sympathetic pathways. Measures are available to prevent certain of the functional disorders which cause syncope. The chances of postural syncope can be reduced by warning the sufferer to avoid standing too quickly and by training him to take other measures to augment venous return before standing. Explanation, and perhaps the use of tranquillisers, may help persons who faint at emotional stimuli (e.g. the sight of blood). Micturition syncope is unlikely to occur if the sufferer learns to urinate in the sitting position. The chances of cough syncope are lessened if the patient is instructed to avoid taking a series of coughs without a breath and if measures are taken to relieve the cause of the cough. Carotid sinus syncope may be prevented by avoiding anything that presses on the side of the neck (e.g. tight, stiff collars) and by inactivating carotid sinus reflexes pharmacologically (e.g. by atropine or by surgical denervation.

Particularly in emotional or postural syncope, but sometimes in syncope from other causes, attempts to relieve the cause of the disorder may fail to stop fainting attacks. If the attacks are frequent enough, or disabling enough, it may be necessary to consider treating the syncope symptomatically by attempting to raise blood pressure or augment venous return. Sympathomimetic agents may be used to raise arterial blood pressure, monoamine oxidase inhibitors may be employed to augment the effects of circulating catecholamines, fludrocortisone to retain enough salt to expand plasma volume, ergotamine or its congeners to promote venous contraction, and elastic stockings or similar devices to compress the venous circulation of the lower limbs, thus diminishing the blood volume of the venous system in the lower limbs.

Drugs Used in Treating Syncope

Most of the drugs used in treating syncope have already been discussed:

atropine p.104
ergotamine p.260
fludrocortisone p.33
levodopa p.87 and monoamine oxidase inhibitors p.270.

(This combination of levodopa and monoamine oxidase inhibitors is used to supply catecholamines, and to delay their catabolism, thus prolonging their actions).

The one group of drugs used in treating syncope which is not considered elsewhere is the sympathomimetic amines (particularly the α-adrenergic agonists). In practice these drugs are not particularly effective in preventing syncope, though they are sometimes used for long term treatment.

Of the sympathomimetics suitable for oral use, amphetamine and methylamphetamine are best avoided because of their potential for producing cerebral stimulation and drug dependence. Probably ephedrine is the sympathomimetic agent most often used to prevent syncope, though its efficacy is open to question.

Ephedrine has some central stimulating effects and peripherally is both an α- and a β-adrenergic agonist. The peripheral actions are partly due to direct receptor stimulation and partly to displacement of noradrenaline from axon terminals. Ephedrine raises blood pressure, by cardiac stimulation and, to some extent, peripheral vasoconstriction. It is a bronchodilator, and may produce some hyperglycaemia. The elimination of ephedrine varies with urine pH, some 88% of a dose being excreted unchanged in acid urine and less if urine is alkaline. With acid urine the half-life is 3.03 hours (Wilkinson and Beckett, 1968). Side effects include excessive central stimulation, insomnia and palpitations.

Treatment of Syncope

The possibilities for treating the cause of syncope have been outlined above and will not be considered further. In the majority of instances correction or avoidance of the factors which provoke syncope will provide sufficient relief of a tendency to syncope and drug therapy is then unnecessary. Where these measures fail, and episodes of fainting are troublesome enough, treatment with oral ephedrine 15mg 3 times a day may be tried. Higher doses may be used later, if necessary and if tolerated. Other measures have been suggested (e.g. the regular use of ergotamine, or the use of levodopa plus monoamine oxidase inhibitors) but one must be careful that the benefits of such therapy are not outweighed by drug side effects. A more acceptable alternative may be to use oral fludrocortisone in doses just below those which produce oedema, with the intention that the resultant fluid retention may raise blood pressure sufficiently to prevent fainting. A dose of 0.1 to 0.2mg per day might be needed. If these measures, singly and in combination, fail, the wearing of elastic stockings and elastic abdominal binders, or the wearing of so-called 'G' suits, may become necessary. The combination of fludrocortisone and levodopa (to provide a source of catecholamines) has been used to treat orthostatic hypotension in the Shy-Drager syndrome (Steiner et al., 1974). Kochar and Itskoritz (1978) found that indomethacin controlled postural hypotension in this disorder.

Chapter VII

Pain

Principal Disorders and Drugs Discussed

Pain in general
Aspirin
Paracetamol
Dextropropoxyphene
Pentazocine

Migraine
Ergotamine
Methysergide
Pizotifen, cyproheptadine, methdilazine
Clonidine

Cluster headache
Ergotamine

Contraction headache
Amitriptyline
Diazepam (see also chapter VI)

Trigeminal neuralgia
Anticonvulsants (see also chapter VI)

There are a number of pain syndromes (e.g. migraine, tic douloureux) customarily regarded as the special province of the neurologist. However, in clinical practice the neurologist may also be involved in the diagnosis and management of pain of uncertain origin and in the attempt to provide relief from intractable pain which is not due to primary neurological disease. Therefore the question of pain in general will be considered before primarily neurological pain disorders.

Disordered Mechanisms

The numerous disease processes which cause pain do so by activating somatic and/or visceral pain receptors or by activating the pain pathway itself. The first neurone in this pathway has its cell body in the dorsal root ganglion or an equivalent ganglion of a cranial nerve (e.g. the Gasserian ganglion). The thinly myelinated fibre of this neurone runs from the peripheral receptor to the dorsal horn of the spinal cord (or, for example, to the nucleus of the spinal tract of the trigeminal) where it synapses. The number and temporal pattern of impulses arriving in this region of the dorsal horn may determine whether the sensory input from pain receptors is experienced as pain (the 'gate-control' theory of pain of Melzack and Wall, 1965). The second neurone in the pain pathway extends from the synapse in the dorsal horn (or in the analogous cranial nerve nucleus) to the relevant sensory relay nucleus of the thalamus on the opposite side, running in the lateral spinothalamic tract (or the analogous pathway from a cranial nerve nucleus). The third sensory neurone with its cell body in the thalamus, projects to the post-Rolandic sensory cortex.

Correction of Disordered Mechanisms

Leaving aside the correction of the disease process responsible for pain, there are a number of possibilities for relieving pain by altering the function of the pain pathway. The biochemistry of the pain pathway and the synaptic transmitters involved in this pathway are little understood. Consequently the symptomatic chemical relief of pain is largely based on empirical data or on producing mechanical interference with the pain pathway.

First Sensory Neurone

In localised pain the entry of pain impulses into the spinal cord can be prevented by nerve root section at the appropriate level. Motor function is spared but all modalities of sensation are impaired. However the local deposition of neurotoxic chemicals (e.g. alcohol or phenol) via intrathecal injection, may tend to produce relatively selective damage to thinly myelinated pain fibres in dorsal roots, while sparing the thicker myelinated proprioceptive fibres. Neuropathological studies tend to show that the damage produced by these chemicals is not very selective (Berry and Olszewski, 1963).

A few peripheral spinal nerves have purely sensory functions (e.g. the saphenous). Such nerves can be sectioned to provide relief of local pain without producing weakness. Sympathetic or parasympathetic fibres from the viscera may be divided surgically to help relieve visceral pain, though some disturbance of visceral motor function may result.

Bombardment of the dorsal horn at the appropriate level with electrical impulses of certain frequencies and intensities may produce local pain relief by altering the 'gate-control' which determines the number of pain impulses which ascend in the second sensory neurone.

Second Sensory Neurone

Because pain impulses run in a discrete pathway in the spinal cord and brain stem, operations such as spinothalamic or quintothalamic tractotomy, or intra-medullary section of the pain pathway, can relieve pain in a limb, in one side of the body or the face, without greatly altering other modalities of sensation or motor function.

It is not clear whether the technique of spinal intrathecal irrigation with cold isotonic or hyperosmolar saline relieves intractable pain of, for example, terminal malignancy, by affecting the primary or secondary sensory neurones, or both (Savitz and Malis, 1973).

Third Sensory Neurone

Some analgesic drugs appear to act at a thalamic level. The third sensory neurone mediating pain can be interrupted in the thalamus by stereotaxic operations, relieving pain in the opposite side of the body.

It is also possible to alter the patient's reaction to pain, thereby lessening suffering, by altering the psychological reaction to pain. Thus sedative and psychotrophic drugs (e.g. phenothiazines) may be used. Prefrontal leucotomy, the operative procedure which disconnects the frontal lobes from the thalamus on each side, is still sometimes employed.

Drugs Used in Relieving Pain

Only a selection of the available analgesic drugs will be considered here. This selection covers most of the range of non-narcotic analgesic potency. It is hoped to provide a description of a sufficient number of drugs to meet the neurologist's therapeutic requirement.

Acetylsalicylic Acid (Aspirin)

Aspirin is extensively used as an analgesic for mild to moderate forms of somatic pain. It is also used for its antipyretic and anti-inflammatory effects, particularly in the treatment of rheumatic fever, rheumatoid disease and osteoarthritis. Recently there has been interest in using aspirin with the aim of preventing thrombotic arterial disease.

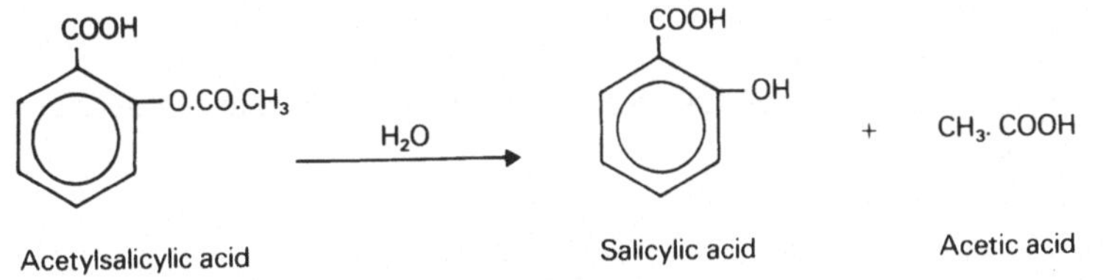

Fig. 7.1. Acetylsalicylic acid and the products of its hydrolysis.

Chemistry

Acetylsalicylic acid (aspirin) is the acetyl ester of salicylic acid. Its molecular weight is 180.15. In the presence of moisture aspirin may hydrolyse to salicylic and acetic acids (fig. 7.1). Aspirin is a rather weaker acid than salicylic acid (pKa values of 3.5 and 3.0 respectively).

Pharmacology

Biochemical Pharmacology
Aspirin has a number of known biochemical actions. It:

1) Inhibits prostaglandin synthesis (among their numerous actions prostaglandins increase local tissue sensitivity to mechanical and chemical pain-producing mechanisms)

2) Acetylates proteins when acetyl groups are freed after hydrolysis of aspirin. This is thought to be how aspirin decreases platelet adhesiveness (Mustard and Packham, 1973)

3) Blocks the enzymatic conversion of arachidonic acid to an as yet uncategorised labile substance which stimulates platelet aggregation (Willis, 1974)

4) Uncouples oxidative phosphorylation in mitochondria.

Pharmacodynamics
Aspirin has the following actions:

1) Analgesic: the drug has a central pain-relieving effect and may also produce analgesia by virtue of its anti-inflammatory properties

2) Antipyretic: it inhibits the synthesis of prostaglandin E, which acts on the hypothalamus to produce pyrexia

3) Anti-inflammatory

4) Uricosuric

5) Central nervous system stimulatory, then depressant. Thus it may cause:
   a) cochlear irritation
   b) irritation of the medullary chemoreceptor trigger zone, producing nausea and vomiting
   c) respiratory stimulation

6) Anti-thrombotic and platelet-inhibiting. Aspirin:
   a) inhibits the ADP release from platelets (this ADP release promotes platelet aggregation)
   b) diminishes platelet adhesiveness
   c) inhibits 5-hydroxytryptamine release from platelets (Zucker and Peterson, 1968)
   d) inhibits prostaglandin synthesis in platelets
   e) in high dose inhibits prothrombin formation

7) Gastric irritation, sometimes causing nausea and vomiting

8) Alteration of blood chemistry, due to a mixture of respiratory alkalosis from central respiratory stimulation and metabolic acidosis from uncoupling oxidative phosphorylation, particularly in muscle.

Pharmacokinetics

Absorption and bioavailability: Aspirin is usually given by mouth. Since it is an acid it tends to be in a relatively non-ionised state in the stomach, and some absorption may occur at gastric level. However the greater part of an aspirin dose appears to be absorbed from the small intestine rather than from the stomach. Seemingly the less favourable pH conditions of the small intestine (from the point of view of increased molecular ionisation and hence decreased absorption) are more than counterbalanced by the extent of the absorptive surface of the small intestine. Aspirin absorption from mixtures and tablets is reasonably rapid, peak plasma salicylate levels often occurring about 2 hours after dosage.

The absorption rate of aspirin varies with a number of factors which have been investigated experimentally e.g. tablet disintegration time, aspirin particle size, aggregation of aspirin after tablet disintegration, aspirin dissolution rate, gastric pH (and the influence of antacids) and rate of gastric emptying (Saunders, 1974). The most important of these factors appears to be rate of solution of the aspirin. Antacids facilitate the absorption of aspirin from tablets by causing more rapid solution of drug in a less acid aqueous environment. This more than offsets the higher degree of ionisation and hence lessened absorption rate of the drug relative to the total amount of aspirin in solution. However, if aspirin is given already in solution, antacids decrease its rate of absorption because they then decrease the fraction of the dose that is non-ionised (Saunders, 1974). If aspirin is given by mouth, and a rapid effect is desired, there may be advantages in using one of the rapidly dissolving types of buffered aspirin tablet and dissolving it in water prior to intake.

Aspirin is a local gastric irritant and to avoid this effect enteric-coated preparations have been developed. Some of these (Day et al., 1976) have been shown to provide the drug in an almost completely bioavailable form. Aspirin in enteric-coated preparations may be at times unsuitable for the relief of acute pain because of slowed absorption of the drug. However for continued use the enteric-coated preparations should provide a satisfactory means of consistent aspirin intake.

Suppositories containing aspirin have been used rectally to obviate the local gastric irritant effects of the drug. The bioavailability of aspirin from even the best of these suppositories is comparatively poor (Gibaldi and Grundhofer, 1975).

Distribution: Because of the rapid hydrolysis of aspirin in the body it is more relevant to consider the distribution of the derived salicylate.

The V_D of salicylate is 0.10 to 0.18L/kg, suggesting that the substance is distributed throughout extracellular water. Albumin binds 50 to 90% of the salicylate present in plasma. The percentage of salicylate bound to plasma protein decreases as plasma salicylate level increases (Davison and Smith, 1961). Salicylate competes for albumin binding sites with a number of anionic drugs (e.g. phenytoin, phenylbutazone, warfarin, penicillin, thiopentone) and also with thyroxine and bilirubin. Exposure to aspirin causes acetylation and permanent alteration of human serum albumin. Salicylate can be found in synovial, cerebrospinal and peritoneal fluid, in milk and in saliva (where its level is about 3% of that of plasma, according to Graham and Rowland, 1972).

Salicylate, like certain other anions, is actively transported out of CSF by an enzymatic mechanism in the cells of the choroid plexus. Salicylate concentrations in cat brain are increased by exposure of the animals to 25% CO_2 gas (Goldberg et al. 1961).

Elimination: Acetylsalicylic acid is thought to undergo rapid hydrolysis in man, the reaction being catalysed by esterases in the intestinal wall and liver. The plasma half-life of aspirin in man is 13 to 20 minutes (Rowland et al., 1972). The resulting salicylic acid has a dose-dependent half-life, ranging in the same subjects from 2.9 hours at low doses to 22 hours at high salicylate levels (Levy, 1965). The biotransformation pathway is shown in figure 7.2. These metabolic reactions occur in many tissues but principally in the liver. The biotransformations of salicylic acid to salicyluric acid and salicyl phenolic glucuronide are capacity-limited under conditions of therapeutic aspirin dosage. The remaining elimination pathways for renal excretion of salicylacyl glucuronide and unchanged salicylic acid are not saturable under these conditions and follow first order kinetics. (The formation of the various hydroxy-acids accounts for very little salicylate elimination). Thus the elimination of both acetylsalicylic acid and salicylic acid involves two processes which follow

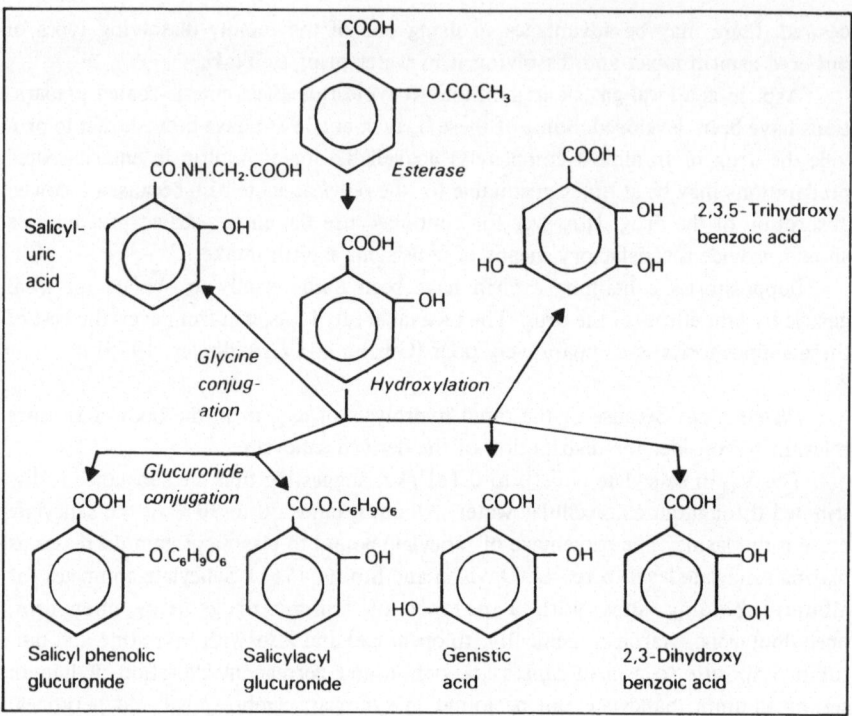

Fig. 7.2. The biotransformation of aspirin.

Michaelis-Menten kinetics and other simultaneous processes which follow first order kinetics. This explains the overall dose-dependent kinetics of the drug (Levy and Tsuchiya, 1976; Levy et al., 1972).

In man, about 14 % of a dose of salicylic acid is excreted unchanged in urine and 75 % appears as salicyluric acid, 10 % as the phenolic glucuronide and 5 % as the acyl glucuronides. However, these proportions alter with drug dose, as explained above. Further, alkalinisation of urine increases salicylate excretion by increasing the ionisation of salicylic acid and salicyluric acids in the distal renal tubules, hence reducing the back diffusion of these substances from urine. In alkaline urine a substantial amount of a salicylate dose may be excreted unchanged. The glucuronide conjugates are actively secreted into the proximal renal tubular lumen and are too water soluble for much back diffusion to occur. Overall, renal excretion of salicylate and its products is facilitated by a high urine volume and alkalinisation of urine.

Plasma level correlations: Plasma salicylate levels over 270μg/ml are likely to be associated with nausea and vomiting. There is said to be no correlation between plasma salicylate level and analgesic effect (Smith and Smith, 1966).

Interactions

Pharmacodynamic interactions: Aspirin and other salicylates are involved in certain interactions which may cause bleeding. Thus intake of alcohol can increase gastrointestinal blood loss due to aspirin. It appears likely that only direct local effects on the gastric mucosa are involved in such instances. Aspirin may increase the anticoagulant effect of warfarin by further depressing prothrombin levels. Aspirin also increases bleeding time, increasing the risk of iatrogenic haemorrhage. (In addition there is the at least theoretical possibility that aspirin may be involved in a pharmacokinetic type of interaction with warfarin, displacing the latter from protein binding sites and increasing its biological effect). Aspirin may also increase the overall anticoagulant effect if given together with heparin.

Pharmacokinetic interactions: Aspirin, and more particularly salicylate, may compete with other anions for plasma protein and perhaps tissue protein binding sites. Anionic drugs which may have their plasma water levels, and thus their biological actions, altered by such a mechanism include penicillin, warfarin, phenytoin, phenylbutazone, chlorpropamide, tolbutamide and methotrexate. The clinical importance of some of these interactions is open to doubt. Even when definite interactions between aspirin and the other drugs occur, other mechanisms may be involved (e.g. in the increased antidiabetic effect of the chlorpropamide-aspirin combination). The interaction between salicylates and methotrexate, increasing the actions of the latter, appears to involve both displacement of methotrexate from plasma protein binding sites and inhibited renal tubular secretion of methotrexate.

Salicylates are involved in interactions at the proximal renal tubular excretory mechanism for organic anions. Here salicylates inhibit the uricosuric actions of sulphinpyrazone and have their own uricosuric effects impaired by phenylbutazone.

Para-aminobenzoic acid is known to inhibit the biotransformation of salicylate to salicyluric acid but this interaction does not appear to be clinically significant.

Antacid intake may alter the rate of aspirin absorption, as indicated above. Urine pH and urine volume may influence the rate of salicylate excretion. Plasma salicylate levels may be changed by these factors.

It is known that concurrent corticosteroid administration depresses plasma salicylate levels, but the mechanisms involved are uncertain. The mechanism whereby salicylates reverse the Na^+ loss produced by spironolactone also is unknown.

Toxicity

Idiosyncratic Toxicity

Hypersensitivity to aspirin occurs occasionally. It may cause acute angioneurotic oedema (often of the face, mouth and alimentary tract), bronchospasm, and laryngeal swelling. Skin rashes may occur. Cross hypersensitivity to indomethacin may occur, but cross hypersensitivity between aspirin and other salicylates is not common.

Dose-related Toxicity
The following are among the recorded toxic effects of aspirin:

1) Local gastrointestinal irritation and bleeding
2) A bleeding tendency
3) 'Salicylism', with headache, dizziness, tinnitus, deafness, dim vision, confusion, drowsiness, sweating, hyperventilation. At higher plasma salicylate levels more severe mental disturbance may occur and electrolyte disturbance from respiratory alkalosis with later an added metabolic acidosis
4) Analgesic nephropathy — the extent to which aspirin is responsible for this syndrome is arguable.

Dysmorphogenicity
High doses of salicylates are dysmorphogenic in rats and mice. Tuchmann-Duplessis (1975) regards as unresolved the question as to whether therapeutic doses of salicylates cause fetal abnormalities in man and advises caution in prescribing salicylates for pregnant women.

Paracetamol

Paracetamol (acetaminophen) is widely used as a mild analgesic with antipyretic properties. Its analgesic potency is roughly equivalent to that of aspirin, though it lacks some of aspirin's therapeutic properties and some of its side effects.

Chemistry

N-acetyl-p-aminophenol (paracetamol; acetaminophen) has a molecular weight of 151.16. It is a neutral compound, unlike aspirin, and is a de-ethylated derivate of phenacetin.

Pharmacology

Biochemical Pharmacology
Paracetamol is an inhibitor of prostaglandin synthesis.

Pharmacodynamics

Paracetamol relieves pain of mild to moderate severity. Its site of analgesic effect is uncertain. It has an antipyretic effect by blocking the action of pyrogens on the hypothalamus.

Pharmacokinetics

Absorption and bioavailability: The absorption of paracetamol is rapid and reasonably complete after oral administration. Peak plasma levels occur 0.5 to 1 hour after dosage. McGilveray and Mattock (1972) calculated an absorption rate constant of 5.6/hour for fasting subjects. The absorption rate was slowed if the drug was taken with meals, particularly high carbohydrate meals, but absorption remained essentially complete. However Rawlins et al. (1977) found the bioavailability ranged between 63% for a dose of 500mg, and 89% for a dose of 1000mg.

Distribution: The drug is said to have a fairly uniform distribution through the various body fluids. Its volume of distribution is 1.03L/kg, a high enough value to suggest a selective accumulation in some tissues.

Rawlins et al. (1977) interpreted the distribution of paracetamol as involving an inner compartment with an apparent volume of 0.6L/kg and an outer compartment with an apparent volume of 0.35L/kg. At toxic concentrations 20 to 50% of the drug in plasma is protein-bound.

Elimination: According to Rawlins et al. (1977) the plasma half-life of paracetamol lies in the range 2.24 to 3.0 hours (2.0 ± 0.1 hour — Prescott et al., 1971). The former authors calculated that the clearance was 352 ± 40ml per minute. Paracetamol overdosage often causes liver damage. In this case the half-life tends to be prolonged to greater than 4 hours (Prescott et al., 1971).

About 2% of a paracetamol dose is excreted unchanged in urine (Albert et al., 1974). About 80% is excreted as conjugates (mainly the glucuronide, but also the sulphate and a cysteine conjugate). Hydroxylated and deacetylated metabolites have been detected. Some of the hydroxylated metabolites are hepatotoxic. The analgesic salicylamide competitively inhibits the biotransformation of paracetamol to its glucuronide and sulphate derivatives.

Plasma level correlations: The maximum analgesic effect of paracetamol occurs some 2.5 hours after dosage, which is rather later than the usual time of maximum plasma level. Nelson and Morioka (1963) found that the course of the analgesic effect of the drug did not correlate well with the course of its plasma level. Plasma paracetamol levels in excess of 300µg/ml 4 hours after dosage are associated with a high risk of liver damage (Prescott et al., 1971; James et al., 1975).

Interactions

Pharmacodynamic interactions: Paracetamol may slightly increase the anti-coagulant effect of warfarin. The mechanism involved is uncertain.

Pharmacokinetic interactions: Paracetamol does not appear to produce a clinically significant induction of the hepatic microsomal enzyme system.

Toxicity

Idiosyncratic Toxicity

Occasional skin rashes and other allergic reactions have occurred. Rarely, depression of leucocytes and drug fever have been recorded.

Dose-related Toxicity

Hepatic necrosis from paracetamol overdosage, or suicide attempt, is becoming an increasing problem. A single dose of 10 to 15g may be hepatotoxic and a dose of 25g potentially fatal. The onset of symptoms may be delayed for some hours and manifestations of progressing liver failure may appear by the second day.

Methaemoglobin formation and analgesic nephropathy have been attributed to paracetamol though the role of paracetamol in the latter is questionable.

Dysmorphogenicity

There is no evidence that paracetamol is dysmorphogenic in man and it does not produce malformations in rats and mice (Tuchmann-Duplessis, 1975).

Dextropropoxyphene

Dextropropoxyphene is used as an analgesic. Its potency is roughly equivalent to that of codeine but it has rather less potential for abuse and drug dependence.

Chemistry

Only the dextrorotatory isomer of propoxyphene has analgesic activity. This synthetic drug is structurally related to the more potent methadone, a narcotic analgesic (fig. 7.3). The molecular weight of propoxyphene is 339.48. Dextropropoxyphene is a base with a pKa value of 6.3. It is available as the hydrochloride or napsylate salts (65mg of the former is equivalent to 100mg of the latter). The hydrochloride is water-soluble but the napsylate is not.

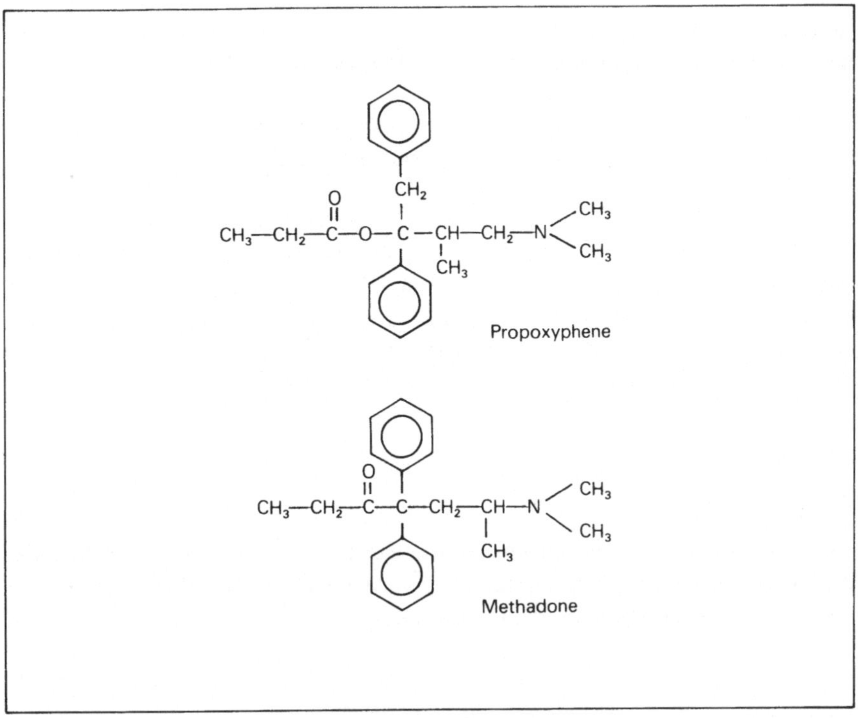

Fig. 7.3. Structural formulae of propoxyphene and methadone.

Pharmacology

Biochemical Pharmacology
No information is available.

Pharmacodynamics
Dextropropoxyphene is a centrally acting analgesic with a tendency to produce sedation, constipation and nausea. The combination of dextropropoxyphene and aspirin has an additive analgesic effect.

Pharmacokinetics
Absorption and bioavailability: Dextropropoxyphene is fairly rapidly absorbed after oral administration. The hydrochloride is more water-soluble than the napsylate and tends to be absorbed more quickly. Measurable plasma concentrations occur 1 hour after dosage and peak levels occur 2 to 3 hours from dosage (Wilson et al., 1976) or 1.5 to 3.6 hours from dosage (Welling et al., 1976). The bioavailability of

the drug from oral suspensions or solution is similar (Wilson et al., 1976). Food intake tends to delay absorption of the drug (Welling et al., 1976).

Distribution: Little detailed information is available. The drug is said to undergo rapid tissue binding, especially to lung, liver, kidney and brain.

Elimination: The plasma half-life of dextropropoxyphene is 1.6 to 4.1 hours (Verebely and Inturrisi, 1974), 3.5 hours, though with a β value of 7.9 hours (Wilson et al., 1976), or 6.57 + 1.53 hours (Wagner et al., 1972). An average of 1.5% of the dose is excreted unchanged in urine; the remainder is biotransformed, chiefly to the *N*-desmethyl derivative norpropoxyphene, which is excreted in urine. Norpropoxyphene has a half-life of 16 hours (Welling et al., 1976).

Plasma level correlations: Data are lacking.

Interactions

Pharmacodynamic interactions: Aspirin and paracetamol appear to interact additively with dextropropoxyphene in so far as analgesia is concerned. Alcohol potentiates the central depressant effects of dextropropoxyphene.

Pharmacokinetic interactions: None has been traced, apart from Kutt's (1971) report that the drug raised plasma phenytoin levels.

Toxicity

Idiosyncratic Toxicity

Such reactions have not been commonly reported. Wiederholt et al. (1967) encountered a patient with decreased renal function who developed episodes of hypoglycaemia when fasting and taking propoxyphene.

Dose-related Toxicity

The following have been reported:

1) Nausea, vomiting and constipation
2) Central nervous system and respiratory depression; confusion and hallucination; convulsions (nalorphine may sometimes antagonise these central toxic effects)
3) Dependence (this is uncommon).

Dysmorphogenicity

Data are lacking.

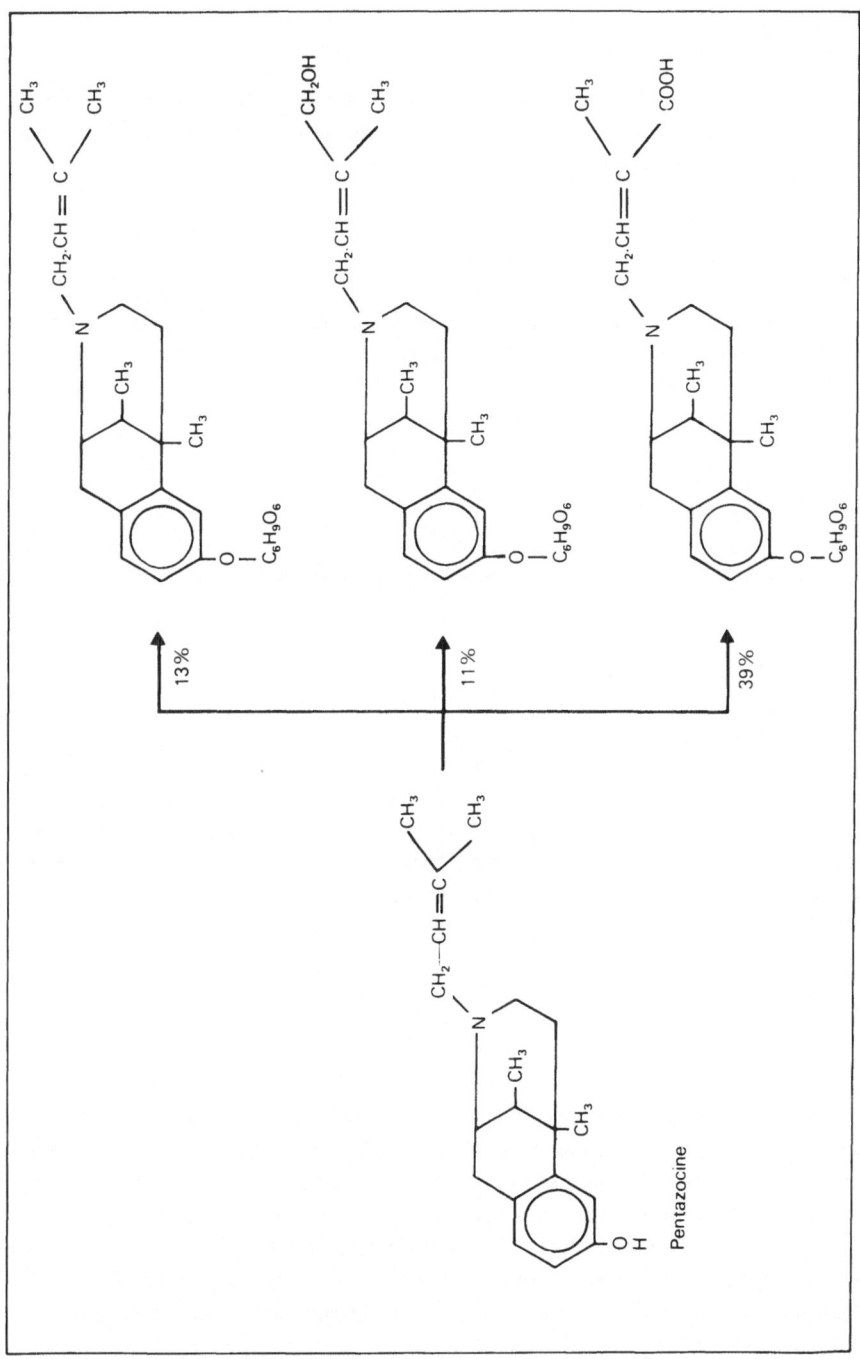

Fig. 7.4. The metabolic pathway of pentazocine.

Pentazocine

Pentazocine may be employed to produce moderately strong analgesia, where a drug with low abuse potential is required. As an analgesic 30 to 50mg of parenteral pentazocine is equivalent to 10mg morphine.

Chemistry

Pentazocine is a synthetic analgesic, molecular weight 285.44, with the structural formula shown in figure 7.4. The compound's analgesic activity resides mainly in the *l*-isomer.

Pharmacology

The pharmacology of the drug was reviewed by Brogden et al. (1973).

Biochemical Pharmacology
No data are available.

Pharmacodynamics
Pentazocine is a fairly potent analgesic with sedative and respiratory depressive properties similar to those of morphine. Unlike morphine, pentazocine produces a slight rise in blood pressure and heart rate. It delays gastric emptying and decreases intestinal motility. Pentazocine does not cause pupillary constriction. It increases uterine activity. Though it does not directly raise intracranial pressure pentazocine may cause an increased pCO_2 from respiratory depression, and this in turn may cause an increase in intracranial pressure.

Pharmacokinetics

Absorption and bioavailability: Pentazocine is well absorbed from the gastrointestinal tract and from injection sites. The T_{max} after oral intake is 1 to 3 hours, but 15 to 60 minutes after intramuscular injection (Berkowitz, 1971). Plasma pentazocine levels are lower after oral than after parenteral administration of the drug (75mg orally is about equivalent to 40mg intramuscularly). There is some evidence suggesting that this difference in bioavailability is due to first-pass metabolism of the drug. This bioavailability difference is a relevant consideration in determining dosage when the drug is given by different routes.

Distribution: The V_D of the drug is about 3L/kg (Agurell et al., 1974), implying considerable tissue binding of the drug. The drug distributes evenly between plasma and red cells (Agurell et al., 1974). Pentazocine readily crosses the blood-brain barrier in cats. Levels of isotope-labelled drug (possibly including metabolites) tend to be high in the liver, lung and gastrointestinal tract. Brain concentrations tend to exceed plasma concentrations. Pentazocine crosses the human placenta. Plasma protein binding data are not available but CSF levels of the drug are about 30 to 40 % of total plasma level (Agurell et al., 1974).

Elimination: Pentazocine has a plasma half-life of about 2 hours (Berkowitz, 1971; Agurell et al., 1974) or 2.5 to 6.0 hours (Beckett et al., 1970). Some 8 to 24 % of a dose is excreted unchanged in urine (when pH conditions are such as to facilitate its excretion) and less than 2 % in faeces. The majority of a pentazocine dose is excreted after biotransformation to a glucuronide conjugate or after the alkyl side-chain is oxidised to alcohol or acid metabolites, which then form phenolic glucuronide conjugates (Berkowitz, 1971). The metabolic pathway is seen in figure 7.4. Approximately 60 % of a pentazocine dose is excreted in urine in the 24 hours after its administration. The pattern of drug metabolism to some extent depends on the mode of administration. After oral intake as much as 25 % of the drug in plasma may be present as metabolites (due to first-pass metabolism). By contrast, metabolites could not be detected in plasma after intramuscular injection of pentazocine in man (Berkowitz et al., 1969).

Plasma level correlations: Analgesic and sedative effects of pentazocine tend to parallel its post-distributional plasma concentrations (Berkowitz et al., 1969).

Interactions
Pharmacodynamic interactions: Alcohol and phenothiazines may potentiate the central depressant actions of pentazocine.

Pharmacokinetic interactions: None are known.

Toxicity

Idiosyncratic Toxicity
Reports cannot be traced.

Dose-related Toxicity
The following reactions have been recorded:

1) Nausea and vomiting
2) Euphoria, hallucinations, delusions, confusion and disorientation

3) Sedation
4) Respiratory depression
5) Sweating, dry mouth, hot flushes, tachycardia, mild hypertension
6) Urine retention
7) Drug dependence (the risk appears relatively small)
8) An instance of myopathy (Steiner et al., 1973).

Dysmorphogenicity
Pentazocine does not appear to be dysmorphogenic in rabbits or rats.

Treatment of Pain in General

When pain cannot be relieved by removing or correcting its cause, and while the cause of pain is itself being determined and then treated, it may be necessary to relieve the pain by prescribing analgesics. If the cause of the pain is untreatable, and the pain is likely to persist, the neurologist may have to consider whether to continue prescribing analgesics, with their general tendency to depress cerebral function, or to recommend a surgical procedure designed to relieve pain if the patient's condition, and prospects for the duration and quality of survival, warrant it. Such matters can be discussed here only in very general terms: the problems of pain are always individual and the treatment policy must be varied to meet the individual patient's needs.

Short Term Pain Relief

In the short term, the symptomatic treatment of pain requires the prescription of an adequate dose of analgesic, at sufficient frequency, to keep the patient comfortable without unduly depressing consciousness or producing other unacceptable side effects. Since pain is so subjective an experience it is difficult to predict the requisite analgesic dose for a particular patient. However in the individual patient, if analgesics have to be repeated, the appropriate dose generally can soon be found by trial, unless the pain severity changes. Milder analgesics (e.g. aspirin or paracetamol) suffice for milder pain, while stronger analgesics (e.g. pentazocine), are required for more severe pain. The need to relieve severe pain quickly, or the associated presence of vomiting may make parenteral administration of analgesics desirable. In these circumstances, if rapid relief of severe pain is sought, intravenous rather than intramuscular injection should be considered. The intravenous injection is preferably given slowly over several minutes to reduce any risk of central depression from high brain levels of drug during the distribution phase. For the types of pain the neurologist is likely to encounter in practice, the drugs considered above will probably provide a sufficient range of analgesic potency.

If repeated dosage is necessary this will generally be given orally or in-tramuscularly at about 4-hourly intervals (perhaps sooner after an initial intravenous injection, since a lower intravenous dose than that given orally or intramuscularly will tend to produce equal early pain relief, but the effect of this lower dose will tend to wear off sooner). Naturally, the higher the intravenous dose used, the longer plasma drug levels will remain above the minimal therapeutic threshold and the longer analgesia will persist. However the size of the dose is limited by the extent of cerebral depression that occurs at the time of peak plasma drug levels.

Long Term Pain Relief

There is no sharp dividing line between short and long term pain relief. If re-peated analgesic prescribing is necessary for more than a few days the neurologist will undoubtedly want to review the patient's situation and perhaps the diagnosis. The neurologist may then need to consider the possibility of having to provide pain relief over many weeks, months or even years, and the risk of becoming embroiled in the problems of drug (narcotic) dependence and tolerance. The milder analgesics may not provide adequate long term relief for the types of pain the neurologist encounters. Sometimes there is no acceptable alternative to the continued use of strong analgesics, because of the nature of the underlying disease. However, particularly for localised pain, and especially when the patient has a reasonable life expectancy, the various surgical measures which influence function in the pain pathway should be con-sidered.

Headache

Headache is the most common symptom encountered in neurological practice. While the majority of headaches appear to be migrainous, it is convenient to consider muscle contraction headache before migraine is discussed here. The contraction headache mechanism tends to become involved as a secondary event in severe head pain from any cause, including migraine.

Contraction Headache

The term 'contraction headache' was used in the American Neurological Association's classification of headache (1962), to avoid the ambiguities inherent in the older term 'tension headache', since the word 'tension' could be taken to refer either to emotional tension, or to muscle tension.

Disordered Mechanisms

A state of continued excessive contraction can develop in the muscles of the back of the neck as a result of:

1) Local injury to these muscles
2) Disease of the cervical spine, discs and ligaments
3) Disease around the shoulder joint, setting up spasm in the trapezius and neighbouring muscles
4) Intracranial or intraspinal disease (e.g. cervical cord tumours, cerebellar tonsillar herniation), apparently causing reflex muscle spasm
5) Head pain, particularly pain at the back of the head, however this is caused (e.g. by migraine)
6) Emotional stress.

Excessive tightness of posterior neck muscles may be symmetrical or asymmetrical. The posterior neck muscles, which insert into the occipital bones below the

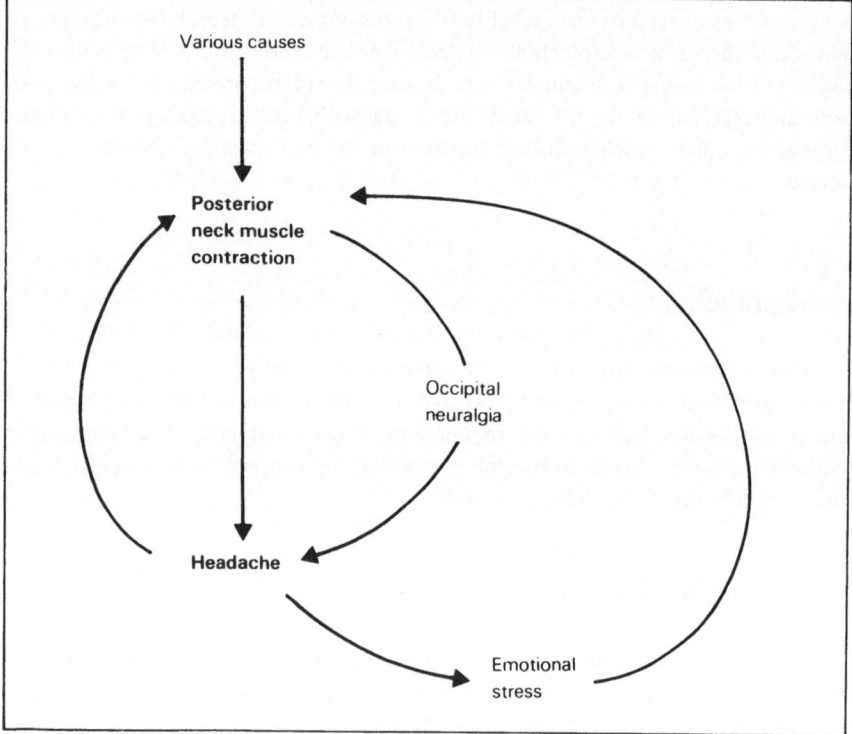

Fig. 7.5. The cycle of cause and effect in contraction headache.

superior nuchal lines, also interdigitate with the epicranial aponeurosis which takes origin from the occipital bones. Hence contraction of the posterior neck muscles exerts traction on the epicranial aponeurosis which is free to move on the skull. Thus traction may be exerted on the aponeurosis as far forward as the eyebrow. To overcome the tendency of the eyebrows to be drawn backward there may be compensatory contraction of the upper facial muscles, including the frontalis. The contraction in the facial muscles and frontalis, and the tightness in the epicranial aponeurosis can reach a stage at which anterior pain is felt, even though the posterior neck muscle tightness has not yet reached a level at which posterior head pain is experienced. Excessive neck muscle tightness tends to produce pain in the scalp rather than in the neck. However this head pain, like any other form of head pain, may cause further reflex tightening of the posterior neck muscles. Thus a vicious circle may be set up. Further, the patient may become apprehensive about his headache and its implications. His fears and anxieties may increase his posterior neck muscle spasm and add a further dimension to the vicious circle mechanism (fig. 7.5).

Neck muscle contraction headache is described by sufferers as being like a tight band or constriction round the head, or like a sense of pressure on the head or an expansion within it. The sensation may be unilateral if the neck muscle contraction is dominantly unilateral.

The greater occipital nerve on each side runs through the upper part of the muscle mass of the back of the neck to enter the scalp at the superior nuchal line. Persisting neck muscle contraction can compress this nerve and make it hypersensitive, with resulting hyperalgesia and dysaesthesia in its territory of supply. Sometimes occipital neuralgia ensues.

Correction of Disordered Mechanisms

Although the disorders which trigger the contraction headache mechanism are themselves often amenable to treatment, such treatment may not necessarily relieve an established contraction headache. The headache mechanism may have reached the stage where it will perpetuate itself through the vicious circle mechanisms mentioned, even though the primary cause is removed. Therefore treatment of contraction headache in its own right is often necessary, even when its cause is cured, or ceases to act. However, treatment of the contraction headache mechanism alone is not likely to give permanent relief if the underlying cause persists.

Treatment of the contraction headache itself is most usefully directed at its final common pathway *viz* excessive posterior neck muscle tightness. This tightness can be relieved by:

1) Application of local heat
2) Massage, shortwave diathermy

3) Relaxation exercises

4) Infiltration of tender areas in the muscles, and their motor points, with local anaesthetic

5) Use of muscle relaxing drugs.

In addition the secondary (vicious circle) mechanisms may be treated by:

1) Using analgesics to lessen the overall pain, thus decreasing secondary neck muscle spasm induced by pain

2) Overcoming anxiety and fear by means of appropriate reassurance and explanation following thorough clinical examination

3) In those instances where occipital neuralgia is present, and persists despite attempts at muscle relaxation, infiltrating the occipital nerves with local anaesthetic and, if this gives temporary benefit, considering possible surgical section of these nerves.

Drugs Used in Treating Contraction Headache

The drugs used are analgesics and muscle relaxants. The relaxants in contemporary use are diazepam (discussed on page 200) and orphenadrine (discussed on page 104, though of dubious value in contraction headache). The extent to which the tranquillising effect of diazepam contributes toward the relief of contraction headache is uncertain. Amitriptyline, widely used as an antidepressant, appears useful in relaxing neck muscle tightness in chronic contraction headache. It is uncertain if amitriptyline is a primary relaxant of neck muscles, but it appears to benefit patients with contraction headache who are not clinically depressed (Lance, 1973). Amitriptyline is discussed below.

Amitriptyline

Amitriptyline is widely used as an antidepressant and is useful in the treatment of contraction headache and in the prophylaxis of migraine. Whether other tricyclic antidepressants are useful in contraction headache is not known, as amitriptyline appears to have been the only derivative adequately tested.

Chemistry

Amitriptyline (MW 277.39) is a tricyclic molecule with a tertiary amine side-chain (fig. 7.6). It is a base with a pKa value of 9.4. Its N-desmethyl metabolite, nortriptyline, is also an antidepressant.

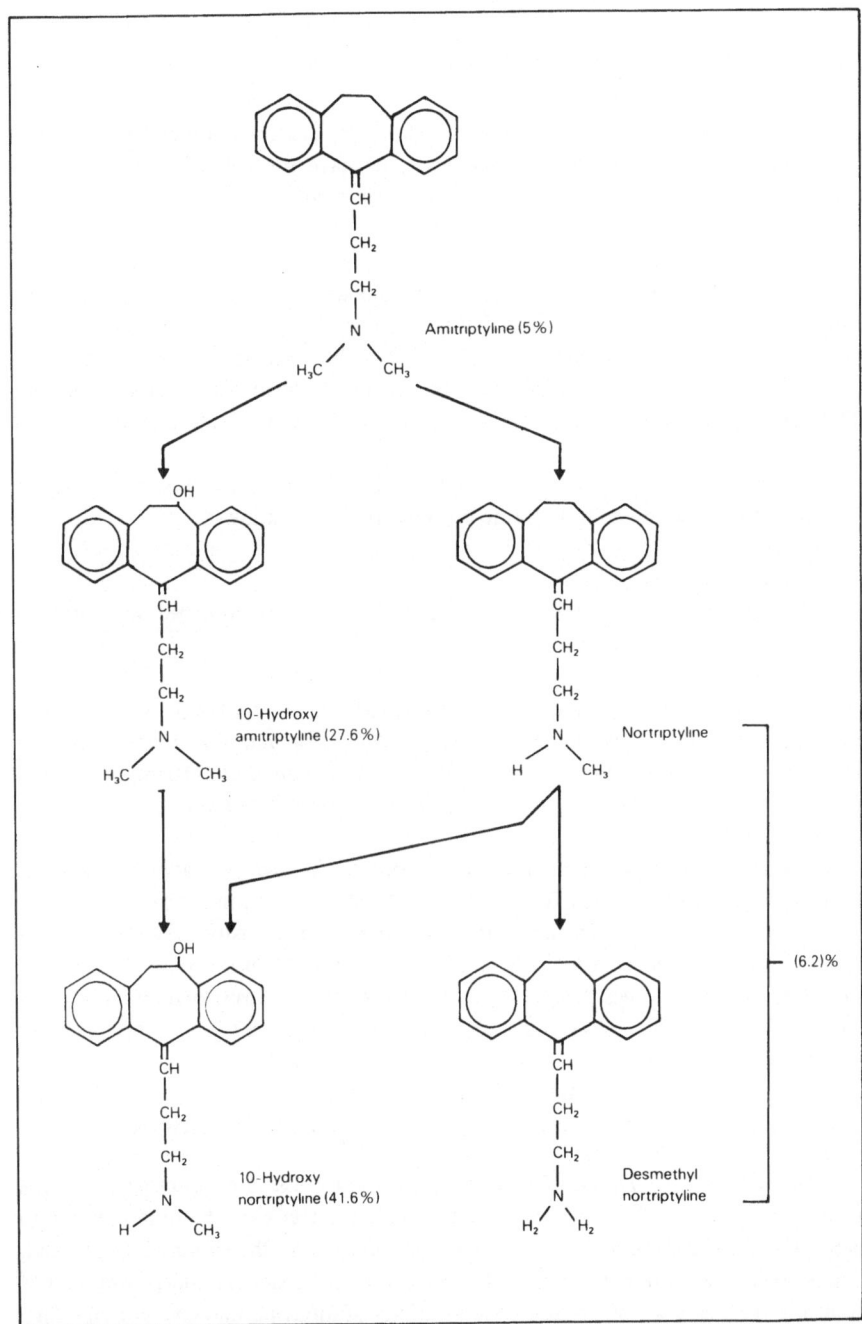

Fig. 7.6. The metabolites of amitriptyline.

Pharmacology

Biochemical Pharmacology

Amitriptyline blocks the uptake of noradrenaline at catecholamine terminals and also inhibits serotonin re-uptake. These actions have the net effect of increasing catecholamine and serotonin concentrations at synapses.

Pharmacodynamics

Tricyclic antidepressants do not elevate mood in normal persons but, if administered continuously, after about 2 weeks relieve endogenous depression and thus elevate the mood of depressed persons. These drugs have sedative properties and anticholinergic actions (e.g. dry mouth, blurred vision, constipation and urine retention). The drugs tend to produce orthostatic hypotension, tachycardia and cardiac arrhythmia.

The mechanism of action of amitriptyline in relieving neck muscle contraction headache and in acting as a migraine preventative is not known.

Pharmacokinetics

Absorption and bioavailability: Amitriptyline is rapidly absorbed after oral intake. Quantitative data are not available.

Distribution: Amitriptyline in plasma is 82 to 96 % protein-bound. Its metabolite nortriptyline is 94.5 % bound (Borga et al., 1969). Few data for amitriptyline distribution are available but the apparent volume of distribution of nortriptyline is very high (18 to 57L/kg, Sjoqvist, 1974), suggesting considerable tissue binding.

Elimination: The plasma half-life of amitriptyline is said to be approximately 40 hours (Lader, 1974), though Jorgensen and Hansen (1976) found that its terminal half-life was 17.1 hours. The drug undergoes hepatic biotransformation to nortriptyline, which has a plasma half-life of 26.8 ± 7.1 hours (Alexanderson, 1972). Santagostino et al. (1974) described the pattern of excretion of amitriptyline metabolites in urine (fig. 7.6). In animals and man (Gram and Overo, 1975) nortriptyline, after oral intake, undergoes extensive first-pass hepatic metabolism. An average of only 2 % of a dose is excreted unchanged in urine (Alexanderson and Borga, 1973) the remainder undergoing ring hydroxylation and conjugation before excretion.

Plasma level correlations: The onset of the antidepressant effect of amitriptyline is delayed for some 10 to 14 days, which is a little longer than the time required to achieve steady-state plasma concentrations, as judged from the elimination rate data. There do not appear to have been studies correlating the onset of antidepressant effect with the time courses of plasma concentrations of amitriptyline and nortriptyline. Steady-state plasma concentrations of nortriptyline correlate poorly with the oral dose of this drug (Alexanderson et al., 1969). It has been suggested that there is no relationship between steady-state plasma nortriptyline level and antidepressant effect (Burrows et al., 1972) but also that steady-state nortriptyline concentrations of 50 to 140ng/ml are associated with an optimal antidepressant effect, while higher levels are of little therapeutic benefit (Asberg et al., 1971; Kragh-Sorensen et al., 1973). However Ziegler et al. (1976) found that recovery from depression increased as plasma tricyclic levels rose above 250ng/ml.

Plasma amitriptyline and nortriptyline levels have not been studied in relation to contraction headache.

Interactions

Pharmacodynamic interactions: Amitriptyline interacts additively with other drugs with sedative effects (e.g. alcohol, chlordiazepoxide) and with other agents which have anticholinergic actions, including phenothiazines. The actions of amitriptyline and nortriptyline in blocking re-uptake of biogenic amines leads to additive interactions with sympathomimetic agents (e.g. amphetamine) and with agents which prolong the actions of catecholamines and serotonin (e.g. monoamine oxidase inhibitors). In this connection it should be remembered that the actions of monoamine oxidase inhibitors may persist for 10 to 14 days after intake of these drugs ceases. The antihypertensive effects of ganglion-blocking agents (e.g. guanethidine, bethanide, and debrisoquine) may be prevented by the sympathetic stimulating effects of tricyclic agents.

Thyroxine potentiates the effects of tricyclic antidepressants. The tricyclic drugs, because of their tendency in high dosage to produce epilepsy, may antagonise the effects of anticonvulsants.

Pharmacokinetic interactions: Urinary acidification is likely to increase the renal excretion of the unmetabolised bases amitriptyline and nortriptyline. However this effect is unlikely to be of practical importance since very little of the elimination of these substances occurs by means of renal excretion of unmetabolised drug. Barbiturates, oral contraceptives and methylphenidate are known to induce the hepatic drug metabolising enzyme system and to increase the biotransformation of tricyclic antidepressants, lowering their plasma levels. Aspirin, chloramphenicol, haloperidol and phenothiazines cause increased plasma nortriptyline levels, while diazepam therapy raises plasma amitriptyline levels (Avery, 1976).

Nortriptyline diminishes the metabolism of dicoumarol, thereby increasing the risk of an excessive anticoagulant action.

Toxicity

Idiosyncratic Toxicity
Idiosyncratic side effects are rare.

Dose-related Toxicity

Such toxic manifestations include the following:

1) Anticholinergic effects:

   dry mouth, blurred vision, constipation, tachycardia, palpitation, urine retention, excess sweating (mechanism unknown)

2) Other effects:

   sedation, headache, tremor, weakness and fatigue, convulsions (in high
   dosage).

In acute overdosage amitriptyline may produce hyperpyrexia, hypertension,
seizures, coma and cardiac arrhythmia; physostigmine, an anticholinesterase which
crosses the blood-brain barrier, can rapidly reverse the central anticholinergic effects
of tricyclic overdosage.

Dysmorphogenicity

There appears to be no good evidence of human dysmorphogenicity from these
tricyclic agents.

Treatment of Contraction Headache

It is unlikely that a patient's contraction headache can be permanently relieved if
the underlying cause continues. Failure of the measures designed to relax neck
muscles, if these measures have been carried out for a sufficient time, suggests that
the underlying cause of the patient's contraction headache has not been dealt with. In
practice, such failure of treatment often proves due to underlying recurrent migraine
which has been masked by the superadded contraction headache and which has not
been recognised because the whole natural history of the headache disorder has not
been elicited. However, sometimes the initiating cause of the contraction headache
may have ceased (e.g. a single severe migraine attack) but a contraction headache persists because of its own self-perpetuating mechanisms. In these circumstances relaxation of the posterior neck muscles may solve the whole problem, though the underlying cause, long forgotten, may not have been recognised or treated.

Hence, in managing patients with contraction headache, the underlying cause
should be identified and treated if possible. Any anxiety should be dealt with by explanation and reassurance. If neck muscle relaxation is to be achieved, this will
usually be attained by physical means (e.g. by the frequent and prolonged application
of heat to the back of the neck and shoulders). The use of a hot water bag, refilled every 20 or 30 minutes, and applied to the back of the neck and shoulders for 2 or 3
hours every evening, may often produce adequate neck muscle relaxation over 2 to 4
weeks. More complicated methods of applying heat (e.g. use of infra-red lamps) may
also be effective. However patients often abandon these more complex devices too

quickly, because they are less convenient to use than hot water bottles. If the headache has been chronic, to avoid relapse it is generally desirable to continue the application of heat to the neck for 1 or 2 weeks after the contraction headache appears adequately relieved. Massage and other forms of physiotherapy can also assist in producing neck muscle relaxation.

Should these local physical measures fail to relieve contraction headache, and should the diagnosis still appear correct, muscle relaxant drugs may be prescribed. Both diazepam and amitriptyline have slow enough eliminations for there to be little reason to give them more often than once a day, so long as the dose is sufficient. Thus 5 to 15mg of diazepam, or 50 to 100mg amitriptyline may be given in the evening every day. If such treatment is to help in chronic contraction headache it often must be taken for several weeks, though if the headache has been present for a relatively short time a shorter course may suffice.

Other measures that may occasionally be necessary in refractory cases include:

1) Infiltration of the motor points of the posterior neck muscles with local anaesthetic once or twice daily, to achieve muscle relaxation which is then maintained by the continued use of heat on the back of the neck and shoulders.

2) Infiltration of the greater occipital nerves with local anaesthetic, and later possible section of these nerves, if there is an element of greater occipital neuralgia which is not relieved by attempts to relax the posterior neck and shoulder muscles.

3) Referral for psychiatric advice.

The weaker analgesics may be used to help diminish the discomfort of contraction headache while attempts are made to interrupt its mechanism. The authors' experience has been that in chronic contraction headache these minor analgesics almost always fail in their intended purpose. In fact the patient has almost always already failed to gain relief from them before seeking medical advice. In general it would seem unwise to use any analgesic more potent than dextropropoxyphene for contraction headache. If the powerful drugs relieve the pain the patient is likely to neglect the physical measures which will relax his neck muscles. Consequently his pain may keep recurring once the analgesic effect wears off. The analgesics may then have to be continued and problems of tolerance and drug dependence may occur. In dealing with chronic contraction headache it is wise not to use analgesics for more than short term pain relief, while physical treatments alone or combined with muscle relaxing drugs, are given time to work.

Migraine

Migraine, in all its variety, is an exceedingly common disorder. Surveys have suggested that up to 15 to 20 % of the adult male population, and up to 23 to 29 % of the adult female population, are affected during their lives (Waters and O'Connor, 1975), though possibly less than a quarter of these numbers are ever likely to seek medical advice about their headaches. There is, as yet, no generally agreed definition of migraine. Here the word is taken in a broad sense of recurrent vascular headache, without there being any requirement that the headache be unilateral, or that a visual 'aura' be present.

The American Neurological Association's Classification of Headache (1962) sets out several subtypes of migraine, chiefly 'classical' and 'common' migraine but, with the exception of cluster headache (or migrainous neuralgia), which is dealt with separately, these variants of migraine are considered together in the present text.

Disordered Mechanisms

The typical migraine attack involves three stages which to some extent overlap in time.

Stage I: Initially there is arterial constriction in the scalp and brain. The scalp vasoconstriction is clinically silent. The cerebral arterial narrowing also often produces no definite clinical manifestation but may cause enough cerebral ischaemia to initiate a migraine 'aura', usually visual, but sometimes somatic, sensory, dysphasic or vertiginous.

Stage II: Dilatation of scalp and brain arteries, often with arteriolar constriction in the scalp and arterio-venous shunting of blood. The restoration of cerebral blood flow terminates the migraine aura but the scalp arterial dilatation may cause headache.

Stage III: Migraine headache may initiate secondary neck muscle contraction headache, as explained earlier.

These events can be at least partly explained by a number of biochemical changes which have been detected in persons with migraine attacks. The initial event appears to be the release of serotonin (5-hydroxytryptamine) from platelets, and perhaps from nerve terminals in the upper brain stem and hypothalamus (Sicuteri, 1972). Platelets from migraine sufferers differ from platelets from normal persons. Platelets from migraine sufferers tend to take up more serotonin but their surface receptors retain it less efficiently (Hilton, 1971). The released serotonin produces vasoconstriction generally, increased capillary permeability (Fanchamps, 1975) and perhaps alterations in hypothalamic and limbic function (e.g. mood changes) which may occur in the early stages of migraine attacks. However, various experimental studies have given somewhat conflicting findings as to the effect of serotonin on external carotid blood flow. Vidrio and Hong (1976) suggested that the underlying state of neurogenic and non-neurogenic vascular tone might determine whether or not serotonin caused external carotid vasodilatation. Released serotonin may trigger release of vasoconstrictor prostaglandins from the lungs. However serotonin, released into the circulation and no longer protected in storage granules in platelets and nerve terminals, is then liable to degradation by the enzyme monoamine oxidase. Thus the stage of abnormal vasoconstriction, due to excess free serotonin circulating in plasma water, is succeeded by a period of relative serotonin depletion, leading to dilatation of the vasculature and headache. The changes in biogenic amine concentration at hypothalamic synapses may be responsible for the nausea and vomiting of migraine and other effects such as hypotension. Sicuteri (1971) suggested that released serotonin might cause an increased central sensitivity to pain. Chemicals which increase local pain sensitivity (e.g. the 9 amino acid-containing peptide, bradykinin, and also prostaglandins), appear around the dilating scalp arteries, perhaps after leaking through capillary endothelium which is abnormally permeable due to serotonin effects (Fanchamps, 1975). These chemicals augment the local pain response. The scalp pain appears to trigger secondary neck muscle spasm through neurogenic mechanisms, as explained earlier in this chapter.

The tendency to migraine is inherited, but a number of factors are known to precipitate attacks in predisposed persons. Among these factors are:

1) Emotional strain, anxiety and fatigue, which may act on the hypothalamus via limbic circuits.

2) Menstruation, when falling plasma oestrogen levels may trigger attacks (Somerville, 1975a).

3) Intake of oral contraceptives, particularly those with a relatively high oestrogen content.

4) Alcohol intake: in some instances alcohol may act simply as a vasodilator to augment an otherwise subclinical migraine attack; on other occasions specific forms of alcohol (e.g. red wines, with high amine contents) may trigger attacks because the amines are taken up by platelets and perhaps axon terminals and competitively displace serotonin from amine storage granules.

5) Intake of food in certain individuals: dairy food intake may activate migraine in some people because raised plasma free fatty acid levels occur, and possibly cause attacks by releasing serotonin. In other persons chocolate may cause attacks because of its content of phenylethylamine, which competitively displaces serotonin from storage granules. Phenylethylamine is a specific substrate for brain type B monoamine oxidase (Yang and Neff, 1973). This and other structurally similar amines release prostaglandin from the lungs (Sandler, 1972). There is evidence that certain patients with migraine have a defective capacity to metabolise phenylethylamine (Sandler et al., 1974).

6) Intake of drugs (e.g. reserpine) which block serotonin re-uptake into platelets after its release (Curzon et al., 1969).

There are other precipitants of migraine (e.g. scalp trauma, exercise, lack of sleep or prolonged sleep). The biochemical modes of action of these precipitants are not yet readily explained.

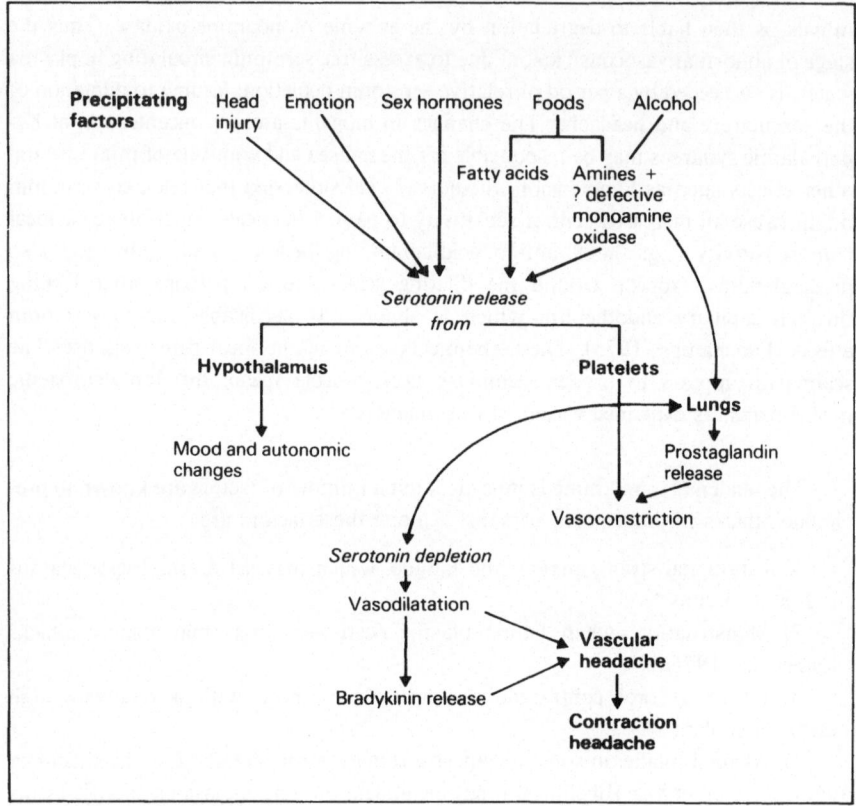

Fig. 7.7. The mechanisms of migraine.

Thus the mechanisms of migraine can be schematised as in figure 7.7. An account of the biochemistry of migraine is given by Bruyn (1976).

Correction of Disordered Mechanisms

Acute Attacks

In the individual migraine attack, the patient is nearly always more disturbed by the headache than by the aura, if any. Therefore if the migraine mechanism can be interrupted prior to the stage of serotonin depletion, the headache may be averted and the patient is likely to regard his treatment as successful. Attempts to shorten the aura by giving vasodilating agents are likely to hasten the onset of the headache and make it more severe.

During the aura it may be possible to give a drug such as aspirin, which inhibits serotonin release from platelets (Zucker and Peterson, 1968) or ergotamine, which prevents scalp arterial dilatation. Such treatment may prevent headache developing or may reduce its severity. At an early stage in the evolution of the headache itself a single oral dose of aspirin may still abort the attack. This benefit may involve more than a simple analgesic effect. Perhaps serotonin and prostaglandin release are still going on early in the attack and the action of aspirin on these mechanisms may be enough to interrupt this.

If the migraine mechanisms cannot be interrupted early in their evolutions, the two main therapeutic possibilities for relieving the headache are:

1) Antagonising the vasodilatation in the scalp by the use of a vasoconstrictor agent (e.g. ergotamine)
2) Using analgesics of adequate potency.

It is often necessary to deal with other consequences of the migraine, principally the nausea and vomiting, by the use of anti-emetic agents (phenothiazines and anti-cholinergic antihistaminics). Nausea and vomiting are very important aspects of migraine. They are associated with gastric atony and delayed gastric emptying. Clinicians have long suspected that vomiting in migraine may prevent the absorption of orally administered drugs. It has also been noted that drugs given by mouth in migraine attacks usually are relatively ineffective in patients who have nausea. Volans (1975) demonstrated the delay in absorption of orally administered aspirin during migraine attacks and showed that metoclopramide-induced gastric emptying hastened aspirin absorption during migraine attacks and improved the therapeutic response.

Neck muscle contraction headache often develops during migraine attacks. As time passes, if the attack is not aborted, and particularly if the migraine has occurred towards the back of the head, the posterior neck muscle contraction mechanism may become the chief factor in the overall headache. It may therefore be necessary to treat the secondary contraction headache along the lines already indicated.

Prevention of Attacks

Migraine is a recurrent disorder. Hence the prevention of attacks would be desirable. Since there is no possibility of altering the underlying genetic tendency to migraine, the therapeutic possibilities are:

1) The avoidance of precipitating factors, if possible. Thus culprit foods and certain varieties of alcohol may need to be avoided. Stress and anxiety may need to be reduced.

2) The use of agents which alter serotonin action:

a) antiserotonin agents (e.g. methysergide) and certain antihistamines (e.g. cyproheptadine, pizotifen, methdilazine). These agents, which have similar molecular structures to serotonin, may conceivably also act as serotonin replacements (rather than antagonists) in states of serotonin depletion

b) monoamine oxidase inhibitors, which will reduce the amount of serotonin degradation

c) amitriptyline which, at least in the central nervous system, inhibits re-uptake of released serotonin.

The net effect of all these agents may be to provide increased free serotonin, or serotonin-like activity, at receptors, though monoamine oxidase inhibitors and amitriptyline may also increase catecholamine concentrations at the appropriate receptors.

3) Use of agents which tend to enhance peripheral vasoconstrictor tone:

a) α-adrenergic agonists — clonidine and ergotamine, both of which have mixed agonist and antagonist effects

b) β-adrenergic blocking agents — propranolol; pindolol.

4) The use of phenytoin, and other anticonvulsants. Empirically it has been found that these agents tend to prevent childhood migraine and certain uncommon varieties of adult migraine. The mode of action is obscure.

Drugs Used in Treating Migraine

Of the drugs used in treating migraine attacks, ergotamine will be considered below. The analgesics were dealt with (p.232-246) and the antinauseants on pages 156-159. Certain of the migraine prophylactics have already been considered (amitriptyline p.250-254; β-blockers p.146-150; and anticonvulsants on pages 168-215). The remaining drugs used for this purpose are discussed below. The pharmacology of many of these agents, with particular relevance to their use in migraine, is well surveyed by Fozard (1975).

Ergotamine

Ergotamine has been used since 1884 to treat migraine attacks (Wolff, 1963). This is virtually its only clinical use.

Chemistry

Ergotamine is an alkaloid derived from the fungus *Claviceps purpurea*, which grows on rye and other grain crops. The molecule has been synthesised (Stoll, 1950).

Ergotamine (MW 581.65) is a base with a pKa value of 6.25 (Maulding and Zoglio, 1970). The molecule comprises a lysergic acid moiety joined from the 8C position through a peptide bond to 3 amino acid residues (fig. 7.8). Only the *l*-isomer of ergotamine is biologically active. On standing in solvents containing hydroxyl groups ergotamine converts to a poorly soluble isomer, ergotaminine (Stoll and Hofmann, 1965). Ergotamine is generally prescribed as the tartrate salt.

Pharmacology

Biochemical Pharmacology

Ergotamine is a partial α-adrenergic agonist with some α-adrenergic blocking activity at supratherapeutic doses. Portion of the lysergic acid moiety bears structural resemblances to noradrenaline and to serotonin (fig. 7.8). Hilton and Zilkha (1974) suggested that ergotamine may occupy serotonin uptake sites on platelets and vessel walls, thus leaving more serotonin available to activate vasoconstrictor receptors.

Pharmacodynamics

Ergotamine is a potent vasoconstrictor agent which in overdoses can produce toxic damage to capillary endothelium. It also augments uterine contraction. It has an emetic action by stimulating the medullary chemoreceptor trigger zone. At levels in the therapeutic range (following doses of 3 to 14μg/kg) Fozard (1975) stated that ergotamine has a selective vasoconstrictor effect in the carotid bed, potentiates vasoconstrictor agents including catecholamines, and blocks serotonin-induced vasoconstrictor responses. Regional cerebral blood flow studies in man suggest that therapeutic doses of ergotamine do not constrict the internal carotid vascular bed though they do constrict the external carotid system (Enmeads et al., 1976).

Pharmacokinetics

Despite the long history of the use of ergotamine in medicine, pharmacokinetic data on the drug are scanty, largely because of the low dose used and consequent difficulty in obtaining a sufficiently sensitive assay.

Absorption and bioavailability: No direct data in man are available, except for the isotopic study of Aellig and Nuesch (1977). These authors showed an absorption half-time of 0.38 ± 0.08 hours after oral administration, and a T_{max} of 2.1 ± 0.8 hours. The considerable discrepancy between the effective oral (2 to 4mg) and intravenous (0.25 to 0.5mg) doses in migraine suggests poor absorption of the drug from the alimentary tract and/or substantial first-pass metabolism in the gut wall and liver. The work of Nimmerfall and Rosenthaler (1976) in monkeys suggested that an average of only 32% of an oral dose of ergotamine is absorbed. Berde et al. (1970) and Schmidt and Fanchamps (1974) obtained some evidence that ergotamine absorp-

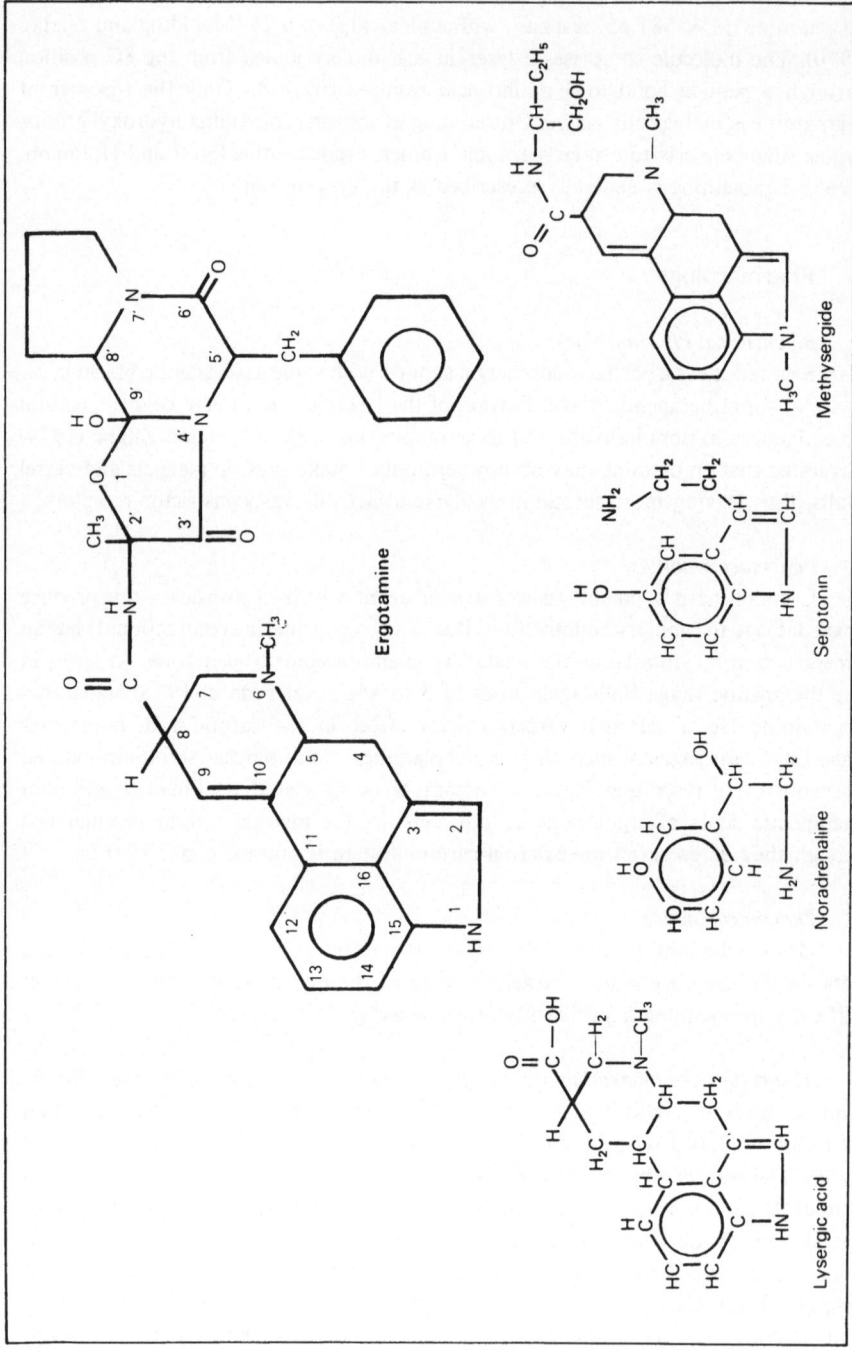

Fig. 7.8. Ergotamine; the lysergic acid moiety has structural resemblances to noradrenaline, serotonin and methysergide.

tion from the alimentary tract of man was enhanced by the simultaneous presence of caffeine. Complexing of another ergot compound, ergotoxin, with xanthine derivatives increased absorption of the ergotoxin from the gut (Zoglio and Maulding, 1970). Working with isotopically labelled ergotamine in man, Aellig and Nuesch (1977) calculated that about two-thirds of the dose was absorbed after oral administration, but from their data one would have suspected that the fraction absorbed was a good deal lower. Sutherland et al. (1974) found that buccal absorption of ergotamine in man was an inefficient process and unlikely to yield a therapeutic intake of the drug into the circulation. Quantitative data for rectal absorption are not available but clinical experience suggests the process often is inefficient. The rate of absorption from intramuscular injection sites and from inhaled aerosols has not been adequately studied. Clinically the authors have the impression that ergotamine aerosols usually fail to relieve migraine.

Distribution: No information is available.

Elimination: No adequate terminal half-life data are available. Using isotopically labelled drug, so that metabolites may have been measured as unchanged drug, Aellig and Nuesch (1977) found that ergotamine had an α-phase half-life of 1.9 ± 0.6 hours, and a β-phase half-life of 21 ± 4 hours. Eadie (1972) found very rapid decline in plasma ergotamine levels after intravenous dosage in what was probably an α-phase, but if so the assay method used was not sensitive enough to determine β-phase data. Eadie's studies (1972) provided some tentative evidence that ergotamine was metabolised extensively. The animal studies of Nimmerfall and Rosenthaler (1976) showed most of the ergotamine absorbed was subsequently excreted in bile. Meier and Schreier (1976) found that only 4.23 % of a dose of radioactive ergotamine appeared in human urine. The pattern of decline of plasma radioactivity after dosage suggested a 'fast' half-life of 5 to 6 hours, and a 'slow' half-life of 30 to 35 hours.

Plasma level correlations: Practically no data are available. Eadie's (1972) findings raised the possibility that the antimigraine effect of ergotamine might correlate better with levels of ergotamine metabolite(s) than with levels of the drug itself, but the assay used was neither sensitive nor specific enough to permit firm conclusions.

Interactions
Pharmacodynamic interactions: Ergotamine may interact with other vasoconstricting agents (e.g. methysergide) to produce dangerous peripheral or coronary arterial constriction. Baumrucker (1973) reported a possible interaction between ergotamine and propranolol which caused painful cyanosis of the feet of a patient.

Pharmacokinetic interactions: None has been well documented, though it has been suggested that triacetyloleandomycin may delay the hepatic biotransformation of ergotamine and thus increase the vasospastic action of the latter (Bigorie et al., 1975).

Toxicity

Idiosyncratic Toxicity

Rarely the manifestations of ergotamine overdosage (e.g. gangrene of the extremities) may occur after such low dosage of ergotamine that one suspects the presence of a metabolic peculiarity. Allergic reactions (itching and oedema) seem to be very uncommon.

Dose-related Toxicity

Such toxic effects include:

1) Nausea and vomiting
2) Cramps in the legs and sometimes in the abdomen
3) Excessive peripheral artery spasm, sometimes causing gangrene of the extremities; coronary artery spasm
4) Venous thrombosis
5) Thirst, confusion and unconsciousness in severe overdosage.

It is said that over-frequent ergotamine dosage can itself cause further vascular headache which may be treated with more ergotamine if its cause is not recognised (Rowsell et al., 1973; Legg, 1974; Anderson, 1975). However, it is possible that this headache may at least in part be due to the caffeine which is contained in many commercial ergotamine preparations, rather than to ergotamine itself.

Dysmorphogenicity

Ergotamine has an oxytocic effect. Therefore, there is a theoretical risk that the drug, taken in pregnancy, might cause fetal damage because of its tendency to induce abortion (and also premature labour). The general tendency of migraine to remit during pregnancy reduces this risk and there is no clear evidence that ergotamine is dysmorphogenic in man.

Methysergide

The main use of methysergide is as a migraine prophylactic. Rarely it is used to relieve serotonin-induced symptoms in patients who have carcinoid tumours with hepatic metastases. There are reports that the drug may be useful in progressive supranuclear palsy (Rafal et al., 1977) and narcolepsy (Wyler et al., 1975).

Chemistry

Methysergide (MW 353.48) is a lysergic acid derivative, bearing a structural resemblance to ergotamine (fig. 7.8) but having a simple aliphatic side-chain attached to the peptide bond linked to C8. The drug is a weak base with a pKa value of 6.62 (Maulding and Zoglio, 1970).

Pharmacology

Biochemical Pharmacology

Methysergide is a serotonin antagonist, except in the carotid vascular bed (Fozard, 1975). It inhibits the serotonin-induced release of spasmogens (mainly prostaglandins) from the lung. Methysergide occupies serotonin uptake sites on platelets, and possibly on vessel walls (Hilton and Zilkha, 1974).

Pharmacodynamics

Methysergide inhibits the release of serotonin (5-hydroxytryptamine), and also its vasoconstrictor and pressor effects, and relieves the increased alimentary motility of patients with carcinoid tumours. Methysergide in therapeutic doses produces a selective peripheral vasoconstriction in the carotid tree. The drug potentiates the effects of catecholamines (Fanchamps, 1975).

Methysergide prevents migraine, though the exact mode of action is not well understood. It has been suggested that in migraine it may act as a serotonin agonist, rather than an antagonist (Curran et al., 1965). Direct carotid vasoconstriction, and impaired prostaglandin release, may be involved.

Pharmacokinetics

Absorption and bioavailability: Bianchine and Friedman (1970) suggest that peak plasma levels of the drug occurred at about 2 hours after oral administration.

Distribution: Clinical data suggest that the drug enters the brain, since it may produce relief in progressive supranuclear palsy.

Elimination: The half-life of the drug in man is 90 minutes (Bianchine, 1968) or about 2 hours (Bianchine and Friedman, 1970). Most of the material present in urine after methysergide dosing is its 1-*N*-desmethyl derivative. Meier and Schreier (1976) found 56.4% of a methysergide dose was excreted in urine.

Plasma level correlations: No data are available.

Interactions

Pharmacodynamic interactions: The vasoconstrictor effect of methysergide might be increased by sympathomimetic agents and by ergotamine.

Pharmacokinetic interactions: None is recognised.

Toxicity

Idiosyncratic Toxicity

There do not appear to be well documented ,idiosyncratic toxic effects.

Dose-related Toxicity

The dose-related toxic effects of methysergide include:

1) Gastrointestinal: nausea, vomiting, abdominal cramps, diarrhoea, anorexia and sometimes weight gain if migraine is controlled
2) Central nervous: drowsiness, weakness, faintness, confusion, euphoria and hallucinations
3) Loss of scalp hair
4) Fibrosis — retroperitoneal (perhaps causing ureteric obstruction), pleural, pericardial and cardiac valvular. This fibrosis may regress to some extent after drug withdrawal. Its occurrence relates to continuous use of the drug for periods of over 6 months, and to high dosage
5) Hypertension or hypotension
6) Vasospastic: angina pectoris and intermittent claudication.

Dysmorphogenicity

There is no definite evidence of dysmorphogenicity in man.

Antiserotonin-Antihistaminic Agents

At least three antiserotonin agents with antihistaminic (and weak anticholinergic) actions have come into reasonably common use for migraine prophylaxis. The chemical structures of these agents (pizotifen, cyproheptadine and methdilazine) are reasonably similar, and clinically their potencies in preventing migraine appear comparable. Therefore they are discussed together.

Pizotifen: Cyproheptadine: Methdilazine

These drugs are used as migraine preventatives (Lance et al., 1970); cyproheptadine and methdilazine are also employed as antihistamines, and sometimes to allay itching. Cyproheptadine has also been advocated as a means of increasing appetite and producing weight gain in children. There are suggestions that cyproheptadine may be used in treating manifestations of carcinoid syndrome, by virtue of its antiserotonin effect. Pizotifen was reviewed in some detail by Speight and Avery (1972).

Chemistry

Pizotifen (MW 295.45) has a pKa value of 6.95. Cyproheptadine (MW 287.39) is a base, usually administered as the hydrochloride. Methdilazine (MW 296.43) is somewhat soluble in water at pH 7.4. The drug is usually supplied as its hydrochloride. The structural formulae of the three drugs are shown in figure 7.9.

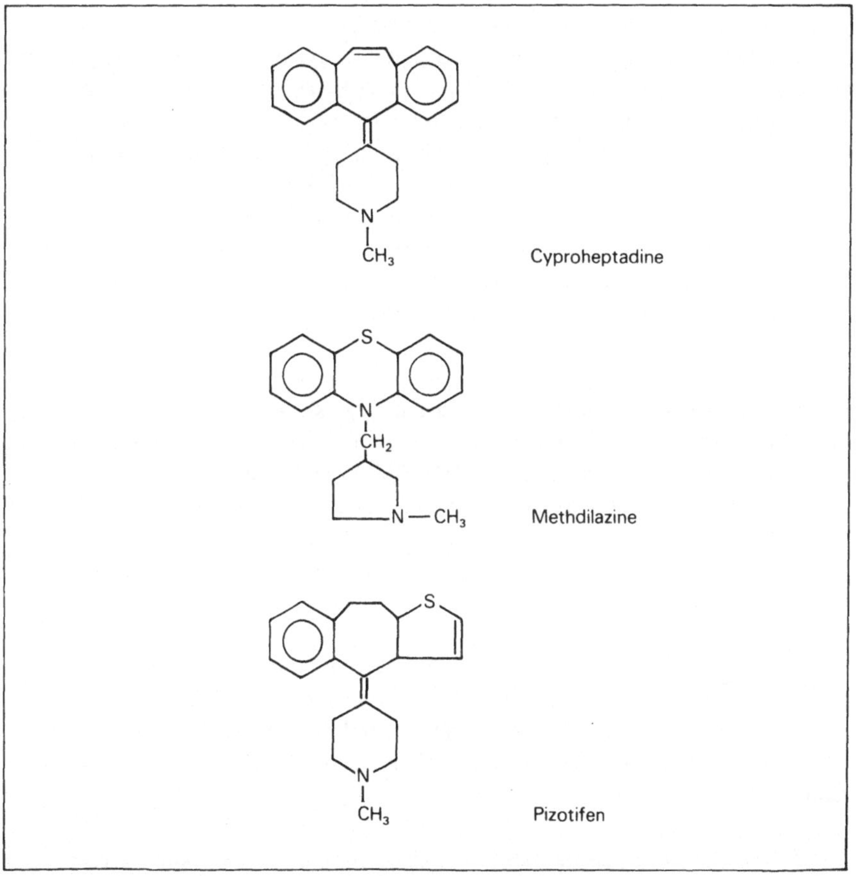

Cyproheptadine

Methdilazine

Pizotifen

Fig. 7.9. Antiserotonin-antihistamine migraine prophylactic drugs.

Pharmacology

Biochemical Pharmacology

The three drugs are serotonin and histamine blocking agents with anti-cholinergic and varying degrees of antibradykinin activity. Cyproheptadine blocks receptors to serotonin, dopamine and tryptamine in the canine arterial wall (Gilbert and Goldberg, 1975) and diminishes growth hormone secretion (Smythe and Lazarus, 1974).

Pharmacodynamics

As well as being antihistaminics and anticholinergics, these drugs are anti-serotonin agents at the concentrations which are likely to be used in migraine prophylaxis. Cyproheptadine does not block the action of serotonin in inducing vasoconstriction in the carotid tree.

Pizotifen has some antidepressant properties. All three drugs are sedatives. Pizotifen and cyproheptadine have some action in correcting experimentally produced atrial arrhythmias in dogs. Pizotifen has a slight hypoglycaemic effect in man.

Pizotifen has little antibradykinin effect (Sicuteri et al., 1967) but potentiates the effects of catecholamines. Cyproheptadine has a greater antibradykinin effect and methdilazine is a reasonably potent antibradykinin agent.

In humans with migraine, pizotifen 0.5mg 3 times a day given for 10 days does not protect against glyceryl trinitrate-induced headache. After 20 days of therapy there is some protection and this protection increases for at least another 10 days (Sicuteri et al., 1970).

Pharmacokinetics

Absorption and bioavailability: Studies in dogs show that ^{3}H-pizotifen is fairly well absorbed from the gastrointestinal tract. In man ^{3}H-pizotifen does not appear in plasma till 2 hours after oral dosage and the T_{max} is 5 to 7 hours.

Some 95 % of an oral dose of ^{14}C-cyproheptadine is absorbed. The T_{max} is 4 to 8 hours.

Methdilazine is said to be fully and quickly absorbed from the gastrointestinal tract (Weikel et al., 1960).

Distribution: Pizotifen in plasma is 89 % protein-bound and its apparent volume of distribution is 6.9L/kg, suggesting a high degree of tissue binding.

Corresponding data for cyproheptadine and methdilazine are not available, though Wold and Fischer (1972) found high tissue to plasma level ratios of cyproheptadine.

Elimination: The plasma half-life of pizotifen is 22 to 26 hours. According to Speight and Avery (1972) some 24 % of an oral dose is excreted in faeces, probably mostly as metabolites. Meier and Schreier (1976) found that 44.1 % of the dose was excreted in urine, but the nature of any metabolites is not known.

Data for the elimination rate of cyproheptadine are not available. However, after ^{14}C-cyproheptadine is given only 34 % of the radioactivity in faeces is due to unchanged drug. About 2 to 20 % of the total drug dose is lost in faeces and at least 40 % in urine. In cats several metabolites have been identified (Hucker et al., 1973). The molecule appears to undergo hydroxylation at the 10-11 double bond, N-dealkylation and N-oxide formation.

Frigerio et al. (1974) have described the presence of epoxide metabolites of cyproheptadine and its N-desmethylated derivative in rat urine. Possibly these epoxides are metabolic intermediates in the formation of 10,11-dihydroxy derivatives.

Few data are available for methdilazine. It is said to form a sulphoxide metabolite (Weikel et al., 1960).

Plasma level correlations: No adequate data are available for any of these drugs in relation to their use in migraine prophylaxis.

Interactions
Pharmacodynamic interactions: These drugs are likely to interact additively with sedatives, including alcohol. Cyproheptadine is said to permit a reduction in dosage of anti-thyroid drugs in treating thyrotoxicosis (Francini et al., 1968).

Pharmacokinetic interactions: No definite examples are recognised.

Toxicity

Idiosyncratic Toxicity
Idiosyncratic toxicity to these drugs appears uncommon.

Dose-related Toxicity
Manifestations include:

1) Drowsiness
2) Weight gain (possibly least with methdilazine)
3) Dizziness
4) Dry mouth
5) Nausea and vomiting.

Dysmorphogenicity
Pizotifen does not appear to be dysmorphogenic in rats or rabbits.

Monoamine Oxidase Inhibitors

There have been reports that monoamine oxidase inhibitors are of benefit in preventing otherwise intractable migraine (Anthony and Lance, 1969). However the main use of these drugs is in treating refractory psychotic depression and phobic-anxiety states. Potentially the monoamine oxidase inhibitors are very dangerous drugs. They are irreversible inhibitors of the enzyme monoamine oxidase which inactivates biogenic amines (e.g. adrenaline, noradrenaline, dopamine and serotonin). Monoamine oxidase also inactivates amines of dietary origin. If monoamine oxidase in the intestinal wall is inhibited, dietary amines (notably tyramine) may be absorbed intact and competitively displace biogenic amines from storage sites. Some dietary amines if absorbed intact also may have a direct hypertensive effect. If foods with a high amine content (e.g. certain cheeses, meat extracts) are eaten by a patient taking monoamine oxidase inhibitors there is a serious risk of catecholamine-induced severe hypertension, which has sometimes resulted in fatal brain haemorrhage. Further, the monoamine oxidase inhibitors are irreversible inhibitors of the enzyme. Therefore their effects persist for up to 2 weeks after dosage is discontinued (until there has been time for the synthesis of new enzyme protein). There may also be dangerous interactions between monoamine oxidase inhibitors and certain drugs (e.g. levodopa).

Because of these risks, monoamine oxidase inhibitors are likely to be used very little in the prophylaxis of migraine and used only in patients who can be relied on to observe appropriate dietary restrictions, not to take medicines except on advice, and who can remain under close supervision.

The subject of monoamine oxidase inhibitors was reviewed by Pscheidt (1964). Some brief details of one inhibitor, phenelzine, are given below.

Phenelzine

Phenelzine has a mood elevating effect and tends to lower blood pressure and relieve angina pectoris. The drug is absorbed quickly. Since it acts irreversibly its duration of biological action is not related to its plasma level. However the drug is metabolised by acetylation and therefore greater maximal effects might be expected in slow acetylators.

The monoamine oxidase inhibitors interact additively with sympathomimetic amines, particularly indirectly acting ones (e.g. amphetamine and tyramine) and with amine precursors (levodopa and tryptophan). The inhibitors interfere with the inactivation of certain drugs (e.g. central depressants including alcohol, narcotics, tricyclic antidepressants and centrally acting anticholinergics). Amine-containing foods (certain cheeses, red wine, beer, pickled herring, chicken liver, yeast, coffee, yoghurt, broad bean pods, canned figs, meat extracts and vegetable extracts) should be avoided.

Toxic effects from phenelzine and other monoamine oxidase inhibitors include agitation, hallucinations, fever, convulsions, hypotension or hypertension, headache, urine retention and inhibition of ejaculation.

Clonidine

Clonidine is used in higher dosage as an antihypertensive agent, and in lower dosage as a migraine prophylactic (Stensrud and Sjaastad, 1976).

Chemistry

Clonidine hydrochloride (MW 266.57) is an imidazoline derivative. The hydrochloride is soluble in water and in the more polar organic solvents.

Pharmacology

Biochemical Pharmacology

Clonidine is an α-adrenergic stimulating agent which also has α-adrenergic blocking activity. In different peripheral tissues it appears to inhibit noradrenaline and acetylcholine release from nerve terminals. In the rat brain stem it increases concentration of serotonin (Maj et al., 1973).

Pharmacodynamics

Low clonidine doses (below 10µg/kg) in cats appear to lower blood pressure by a direct vasodilating effect on vascular smooth muscle (Zamis and Hanington, 1969). However there is also evidence of an immediate vasoconstrictive action due to α-adrenergic stimulation (Anden et al., 1970). With higher doses medullary and hypothalamic level effects occur, leading to reduction of sympathetic nervous system activity, producing hypotension. The vasoactive properties of the drug led to a trial of its use in migraine.

Pharmacokinetics

Absorption and bioavailability: The data of Dollery et al. (1976) indicate that measurable quantities of clonidine appear in plasma 30 minutes after oral dosage and that peak plasma levels occur 1.5 hours after dosage. Rehbinder and Deckers (1969) stated that oral clonidine had a bioavailability of 65 to 95%.

Distribution: The mean apparent V_D in man is $3.94 \pm 0.94L/kg$, suggesting substantial binding of the drug to tissues. About 20% of the drug in plasma is said to be protein-bound.

Elimination: The plasma half-life of clonidine in man is 12.7 ± 7 hours and its clearance $22.44 \pm 9.12L/hour$ (Dollery et al., 1976). The latter values suggest that elimination of clonidine in man involves either biotransformation or active renal tubular excretion, or both, but little detail is available. Some two-thirds of a clonidine dose is said to be excreted in urine (53% unchanged) and one-third in faeces.

Interactions

Pharmacodynamic interactions: Tricyclic antidepressants antagonise the antihypertensive actions of clonidine by blocking its uptake at receptors and other sites (Connolly, 1973). The effect of tricyclic antidepressants on the migraine-preventing action of clonidine is unknown.

Pharmacokinetic interactions: No information is available. Thus far clonidine plasma levels have been measured only by GC-MS techniques, and these are not widely available.

Toxicity

Idiosyncratic Toxicity

Allergic reactions including rashes, pruritus and angioneurotic oedema, have been recorded.

Dose-related Toxicity

The more common side effects of clonidine, when the drug has been used in low dosage for migraine prophylaxis, are:

a) drowsiness
b) dry mouth
c) nausea and vomiting
d) agitation
e) depression
f) palpitation; flushing
g) faintness and hypotension.

Rebound hypertension may occur if clonidine therapy for hypertension is stopped abruptly (Conolly, 1973). This problem does not appear to have been recorded in relation to the lower drug doses used in migraine prophylaxis.

Dysmorphogenicity
No data are available as to human dysmorphogenicity of the drug.

Treatment of Migraine

Treatment of Acute Attacks

The neurologist may sometimes be called on to treat a patient *during an acute at-tack of migraine.* If the patient is seen at an early phase of the attack, and previous attacks have been severe, an intravenous or intramuscular injection of 0.25mg ergotamine (or 0.5mg if the patient has tolerated this dose before) may produce speedy relief. The intravenous route is likely to be more effective than the intramuscular. If nausea and/or vomiting are severe, an intramuscular injection of 12.5mg prochlorperazine or 50mg cyclizine may be necessary.

More often the patient is seen when severe headache has already been present for several hours. In general, the longer the headache has been present before the patient is seen, the more likely it is that the vasodilatation mechanisms will have given way to neck muscle contraction as the dominant factor in causing the headache. Consequently parenteral ergotamine is less likely to be effective, and it may be necessary to use strong analgesics to provide relief (e.g. intramuscular pentazocine 60mg). If at all possible other narcotics should be avoided because of the fear that their successful use may set the patient on the pathway to narcotic dependence.

As well as providing adequate analgesia in a rapidly available form when the patient has endured severe migraine for several hours, it is often wise to sedate the sufferer so that he can sleep through the remainder of the attack. Parenteral diazepam 5 to 10mg may be used or, if there is much nausea, parenteral chlorpromazine 50 to 100mg or a sedative antihistaminic with anti-emetic actions (e.g. intramuscular promethazine 50mg). In trying to relieve a severe migraine attack parenteral therapy is nearly always needed as the absorption of orally administered drugs cannot be relied on, as explained earlier.

In a very much more commonly encountered situation the neurologist is called on to advise the patient how to manage acute attacks of migraine when the patient is *seen during a headache-free interval.* Probably the most important point is to ensure that the patient understands the need to treat his attacks as early as possible. There is a widespread belief among the general public that analgesic drugs should not be taken unless pain is so severe that relief is imperative. For pain in general this belief may be valid, but in migraine it very often leads to therapeutic failure: increasingly frequent migraine develops and may lead to excessive analgesic intake, sometimes with consequent renal damage.

Migraine attacks may be treated with analgesics or with ergotamine. An analgesic such as aspirin probably does not function only as an analgesic in migraine;

it may also interrupt facets of the migraine mechanism (e.g serotonin release from platelets, prostaglandin synthesis in various sites). Therefore the earlier aspirin is taken the greater the chance it may interrupt the migraine mechanism before that mechanism has become so advanced that the attack must run its course. Early ergotamine administration also is desirable, since this drug may also have effects on serotoninergic mechanisms. The earlier ergotamine is used during the vasodilating phase of migraine the lower the ergotamine dose that is likely to be effective. Further, as explained above, the development of gastric atony as a migraine attack evolves can seriously delay oral therapy from reaching the absorptive surfaces of the small intestine. Hence therapy early in the attack is desirable to increase the chances of efficient drug absorption, allowing interruption of the migraine mechanism.

Aspirin

When the patient treats his own migraine attacks the drug of first choice is probably aspirin. Speed of action is essential. Therefore use of one of the soluble aspirins is preferable and there may be some value in dissolving the drug in a small volume of water before swallowing it. The patient should take the aspirin as soon as he recognises a migraine attack has begun. At this stage the headache is often mild and the patient may consider that only a small dose of aspirin (e.g. 300mg) would be necessary for analgesia. However he should be made to realise that aspirin is not being used merely as an analgesic in these circumstances and that if a sufficient portion of this first aspirin dose is not absorbed there is little chance that enough aspirin will be absorbed from subsequent doses to relieve the migraine at a more advanced stage of its evolution. Therefore the patient should take a larger initial aspirin dose (e.g. 600 to 900mg or more) than appears necessary in relation to the severity of the pain at the time of dosage. He should recognise that there is probably little point in his attempting to take subsequent aspirin doses during the attack.

One wonders whether the problems of analgesic nephropathy in persons with recurrent headache are due to low initial analgesic doses at the onset of migraine, with repeated larger doses which fail to be absorbed during the next few hours. Finally, when the migraine is over and alimentary motility returns, there may be absorption of the whole accumulated dose (unless some has been vomited). This intake of analgesic may overload the liver's biotransformation capacity for a time and there may be large amounts of unmetabolised analgesic (e.g. salicylate) excreted into the renal tubular fluid. The patient may also be rather dehydrated after not having taken any fluids for many hours because of his nausea during the migraine. Because of this dehydration and the consequent conservation of water, there may be very high concentrations of salicylic acid and other analgesics in the distal renal tubules and collecting tubules, with the risk of chemically induced renal damage.

Anti-emetics

Because many patients with migraine regularly have troublesome nausea (and vomiting) during their attacks, it may be useful to prescribe an oral anti-emetic (e.g.

metoclopramide 10mg; prochlorperazine 10mg; thiethylperazine 6.5mg or meclozine 25mg) at the time the initial aspirin dose is taken. Metoclopramide probably has advantages over the other centrally acting anti-emetics in these circumstances. If the drug is absorbed it will increase gastric motility and hence expedite the passage of aspirin to the small intestine, where it can be absorbed. Volans (1975) has shown that intramuscular metoclopramide is useful in this way, though intramuscular thiethylperazine is not (Wainscott et al., 1976). However intramuscular injection usually is not a practicable route of treatment when the patient has to manage his own therapy. From experience one suspects that orally administered metoclopramide often fails to be absorbed quickly during attacks of migraine. Gastric atony probably delays its entry to the small intestine and, being a base, metoclopramide is unlikely to be absorbed till it reaches the non-acidic pH of the small intestine. In this circumstance metoclopramide would be less likely to be absorbed than aspirin. In theory aspirin would be absorbed to some extent from the acidic environment of the stomach, though its relatively low solubility at acid pH reduces the amount of non-ionised drug in solution and thus available for absorption. Information is needed on the absorption characteristics of metoclopramide during migraine and the possibilities of its sublingual and rectal absorption might be worth exploring.

Ergotamine

Should oral aspirin fail to stop the patient's migraine attacks (or oral paracetamol in patients intolerant of aspirin) it will probably be necessary to use ergotamine. This drug should be used with caution, particularly in patients with peripheral or coronary arterial disease, and it is wise to use a low dose (e.g. 1mg orally) the first time it is taken, in case the patient is one of those rare individuals whose vasculature is hypersensitive to the vasospastic effects of the drug. When oral ergotamine is used the considerations which apply are very similar to those which apply for aspirin. The initial dose should be taken as early as possible in the attack and should be taken in the knowledge that it is this dose of ergotamine that is most likely to be effective in that attack. Patients are often told to take 1 or 2mg ergotamine orally (alone, or in a combined preparation with caffeine and/or an anti-emetic) at the onset of migraine, with repeated 1mg doses every 30 to 60 minutes, usually to a limit of 4 or 6mg ergotamine. Such patients almost always report that either the first dose works, or that the whole regimen fails (or produces such delayed benefit that one suspects the migraine has simply followed out its natural history). The patient should find by experience the initial oral ergotamine dose that is usually effective for his migraine. Thereafter he should take this dose as soon as he realises that an attack has begun. This dose usually proves to lie between 2 and 4mg. If this ergotamine dose fails in a particular attack it is unlikely that the patient will be able to do much more to relieve that attack. If preparations are used in which ergotamine is combined with caffeine and perhaps with an antihistamine, it is sometimes found that a sufficient ergotamine dose cannot be taken because of side effects of the other drugs in the preparation. In this circumstance use of separate preparations of the various drugs permits dosage flexibility and may produce a better therapeutic effect.

It appears logical to combine oral ergotamine with an oral non-narcotic analgesic (e.g. aspirin, paracetamol, dextropropoxyphene) in an attempt to relieve pain by more than one method. Oral anti-emetics may be added to ergotamine therapy. Metoclopramide has theoretical advantages, but the same considerations apply as were discussed above in relation to the use of metoclopramide with aspirin. It is sometimes said that oral ergotamine intake should not exceed 12mg per week. The validity of this figure is open to doubt, but if the policy is adopted of using a single 2 to 4mg ergotamine initial dose and not repeating it in the attack there is little chance that as much as 12mg will be taken in any one week.

Alternatives to Oral Drugs

Some patients with migraine rapidly develop nausea and vomiting, either as soon as their attacks begin or immediately they swallow medication. Others wake with attacks already well established or, for various reasons, do not start therapy immediately the attack has begun. In such patients oral treatment is unlikely to be successful because of drug absorption problems. However ergotamine can be given as a rectal suppository. The rectal route should avoid the problems of poor absorption associated with nausea and vomiting and should reduce the amount of any first-pass hepatic metabolism of the drug. Sometimes suppositories are effective when oral therapy is not, but often rectal ergotamine proves unsatisfactory and this mode of administration is inconvenient. The scanty experimental data suggest that ergotamine is poorly absorbed from the small intestine and it seems likely that rectal absorption would be even less efficient. Aspirin absorption from the rectum is known to be poor, so that rectal therapy by no means answers the problems raised by altered alimentary motility and vomiting in migraine.

To overcome these problems attempts have been made to administer ergotamine sublingually, or by inhalation. These routes of administration avoid any first-pass hepatic inactivation of part of the dose which might occur when the drug is swallowed. Unfortunately there is no evidence that ergotamine is efficiently absorbed from either of these routes. Both methods of administration could lead to much of the dose finally being swallowed and eventually being absorbed from the small intestine. Sublingual and inhaled ergotamine sometimes appear effective but usually in those patients in whom oral ergotamine is useful.

Secondary Contraction Headache

If the above therapy fails to relieve a patient's migraine attack he has the alternatives of enduring his pain till it subsides or of seeking further treatment from his doctor, as discussed earlier. It is worth telling the patient that the vascular events of migraine have nearly always run their course within 24 hours of the onset of headache. Any pain which persists longer than this is usually due to secondary neck muscle contraction headache. This will not respond to migraine therapy but is likely to respond to measures designed to relieve contraction headache, as discussed previously (p.254-255). Use of these measures may avoid the need to give narcotics. Contraction headache may become the dominant source of pain much earlier in the migraine attack.

Prevention of Migraine

The above measures may be successful in relieving a patient's migraine attacks; not infrequently they fail. If so, and if the cause of the failure cannot be remedied, the neurologist should consider the question of prophylactic therapy. While non-pharmacological preventative measures should be explored, even in infrequent migraine, attacks which are not relieved by treatment and which recur more often than once or twice a month usually warrant continuous preventative drug therapy, or, occasionally, preventative drug therapy restricted to times of high risk.

Non-pharmacological Measures

Some of the factors which may precipitate migraine attacks in susceptible persons have been mentioned already (p.257). If such factors can be identified in a patient, and it is possible for him to avoid them, he may have less migraine. Thus a patient may be willing to forgo eating foods such as chocolate, cream, oranges or nuts, or to deny himself red wine, or alcohol in general. A woman may seek an alternative to using a hormonal contraceptive pill, particularly avoiding one with high oestrogen content. However it is often difficult to alter the various 'stress' situations which may precipitate migraine without radical alterations in the patient's life style. The neurologist who recommends a change of employment in the hope of alleviating a patient's migraine takes a heavy burden of responsibility on himself.

In practice, the attempt to seek out and remove precipitating factors does not often appear to help patients with migraine.

Intermittent Preventative Drug Therapy

A minority of patients with migraine get their attacks, or most of their attacks, at times which they come to recognise as their own peculiar high risk ones. Examples are migraine provoked by strenuous exertion (e.g. football), by circumstances where excitement is likely, and menstrual migraine. If individuals with such patterns of migraine take a relatively low dose of aspirin (e.g. 300mg) or ergotamine (1mg) orally an hour or so before exposure to the precipitating circumstance, often the expected migraine will not develop. If the timing of the precipitant cannot be so accurately determined (e.g. in menstrual migraine) repeated doses of aspirin or ergotamine may be given 3 times a day for 2 to 4 days around the time of high risk. This method of prevention is perhaps less successful than prevention when the time of risk can be more exactly determined. Sometimes it seems merely to postpone the migraine till prophylaxis ceases. Somerville (1975b) has shown that it is possible to prevent menstrual migraine by implanting oestrogens so that ovulation is suppressed. However some subjects got more migraine overall, while using this therapy. The problems that arise from continued oestrogen (or progesterone) therapy are such that hormonal treatment would rarely be an acceptable method of managing menstrual migraine.

Continuous Drug Prophylaxis of Migraine

In most patients, if migraine attacks occur frequently they also occur unpredictably. In such circumstances prophylactic drugs should be taken continuously. The drugs discussed below are dealt with in the order in which a neurologist might choose to use them in practice.

Antiserontonin antihistaminics: For many patients methdilazine, cyproheptadine and pizotifen appear roughly equivalent as migraine preventatives. In some, one drug is clearly preferable to the others but on the whole methdilazine may have slight advantages in that it is the cheapest and probably has the least tendency to increase appetite. The approximate equivalent doses are methdilazine 4 to 8mg, cyproheptadine 4mg and pizotifen 0.5mg. There is too little pharmacokinetic knowledge about the drugs to develop rational therapeutic routines. The drugs usually are given as one dosage unit 2 or 3 times a day. They are certainly not always successful (Hubbe, 1973).

If benefit occurs it often seems to require 2 to 4 weeks of continuous dosage first. There is therefore a risk that therapy may be terminated before it has had time to work. Further, the dose which produces benefit varies widely from patient to patient, usually lying between 2 and 8 dosage units each day. It seems reasonable practice with these drugs to increase the dose by one dosage unit each month till such time as migraine comes under an acceptable degree of control, or until side effects (mostly drowsiness) become unacceptable. This process of slow dosage increase minimises the risk of using unnecessarily high doses, but can mean that there is a delay of several months till benefit occurs. However, till proper plasma level-therapeutic response correlations are established for these drugs it is difficult to rationalise their use further. If the drugs are used in standard dosage regimens of one tablet 3 times a day there will be many therapeutic failures, but if dosages are increased slowly the ultimate response often is a good deal better. If one drug fails to relieve a patient's migraine when the dose is taken to its limit of tolerance, it is worth trying a second member of this group before using drugs with different mechanisms of action. If these antiserotonin agents control a patient's migraine for 2 or 3 months it may then be possible to find a new minimum dose which continues to hold the migraine in check. Because benefit seems to carry over for about 4 weeks after a dose reduction it is unwise to reduce the dose too rapidly or the migraine may flare into activity unexpectedly.

When patients begin taking these agents they should be warned that the treatment may increase appetite and lead to weight gain. If patients deliberately restrain their food intake during the first 2 or 3 weeks of therapy the increased appetite seems to subside and weight gain is avoided.

Clonidine: If the antiserotonin antihistaminics fail, clonidine might well be the next drug tried, though the authors' experience with it has not been very encouraging when the antiserotonin drugs have failed. Anthony et al. (1972) also did not appear to find the drug particularly impressive and Ryan et al. (1975) and Sillanpaa (1977) found it little or no better than a placebo. In the doses used to treat migraine, clonidine appears to be a very safe drug with relatively mild side effects (e.g. drowsiness, dry mouth). The initial clonidine dose is 25µg 3 times a day or 50µg twice daily. At intervals of 2 to 3 weeks, or longer, doses are increased by 25µg daily to a limit of 150µg daily, beyond which it is said further benefit does not occur (Wilkinson, 1972). The study of Stensrud and Sjaastad (1976) suggested that the beneficial effects of clonidine decreased with time.

β-Adrenergic blockers: Propranolol (Ludvigsson, 1974; Borgesen et al., 1974; Stensrud and Sjaastad, 1976a) and pindolol (Anthony et al., 1972) have been found useful in migraine prophylaxis. Either drug is given 2 or 3 times a day, initially in total daily doses of 60 or 80mg for propranolol, or 10 to 15mg for pindolol. In children Ludvigsson (1974) used propranolol in a dose of 1mg/kg 3 times a day. Every week or fortnight dosage may be increased as necessary to control migraine, or until side effects preclude further increase. Little has been published on the upper dosage limits for β-blockers in the treatment of migraine or on the correlation between their plasma levels and the degree of migraine prevention. Till this knowledge is available migraine prophylactic therapy with β-blockers must be adjusted on clinical grounds only.

Amitriptyline: There have been at least two reports that this drug is an effective migraine preventative (Gomersall and Stuart, 1973; Couch et al., 1976). The average dose used by the latter authors was 75mg at night, though Gomersall and Stuart (1973) found 10 to 60mg at night adequate. Pharmacokinetic knowledge about the tricyclic antidepressants, and the wide scatter of plasma drug levels at any given dose, suggest that higher or lower doses might confer greater benefit in migraine prophylaxis. It seems likely that the drug would need to be used for several weeks to produce benefit.

While amitriptyline is a dangerous drug in overdosage (p.254), it has been widely used for some years as an antidepressant. Therefore it might be reasonable to use amitriptyline in migraine if the migraine preventatives already mentioned have failed.

Methysergide: Though methysergide is an antiserotonin agent its side effects are both more frequent and potentially very much more severe than those of the antiserotonin antihistaminics. The more vigorously antiserotonin antihistaminics are used in migraine prophylaxis, the less often it appears necessary to use methysergide, though the latter is probably more effective as a migraine preventative (Lance et al., 1970). The initial methysergide dose is 1mg 2 to 4 times a day. As with the other antiserotonin agents, dosage increases should be made not more frequently than at 3 or 4-week intervals. Dosage is increased till migraine control is obtained or until side effects preclude further increase. Patients taking methysergide should be followed closely, their blood pressures checked, and evidence of cardiac or renal damage sought. The drug should not be used for more than 6 months continuously without being withdrawn for 1 to 2 months. If methysergide has conferred benefit it is often possible to replace the drug with an antiserotonin antihistamine and maintain the benefit. When methysergide produces benefit its dosage should be reduced as soon as possible, to try to find the minimum dose that will maintain migraine control. Dose reductions are best made at monthly intervals.

Monoamine oxidase inhibitors: If all the above drugs fail one may have to consider using a monoamine oxidase inhibitor such as phenelzine 15mg 3 times a day. In the authors' view such a drug should be used only in reliable patients who will follow the necessary restrictions as to diet and intake of other drugs, and who can be kept under close supervision.

Treatment of Certain Migraine Situations

Mixed Headache

Sometimes patients present with a history of months or years of increasingly frequent migraine attacks which have culminated in the situation where the neck muscle contraction headache which follows one migraine attack does not have time to settle before the next migraine arrives. Such patients complain of continuous headache, sometimes with exacerbations, but it is only when the earlier history of migraine attacks is obtained that the true nature of the situation is likely to be recognised *viz* that the patient has 'mixed' headache i.e. migraine plus contraction headache.

Therapy requires separate measures designed to deal with each of the types of headache. The contraction headache is treated along the lines already indicated (p. 254-255), while aspirin and/or ergotamine are used for any headache exacerbations, as these are likely to be migrainous. While such a combined regimen may provide perfectly satisfactory results commonly, as the contraction headache settles (or fails to settle if there is too much migraine exacerbating the situation), it becomes apparent that there are many more migraine attacks than had appeared likely earlier. It is then necessary to apply migraine prophylactic measures as well in order to control the overall situation.

Migraine in Childhood

Children with migraine are often brought to the neurologist for diagnosis rather than for treatment. The public in general is not aware that children can get migraine. Children's migraine attacks are frequently relatively short lived and treatment with oral aspirin or paracetamol is often all that is required. It is practically never necessary to use ergotamine.

When attacks are frequent enough, and severe enough, preventative treatment may be necessary. While drugs employed for preventing adult migraine could be used, there are reservations about using antiserotonin agents in children because they may inhibit growth hormone release (Smythe and Lazarus, 1974) leading to possible growth suppression. In general one would prefer to use drugs with the least likelihood of side effects and the least severe side effects. However anticonvulsants, notably phenytoin, alone or in combination and in doses comparable to those used in treating epilepsy (p. 220), often prove effective in preventing childhood migraine and make the use of other agents unnecessary. Curiously, this migraine-preventing action of anticonvulsants seems to cease to apply after the age of about 12 years, except in a few rather uncommon varieties of migraine, discussed below.

Some years ago, prochlorperazine (5 to 10mg daily, depending on body weight), enjoyed a vogue as a migraine prophylactic, particularly in childhood, but there seems to have been little recent interest in its use.

Continuing Migraine

Rarely the vasodilatation element in a migraine attack persists for several days or weeks (or one migraine attack succeeds another at such short intervals that the patient appears to have a continuous vasodilatation headache). This situation should be distinguished from the much more common one of mixed migraine and contraction headache. Continuing migraine may at times respond to a sufficient dose of intramuscular or intravenous ergotamine, but the degree of local oedema and inflammatory response in and around the dilated scalp vessels may make anti-inflammatory agents necessary. At times aspirin or indomethacin may produce relief but corticosteroids appear to offer more reliable benefit. Bearing in mind the degree of discomfort commonly experienced in continuing migraine, it is probably reasonable to give oral prednisone 10mg 3 or 4 times a day, or equivalent doses of another steroid, once the diagnosis of continuing migraine is made and an intravenous dose of ergotamine fails to bring relief. Analgesics of adequate strength are needed till the steroids have time to work. Once the continuing migraine is controlled (usually in 1 to 3 days), steroid dosage can be reduced fairly rapidly and the question of migraine prophylaxis considered if the past history of migraine indicates it.

'Hemiparaesthetic' Migraine

This variety of migraine is sometimes called 'hemiplegic' migraine, though this is a misnomer except in the occasional instance when true paralysis occurs. The aura comprises manifestations of ischaemia in the middle cerebral artery territory of supply (paraesthesia in the contralateral hand, spreading to the face, with expressive dysphasia if the dominant hemisphere is involved) with or without consequences of ischaemia in the posterior cerebral artery (contralateral visual field disturbances).

Patients with this type of migraine often present for diagnosis, rather than for treatment. Some writers have had reservations about the use of ergotamine in this type of migraine, fearing that the vasospastic action of the drug may convert temporary brain ischaemia into permanent cerebral infarction (Dunlop, 1969). Whether these fears are justified is uncertain, but Weil (1952) showed that rapidly acting barbiturates may shorten attacks of migraine of this type. Oral quinalbarbitone (50 or 100mg) at the onset of such attacks avoids the potential problems of ergotamine and is often effective.

Oral anticonvulsants, particularly phenytoin, taken regularly in doses comparable with, or rather lower than those used for epilepsy, nearly always provide highly effective prevention of this type of migraine.

Basilar Artery Migraine

Migraine with a visual aura (due to posterior cerebral artery territory ischaemia) is a manifestation of migraine within the territory of supply of the basilar artery. However in practice the term 'basilar artery migraine' is usually applied to those varieties of migraine in which the aura comprises consequences of brain stem ischaemia, notably vertigo. For such migraine, prophylaxis with anticonvulsants, or anticonvulsant combinations, often proves effective.

Migraine in Which the Main Problem is the Aura

Occasionally a patient has little or no headache in his migraine attacks but is distressed by his aura and seeks treatment for it. In these circumstances a rapidly acting vasodilator (e.g. sublingual glyceryltrinitrate 100 or 150µg) may terminate the aura quickly, though sometimes at the cost of exaggerating the subsequent headache.

Periodic Migrainous Neuralgia — Cluster Headache

Although this disorder bears a close affinity to migraine there are certain features which suggest that it is a separate entity e.g. its peculiar temporal profile, its seemingly different biochemical background, and its much less definite genetic background (Sutherland and Eadie, 1973).

Disordered Mechanisms

The factors which produce the peculiar time pattern of the clusters of attacks of migrainous neuralgia are uncertain. They are discussed by Anthony (1972). In individual attacks it is believed there is an initial phase of intense spasm in the infraclinoid section of the internal carotid artery on one side. This may cause temporary paralysis of the cervical sympathetic supply, producing a Horner's syndrome. This vasospastic phase, itself often clinically silent, is followed by relatively sudden vaso-dilatation in the carotid branches supplying the forehead and temple on the same side. This may cause severe headache which usually lasts between 0.5 and 3 hours. When clusters are present, but not at other times, attacks are consistently produced by the intake of alcohol, or by the injection of histamine. Anthony and Lance (1971) have shown that plasma histamine levels increase during attacks of migrainous neuralgia (though not in migraine attacks).

Correction of Disordered Mechanisms

Precipitating causes, in particular alcohol, can be avoided. Antihistamines were said not to be useful as they do not influence tissue histamine levels (Anthony, 1972). However, more recent work suggested that both histamine type I blocking agents (e.g. mepyramine), and type II blocking agents (e.g. cimetidine) might relieve migrainous neuralgia in some, but not in all, patients (Piper et al., 1977). Ergotamine given parenterally, and occasionally orally, may abort attacks if given at their commencement.

Attacks of migrainous neuralgia usually develop very rapidly and are relatively short lived. Therefore patients nearly always find that self-administered drug treatment taken at the onset of their attacks usually is of no value. Empirically it has been found that the regular intake of ergotamine, or of antiserotonin agents, will protect against attacks. Recently it has been claimed that prednisone therapy is effective (Jammes, 1975). How these various agents interrupt the migrainous neuralgia mechanism is not known.

Drugs Used in Migrainous Neuralgia

The majority of these drugs have been dealt with earlier in the present chapter (ergotamine, methysergide, the antiserotonin antihistaminics), and prednisone was considered on page 33.

Drug Treatment of Migrainous Neuralgia

As previously mentioned, the treatment of migrainous neuralgia is essentially prophylactic.

Symonds (1956) popularised the use of ergotamine in preventing attacks of migrainous neuralgia, though Ekbom (1947) had earlier suggested this treatment. Symonds recommended that ergotamine should be given intramuscularly 3 times a day and, when attacks had been prevented for 5 to 7 days, therapy should be omitted to see if the cluster was over. If not, attacks were controlled with ergotamine for another week and then the effect of ergotamine withdrawal was ascertained. This process continued till the patient remained free from attacks. It is usually unnecessary to inject ergotamine (Sutherland and Eadie, 1972). If the patient with migrainous neuralgia is treated before his attacks have been present for too long, in the majority of instances an oral ergotamine dose of 1mg 3 or 4 times a day will stop the attacks promptly. After one week of treatment the ergotamine can be withdrawn, often without relapse of the pain. If the pain recurs, oral ergotamine is used for another week or so. The protective action of an ergotamine dose appears to last for about 6 hours in migrainous neuralgia. Sometimes higher ergotamine doses are needed. Occasionally, if attacks occur at a fixed hour each day, as they may do, a single 2mg ergotamine dose 1 or 2 hours before the expected attack may be all that is required. Naturally the patient should be watched for ergotamine side effects, but these are quite infrequent when one considers the extent of ergotamine intake.

Should ergotamine fail to control migrainous neuralgia, as sometimes occurs when treatment of a cluster has been delayed for many months, various antiserotonin migraine prophylactics may be used in the same way in which they are used in migraine. These agents do not appear to be as effective as ergotamine in preventing attacks of migrainous neuralgia. The present authors have found oral ergotamine generally satisfactory and do not have the experience to assess the report of Jammes (1975) that prednisone will prevent attacks of migrainous neuralgia and that, in some cases, a single 30mg dose will give relief for over 60 days. However the possibility of using this drug should be considered in recalcitrant cases. There are recent reports that long term lithium therapy may benefit chronic migrainous neuralgia (Ekbom, 1977; Kudrow, 1977).

It is worth pointing out that the use of strong analgesics, or narcotics, to relieve the pain of migrainous neuralgia is fraught with the danger of producing drug dependence.

Trigeminal Neuralgia

Disordered Mechanisms

Trigeminal neuralgia arises from processes which irritate the trigeminal nerve. The majority of cases are idiopathic (tic douloureux) though there have been increasing suggestions in neurosurgical literature that compression of the trigeminal root by aberrant blood vessels or arachnoid adhesions accounts for many of these instances. Pain similar to that of idiopathic tic douloureux can arise from a true trigeminal neuritis, from compressive lesions in the cerebello-pontine angle (e.g. acoustic neurinoma) and from disease affecting trigeminal fibres in the brain stem (e.g. multiple sclerosis).

Correction of Disordered Mechanisms

If trigeminal neuralgia is due to a lesion which requires treatment in its own right (e.g. an acoustic neurinoma) that lesion should be treated appropriately. In idiopathic cases measures which decrease the trigeminal afferent input into the trigeminal sensory nuclei appear to provide pain relief. Such measures include:

1) Use of the anticonvulsants carbamazepine, phenytoin or clonazepam (at least the first two of these inhibit trigeminal sensory conduction)
2) Damaging the trigeminal sensory root by:

   a) injection of alcohol locally
   b) direct surgical section.

Drugs Used in Treating Trigeminal Neuralgia

These were considered in the section on epilepsy (chapter VI).

Treatment of Trigeminal Neuralgia

Once it has been established that the patient's trigeminal neuralgia is idiopathic i.e. there is no causative process requiring treatment in its own right, the treatment of first choice for tic douloureux is carbamazepine. For the average adult an initial dose of 100mg 3 times a day may be rapidly increased over 3 or 4 days to 200mg thrice daily. Beyond this stage, pharmacokinetic considerations suggest that dosage should increase every 5 to 7 days as necessary to obtain pain relief. More frequent dose increments make it likely that the steady-state from one dosage had not been reached before dosage was increased again. However the need to control pain quickly may necessitate more rapid dose increases, if the patient is not unduly troubled by side effects. We have not seen tic douloureux controlled by carbamazepine plasma levels lower than 5μg/ml and sometimes much higher levels have been needed. Carbamazepine dosages up to 2000mg per day may be required. It has been suggested that tic douloureux is likely to go into remission once it is controlled by the drug, so that therapy may be discontinued until the disorder becomes active again. However in the authors' experience such a policy has sometimes led to tic douloureux becoming resistant to maximum tolerated carbamazepine doses, whereas if carbamazepine is used continuously from the outset, though the patient adjusts his dose to keep himself just pain free, the risk of later drug failure is lessened.

If patients cannot tolerate carbamazepine, phenytoin may be used in its place, though it is rather less effective. The average dose is 5mg/kg/day, but dosage may be taken to the patient's limit of tolerance if necessary to relieve the pain. Recent reports (e.g. Chandra, 1976; Court and Kase, 1976) suggest that clonazepam may be effective in tic douloureux even after carbamazepine has failed. An initial dose of 1mg twice daily may be increased progressively at intervals of 5 to 7 days till pain control is obtained or till further dose increase produces unacceptable side effects.

Once a patient with tic douloureux requires drug therapy he is likely to need this treatment permanently, though dosage should be kept as low as possible, consistent with adequate pain relief.

If drug treatment fails to relieve tic douloureux, surgical measures need to be considered. At present many surgeons prefer direct surgical exploration and selective section of the trigeminal root, reserving alcohol injection of the gasserian ganglion for very frail patients. Of course, the patient should realise that the operation will produce a degree of facial analgesia, with its attendant problems.

Other Neuralgias and Painful Neuropathies

Glossopharyngeal Neuralgia

Considerations as to aetiology and treatment are as for trigeminal neuralgia (Ekbom and Westerberg, 1966).

Supraorbital Neuralgia

Neuralgic pain in the supraorbital territory is most often due to injury to the nerve where it emerges at the eyebrow. There is no specific drug therapy but analgesics may give temporary relief. For more lasting alleviation surgical section of the nerve, or injection of local anaesthetic or alcohol into it, appears necessary.

(Greater) Occipital Neuralgia

Occipital neuralgia is usually due either to neck injuries or to prolonged severe posterior neck muscle spasm. If it does not respond to measures intended to relax neck muscle spasm (p.254-255) repeated injections of local anaesthetic into the affected nerve at the superior nuchal line may be necessary. If these fail, nerve section may be necessary to afford relief.

Post-herpetic Neuralgia

Such neuralgia may occur in the territory of any posterior root ganglion involved by herpes zoster. Older people are particularly at risk. There is no proven effective drug therapy, although there is a belief that carbamazepine may be helpful. However the evidence is doubtful (Killian and Fromm, 1968). Galbraith (1973) found that amantadine 100mg twice daily, given for 28 days from the onset of the rash, decreased the incidence of pain persisting for more than one month. In the first 6 months of the neuralgia a number of measures may be useful. The later the treatment is attempted the less satisfactory is the result. Measures such as local x-ray therapy, injections of vitamin B_{12} and the use of steroids have all enjoyed some vogue, but at the present time probably the most useful measures appear to be:

1) Repeated percussion of the tender areas (not the anaesthetic central zone, but its hyperaesthetic margins) for 10 minutes 4 times a day for several weeks
2) Repeated use of a vibrator on the tender areas for similar periods
3) Spraying the painful area repeatedly with cooling sprays e.g. ethyl chloride (Taverner, 1960) or certain fluorocarbon derivatives
4) Regional sympathetic blocks with local anaesthetic, and if these blocks are successful, regional sympathectomy
5) Operative procedures to relieve pain at a more central level.

Nathan and Wall (1974) have reported benefit in some cases from prolonged self-administered electrical stimulation, using a portable apparatus.

Painful Nerve Root Compression

This is most often due to herniated cervical or lumbar discs, with or without osteophyte formation, though other types of mechanical lesion may be responsible. The usual management is to prescribe adequate oral analgesics and to apply conservative orthopaedic measures. The results of investigations and the passage of time will determine whether additional orthopaedic and surgical measures are necessary. Green (1975) has reported rapid relief of pain due to proven herniation of lumbar discs by giving high dosage parenteral dexamethasone (60mg on the first day, with the dose decreasing to 8mg daily by the end of a week). It seems likely that oral doses of the same magnitude, or perhaps of a lesser magnitude, would be as useful.

Painful Peripheral Neuropathies

The pain of compression (entrapment) neuropathies can nearly always be relieved by surgical relief of the compression. As an interim measure local injection of a slowly dissolving corticosteroid (e.g. prednisolone methylacetate) may produce several weeks of relief by diminishing any local oedema and inflammatory response.

For all other painful forms of peripheral neuropathy usually all that can be offered are analgesics (avoiding narcotics because of the problems of tolerance and drug dependence) and attempted correction of the underlying disorder, (e.g. diabetes mellitus) if this can be identified. Chakrabarti and Samantaray (1976) reported relief of pain and sensory symptoms in diabetic peripheral neuropathy, following the use of carbamazepine.

Causalgia

Causalgic pain after peripheral nerve or nerve root injuries may at times be relieved by α-adrenergic blocking agents (e.g. phenoxybenzamine). However the disorder often requires regional sympathectomy (if a test regional sympathetic block with local anaesthetic provides temporary relief).

Tabetic 'Lightning' Pains

There are reports that carbamazepine will control these pains (Killian and Fromm, 1968; Ekbom, 1972).

Painful Crises in Fabry's Disease

The painful crises in this condition are said to respond to carbamazepine (Shibasaki et al., 1973). Phenytoin may also be tried.

Temporo-mandibular Joint Pain

Disorders of the symmetry of the bite, often secondary to missing teeth or to persistent grinding down of the teeth on one side, can cause severe continuous pain over the whole temple and masseteric area, though centred on the jaw joint and external ear canal. The definitive treatment of this disorder is based on dental measures to correct the bite disturbance. Medically all that can be offered are explanation and reassurance and the prescription of analgesics and muscle spasm relieving drugs (e.g. diazepam), to help relax the temporalis, masseteric and pterygoid muscle spasm (which causes much of the pain), till the dental measures have time to take effect.

Chapter VIII

Disorders of Sleep

Principal Disorders and Drugs Discussed

Narcolepsy and catalepsy
  Amphetamines
  Imipramine

Insomnia
  Nitrazepam (see also chapter VI)

Sleep disorder is relatively uncommon as a neurological presenting symptom though very many patients complain of incidental insomnia.

Narcolepsy and Insomnia

Disordered Mechanisms

The regulation of alertness appears to be a function of the mesodiencephalic reticular formation, which projects diffusely to the neocortex. When sleep disturbance is due to local disease related to these pathways, that disease is nearly always located in the region around the third ventricle. Sleep disturbance may involve the occurrence of too much sleep, or too little sleep. Other disturbances of brain function may occur in association with alterations of sleep.

The syndromes involving too much sleep include:

1) Narcolepsy. This may be idiopathic, hereditary (in males) or due to disease (e.g. trauma, tumour, or encephalitis) affecting the region around the third ventricle. In narcolepsy, sufferers pass very rapidly from wakefulness to REM sleep, without going through the normal period of non-REM sleep.

2) Various forms of parasomnia or hypersomnia, perhaps associated with hyperphagia (e.g. Klein-Levin syndrome).

Too little sleep (insomnia) has numerous causes, many of them psychological, some of them painful.

The disorders associated with sleep disturbance include cataplexy, sleep paralysis, sleep walking and hypnagogic hallucinations. Cataplexy appears to occur only in association with narcolepsy.

Pharmacological evidence suggests that increased alertness is associated with increased catecholamine-mediated transmission in the mesodiencephalic reticular formation. There is experimental evidence that increased serotonin concentrations in the brain stem can be associated with the production of sleep (Wyler et al., 1975).

Correction of Disordered Mechanisms

It is possible to correct excessive drowsiness, as in narcolepsy, by using agents which increase noradrenaline activity in the mesodiencephalic reticular formation. This effect can be obtained from drugs which displace noradrenaline from storage sites in nerve terminals (e.g. amphetamine), or which prevent the re-uptake of noradrenaline which has already been released (e.g. imipramine). The latter group of agents also prove of some use in relieving cataplexy, perhaps because of their action in blocking serotonin re-uptake by axon terminals. The serotonin antagonist methysergide is also reported to correct narcolepsy (Wyler et al., 1975).

Many agents which depress the function of the nervous system can be used to relieve insomnia. Some of these agents (e.g. nitrazepam) act on amine-mediated transmission at synapses in the regions around the third ventricle.

Drugs Used for Treating Sleep Disorders

Amphetamine and Dexamphetamine

The recommended uses of amphetamine and dexamphetamine are now for treating narcolepsy and cataplexy and hyperkinetic behaviour disorders in children. However, the drugs have also been used to depress appetite and as a stimulant to combat fatigue. These latter uses are discouraged because of the higher risk of drug dependence.

Chemistry

Amphetamine (racemic β-phenylisopropylamine; MW 135.20) (fig. 8.1) is a basic liquid which is slightly soluble in water. The corresponding sulphate is

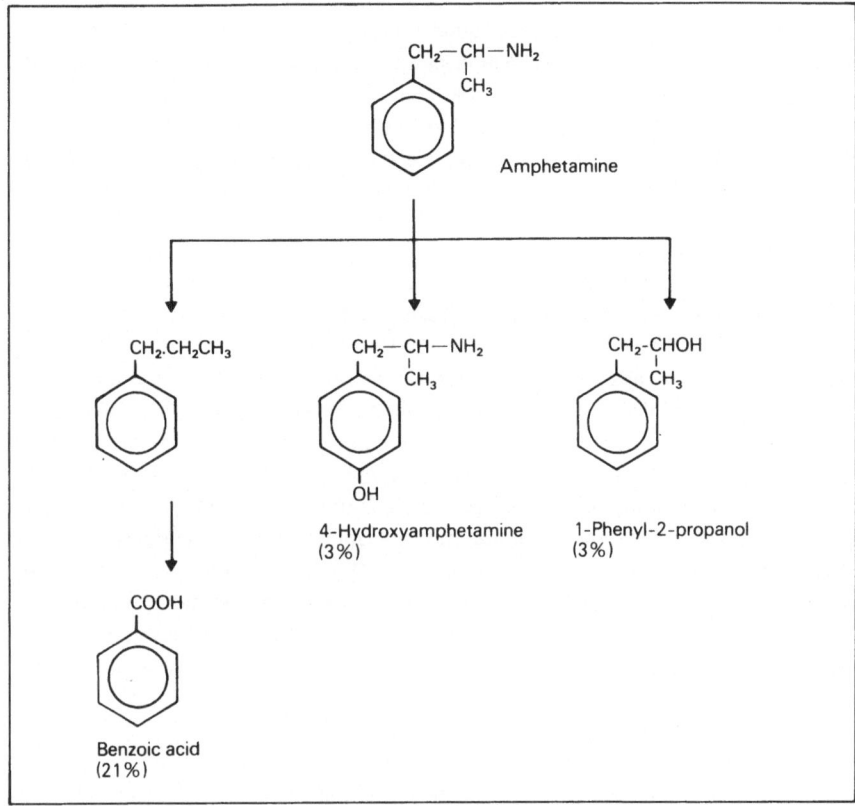

$Fig. 8.1$. The biotransformation of amphetamine (figures in parentheses are those of Dring et. al., 1970).

crystalline. Dexamphetamine is the d-isomer of amphetamine. Dexamphetamine also is usually prescribed as the sulphate, which is crystalline. The pKa of amphetamine is 9.93.

Pharmacology

Biochemical Pharmacology

Amphetamine and dexamphetamine are taken up by the amine-uptake pumping mechanisms in central and peripheral nerve terminals. In terminals these drugs competitively displace catecholamines from storage granules. The release of noradrenaline from noradrenergic neurones is more sensitive to amphetamine than is the release of dopamine from dopaminergic neurones (Azzaro and Rutledge, 1973). D-amphetamine also inhibits dopamine uptake into synaptosomes from certain regions of rat brain (Horn et al., 1974). Amphetamine and dexamphetamine reversibly inhibit the enzyme monoamine oxidase, particularly the A species of the enzyme (Mantle et al., 1976). Amphetamine also inhibits phosphatidylcholine synthesis in brain at the cytidine diphosphorylcholine diglyceride transferase stage (Hitzeman and Loh, 1973).

Pharmacodynamics

Amphetamine and dexamphetamine have α and β-adrenergic agonist actions. They raise systolic and diastolic blood pressure and in high doses may cause cardiac arrhythmia. They have some bronchodilator effect and increase the tone of the bladder sphincter. The drugs stimulate the central nervous system at several levels, producing heightened alertness, increased capacity for mental and physical activity, tremor, restlessness, excitement, mood elevation and agitation and insomnia. In relation to central nervous system stimulation, d-amphetamine has 3 to 4 times the potency of l-amphetamine and therefore 1.5 to 2 times the potency of racemic d-l amphetamine. Amphetamine facilitates monosynaptic and polysynaptic transmission in the spinal cord and may stimulate the respiratory centre which is depressed by drugs. Amphetamine and dexamphetamine act on the hypothalamus to suppress appetite. Amphetamine increases plasma concentrations of free fatty acids in man and at times causes a small increase in oxygen consumption, possibly because it produces restlessness.

Pharmacokinetics

Absorption and bioavailability: Amphetamine and dexamphetamine are absorbed after oral administration. Maximum plasma levels of dexamphetamine occur 1.75 hours after oral administration (Beckett et al., 1969) or after 2 hours (Rowland, 1969).

Distribution: In the dog, plasma and CSF dexamphetamine levels were equal 1 hour after intraperitoneal administration of the drug; brain, liver, lung, kidney and spleen had drug levels 8 to 17 times those of plasma, while amphetamine levels in body fat were lower than those of plasma (Axelrod, 1954). Findings in the rat were reasonably similar (Maickel et al., 1969). Data for plasma protein binding in man are lacking but the findings in the dog cited above suggest there is little binding.

Elimination: The pattern of elimination of amphetamine is highly dependent on urine pH. The drug has a pKa value of 9.9. Hence the more acid the urine the greater the ionisation of any amphetamine in the urine. Ionised amphetamine does not resorb passively as water resorbs in the renal tubules. Under certain conditions the renal clearance of amphetamine can be virtually that of inulin, i.e. 120mg/min (Rowland, 1969). In hyperactive children the half-life of amphetamine averaged 7 hours (range 4 to 32 hours; Firemark et al., 1977). Anggard et al. (1973) showed that, in man, the half-life of amphetamine was 7 to 14 hours when urine pH was below 6.6 and 18 to 34 hours when urine pH was above 6.7. At urine pH values below 6.6 some 67 to 73 % of the amphetamine dose was excreted in urine unchanged, whereas with more alkaline urine 17 to 43 % of the dose was excreted unchanged. That portion of the amphetamine dose which is not excreted unchanged is excreted after biotransformation. The pattern of biotransformation is species dependent but in man appears to follow the pathways shown in figure 8.1.

Plasma level correlations: Clinical observation suggests that the effects of amphetamine usually wear off in about 4 hours, which is a good deal shorter than even the lower values quoted for the half-life of the drug. Perhaps tolerance to the drug develops. These observations raise the possibility that there may be no consistent relationship between plasma levels of amphetamine and its biological effects.

Interactions

Pharmacodynamic interactions: Amphetamine may interact with monoamine oxidase inhibitors (e.g. phenelzine) to produce dangerous manifestations of excessive sympathetic activity, since the noradrenaline released by amphetamine can no longer be degraded by the enzyme.

The hypotensive action of guanethidine and related drugs (bethanidine, debrisoquine) depends on their inhibition of noradrenaline release from peripheral nerve terminals. This action is antagonised by amphetamine.

The central actions of amphetamine are antagonised by phenothiazines (e.g. chlorpromazine) which prevent noradrenaline released by amphetamine from gaining access to its receptors.

Pharmacokinetic interactions: Amphetamine levels in plasma are increased by substances which make urine alkaline (e.g. sodium bicarbonate, thiazide diuretics) and are decreased by acidifying the urine (e.g. with ammonium chloride or ascorbic acid).

Toxicity

Idiosyncratic Toxicity

Rarely, patients develop manifestations of amphetamine overdosage at much lower amphetamine doses than usual.

Dose-related Toxicity

Acute amphetamine overdosage causes tremor, restlessness, hyperactivity, chorea (Klawans and Weiner, 1974b), irritability, insomnia, anxiety, delirium, hallucinations, headache, convulsions, coma, palpitations, cardiac arrhythmias, sweating, hypertension or hypotension, dry mouth, nausea, vomiting and abdominal cramps.

Chronic amphetamine intoxication may produce symptoms similar to the above, but with mental disturbance as the most prominent feature. This disturbance sometimes resembles schizophrenia.

Tolerance to amphetamine may occur, and dependence on the drug. These effects seem to be more frequent when the drug is used to elevate mental performance or wakefulness to supranormal levels, than when the drug is used in the treatment of narcolepsy.

Dysmorphogenicity
We have not traced reports of human dysmorphogenicity.

Methylphenidate

Methylphenidate (MW 233.30) is rather widely used in the USA for the same purposes as amphetamine. Its structure resembles that of amphetamine, and its actions and abuse potential are reasonably similar to those of amphetamine.

Imipramine

Although imipramine (MW 280.40) is a very important tricyclic antidepressant drug, its role in neurology is virtually confined to the treatment of cataplexy, a comparatively rare condition, and certain varieties of intractable pain. Another tricyclic antidepressant, amitriptyline, has been discussed in some detail in relation to the treatment of contraction headache (p.250). In general the dosage forms, biochemical pharmacology (blocking noradrenaline and serotonin re-uptake into nerve terminals), pharmacodynamics, interactions and toxicity of imipramine and amitriptyline are reasonably similar.

Imipramine forms an active N-desmethylated metabolite and a di-desmethyl metabolite. Both parent substance and its desmethylmetabolites undergo hydroxylation and subsequent glucuronide conjugation at the 2 and 10 positions. An N-oxide also forms in man (Parke, 1968). Some pharmacokinetic data are given by Gram and Christiansen (1975). The half-life of imipramine is 8 to 16 hours and that of desmethylimipramine 12 to 54 hours. Some 75 to 95% of the former and 73 to 92% of the latter in plasma are bound to plasma protein. The volumes of distribution are high (20 to 40 and 22 to 59L/kg^{-1} respectively) suggesting considerable tissue binding of both substances. Imipramine undergoes an enterohepatic circulation (Dencker et al., 1976).

Nitrazepam

A considerable number of hypnotic agents are available. Of these, nitrazepam is probably the safest. It is well established in use. The drug is also used as an anticonvulsant, particularly for myoclonic seizures. Its pharmacology has been considered in some detail in chapter VI. Whether the treatment of insomnia should be considered in detail in a book on clinical neuropharmacology might be argued. However if a neurologist were to prescribe a hypnotic it is likely that he would use nitrazepam as his drug of first choice.

Treatment of Sleep Disturbances

Narcolepsy

It should first be established whether or not the narcolepsy is due to any disorder requiring treatment in its own right. If no treatable lesion is found the narcolepsy should be treated symptomatically. A dose of amphetamine or dexamphetamine (either drug is equally suitable) should be found in each patient such that it maintains the sufferer in a normal state of alertness when he needs to be alert. In general the alerting effect of a dose of these drugs lasts some 4 to 6 hours and if a dose is taken within 4 to 6 hours of the patient's bedtime it is likely to interfere with his sleep. If these durations of drug action are kept in mind doses are best taken about 7am, about noon and perhaps about 4pm (if the patient wishes to remain alert in the evening). However, if his intent is to spend a tranquil domestic evening, the late afternoon dose might be omitted, or reduced in amount. In managing a patient with narcolepsy it is important to ensure that he does not increase his amphetamine (or dexamphetamine) dose in order to raise his intellectual performance above what is normal for him, or in order to prolong his period of wakefulness to beyond what is normal for him. If he does this, problems of tolerance and drug dependence may develop, whereas the risk of these problems appears very much less if the patient accepts that his treatment should never be used to lift his performance beyond his norm.

The dose of amphetamine needed to control narcolepsy varies greatly from patient to patient. Therapy may begin with 2.5mg of the drug in the morning and at lunch and the dose be increased at weekly intervals. Since the drug has a half-life of 7 to 14 hours, this regimen will prevent a dosage increase being made before the steady-state from the previous dose has been attained (though this argument may be an uncertain one in view of the probable poor correspondence between plasma amphetamine levels and biological effects). Doses of the order of 20mg twice or more daily, may occasionally be needed but it is important to find the minimum dose that controls the patient's problem. This reduces the risk of drug dependence.

Usually dexamphetamine or amphetamine therapy must be continued permanently. Once a satisfactory dose regimen is found it is unusual for this to need alteration over long periods. If the dose must keep being increased to relieve a patient's symptoms one should suspect that the patient is expecting the drug to lift his mood or performance above normal. Explanation at this stage may prevent the problems of drug dependence.

Some patients find that oral amphetamine or dexamphetamine therapy produces too short a period of alertness which is perhaps followed by rebound fatigue and depression. In such patients the use of a 10 or 15mg sustained release dexamphetamine preparation in the morning may prove more satisfactory.

Cataplexy

If amphetamine therapy of narcolepsy does not adequately relieve associated cataplexy (and it often does not) imipramine may be added (Hishikawa et al., 1966). For an adult the initial dose is likely to be 25mg 2 or 3 times a day, but pharmacokinetic considerations suggest that a single nocturnal dose of 50 or 75 or 100mg may be adequate, and could also have an appropriately timed hypnotic effect. The more recently introduced chlorimipramine may be used instead of imipramine (Guilleminault et al., 1976).

Parasomnia

Some forms of parasomnia occur in relation to acute illness. Here the sleep disturbance does not require treatment and in fact is helpful in that the patient tends to sleep through the period of acute disturbance of brain function.

When parasomnia is present for a longer time (as in the Klein-Levin syndrome) the appropriately timed use of amphetamine may increase the patient's alertness, though other problems of behaviour and mental functioning may remain.

Sleep Paralysis, Somnambulism, Hypnagogic Hallucinations

Drug therapy often is not needed for these disorders. Explanation of their natures, reassurance about their outcome, and attempts to alleviate sources of anxiety and stress in the patient's life are more likely to be helpful in the long term. Imipramine and desmethylimipramine are reported to be useful (Hishikawa et al., 1966).

Insomnia

When it is necessary to treat insomnia, a reasonable course is to prescribe 5mg of oral nitrazepam to be taken about 30 minutes before going to bed. Occasionally 10mg may be necessary. There are, of course, many alternative hypnotics, but it is not proposed to discuss the use of these here. Problems may arise because patients develop a degree of psychic dependence on hypnotics if these are used regularly over a period of more than a few weeks. Therefore, if the patient is genuinely troubled by insomnia, the aim should be to prescribe a sufficient hypnotic dose to produce satisfactory sleep for several nights, without 'hangover' during the day, while the factors which cause insomnia are elucidated and corrected. It is the continued use of hypnotics which should be avoided. Further, patients with insomnia sometimes take other drugs with sedative properties (e.g. antidepressants, antihistamines). Now that more pharmacokinetic data on individual drugs are becoming available, it is sometimes found that such drugs may be taken in a single larger dose in the evening rather than as divided doses during the day, without impairing the primary action of the drug, and with a greater chance of obtaining an appropriately timed sedative effect from it. Sedation seems related more to the rate of rise, and the extent of rise, of plasma levels of the relevant drug, than to the absolute levels finally attained.

Chapter IX

Sphincter Disturbances

Principal Disorders and Drugs Discussed

Urinary incontinence
Propantheline

Urinary retention
Carbachol, bethanecol

Generally speaking, the prospects for correcting neurogenic bladder or rectal disturbance by pharmacological means are not great, but they are sufficient to warrant discussion.

Incontinence and Retention

Disordered Mechanisms

The innervations of the bladder and rectum follow similar principles. Activity of a parasympathetic outflow from the second and third sacral segments causes contraction of the bladder and rectal detrusor muscles and relaxes their sphincters. In the case of the bladder only, activation of the sympathetic innervation from the upper lumbar cord segments has the opposite effects, *viz* it contracts the bladder sphincter and relaxes the detrusor muscles. Local stretch of the bladder wall can set up intramural reflexes which activate bladder contraction with relaxation of its sphincter. Afferent impulses from the bladder and rectal walls pass to the sacral spinal cord via dorsal root ganglia. These impulses may reflexly activate bladder and rectal emptying through spinal cord mechanisms. Onto these spinal reflex arcs descend pathways from the paracentral lobules of the cerebral cortex. These descending pathways provide voluntary control of micturition and defaecation.

Lesions anywhere along these various pathways, *viz* in the afferent limbs of the reflex arcs, in the appropriate cord segments, in the efferent pathways, or in the descending pathways from the cerebrum, can disturb micturition and defaecation. In relation to the rectum the final result is usually constipation, sometimes with overflow incontinence. What happens to bladder function depends on the site of the lesion, on how well the intramural reflex mechanism develops, and also on whether bladder distension, or urinary infection, damages the bladder wall.

Correction of Disordered Mechanisms

It may be possible to correct disordered bladder and rectal function by relieving the pathological process which has caused the disturbance. If not, there is no pharmacological technique for restoring normal activity in the descending pathways from the cerebrum, in the afferent limb of the spinal reflex arcs, or in the spinal cord itself.

Incontinence

The problem of neurogenic incontinence may be alleviated by increasing peripheral sympathetic function or by blocking peripheral parasympathetic function. Sympathomimetic drugs e.g. ephedrine, may help relieve incontinence but their cardiovascular and neurological side effects generally preclude their use in treating the symptom. Therefore in practice the pharmacological treatment of incontinence depends on the use of anticholinergics. Nocturnal enuresis in children is often treated with tricyclic antidepressants. These drugs have sedative and anticholinergic properties.

Retention

Neurogenic retention of urine (or of faeces) may be helped by increasing peripheral parasympathetic activity. This may be achieved by using directly acting cholinergic drugs or by blocking acetylcholinesterase activity e.g. by using anticholinesterases. The side effects of both groups of drug, and in particular the risk of generalised cholinergic weakness from anticholinesterase overdosage, may preclude adequate relief of retention. If used at all, such drugs are employed mainly as short term measures to treat neurogenic retention of urine.

Drugs Used in Treatment

Anticholinesterases have been discussed in relation to myasthenia (chapter III) and centrally acting anticholinergics in relation to Parkinsonism (chapter IV). The anticholinergics most often used to relieve neurogenic urinary incontinence are those synthetic agents containing a quaternary nitrogen atom (e.g. propantheline) which lack central actions. These agents have found their chief use in treating peptic ulcer, though their efficacy for this purpose, if used orally, is suspect. Atropine and the anticholinergic anti-Parkinsonian drugs are probably at least as effective as the quaternary nitrogen-containing compounds in relieving incontinence. However the latter compounds do not cross the blood-brain barrier, whereas the former do. Hence use of the quaternary nitrogen-containing anticholinergics, despite their relatively inefficient absorption after oral administration, offers the advantage of avoiding central neurological side effects if they must be given in high dosage to control urinary incontinence.

Two cholinergic agents, carbachol and bethanecol, are sometimes used to relieve neurogenic retention of urine.

Anticholinergics: Propantheline

A number of quaternary nitrogen-containing anticholinergics are marketed. Adequate quantitative data for these agents are lacking, particularly in relation to their relatively limited use in neurology. Hence only one agent, propantheline, will be considered here.

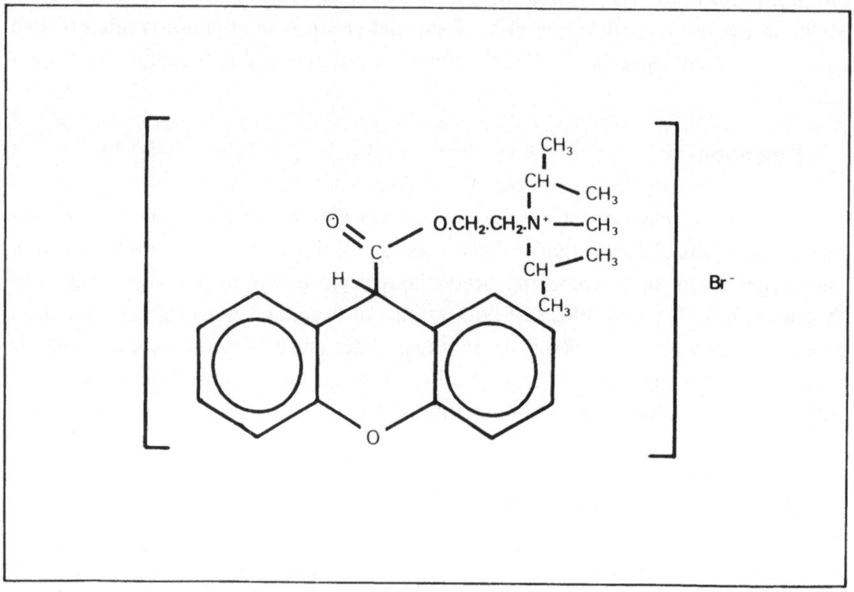

Fig. 9.1 Structural formula of propantheline bromide.

The chief use of propantheline in neurology is in treating urinary incontinence. In general medicine it has been widely used for treating peptic ulcer, 'spastic' disorders of the colon and uterus, and occasionally for ureteric and biliary colic.

Chemistry

The structural formula of propantheline bromide (MW 448.42) is seen in figure 9.1.

Pharmacology

Biochemical Pharmacology
Propantheline blocks the muscarine-like and nicotine-like effects of acetylcholine at sites to which it can gain access (i.e. sites outside the central nervous system).

Pharmacodynamics
Propantheline has antimuscarinic effects which tend to spare the central nervous system and to a lesser extent the eyes. The antimuscarinic action includes:

1) Eyes: mydriasis; paresis of accommodation; worsening of narrow angle glaucoma
2) Heart: tachycardia
3) Respiratory system: decreased secretion
4) Gastrointestinal system: decreased salivation, decreased gastric secretion and acidity, decreased alimentary tract motility
5) Urinary tract and bladder: decreased motility
6) Sweat glands: decreased sweating.

Propantheline also has antinicotinic actions which can produce postural hypotension and impotence. In overdosage propantheline can cause curariform neuromuscular blockade.

Pharmacokinetics
Absorption and bioavailability: Like other quaternary nitrogen containing molecules, propantheline is poorly and unpredictably absorbed after oral administration. Its bioavailability after oral administration is about 10% (Moller and Rosen, 1968). The drug tends to decompose in the upper small intestine (Beermann et al., 1972).

Distribution: Quantitative data are lacking but propantheline has very little capacity for penetration across the blood-brain barrier and enters the eye more slowly than does atropine.

Elimination: The terminal half-life of propantheline is 2.2 to 3.7 hours and clearance 79L per hour (Vose et al., 1979).

Plasma level correlations: No data are available.

Interactions

Pharmacodynamic interactions: Propantheline might be expected to interact additively with other agents which have anticholinergic properties (e.g. procainamide, quinidine, tricyclic antidepressants). The bradycardia due to β-adrenergic blockade from propranolol might be antagonised by the anticholinergic effect of propantheline.

Pharmacokinetic interactions: The effect of propantheline in delaying gastric emptying and diminishing intestinal motility may increase the absorption and plasma levels of a poorly absorbed drug such as digoxin (Manninen et al., 1973).

Toxicity

Idiosyncratic Toxicity

No definite idiosyncratic side effects have been traced.

Dose-related Toxicity

As propantheline dose is increased side effects such as a dry mouth, blurred vision from paresis of accommodation, and urine retention become more common. Postural hypotension and impotence may occur from blocking of cholinergic transmission in sympathetic ganglia. At high drug doses skeletal muscle weakness from neuromuscular junction blockade may develop.

Dysmorphogenicity

Reports of human dysmorphogenicity from the drug have not been traced.

Cholinergic Agents: Carbachol, Bethanechol

The cholinergic agents usually employed to promote micturition in cases of neurogenic retention are carbachol and bethanechol. These drugs are used to increase motility of the urinary tract and, rarely, of the gastrointestinal tract.

Chemistry

Carbachol (MW 182.65) and bethanechol chlorides (MW 196.68) resemble acetylcholine in structure, though they are amides rather than esters (fig. 9.2). They are both water-soluble compounds.

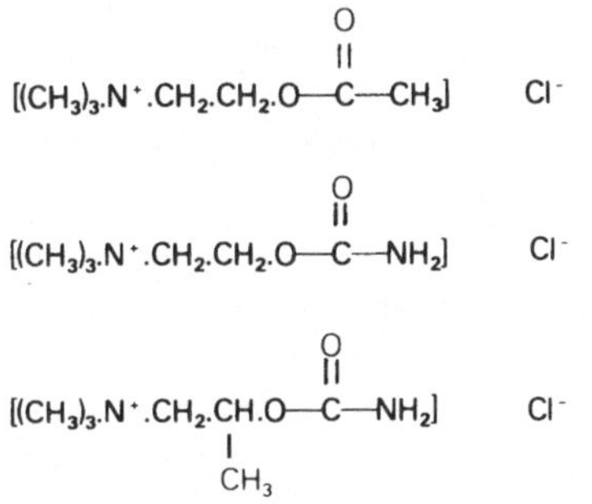

O
||
[(CH₃)₃.N⁺.CH₂.CH₂.O—C—CH₃]   Cl⁻   Acetylcholine chloride

O
||
[(CH₃)₃.N⁺.CH₂.CH₂.O—C—NH₂]   Cl⁻   Carbachol chloride

O
||
[(CH₃)₃.N⁺.CH₂.CH.O—C—NH₂]   Cl⁻   Bethanechol chloride
                    |
                   CH₃

Fig. 9.2. The cholinergic drugs carbachol and bethanechol.

Pharmacology

Biochemical Pharmacology

Both drugs are acetylcholine agonists at the muscarinic cholinergic receptors to which they can gain access and carbachol has a nicotine-like action on autonomic ganglia. The drugs may act by displacing acetylcholine from its storage sites within nerve terminals.

Pharmacodynamics

Given orally or subcutaneously in therapeutic dosage carbachol and bethanechol act rather specifically on the smooth muscle of the bladder and gastrointestinal tract, increasing its contractility. In ordinary dosage they have little effect on the cardiovascular system though they produce a transient fall in diastolic blood pressure and a slight tachycardia. Potentially they can cause bronchospasm. There is some tendency to cause increased bronchial, lachrymal, salivary, digestive and sweat gland secretion. If instilled into the conjunctival sac they produce miosis. These drugs have no central nervous system effects as they are too polar to cross the blood-brain barrier readily.

Pharmacokinetics

Absorption and bioavailability: Though these drugs are absorbed after oral administration their polar natures, and the fact that their parenteral doses are 15 to 50 % of their oral ones, suggest the possibility that their bioavailability is incomplete.

Distribution: Neither drug crosses the blood-brain barrier in significant quantities, so that they have no central effects if given in ordinary dosage. Detailed quantitative data regarding their distributions are not available.

Elimination: Neither drug is hydrolysed by acetylcholinesterase or by nonspecific esterases. Details of their elimination are not available.

Plasma level correlations: No data are available.

Interactions
Pharmacodynamic interactions: Quinidine and procainamide antagonise the effects of these cholinergic agents and atropine and other anticholinergics selectively block them.

Pharmacokinetic interactions: No data are available.

Toxicity

Idiosyncratic Toxicity
No instances have been traced.

Dose-related Toxicity
Given intravenously or intramuscularly the relative selectivity of action on the urinary and alimentary systems of the drugs is said to be lost. They can then cause blurred vision, salivation, bronchospasm and hypotension, nausea and vomiting, abdominal cramp, substernal distress, syncope, asystole and unconsciousness.

Dysmorphogenicity
Data are lacking.

Treatment of Disturbed Sphincter Function

Urine Incontinence

Mild neurogenic urinary incontinence may be helped by the use of anticholinergic drugs e.g. propantheline 15mg 3 times a day initially. Later higher doses, increased to the limit of the patient's tolerance, may be used if necessary. Sometimes such treatment, combined with deliberate bladder emptying every 2 or 3 hours to prevent bladder distension, which triggers local reflex bladder contraction, can make the sufferer's life very much more acceptable. If such pharmacological treatment fails, the use of some form of mechanical urine collection device may become necessary.

Urine Retention

Acute neurogenic retention of urine, in the absence of structural bladder neck obstruction, may be treated initially by the subcutaneous injection of 0.25mg of carbachol, or 5mg bethanechol, repeated after 30 minutes, if necessary. If this is successful, but the retention recurs, oral carbachol 2mg, or bethanechol 10mg, 3 times a day, may permit bladder emptying for a few days till a sufficient degree of neurological recovery occurs. Injection of these drugs may promote defaecation, particularly if the bowel is full.

Should these measures fail to relieve urine retention, catheterisation is likely to be necessary and the further management of the problem becomes a matter for a urologist.

Faecal Retention

In its own right constipation of neurogenic origin is not ordinarily treated by systemic drug therapy. However such therapy, if used for concurrent urine retention, may help constipation. Neurogenic constipation is usually treated by means of local measures such as bulk laxatives, faecal wetting agents (e.g. sodium diocytlsulphosuccinate), enemas and, if necessary, manual removal of faeces.

Chapter X

Vascular Disease

Principal Disorders and Drugs Discussed

Intracranial haemorrhage
  Intracranial pressure-reducing agents (see also chapter II)

Subarachnoid haemorrhage
Brain ischaemia and infarction
  Heparin
  Warfarin, phenindione
  Dipyridamole
  Sulphinpyrazone
  Dextrans

The main consequences of vascular disease of the central nervous system are haemorrhage and ischaemia (with or without infarction). Though haemorrhage and ischaemia may co-exist, it is convenient to discuss these topics separately.

Intracranial Haemorrhage

Disordered Mechanisms

Intracranial haemorrhage produces two major patterns of clinical picture, that of a mass lesion (extradural, subdural, or within the nervous tissue) and that of a diffuse, or extensive, subarachnoid haemorrhage. Both types of picture may sometimes be present simultaneously in the one patient.

The major causes of intracranial haemorrhage are:

1) Trauma to the head
2) Arterial hypertension

3) Blood vessel defects e.g. aneurysms, arteriovenous malformations and angiomas

4) Bleeding disorders e.g. thrombocytopenic purpura

All these conditions may lead to escape of blood from the vascular lumen into its surroundings. Blood that enters the cerebrospinal fluid may spread extensively. Otherwise blood tends to accumulate locally around the bleeding site. The extent and pattern of its spread is then determined by local anatomical factors and local tissue tension, and by the pressure under which the blood escapes from the vessels. The local blood collection (extradural, subdural or intracerebral) constitutes a mass lesion raising intracranial pressure. This mass lesion may cause ischaemia and oedema in the surrounding brain, producing a further deficit in brain function. Subarachnoid bleeding not infrequently causes cerebral vasospasm (Heros et al., 1976) with brain ischaemia. The behaviour of mass lesions has been discussed further in chapter II.

Correction of Disordered Mechanisms

Intracranial Haematoma

The therapeutic possibilities for correcting the mass lesion aspects of an intracranial haematoma, including the possibility of surgical drainage, have been considered in chapter II. The question of dealing with the causative process must also be considered. If the causative process persists there is risk of further bleeding.

Sometimes an acute temporary rise in blood pressure occurs after a cerebral vascular ictus. Significant hypertension should be controlled but how rapidly this control is achieved may involve some nicety of judgement. Rapid reduction of the systemic arterial pressure in the presence of a raised intracranial pressure may decrease brain perfusion and increase brain injury from ischaemia. However to leave cerebral arterial pressure too high increases the risk of further haemorrhage which may also damage the brain. Further, severe hypertension may precipitate cardiac failure, with consequent possibilities of brain hypoxia.

Leaving aside the question of malignant hypertension, where blood pressure reduction is indicated, the authors know of no good evidence of help in deciding the critical level of blood pressure above which it is desirable to take steps to control hypertension rapidly in a patient with a recent intracranial haematoma. Their practice is to treat previously untreated hypertension in the acute situation only when the patient's cardiac state suggests that this is desirable. Such an attitude is in general agreement with the view of Marshall (1976). Once the acute effects of the intracranial haematoma have stabilised or are improving, either spontaneously or as the result of therapeutic endeavour, more gradual control of hypertension can be attempted in the light of the patient's general cardiovascular state and the extent of residual brain function.

It may be possible to correct aneurysms or arteriovenous malformations surgically, or to excise them. Appropriate steps can be taken to remedy many types of bleeding disorder once the exact nature of the condition is defined.

Subarachnoid Haemorrhage

Unless an associated intracranial haematoma exists there is no mass lesion problem in cases of subarachnoid haemorrhage though the intracranial pressure may rise. Secondary arterial spasm may occur and may produce brain ischaemia. The consequences of spasm and ischaemia may require medical treatment (p.310-326). Otherwise the management of subarachnoid haemorrhage involves the relief of associated headache with analgesics, supportive therapy and nursing care as indicated. Surgical attempts to remedy the cause of the bleeding will need to be considered (e.g. clipping the neck of a cerebral aneurysm).

Drugs Used in Treating Intracranial Haemorrhage

The drugs used in treating intracranial bleeding (drugs which lower intracranial pressure) have been discussed elsewhere (mostly in chapter II).

Treatment of Intracranial Haemorrhage

Extradural Haematoma

The mass lesion effects of extradural haematoma usually develop so quickly that attempts to reduce intracranial pressure by medical measures do not have time to work before brain displacement kills the patient. The extradural blood should be removed and the bleeding artery occluded.

Subdural Haematoma

In acute rapidly progressing subdural haematoma the considerations are as for extradural haemorrhage (see above). In patients with chronic subdural haematoma the medical measures capable of reducing intracranial pressure rapidly (e.g. IV glycerol or mannitol, and corticosteroids) can produce useful improvement in the patient's condition but almost inevitably surgical drainage of the haematoma will be required. Rarely, one sees a patient who has a very long standing subdural haematoma and who has no clinical symptoms or signs.

Haematomas Within the Brain Substance

While such lesions are generally related to hypertension they sometimes may be due to trauma, to aneurysms, vascular malformations or a bleeding disorder. The surgical considerations involved in treating vascular lesions, and the detailed medical management of the various types of bleeding disorder, will not be dealt with here. As discussed earlier in this chapter the question of blood pressure reduction in the acute stage of management of a patient with an intracerebral haematoma is contentious. The authors' practice is not to institute antihypertensive therapy at this acute stage unless it seems likely that the degree of left ventricular overload will produce cardiac failure. If the patient survives the acute illness and has reasonable prospects of continued useful life any residual hypertension can then be dealt with on its merits.

In essence, the medical treatment of a haematoma within the brain substance is aimed at reducing intracranial pressure and minimising secondary effects of a mass lesion for a few days. If this can be done, and further bleeding does not occur, the patient's prognosis for survival and for neurological recovery improves. The prospects of successful surgical removal of clot, and liquid blood, without subsequent rebleeding, are improved and the operative mortality is lowered the longer surgery can be delayed. Further, if the patient's condition improves as a result of medical treatment of the mass lesion effect, and does not deteriorate when this treatment is discontinued, surgery can usually be avoided. In general, haematomas in the internal capsule region, or in the pons, carry very high operative mortalities. Prospects for survival are better in the case of external capsule, frontal or temporal lobe, or intracerebellar haematomas (McKissock et al., 1959).

Once the patient with intracerebral haematoma presents and the diagnosis is established, the medical treatment for raised intracranial pressure should be instituted and the collaboration of a neurosurgeon sought, unless it is obvious that the patient has no hope of survival.

Subarachnoid Haemorrhage

In uncomplicated subarachnoid haemorrhage management comprises keeping the patient comfortable with analgesics (e.g. aspirin, dextropropoxyphene or pentazocine) for as long as is necessary. The cause of the bleeding should be investigated and, if possible, corrected. This correction is likely to involve neurosurgery. When subarachnoid haemorrhage is complicated, the complicating factor is likely to be an intracranial haematoma, the management of which is discussed above, or cerebral arterial spasm, with ischaemia, the management of which is considered in the following section of this chapter.

Patients with the various forms of intracranial bleeding discussed above require a considerable amount of skilled nursing care. Some patients may be unconscious, in which case their airway must be kept patent, their fluid and electrolyte balance maintained and their bladder and bowel functions cared for. Complications e.g. epilepsy, leg vein thrombosis, pulmonary embolism, chest infection, require appropriate therapy. During recovery extensive physiotherapy, occupational therapy and speech therapy may be needed.

Brain Ischaemia and Infarction

Disordered Mechanisms

Ischaemia and infarction of the brain usually result from inadequacy of its arterial blood supply. The adequacy of the brain's blood supply depends chiefly on the patency of the lumina of brain arteries and on the arterial blood pressure. While brain ischaemia may be caused by arterial hypotension, severe narrowing or blockage of the lumina of brain arteries is a much more frequent cause. At times both factors may operate simultaneously.

The lumina of brain arteries may be narrowed or occluded by:

1) Atheroma, with or without local thrombosis
2) Various forms of arteritis (due to tuberculosis, syphilis, polyarteritis nodosa, temporal arteritis etc.)
3) Embolism, of sterile or infected blood clot, of platelets, of cholesterol from atheromatous plaques and possibly of fat (though the fat found in the brain in so-called fat embolism may not be of embolic origin, according to Sevitt, 1962).
4) Arterial spasm e.g. in relation to a recently ruptured cerebral aneurysm.

Local ischaemia may cause reduction in or suppression of local neuronal function, perhaps after a stage of heightened excitation. The effects of ischaemia may be brief, as may happen if:

1) The ischaemic portion of brain is small and a collateral circulation develops rapidly,
2) An embolus, after lodgement, breaks up and moves on, or
3) A temporary fall in blood pressure, which has further reduced blood flow through a narrowed artery, is corrected.

If ischaemia persists, and is severe enough, some brain tissue may become infarcted. With extensive enough infarction and breakdown of the blood-brain barrier, local swelling of the damaged and dead brain tissue may produce a significant mass lesion effect. Anoxic damage to capillary walls in the margins of the affected area, where the collateral circulation maintains some blood flow, may lead to escape of blood cells into the brain so that the margins of the infarct may become haemorrhagic. Thus the initial cerebral deficit due to ischaemia and infarction may be increased by the consequences of ischaemic brain swelling and local haemorrhage. If the patient survives this acute phase and the mass lesion effects of ischaemic swelling and perhaps haemorrhage wear off, there is likely to be some recovery of function if previously ischaemic neurones resume their normal activities, though some permanent deficit is likely if neurones have died from the ischaemia.

Though it is relatively uncommon, cerebral infarction may also occur because major cerebral veins become occluded by clot. When venous infarction occurs it is often in patients who are dehydrated or who have local intracranial or cranial infections. If brain becomes ischaemic because its venous outflow is blocked, there will very probably be local oedema and capillary haemorrhage also, so that venous infarction is even more likely than arterial infarction to be associated with bleeding into the brain substance and cerebrospinal fluid.

Correction of Disordered Mechanisms

The possibilities for correcting the disordered mechanisms of brain ischaemia are:

1) Correcting the causative process
2) Promoting the collateral circulation
3) Relieving mass lesion effects and the consequent raised intracranial pressure.

Correcting the Causative Process

If the causative process can be corrected quickly enough, ischaemic neurones may be saved from irreversible damage or necrosis. Even if the correction is slower, extension of the infarction, or development of new areas of ischaemia, may still be avoided.

Apart from surgical excision and blood vessel reconstruction, there is no satisfactory method of dealing with an atheromatous lesion quickly, whether or not there is associated local thrombosis. An acute thrombus might be removed surgically, but such surgery carries substantial hazards (Marshall, 1976). Thrombosis might also be treated with anticoagulants to prevent its extension. If the ischaemic area is haemorrhagic the use of anticoagulants may increase the brain haemorrhage. Use of long term anticoagulants to prevent further ischaemic brain damage in patients with established cerebrovascular disease has not been successful (Hill et al., 1962; Enger and Boyersen, 1966).

Specific chemotherapy is available for certain forms of arteritis, (e.g. cortico-steroids for temporal arteritis, penicillin for syphilitic endarteritis).

The source of emboli may be removed or corrected surgically. The risk of emboli due to bacterial endocarditis may be reduced by using appropriate antibiotics. Anti-coagulants may be used in the hope of preventing further clot formation at the site of origin of emboli (at the possible cost of increasing the extent of any haemorrhagic brain infarction which has occurred from recent emboli). The risk of platelet emboli may be reduced by the use of agents which decrease platelet adhesiveness (e.g. aspirin, possibly dipyridamole and sulphinpyrazone). Dietary measures and drug therapy to reduce hyperlipidaemia may lessen the risk of cholesterol emboli in the long term, but there is no medical treatment which can have a significant immediate effect on the atheromatous ulcers, which are the source of cholesterol and lipid debris emboli.

The drug treatment of cerebral arterial spasm is still largely experimental. The subject has been reviewed by Norwood (1977). Serotonin appears the most likely agent to initiate arterial spasm after subarachnoid haemorrhage. Serotonin activates the enzyme guanyl cyclase, which catalyses the formation of cyclic guanosine monophosphate (cGMP), which in turn promotes contraction of smooth muscle. Cyclic adenosine monophosphate (cAMP) has the opposite action on smooth muscle. Certain drugs (e.g. the β-adrenergic agent salbutamol) which stimulate adenyl cyclase, the enzyme which catalyses cAMP formation, and drugs which inhibit phos-phodiesterase, the enzyme which catalyses the breakdown of cAMP, might be ex-pected to relieve cerebral arterial spasm. However phosphodiesterase inhibitors (e.g. papaverine, methyl xanthines, chlorpromazine, reserpine, hydrallazine and diazoxide) do not abolish experimental cerebral arterial spasm. The combination of phos-phodiesterase inhibition (with aminophylline) and adenyl cyclase stimulation (with salbutamol), does relieve cerebral arterial spasm in monkeys. Inhibition of guanyl cyclase activity might be expected to be therapeutically useful. Such inhibition might be produced by nonspecific inhibitors (e.g. phenoxybenzamine), α-adrenergic blocking agents (e.g. phentolamine), or serotonin blocking agents (e.g. methysergide). It is un-certain whether such pharmacological considerations in experimental animals would be applicable in man.

Correction of arterial hypertension may prevent, or delay, the ischaemic conse-quences of cerebral arteriosclerosis. However, iatrogenic hypotension should be avoided, particularly if there is arterial stenosis, lest treatment reduce cerebral blood flow. Haemodynamic factors which reduce cerebral blood flow or oxygenation should be corrected, as far as is possible. Thus cardiac arrhythmia, anaemia and polycythaemia, if present, should be treated.

In view of the probable association between oral contraceptive intake and cerebral arterial occlusion in younger women (Bickerstaff and Holmes, 1967) these agents are best avoided if ischaemic manifestations have occurred.

Promoting the Collateral Circulation

It seems likely that the metabolic products of local ischaemia in many instances will have caused maximal possible dilatation of the potential collateral circulation. Therefore the use of vasodilating drugs, even if they had an effect on the cerebral arteries, might merely dilate vessels in normal brain tissue and divert blood from the ischaemic area. However, in local brain ischaemia of moderate degree, insufficient to produce infarction, the collateral circulation may not be maximally dilated. Here the use of a vasodilating agent such as 5 % carbon dioxide gas (inhaled for a few minutes each half hour), or blockade of the cervical sympathetic trunk with local anaesthetic, may produce a temporary improvement in the impaired brain function. Agents which decrease the viscosity of the blood may also facilitate blood flow in the collateral circulation.

Reduction of cerebral oedema (see below) may permit the collateral circulation to open further by reducing the intracranial pressure.

Relieving Mass Lesion Effects

This was discussed in chapter II. If raised intracranial pressure due to brain oedema can be reduced so that the collateral circulation is improved in the ischaemic area, the consequent reduction in ischaemia may further decrease the local swelling and break the vicious circle involved in ischaemic swelling. Cerebral oedema is more likely to be important with extensive infarcts than with smaller ones. Thus, while Patten et al. (1972) found that high dose dexamethasone, given in the acute phase of stroke, improved the recovery of function, the benefits were greater in patients with the more severe strokes.

Drugs Used in Treating Brain Ischaemia

The drugs used for this purpose include: anticoagulants, platelet-inhibiting drugs, agents which reduce blood viscosity, and drugs which lower intracranial pressure. Of the platelet-inhibiting drugs aspirin was considered in chapter VII, and the drugs used in reducing intracranial pressure in chapter II. Antihypertensive drugs will not be considered here.

Anticoagulants

Among the anticoagulants, intravenous heparin is used when an immediate effect is required. Anticoagulants are often given for periods of weeks or months and orally effective coumarin or indanedione derivatives are then used. One widely used member of each family of drugs is considered below.

Heparin

The major therapeutic use of heparin is as an anticoagulant agent.

Chemistry

Heparin is a mucopolysaccharide of heterogeneous composition. Its source to some extent determines its physical, chemical and pharmacological properties. The main commercial sources of heparin are the intestinal mucus and mucosa of the pig, sheep and ox. The heparin molecule comprises repeated partly sulphated units of the sugars α-D-glucuronic acid and 2-amino-2-deoxy-α-D-glucose, connected by a 1-4 or 1-6 glycosidic link. The molecular weight of heparin may vary between 3000 and 37,500. Heparin is a strong organic acid. The drug is available commercially as its sodium and calcium salts. Strengths of heparin solutions are measured in International Units.

Pharmacology

Biochemical Pharmacology
In the presence of an α-globulin co-factor, heparin forms an active complex which blocks the conversion of prothrombin to thrombin. It thereby interferes with blood clotting processes. Heparin may inhibit blood factors required for the formation of thromboplastin. Heparin enhances thrombolysis and may possibly enhance platelet aggregation.

Heparin causes the release of a lipase from tissues and this can lead to clearing of lipaemic plasma, with elevation of plasma free fatty acid concentrations.

Pharmacodynamics
The anticoagulant effect of heparin begins as soon as the drug enters the circulation. Coagulation time is prolonged though bleeding time is usually unchanged. Heparin prevents venous thrombosis after surgery and in other high risk situations e.g. after myocardial infarction. With excessive dosage there is risk of haemorrhage.

Pharmacokinetics
Absorption and bioavailability: In therapeutic as distinct from prophylactic use, heparin is nearly always given intravenously. In this case absorption is immediate.

The drug is not effective after oral or sublingual administration. Heparin is absorbed after subcutaneous administration. Local haematomas may form around the injection site.

Distribution: The apparent volume of distribution is 0.06L/kg. The drug is not bound to plasma proteins.

Heparin is concentrated in blood vessel endothelium. It tends to be taken up by cell membranes and other surfaces with which it comes in contact. The drug does not cross the placenta, nor enter milk.

Elimination: The plasma half-life of the drug varies in individuals between 41 and 149 minutes (Estes et al., 1969). The half-life may be dose-dependent (Olsson et al., 1963). The drug undergoes some metabolism in the liver. Some unchanged heparin may be found in the liver.

Plasma level correlations: Since the therapeutic effect of heparin can be assessed by measuring coagulation time, correlations between plasma drug level and effect are of little practical importance.

Interactions

Pharmacodynamic interactions: Heparin interacts additively with oral anti-coagulants of the coumarin or indanedione class. The platelet-inhibiting actions of aspirin, dipyridamole or sulphinpyrazone may reinforce the anticoagulant action of heparin. The actions of heparin on blood clotting are antagonised by protamine.

Pharmacokinetic interactions: None are known.

Toxicity

Idiosyncratic Toxicity

Heparin rarely causes hypersensitivity reactions and anaphylaxis. Thrombocytopenia has occurred (Babcock et al., 1976).

Dose-related Toxicity

Heparin overdosage may cause bleeding. Prolonged heparin dosage of over 15000 units per day may lead to osteoporosis (Griffiths, 1965).

Dysmorphogenicity

There is a possibility that heparin-induced bleeding on the maternal side of the placenta may cause anoxic fetal damage.

Warfarin and Phenindione

The only therapeutic use of these drugs is as anticoagulants.

Chemistry

Warfarin (MW 308.32) is a coumarin derivative; it is an acid with a pKa of 5.05. It is usually administered as its sodium salt. There are R and S enantiomorphs, the latter having a higher intrinsic anticoagulant activity. Phenindione (MW 223.23) is derived from indanedione, and is also an acid drug. The molecular structures of these two compounds are shown in figure 10.1.

Pharmacology

Biochemical Pharmacology

Warfarin and phenindione are competitive inhibitors of vitamin K. They therefore inhibit the effect of vitamin K on the hepatic synthesis of certain blood clotting factors (prothrombin, factors VII, IX, X).

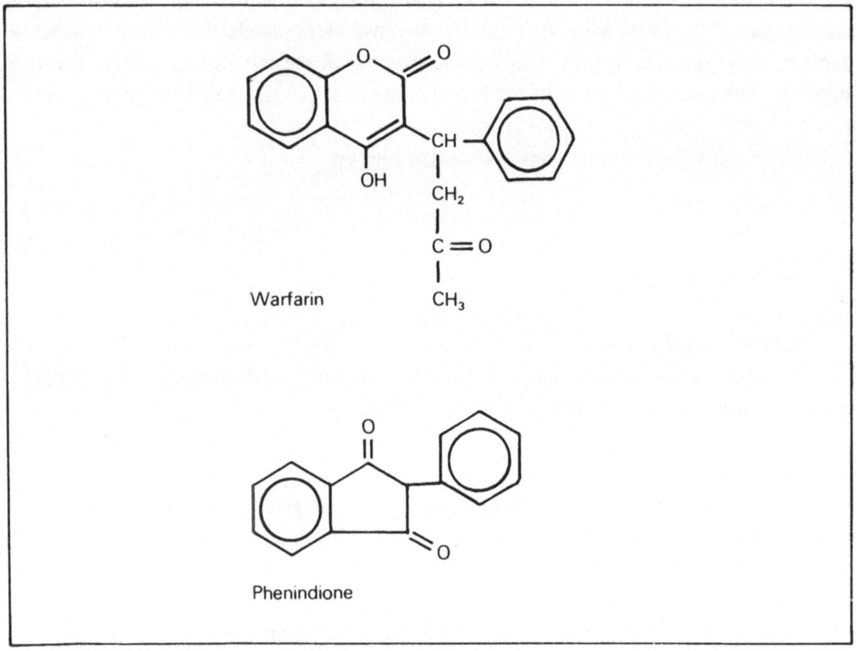

Fig. 10.1. Structural formulae of the anticoagulants warfarin and phenindione.

Pharmacodynamics

These drugs inhibit blood clotting, with a latent period of at least 12 to 24 hours after their administration. This latent period occurs because, although inhibition of synthesis of clotting factors commences immediately the drug is absorbed and reaches the liver, some time is required for the disappearance of the circulating clotting factors that are already formed. The delay in anticoagulant effect of warfarin and its duration of action, are shorter than those of phenindione. With phenindione, therapeutically effective prothrombin times can be achieved in 1 to 2 days, and when therapy is discontinued prothrombin time returns to normal in 1 to 4 days.

Pharmacokinetics

Absorption and bioavailability: Warfarin is almost completely absorbed from the alimentary tract.

Distribution: In plasma warfarin is 97 % bound to plasma protein. The apparent volume of distribution of warfarin is about 0.1 L/kg, suggesting that the drug's distribution extends through part of the volume of extracellular water. These anticoagulant drugs pass through the placenta and also appear in milk.

Elimination: The half-life of warfarin is 30 to 50 hours (R enantiomorph 58 ± 5 hours, S enantiomorph 33 ± 4 hours according to O'Rielly, 1974), and that of phenindione is 5 to 10 hours. The drugs are hydroxylated in hepatic microsomes to form biologically inert compounds. Less than 1 % of a warfarin dose is excreted unchanged in urine.

Plasma level correlations: As explained earlier, there is a lag between the time course of plasma anticoagulant levels and the effect of these drugs on prothrombin time. Steady-state conditions will occur later with warfarin (1 to 2 weeks) than with phenindione (1 to 2 days). There is also a 1 to 2 day lag between plasma drug level changes and changes in anticoagulant effect for both drugs.

Interactions

Pharmacodynamic interactions: Vitamin K is a competitive antagonist of warfarin and phenindione. Therefore factors which decrease vitamin K absorption (e.g. mineral oil in the diet) increase the effects of oral anticoagulants. Oral antibiotics may inhibit intestinal bacteria, thus decreasing vitamin K synthesis and enhancing the effect of anticoagulants.

Substances with anticoagulant actions (e.g. heparin, salicylates, quinidine) augment the effects of warfarin and phenindione. Thyroid hormone administration may increase the actions of anticoagulants by increasing the degradation of clotting factors.

Pharmacokinetic interactions: Many probable or possible pharmacokinetic interactions of anticoagulants are known or suspected. Cholestyramine and possibly griseofulvin, given with warfarin, may bind the latter drug in the gut and prevent its absorption.

A number of acidic drugs may displace anticoagulants from plasma protein binding sites. The increased amount of unbound drug produces an increased anticoagulant effect. Drugs which act in this way include ethacrynic acid, nalidixic acid, mephenamic acid, trichloracetic acid (derived from chloral hydrate), indomethacin, clofibrate, sulphaphenazole, diazoxide, tolbutamide, phenylbutazone, oxyphenbutazone and certain radiographic contrast media (Sellers and Koch-Weser, 1971).

The biotransformation of warfarin and phenindione can be increased, and their effects lessened, by drugs which induce the hepatic microsomal mixed-oxidase system. Such agents include barbiturates, carbamazepine, phenytoin, griseofulvin, haloperidol and glutethimide.

The biotransformation of warfarin is slowed, and its anticoagulant action is potentiated, by co-trimoxazole, sulphaphenazole, sulphadiazine and sulphamethiazole (Hansen et al., 1975; Hassall et al., 1975). Administration of the benzodiazepines, nitrazepam and diazepam does not alter plasma warfarin concentrations (Orme et al., 1972).

Toxicity

Idiosyncratic Toxicity

Anorexia, nausea, vomiting and diarrhoea occur so uncommonly with warfarin therapy that their pathogenesis may involve idiosyncratic mechanisms of various kinds. Skin lesions, including urticaria and alopecia, may occur at times. Sensitivity reactions are more common for phenindione, and include rashes, pyrexia and leucopenia. This drug may produce fever and malaise. Serious renal damage has also been reported. Hepatitis and agranulocytosis are recorded as uncommon side effects.

Occasional instances of slowed warfarin metabolism, with therapeutic doses causing haemorrhage, have occurred. Such patients may also be slow metabolisers of phenytoin (Bochner et al., 1975).

Dose-related Toxicity

Excessive anticoagulant dosage involves the risk of haemorrhage from various sites, commonly from the gastrointestinal and urinary tracts. Intracranial bleeding may occur. The risk of such haemorrhage necessitates regular measurement of prothrombin times in patients taking anticoagulants. The antidote is vitamin K_1 which, if given intravenously, restores prothrombin time to normal within a few hours as synthesis of clotting factors resumes.

Phenindione may produce a red-orange colour in urine; this is due to a metabolic product and may be confused with haematuria.

Dipyridamole

It is not proposed to discuss this agent in detail. Although it has pharmacological actions which might be expected to benefit patients with cerebral vascular disease, therapeutic trials have usually not substantiated its usefulness (Acheson et al., 1969).

Dipyridamole inhibits the active (saturable) uptake of adenosine and adenine nucleotides into red blood cells and into tissue cells. This inhibition of uptake has the effect of increasing the action of these nucleotides, which produce relaxation of vascular smooth muscle. However dipyridamole also blocks platelet aggregation caused by adenosine diphosphate (Mustard and Packham, 1973). The drug also inhibits the enzyme phosphodiesterase. While the tendency to vasodilatation produced by dipyridamole, and its inhibitory effect on platelet aggregation, might appear to be of potential use in patients with certain forms of cerebral vascular disease, the usual doses given to man (25 to 50mg 2 or 3 times a day) do not appear effective clinically. Side effects from these doses are mild (e.g. nausea, vomiting, diarrhoea, headache, vertigo).

Sulphinpyrazone

Sulphinpyrazone (MW 404.48) is a strong organic acid (pKa 2.8) which is slightly soluble in water. It is a potent uricosuric agent used to treat gout, prophylactically. Packham et al. (1967) showed that the drug prolonged platelet survival in man by inhibiting platelet aggregation provoked by collagen and antigen-antibody complexes. This action causes decreased release of adenosine diphosphate and 5-hydroxytryptamine from platelets. It is not yet clear whether this effect on platelets is therapeutically useful in human cerebrovascular disease.

Sulphinpyrazone is well absorbed from the gastrointestinal tract (Burns et al., 1957). In plasma 98 to 99% is bound to protein and the drug may displace other anionic substances from plasma (and probably tissue) protein binding sites. The half-life of sulphinpyrazone is 4.29 ± 0.25 hours (Kadar et al., 1973). Most of a dose of the drug is excreted unchanged in urine, though a hydroxyphenyl metabolite with a half-life of 1 hour is known (Dayton et al., 1961).

Side effects of the drug include hypersensitivity rashes and fever, and gastrointestinal irritation. At least experimentally, the drug may depress haemopoiesis.

Dextrans

Dextrans are branched-chain polysaccharides containing glucose residues. Those in current therapeutic use have molecular weights of 75,000 and 40,000. Given intravenously, dextrans act as plasma volume expanders and lower blood viscosity (Bochenstein et al., 1966). Up to 50% of an intravenous dose may be excreted into urine, but the remainder is very slowly metabolised. These dextrans coat platelets and thus interfere with platelet function and aggregation. They also coat red cells and prevent rouleau formation and they form complexes with various plasma clotting factors. Collectively these effects reduce the risk of blood sludging and clotting. Usually MW 40,000 dextran is used intravenously in a dose of 10ml of a 10% solution per kg body weight. The dose is given over several hours. The full dose may be repeated every second day, or 5ml/kg may be given daily. Overdosage may lead to haemorrhage or to circulatory overload from excessive expansion of plasma volume. Allergic reactions may occur and are sometimes severe.

Treatment of Brain Ischaemia

It is convenient to discuss the treatment of brain ischaemia in relation to several specific clinical situations which cover the majority of ways in which brain ischaemia presents in neurological practice.

Established Acute Brain Infarction

Correcting the Causative Process

In the acute phase of a brain infarct it is often impossible to know how much of the deficit in function is due to tissue death and how much to ischaemic injury, some of which is at least potentially reversible. It is also difficult to know if the infarct is haemorrhagic. Without computerised axial tomography the clinician is often uncertain whether he is dealing with brain infarction or haemorrhage. Correcting the causative process in ischaemia may prevent this process extending and causing further brain injury; correcting the causative process may also improve blood flow to ischaemic brain and help restore function.

Thrombosis
Most often cerebral infarction is due to thrombosis of a major cerebral artery, or the internal carotid itself, at a site of previous atheroma. No medical treatment is likely to alter the atheroma quickly enough to be clinically useful (even if such treatment could alter the atheroma at all). The use of anticoagulants might prevent the thrombosis extending and causing more brain ischaemia. However, if the infarct is haemorrhagic, or if an intracerebral haematoma has been incorrectly diagnosed as an infarct, the use of anticoagulants may increase haemorrhage and make the situation worse. Experience has tended to show that, at least in carotid territory infarction, the

benefits of using anticoagulants do not outweigh the risks (Marshall and Shaw, 1960). The study of Hill et al. (1962) found that the risks of haemorrhage more than outweighed the benefits of anticoagulant therapy in patients with completed stroke. Similar considerations are likely to apply for the use of other agents that interfere with blood clotting e.g. IV dextran (MW 40,000). Surgical removal of intravascular thrombus, in particular thrombus in the internal carotid artery in the neck, may restore blood flow and relieve ischaemia, if carried out within a few hours of the onset of symptoms. However in an infarcted portion of brain restoration of arterial flow may cause ischaemic arteriolar and capillary walls to give way, causing a haematoma. Bruetman et al. (1963) reported such an event after carotid endarterectomy.

Hypertension

In benign hypertension, unless there is danger of the left heart becoming overloaded, there seems to be little advantage in treating previously untreated hypertension during the acute phase of established brain infarction due to thrombosis.

Embolism

Brain infarction may be due to embolism from a proximal atheromatous site in the carotid or vertebral arterial trees, from the heart valves (as in bacterial endocarditis) or from the chambers of the left heart (as after myocardial infarction). Atheromatous ulcers in the carotid wall, possibly with attached clot, may be removed surgically. The consensus of opinion appears to be that anticoagulants should be used to prevent further emboli in persons who have brain emboli of cardiac origin (Oxbury, 1975), despite the risks of intracranial bleeding. The presence of hypertension is a relative contraindication to the use of anticoagulants. High blood pressure should be reduced before anticoagulants are used. Anticoagulants should be given for at least 6, and preferably 12 months (Adams et al., 1974). This is the period of greatest risk of further emboli in cases of myocardial infarction. In mitral stenosis with persisting atrial fibrillation there is risk of further emboli for 2 years after the first embolus (Carter, 1965). In these circumstances anticoagulant therapy should be continued for 2 years, or longer (Fleming and Bailey, 1971). In suitable cases of mitral stenosis cardiac surgery may be considered.

An account of anticoagulant therapy is given later in this chapter.

If the embolus is infective, (e.g. from bacterial endocarditis) the appropriate antibiotics are indicated.

Arteritis

When brain infarction is due to some form of arteritis (e.g. tuberculous, syphilitic, giant-cell) the appropriate therapeutic agents should be used.

Spasm

As pointed out earlier, there is no established drug therapy for cerebral arterial spasm.

Promoting the Collateral Circulation

If there is a significant amount of ischaemic brain, as well as an infarct, endeavours to produce maximal collateral circulation may at times be useful. Thus inhalations of 5% carbon dioxide in air may be tried for 5 minutes each half-hour. Hutchinson (1976) was not impressed with the results of this therapy. The cervical sympathetic trunk on the appropriate side may be blocked by injection of local anaesthetic (e.g. 1% procaine). If this latter procedure produces benefit it may be repeated. If benefit occurs again, surgical section of the sympathetic trunk may be considered. Whether these various measures do more than accelerate recovery which would have occurred anyway is uncertain. Reduction of intracranial pressure (see below) may improve flow in the collateral circulation.

Relieving Mass Lesion Effects

Sometimes brain infarction may be accompanied by considerable brain swelling, with a significant mass lesion effect and raised intracranial pressure. In these circumstances intravenous glycerol may be given (Meyer et al., 1971; Mathew et al., 1972). The use of glycerol tends to restore brain metabolism (Meyer et al., 1974). This may not be due to a direct metabolic effect of glycerol but to an improved brain circulation as intracranial pressure is reduced. Concurrently with glycerol, intravenous corticosteroids may be used (p.43), also with the aim of reducing intracranial pressure, since these agents appear to reduce the abnormal permeability of capillary endothelium in ischaemic brain.

Whether these pressure-reducing measures should be used when there is no clinically detectable mass lesion effect is arguable. Presumably in these circumstances there still may be a degree of local brain swelling. If this swelling could be reduced there may be an increased collateral circulation, with improved brain function.

The pressure-reducing agents are relatively safe to use, but there is no good statistical evidence that they confer benefit in acute cerebral infarction (Candelise et al., 1974; Norris, 1976). Kaste et al. (1976) reported the failure of the combination of high dose dexamethasone (20mg/day) and intravenous low molecular weight dextran to influence the outcome of acute brain infarction.

While intracranial pressure-lowering agents do not appear to improve average recovery from cerebral infarction, this does not necessarily prove that such agents are of no benefit in some patients whose infarcts have constituted significant mass lesions. When groups of patients are studied, a response in such patients may be concealed by a failure to produce benefit in a larger number of patients who have no significant brain swelling in relation to their infarct.

Although medical measures are available to treat established brain infarction, one must conclude that the results are often far from satisfactory.

Anticoagulant Therapy

When oral warfarin or other coumarin or indanedione derivatives are given, there is 12 to 48 hours delay before an anticoagulant effect occurs. As soon as these drugs are absorbed they competitively antagonise the action of vitamin K. They therefore prevent the formation of certain clotting factors. However, it takes many hours for the supply of pre-existing clotting factors to be exhausted, so that the onset of the anticoagulant effect is delayed. In cerebral embolism, where an immediate anticoagulant effect is usually required, intravenous heparin is therefore used, though the oral anticoagulants are commonly given at the same time. After 48 hours heparin can be discontinued as the anticoagulant effect of the coumarin or indanedione derivative develops. If a delay in the onset of anticoagulant action is acceptable heparin need not be used.

The usual sodium heparin dose is 10,000 units intravenously every 6 hours for 48 hours. 6-hourly intravenous administration does not produce an increased clotting time for the whole duration of the dosage interval. Therefore, even though intermittent heparin therapy in practice usually proves adequate, some might prefer to give heparin by continuous intravenous infusion in 5% glucose or 0.9% saline or similar fluids, so that a heparin dose of 20,000 units is given over 12 hours. When heparin is used in this way for 48 hours it is usually unnecessary to estimate blood clotting time. Should bleeding occur while heparin is being given, an intravenous dose of protamine sulphate, 1mg for each 1000 units of heparin given within the past 6 hours, will counteract any residual heparin effect rapidly.

Initially, warfarin 40mg may be given orally as a single dose, or phenindione 200mg on the first day and 100mg on the second. On the third day prothrombin activity is measured and dosage is then adjusted, as necessary, daily or on alternate days, to keep the prothrombin time at 2.5 to 3 times normal. Bearing in mind the 24 to 48 hour delay between a change in the dose of these anticoagulant agents and the appearance of a changed anticoagulant effect, there is usually little point in measuring prothrombin time and adjusting doses more often than every second day. As time passes most patients can be managed adequately with less frequent prothrombin time measurements and dosage adjustments e.g. fortnightly or monthly. Should bleeding occur, or should it be desired to reverse the anticoagulant effect over 6 to 10 hours, intravenous vitamin K_1 15 to 25mg is given. Oral vitamin K_1 acts a little more slowly.

It should be pointed out that those who have obtained useful results from anti-coagulant therapy in cerebral vascular disease have generally been those interested in managing anticoagulant therapy closely. There are many hazards in long term anti-coagulant therapy, particularly therapy in outpatients e.g. dosage mistakes by the patient, pharmacokinetic interactions between the anticoagulant and other drugs taken. Unless there are special local facilities for the follow-up of anticoagulant thera-py one might wonder how often such therapy is justified in neurological patients.

Persisting and/or Progressing Regional Brain Ischaemia

Sometimes after occlusion of a cerebral artery there is evidence that the cerebral deficit of function is chiefly due to continuing ischaemia rather than established in-farction. Thus the EEG may show a severe and continuing focal disturbance which could arise only from malfunctioning rather than from dead neurones. Angiography may show a reasonable but delayed collateral circulation beyond the block or stenosis in the arterial lumen. In this circumstance the various measures discussed above, which in non-embolic infarction are pursued in the hope of lessening the effects of any attendant ischaemia around the infarct, should again be employed, and the use of anticoagulants should be considered.

When brain ischaemia is increasing locally, as may occur in progressing stroke, there is again a place for measures aimed at correcting the cause of the situation, and for enhancing the collateral circulation. In this circumstance it seems generally agreed that anticoagulants are beneficial if the patient is not hypertensive (Marshall, 1976). Anticoagulant therapy may be continued till the patient's neurological state is stable for several weeks, or more. Hypertension should be treated before anticoagulants are used, or if there is malignant hypertension; otherwise attempts to reduce hyperten-sion at this stage may do more harm than good, by causing decreased perfusion of ischaemic brain. Any factors which might decrease cerebral oxygenation (e.g. anaemia, hypotension) should be corrected.

Transient Ischaemic Attacks

Recurrent small emboli (of platelet aggregates, of thrombus, or of atheromatous debris) from atheromatous sites in the proximal carotid system may produce repeated temporary (less than 24 hours) disturbances of brain, or retinal function, without a permanent deficit. Similar episodes may occur in the vertebro-basilar system. In both these circumstances treatment is directed at relieving the cause of the episodes. If the cause of transient ischaemic attacks is left untreated, there is a greater than 1 in 3 risk of a major stroke within 5 years (Hass, 1972).

Platelet and thrombus embolism may be treated by using various antithrombotic agents and agents active against platelet aggregation. In these conditions anticoagulants may be useful (Marshall, 1976; Ross Russell, 1976) but there are attendant risks of bleeding. Pearce et al. (1965) found that long term anticoagulants did not offer significant benefit in transient ischaemic attacks. However, Toole et al. (1975) found that anticoagulants did prevent further transient ischaemic attacks, but not further strokes. If anticoagulants are to be used hypertension should be controlled first. Anticoagulants probably should be used till the attacks have ceased for a year or so (Marshall and Reynolds, 1965). In recent years treatment with regular prophylactic aspirin has been advocated, and has seemed to reduce the frequency of retinal embolic manifestations (Harrison et al., 1971). Benefit often appears about 2 to 3 days after beginning aspirin therapy and persists while the drug is continued. The usual aspirin dose is 300mg 3 times a day, but as the effect of a single aspirin dose in altering platelet properties lasts about 3 days (Mustard and Packham, 1973), clearly once or twice daily dosage should suffice. Occasional omitted aspirin doses should not impair the therapeutic effect. The drug may be given for years. If aspirin produces gastric irritation, enteric-coated aspirin preparations may be used. The results of treating platelet or thrombus emboli with aspirin are sufficiently satisfactory (Yatsu, 1977) that aspirin, rather than anticoagulants, is tending to become the medical treatment of choice for transient ischaemic attacks. Whether aspirin need be combined with another platelet-inhibiting agent e.g. dipyridamole, is debatable, though the combinations have been rather widely used. In patients who cannot tolerate aspirin there may be a place for oral dipyridamole 100mg 3 or 4 times a day or sulphinpyrazone 400 to 800mg per day.

Until the advent of aspirin prophylaxis, the treatment of choice for transient ischaemic attacks rested between anticoagulants and surgical removal of the source of emboli (usually by carotid endarterectomy). Some may still regard surgery as the preferred treatment and certainly it should be considered very seriously:

1) If aspirin and anticoagulant therapy fail
2) If the emboli consist of cholesterol or other atheromatous debris, or
3) If, in the presence of an atheromatous stenosis of the carotid system, transient brain ischaemia is due to episodic hypotension (as from bouts of cardiac arrhythmia) which cannot be treated adequately.

Mutliple Arteriopathic Infarcts (Lacunes)

Cerebral arteriosclerosis and hypertension may cause multiple small cerebral infarcts (lacunes) over a period of months or years. Usually arteriography shows no single area of narrowing of arterial lumens, but rather evidence of widespread arteriosclerosis. The two most typical clinical pictures produced in this way are multi-infarct dementia and arteriopathic pseudobulbar palsy. In both of these conditions it is usually not a single acute ischaemic event which brings the patient to the neurologist, but an accumulation of several such events. Therefore it is rarely possible to employ the measures discussed above to treat the acute stages of brain infarction. In practice measures designed to correct the possible cause of the disorder (e.g. the use of anticoagulants) rarely seem of much use. The disorder's natural history seems to proceed relentlessly, undisturbed by attempts at treatment. Aspirin, given in the attempt to prevent further episodes, is likely to be safe in the majority of instances. Its efficacy is unproven in these circumstances. Hypertension and hyperlipidaemia should be controlled, though there is no proof that these measures are of benefit in this situation.

Long Term Management After Brain Infarction

Once cerebral infarction has occurred, to what extent are prophylactic measures against further infarction useful, or necessary? The situation in relation to recurrent transient ischaemic attacks has been discussed above. After a solitary major ischaemic episode, unless there is a directly treatable source of further ischaemia (e.g. a carotid stenosis, bacterial endocarditis) there is little evidence that prophylactic measures are of much value. On the whole, control of hypertension is probably useful (Marshall, 1976). Thus Carter (1970) concluded that continuous control of diastolic hypertension (i.e. production of a diastolic blood pressure below 110mm Hg) after the first stroke, in persons under 65 years, reduced the overall mortality and recurrence rate of non-fatal stroke. Bradshaw and Brennan (1975) showed that long term anticoagulation did not improve the outlook, though there had been earlier suggestions that anticoagulation did offer marginal benefit (McDowell et al., 1963). Dietary measures intended to retard the progress of atheroma, and the use of antihypercholesterolaemic drugs, are not of established value in these circumstances. The prescription of regular aspirin to decrease platelet stickiness may be little more than a hopeful, though reasonably innocent, gesture.

Chapter XI

Demyelinating and Autoimmune Disease

Principal Disorders and Drugs Discussed

Multiple sclerosis
  Corticosteroids, corticotrophin (see also chapter II)

Autoimmune disease
  Azathioprine
  Cyclophosphamide
  Methotrexate
  Corticosteroids (see also chapter II)

Primary Demyelinating Disorders

Disordered Mechanisms

A number of neurological disorders appear to have primary demyelination as their common pathological basis. In these disorders the primary pathological event appears to be a local breaking down of myelin in the central and/or peripheral nervous system, with a relative preservation of axis cylinders formerly encased in the affected myelin. Multiple sclerosis is the most common of the primary demyelinating diseases. Despite a great deal of research it is probably fair to say that there is no generally accepted view as to the aetiology of multiple sclerosis, as to how the episodes of demyelination are precipitated, and as to what determines their location in the central nervous system. The main hypotheses now in vogue are that multiple sclerosis is an autoimmune disorder, or is due to 'slow virus' infection. The aetiologies of neuromyelitis optica and Schilder's sudanophil diffuse sclerosis also remain obscure, though one form of the latter, associated with adrenal insufficiency, appears to be inherited as a sex-linked recessive. The animal model of experimental allergic encephalitis provides some basis for understanding the pathogenesis of the primary demyelinating neuritides and radiculopathies (Guillain-Barre syndrome), and the myelinoclastic encephalomyelopathies. The latter may be idiopathic, or para-infectious (associated commonly with measles, varicella, smallpox vaccination). Experimentally, analogous neuropathological appearances of areas of perivenous demyelination can be produced by immunising animals against their own peripheral or central myelin. It is thought that trivial or more major infection, or immunisation, can sometimes make a person 'allergic' to his own myelin.

Thus the primary demyelinating disorders appear to be an aetiologically diverse group of conditions which have some common pathological basis.

Correction of Disordered Mechanisms

Multiple Sclerosis

Because we are ignorant of the mechanisms involved in the pathogenesis of multiple sclerosis it is impossible to design treatment of the disorder based on correction of disturbed mechanisms. Partly because of analogies with experimental allergic encephalitis, there are some grounds for believing that multiple sclerosis may be an autoimmune disorder. Hence attempts have been made to treat multiple sclerosis with measures that suppress immune mechanisms. The authors' impression is that high dose adrenal corticosteroids sometimes shorten exacerbations of multiple sclerosis and perhaps reduce the final disability caused by individual exacerbations. Some controlled studies, certain of which did not employ very high steroid doses (Tourtelotte and Haerer, 1965), have tended to suggest that steroids are of benefit in multiple sclerosis. Corticosteroids have several different modes of action and a response to corticosteroids does not really provide evidence that multiple sclerosis is an autoimmune disorder. Continuous therapy with high dose corticosteroids does not seem to prevent further relapse of multiple sclerosis and bolus alternate day high dosage corticosteroid use, such as is effective in generally accepted autoimmune disorders like myasthenia and polymyositis, does not appear to have much effect on the course of multiple sclerosis. The pattern of corticosteroid use that appears helpful in multiple sclerosis is the regular administration of the drugs in high dosage in the first few days of an exacerbation of the disorder. At the time of writing other methods of immune suppression are being investigated as treatment for multiple sclerosis. For instance Swinburn and Liversedge (1973) showed that 2 years of therapy with azathioprine did not appear to alter the course of multiple sclerosis in 19 patients. Silberberg et al. (1973) drew a similar conclusion from their studies. Drachmann et al. (1975) found that cyclophosphamide did not significantly alter the course of acute exacerbations of multiple sclerosis. There is also interest in the use of diets enriched with linoleic acid, prescribed on the basis that patients with multiple sclerosis have diminished plasma levels of this fatty acid. However Love et al. (1974) showed that reduced plasma linoleate concentrations are not specific for multiple sclerosis, and occur in patients with other diseases. Swank (1970) on the basis of an uncontrolled study of 146 patients with multiple sclerosis followed for a mean period of 17.1 years, claimed that a low fat diet decreased the rate of progression of the disorder and the frequency and severity of exacerbations.

Other Demyelinations

High dose steroids sometimes appear helpful in the acute phase of neuromyelitis optica but no therapy appears of much use in Schilder's disease.

In the myelinoclastic encephalitides our clinical impression is that high dose corticosteroids tend to reduce the severity of attacks, though no firm evidence is available. While the effect of steroids on immune mechanisms may play a part in this type of acute encephalitis, the steroids may produce benefit by reducing raised intracranial pressure due to cerebral swelling.

Although there have been dissenting opinions (Goodall et al. 1974), there is now reasonable evidence that steroids are of benefit in Guillain-Barre polyneuritis, probably because of both anti-inflammatory and anti-immune effects (Heller and de Jong, 1963).

Drugs Used in the Treatment of Demyelinating Diseases

The glucocorticoids, tetracosactrin and corticotrophin are the only drugs of any established value in primary demyelinating disease. They are discussed in chapter II.

Treatment of Acute Primary Demyelination

Multiple Sclerosis

Drug therapy appears of some use in the acute phase of primary demyelination in multiple sclerosis. High dose steroids may be given for 1 to 2 weeks. Dosages may then be reduced in stages over the next 2 or 3 weeks, unless the disorder worsens as dosage falls, in which case higher dosages should be used again for a time. Oral prednisone or prednisolone 100 to 150mg per day, in 3 or 4 divided doses, or dexamethasone 4mg 4 times a day, may be used for the first 7 to 14 days of the acute illness. If the patient cannot swallow, similar doses may be given intravenously at first, and then by intramuscular injection. During withdrawal of therapy it is generally possible to halve the previous steroid dose every third day, and finally when about one-eighth of the initial dose has been taken for 3 days, to discontinue the steroids. With such a relatively short course of steroids, persisting adrenal suppression is unlikely. However some may choose to stimulate the adrenals with 2 or 3 daily injections of tetracosactrin at the end of the course of steroids. If the steroids cause dyspepsia, antacids may be given. Otherwise these relatively short courses of high dosage steroids are not usually associated with serious side effects.

Workers have sometimes used IM corticotrophin (40 units per day) or an equivalent amount of tetracosactrin to treat acute episodes of primary demyelination. Some therapeutic trials have shown these regimens to be helpful (Miller et al., 1961b). However for the reasons suggested in chapter II, the authors prefer to use a known corticosteroid dose rather than depend on an uncertain corticosteroid response to adrenal stimulation, particularly when the response of primary demyelination to corticosteroid seems to depend on the administration of a critical threshold drug dose (for prednisone, about 60 to 80mg per day in many patients). When exacerbations of multiple sclerosis affect the spinal cord the use of single or repeated intrathecal injections of glucocorticoid (e.g. 40mg methylprednisolone acetate) may minimise unwanted systemic steroid effects while improving the neurological disorder. High local steroid concentrations can be achieved in this way (Lehrer et al., 1973). With repeated intrathecal injection of one preparation of methylprednisolone acetate containing polyethylene glycol in its vehicle, there is risk of producing sclerosing spinal pachymeningitis (Bernal et al., 1976).

Over the years numerous other therapies have been employed in multiple sclerosis. None can be recommended with confidence. Intrathecal tuberculin has been proved ineffective in well designed studies (Kelly and Jellinek, 1961; Miller et al., 1962), as have tranylcypromine (Barrow and Rischbieth, 1965; Lance et al., 1965), chloroquine, aspirin and parenteral γ-globulin (Miller et al., 1961a, 1963). A high dietary intake of linoleic acid (17g a day, given as sunflower seed oil or emulsion) may reduce the frequency and severity of relapses, though it has not been proven to change the overall rate of clinical deterioration (Miller et al., 1973).

Once the acute phase of primary demyelination has passed, steroids appear of little or no use. Millar et al. (1967, 1970) found that continued corticotrophin therapy, for at least 18 months, did not appear to alter the course of multiple sclerosis. However, Tourtelotte and Haerer (1965) did obtain some tentative evidence that multiple sclerosis patients taking 8 to 12mg methylprednisolone daily fared a little better than control patients over an 18 month follow-up period. Other drug treatment that is used during multiple sclerosis remissions is essentially symptomatic (e.g. baclofen or diazepam for spasticity, anticholinergics for urine incontinence) and is aimed at helping residual disability.

Other Demyelinations

Neuromyelitis optica, Guillain-Barre polyradiculitis or myelinoclastic encephalitis may be treated with a similar high dose glucocorticoid regimen to that suggested for exacerbations of multiple sclerosis. The controlled study of Bowden et al. (1974) showed that corticotrophin did not improve the outcome in acute optic neuritis, though the earlier work of Rawson and Liversedge (1969) had suggested that corticotrophin did confer some benefit if given in the first month of the illness.

Accepted Autoimmune Disorders

The concept of autoimmune disease is relatively recent and the question of which neurological disorders fit within this category is not yet settled. Some would classify multiple sclerosis and the other primary demyelinations discussed earlier in this chapter as among the autoimmune conditions, though others might have reservations. Therefore the neurologist's traditional classification of the primary demyelinations has been retained in this book. There is good evidence that myasthenia gravis is an autoimmune disorder. However we decided to deal with myasthenia in the section on motor disorders (chapter III).

Considered broadly, the autoimmune disorders that concern the neurologist fall into two categories:

1) Those which are conventionally regarded as primarily neurological including:
   a) certain primary demyelinations, in particular myelinoclastic encephalitis and the Guillain-Barre syndrome
   b) certain rare forms of relapsing peripheral neuritis
   c) myasthenia gravis
   d) polymyositis and dermatomyositis.
2) Those in which the nervous system may be involved as part of a more general process, including:
   a) systemic lupus erythematosus
   b) polyarteritis nodosa
   c) rheumatoid disease
   d) giant cell arteritis
   e) polymyalgia.

Disordered Mechanisms

In the autoimmune disorders some as yet incompletely understood mechanisms cause cells to form antibodies against components of some of the patient's tissues. The interaction between these antibodies and the specific tissue components is responsible for the clinical manifestations of the various disorders.

Correction of Disordered Mechanisms

Treatment of autoimmune disorders may be directed at preventing abnormal antibody formation and/or minimising the consequences of the abnormal antigen-antibody reaction in specific tissues.

Certain cytotoxic agents e.g. azathioprine, methotrexate, cyclophosphamide, act by destroying antibody-producing lymphocytes as these cells proliferate. Corticosteroids interfere with antibody formation and also suppress local inflammatory responses consequent on antigen-antibody reactions.

In myasthenia it may be possible to extirpate surgically the major site of auto-antibody formation *viz* the thymus.

Drugs Used in Treatment

Only a few of the available drugs with immunosuppressive actions will be discussed here.

Azathioprine

Azathioprine is used as an antimetabolite and immunosuppressive agent.

Chemistry

Azathioprine (MW 277.29) is a purine analogue. Within the body it may react non-enzymatically with free sulphydryl groups to slowly liberate 6-mercaptopurine (MW 152.19), the active fraction (fig. 11.1).

Pharmacology

Biochemical Pharmacology

The action of azathioprine is mediated through the 6-mercaptopurine released from it, as explained above. 6-Mercaptopurine is incorporated in a 5'-phosphate ribonucleotide within cells, replacing normal purines in this synthesis. The thio-inosinate so formed inhibits a number of vital metabolic reactions (e.g. the conversion of inosinate to adenylosuccinate, the conversion of inosine monophosphate to xanthylate).

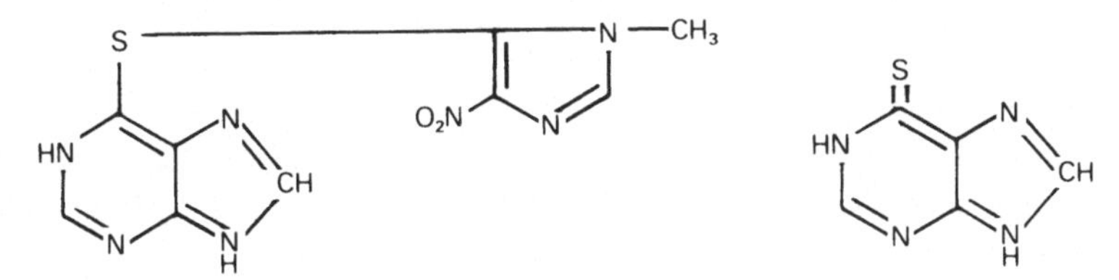

Fig. 11.1. Structural formulae of azathioprine and its active fraction, 6-mercaptopurine.

Pharmacodynamics

The cytotoxic actions of 6-mercaptopurine affect rapidly dividing cells (e.g. the cells of bone marrow, gonads and the gastrointestinal wall) more rapidly and severely than slowly dividing cells. The action of mercaptopurine on dividing lymphocyte precursors reduces antibody production by these cells.

Pharmacokinetics

Absorption and bioavailability: Azathioprine is absorbed after oral administration with a T_{max} of 2 hours (Elion, 1972). In essence, it serves as a pro-drug for 6-mercaptopurine.

Distribution: Data on the distribution of azathioprine are not available, but the derived 6-mercaptopurine enters cells, particularly rapidly dividing cells. Some 30 % of azathioprine in plasma is bound to plasma protein. Azathioprine crosses the placenta (Saariskoski and Seppala, 1973).

Elimination: The half-life of azathioprine is 3 hours or 4.5 to 5.0 hours (Elion, 1972) and that of 6-mercaptopurine averages 21 or 47 minutes (Loo et al., 1968). Approximately 20 % of a 6-mercaptopurine dose is excreted unchanged in urine though if azathioprine is given only 1 % of the dose appears in urine as mercaptopurine (Elion, 1972). The remainder is biotransformed by:

1) Methylation and then oxidation of sulphydryl group, and incorporation of the methyl derivative into nucleotides
2) Oxidation to thiouric acid by the hepatic enzyme xanthine oxidase. This reaction is inhibited by allopurinol.

The metabolism of azathioprine is altered in persons with liver disease (Bach and Dradenne, 1972).

Plasma level correlations: No data are available.

Interactions
Pharmacodynamic interactions: Mercaptopurine has additive effects if given with other cytotoxic agents which act on different aspects of nucleotide and nucleic acid formation.

Pharmacokinetic interactions: Allopurinol, an inhibitor of xanthine oxidase, diminishes the biotransformation of mercaptopurine to the inactive metabolite thiouric acid. This increases the cytotoxic effect of mercaptopurine.

Toxicity

Idiosyncratic Toxicity
Skin rashes may occur.

Dose-related Toxicity
Anorexia, nausea and vomiting occur in an appreciable number of cases. The main side effect is depression of the bone marrow. Jaundice from bile stasis and hepatic necrosis may occur.

Dysmorphogenicity
Because of their relatively selective effects on rapidly dividing cells azathioprine and mercaptopurine are likely to produce fetal injury if given to pregnant women.

Cyclophosphamide

Cyclophosphamide is an alkylating agent used in treating neoplastic disease and in immunosuppression. In neurology the drug has been used to treat polymyositis, various 'collagen' disorders and Guillain-Barre polyneuritis (Rosen and Vastola, 1976).

Chemistry

Cyclophosphamide (MW 261.10) is a nitrogen mustard derivative (fig. 11.2).

Pharmacology

Biochemical Pharmacology

Alkylating agents such as cyclophosphamide provide alkyl groups which attach to desoxyribosenucleic acid molecules, causing cellular damage.

Pharmacodynamics

Alkylating agents exert their effects mainly on rapidly proliferating cells and tissues, though alkyl groups attach to nucleic acids in all cells and tissues. The action on haemopoietic cells appears within 6 to 8 hours of dosage. Amenorrhoea and impaired spermatogenesis may occur and there is likely to be damage to the intestinal mucosa and hair follicles. Cyclophosphamide has relatively less effect on platelet precursors than other nitrogen mustards, but is more likely to damage hair follicles and cause alopecia.

Pharmacokinetics

Absorption and bioavailability: After oral administration cyclophosphamide is well absorbed. Peak plasma concentrations occur 1 hour after oral dosage.

Distribution: After absorption cyclophosphamide enters cells to exert its biological effects. Its V_D is approximately the volume of extracellular water (Bagley et al. 1973). Between 0 and 10% of the drug in plasma is protein-bound; alkylating metabolites occur in plasma and some 56% of these are protein-bound.

Elimination: The mean half-life of cyclophosphamide is 4.9 hours (range 3.0 to 6.5 hrs), 4 to 5.5 hours (Mouridsen et al., 1976) or 6.5 hours (Bagley et al., 1973). An average of 29.6% of the dose is excreted unchanged in urine (Adamson, 1971) though Mouridsen et al. (1976) quoted figures of 10 to 14% and Bagley et al. (1973) found that less than 20% of the dose was excreted unchanged. The drug undergoes metabolism in the hepatic microsomal mixed-oxidase system (Connors et al., 1974) (fig. 11.2). With the exception of phosphamide mustard, the final metabolites are non-toxic. The elimination of the drug may be slowed in the presence of renal failure so that reduced dosage may be necessary (Mouridsen and Jacobsen, 1975).

Plasma level correlations: No data are available in relation to the use of the drug in neurological disease.

Interactions

Pharmacodynamic interactions: Cyclophosphamide may have additive cytotoxic effects if combined with other drugs which affect nucleic acid synthesis by different mechanisms.

Pharmacokinetic interactions: Cyclophosphamide has been reported to increase the hypoglycaemic action of insulin, possibly by inhibiting formation of antibodies against insulin. Cyclophosphamide may also decrease plasma pseudocholinesterase levels and this can lead to an abnormally prolonged effect of administered succinylcholine. Its biotransformation is increased by prednisone administration

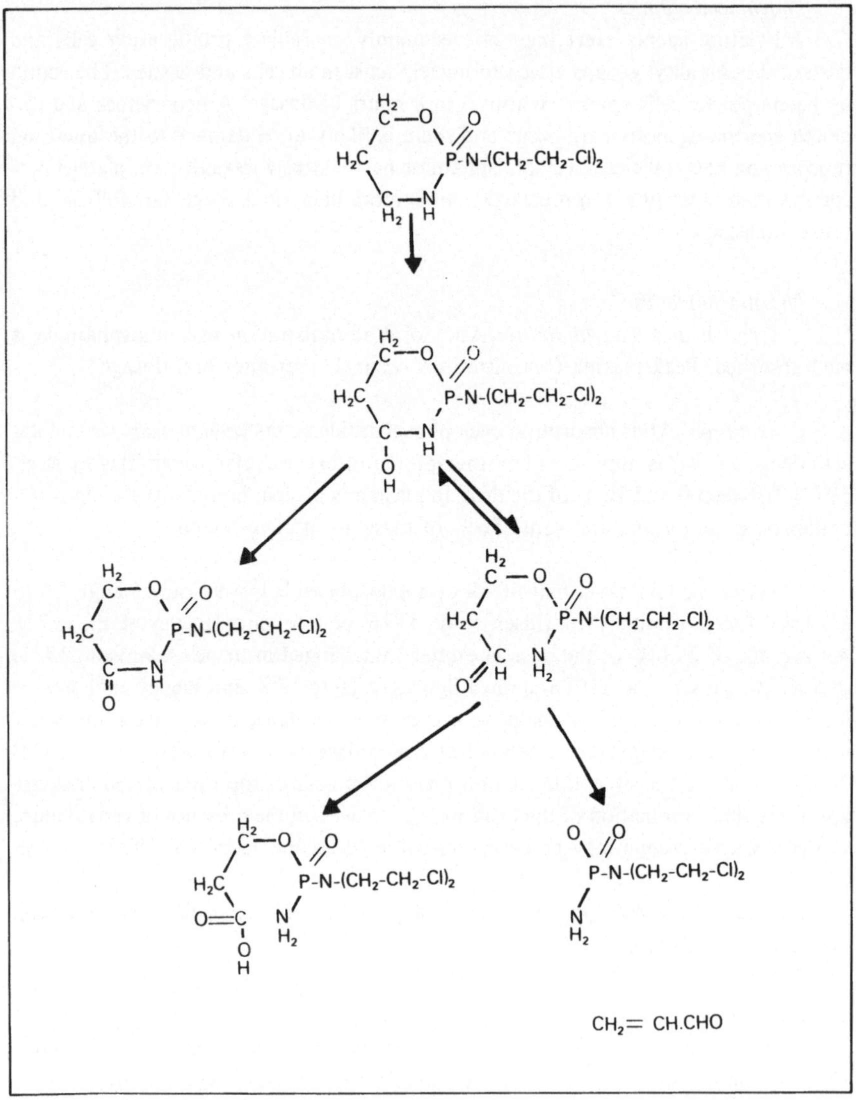

Fig. 11.2. Biotransformation of cyclophosphamide.

(Mouridsen et al., 1976), though Bagley et al. (1973) found that prednisolone did not alter the elimination of cyclophosphamide. The latter authors also stated that allopurinol pretreatment slowed the elimination of cyclophosphamide.

Toxicity

Idiosyncratic Toxicity
Such reactions appear to be uncommon.

Dose-related Toxicity
Manifestations include the following:

a) bone marrow depression
b) nausea and vomiting
c) alopecia
d) mucosal ulceration
e) brief dizziness
f) transverse nail ridging
g) increased skin pigmentation
h) interstitial pulmonary fibrosis
i) hepatic damage
j) aseptic haemorrhagic cystitis
k) inappropriate antidiuretic hormone secretion
l) sterility

Dysmorphogenicity
The mode of action of cyclophosphamide makes it potentially a dysmorphogen.

Methotrexate

Methotrexate is a folic acid antagonist used in treating acute leukaemia, chorionic carcinoma and psoriasis. It is also used as an immunosuppressive agent.

Chemistry

Methotrexate (MW 454.46) is an analogue of tetrahydrofolic acid (fig. 11.3). It has pKa values of 4.3 and 5.5.

Pharmacology

Biochemical Pharmacology

Methotrexate is a 'pseudo-irreversible' inhibitor of the enzyme dihydrofolate reductase. (Despite its very high affinity for the enzyme, methotrexate does not form covalent bonds with dihydrofolate reductase). Concentrations of folic acid that can be attained therapeutically will not reverse the inhibition of the enzyme. This effect of methotrexate can be countered by administration of leucovorin (folinic acid; N^5-formyltetrahydrofolic acid), which has several known actions (it increases reflux of intracellular methotrexate, inhibits a cellular transport mechanism and replaces reduced folate coenzymes). Inhibition of dihydrofolate reductase causes a deficiency in tetrahydrofolate, which is required for the synthesis of thymidylic acid from deoxyuridylic acid.

Pharmacodynamics

Inhibition of tetrahydrofolate reductase causes cytotoxic effects which tend to appear in the most rapidly dividing types of cell. Within 6 hours of dosage, cells of the intestinal mucosa swell and show cytoplasmic vacuoles, and then desquamate. The lesions may go on to a haemorrhagic enteritis. Bone marrow changes occur within 24 hours. There is inhibition of proliferation of erythroid precursors and changes in myelopoiesis which can go on to aplasia of the marrow if a large enough methotrexate dose is given. In lymphatic tissue there is a reduction in the numbers of lymphocytes.

Pharmacokinetics

Absorption and bioavailability: In ordinary doses (0.1 mg/kg) methotrexate is said to be well absorbed from the gastrointestinal tract but the bioavailability of the drug decreases at higher dosage. It is absorbed from intramuscular injection sites.

Distribution: Some 25% to 50% of methotrexate in plasma is bound to plasma protein. The drug may compete with sulphonamides and salicylates for plasma protein binding sites. Methotrexate is a relatively large polar molecule, and its entry into cells depends on specific uptake mechanisms. It is poorly transported across the blood-brain barrier, so that methotrexate levels in CSF are low relative to those in plasma. That portion of a methotrexate dose which binds to the enzyme dihydrofolate reductase is only very slowly released, owing to the tightness of the binding.

Elimination: Methotrexate has a half-life of 1.12 ± 0.19 days (Huffman et al., 1973). Some 80% of the dose is excreted unchanged in urine, though the percentage excreted is less with smaller doses. The drug appears to undergo little biotransformation in man.

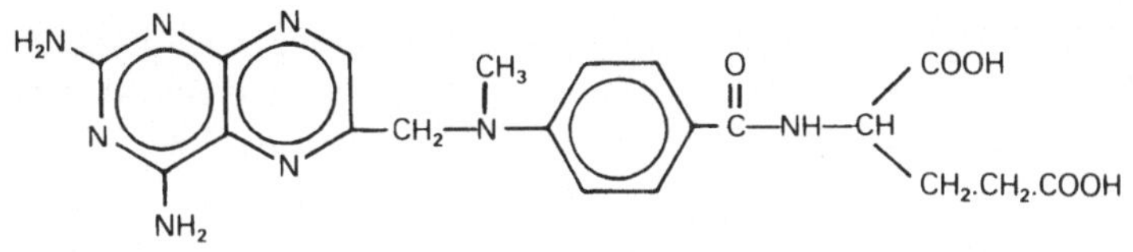

Fig. 11.3. Structural formula of methotrexate.

Plasma level correlations: Methotrexate plasma concentrations are directly proportional to dosage.

Interactions
Pharmacodynamic interactions: Folinic acid is in effect a methotrexate antagonist because it supplies tetrahydrofolate after synthesis of this substance has been blocked by methotrexate. This interaction is really a post-receptor one, rather than an interaction at the receptor.

Pharmacokinetic interactions: Sulphonamides (e.g. sulphisoxazole), salicylates and aminobenzoic acid competitively displace methotrexate from plasma protein binding sites.

Toxicity

Idiopathic Toxicity
Idiopathic toxic reactions appear to be uncommon.

Dose-related Toxicity
Methotrexate may cause the following:

a) stomatitis
b) diarrhoea
c) haemorrhagic enteritis
d) alopecia
e) dermatitis

f) renal damage

g) hepatic dysfunction, sometimes going on to cirrhosis

h) sterility

i) aplasia of bone marrow cellular elements.

Smith (1975) described widespread oligodendroglial destruction in the cerebral and cerebellar white matter in 3 of a series of 10 persons given intrathecal methotrexate. Clinically there were confusion, dementia, unsteadiness and EEG alterations.

Dysmorphogenicity

Therapy with methotrexate in pregnant women may cause abortion, or teratogenesis.

Treatment of Autoimmune Neurological Disorder

At the present time corticosteroids are probably the treatment of choice to suppress immune mechanisms when this is necessary in neurological disease. Simultaneously corticosteroids may reduce the severity of any inflammatory reaction produced by the abnormal immunological reactivity. Until recently immunological disorders were usually treated by regular administration of glucocorticoids in high dosage several times a day, oral prednisone or prednisolone 25mg 4 times a day, or oral dexamethasone 4mg 4 times a day being used initially; this dose should be reduced as quickly as possible, over a number of days, to as low a level as controls the patient's disorder, so as to minimise steroid side effects. It is now increasingly recognised that immunosuppression can be achieved with a single large bolus dose of steroid given every second day. For instance 100mg of prednisone or prednisolone, or 16mg dexamethasone, may be given by mouth every second morning. Used in this way unwanted steroid effects are greatly reduced, and at times may be negligible, even though high steroid doses are given for many months. The ability to reduce steroid toxicity in this way permits their more effective long term use in immunosuppression.

Such bolus corticosteroid regimens are useful in treating myasthenia (chapter III), polymyositis, collagen diseases affecting the nervous system and relapsing forms of polyneuropathy. As pointed out earlier, this regimen appears ineffective for multiple sclerosis.

If steroids fail to achieve an adequate immunosuppressive effect, or cannot be used by virtue of their toxicity, use of an antimitotic agent may be considered. Used for this purpose methotrexate is given in an initial oral dose of 2.5 to 10mg daily. As time passes, the size of the dose is adjusted to achieve control of the underlying disease if this can be achieved without undue toxicity. Regular examination of the peripheral blood provides some protection against excessive dosage. If evidence of undue marrow toxicity develops folinic acid may be given in an attempt to minimise further damage. This antidote may be given in doses of 6 to 9mg, every 4 to 6 hours, by intramuscular injection. Malaviya et al. (1968) reported the use of methotrexate in treating dermatomyositis.

As an alternative to methotrexate, oral cyclophosphamide 2 to 3mg per kg per day initially, may be used to achieve immunosuppression. As time passes the dose may need to be increased, or decreased, to control the patient's disorder. Regular blood counts are imperative if cyclophosphamide is used. Rosen and Vastola (1976) found cyclophosphamide beneficial in the Guillain-Barre syndrome, with reversible hair loss as the only side effect.

In place of methotrexate and cyclophosphamide, immunosuppression may be achieved with oral azathioprine given initially in a dose of 50 to 100mg per day. Subsequent doses are adjusted according to the patient's clinical condition. Bone marrow function should be checked by repeated blood counts during the course of treatment. Yuill et al. (1970) obtained benefit in steroid-refractory polyneuropathy by using azathioprine. Palmer (1965) reported the use of mercaptopurine in treating steroid resistant Guillain-Barre syndrome.

These antimitotic drugs are sometimes referred to as steroid-sparing agents. However, since the advent of intermittent bolus steroid therapy, it seems that there is usually little need to use cytotoxic drugs in autoimmune neurological disorders unless they fail to respond to potentially adequate steroid doses.

Chapter XII

Infections

Principal Disorders and Drugs Discussed

Viral meningitis
  Amantadine (see also chapter IV)
  Cytarabine
  Idoxuridine

Bacterial meningitis
  Penicillins
  Streptomycin, gentamicin
  Chloramphenicol

Tuberculous meningitis
  Isoniazid
  Ethambutol
  Rifampicin
  Streptomycin

Cryptococcal meningitis
  Amphotericin B
  Flucytosine

Hansen's disease
  Dapsone

Cerebral malaria
  Chloroquine

Brain abscess

Neurosyphilis

In most temperate climates infective disease of the nervous system is no longer a common clinical problem, though there are a considerable number of infective agents which may at times involve the nervous system. Because of the diminished frequency of nervous system infections, therapeutic agents which might find only an occasional use in neurological infection will not be discussed. For convenience, infections with different categories of organism will be considered separately.

Viral Infections

Disordered Mechanisms

A number of viruses may infect the nervous system. Some tend to attack the meninges rather selectively to produce the picture of aseptic meningitis, a self-limiting illness with relatively mild leptomeningeal inflammation. Other viruses (and also a few of the viruses which on other occasions cause aseptic meningitis) may attack neurones selectively. Such viruses usually produce the picture of a polioclastic panencephalitis (to be distinguished from the myelinoclastic encephalitides considered in chapter XI). Some viruses, however, may be relatively selective in the groups of neurones that they attack. Thus in herpes zoster the varicella virus exhibits a predilection for neurones in posterior root ganglia. The poliomyelitis virus tends to attack anterior horn and bulbar motor neurones. The virus of herpes simplex sometimes shows some preference for neurones in the temporal lobes. The result of infection with various polioclastic viruses is neuronal injury and death, with local tissue swelling and an inflammatory reaction.

Correction of Disordered Mechanisms

Ideally, treatment should be directed against the causative agent but, in general, antiviral chemotherapy is not sufficiently advanced for this therapeutic approach to have much practical application. Even if adequate antiviral agents were available it would also be necessary to have the means of identifying the causative virus early in the course of the illness, in order that the appropriate drugs might be prescribed at an early enough stage in the disorder to influence its natural history. Progress in achieving early viral diagnosis has been made chiefly in relation to herpes simplex infection, using immunofluorescent techniques. This is the form of viral encephalitis in which there has been some systematic attempt to treat the causative organism, though the efficacy of the treatment remains uncertain. There is a report that pancreatic ribonuclease, 30mg given 4-hourly for 5 to 6 days, is beneficial in Siberian tick-borne viral encephalitis (Glukhov et al., 1976).

Apart from treating the causative agent, the main therapeutic possibilities in viral infections of the nervous system are:

1) Reducing the inflammatory response and cerebral oedema
2) Relieving symptoms (e.g. by prescribing analgesics for headache, anti-emetics for nausea, anticonvulsants for fits).

Adrenal corticosteroids in high dosage may be used to diminish inflammation and oedema of neural tissue, thus reducing the consequences of any raised intracranial pressure. There is concern that steroids used in this way might have a detrimental effect by suppressing immune mechanisms and thus increasing the viral invasion of the nervous system. However, the consensus of contemporary opinion is that steroids should be used when intracranial pressure is raised by viral infection. In this case the benefits of steroids outweigh their risks. There is no point in using steroids in a benign condition, such as aseptic meningitis, and their use and value are not established in localised selective infections such as herpes zoster and poliomyelitis.

Drugs Used in the Treatment of Viral Infections

Amantadine was discussed in chapter IV, in relation to its use in Parkinsonism. Cytarabine and idoxuridine are considered below.

Cytarabine

Cytarabine is used as an antineoplastic and immunosuppressive agent. It has been employed in treating herpes simplex encephalitis (Liversedge, 1976).

Chemistry

Cytarabine (cytosine arabinoside) is a pyrimidine analogue (MW 243.22) with a pKa of 4.5.

Pharmacology

Biochemical Pharmacology
Within the body cytarabine is converted enzymatically to its 5-monophosphate nucleotide, which then interferes with nucleic acid metabolism and hence damages cells and hinders multiplication of viral particles. There may be inhibition of the enzyme ribonucleoside diphosphate reductase and certain forms of virally induced RNA-dependent DNA polymerase.

Pharmacodynamics
Cytarabine exerts its maximum toxicity in rapidly proliferating cells (e.g. bone marrow cells) and cells of the alimentary tract mucosa. It has an immunosuppressive action. By interfering with DNA synthesis it inhibits replication of DNA viruses. Its spectrum of antiviral activity is similar to that of idoxuridine, and includes vaccinia, varicella and herpes viruses, cytomegalovirus, polyoma and SV 40 viruses.

Pharmacokinetics

Absorption and bioavailability: The bioavailability of cytarabine, given orally, is less than 20%. The drug is usually given by intravenous injection or infusion, or sometimes by intrathecal injection.

Distribution: Quantitative data for man are not available, though obviously the drug enters cells.

Elimination: Cytarabine has a mean half-life of 1.85 hours (Ho and Frei, 1971). It appears to undergo extensive biotransformation as an average of only 7.1 % of a dose appears unchanged in urine. The main metabolite is arabinosyl uracil, which is pharmacologically inactive.

Plasma level correlations: Data are not available.

Interactions
Pharmacodynamic interactions: Cytarabine is likely to interact additively if given with other antineoplastic agents which have different modes of action (e.g. methotrexate).

Pharmacokinetic interactions: Data are not available.

Toxicity

Idiosyncratic Toxicity
Descriptions of clear-cut idiopathic side effects are not available.

Dose-related Toxicity
Such side effects include:

a) bone marrow suppression, leading to leucopenia, thrombocytopenia and anaemia
b) gastrointestinal disturbances
c) stomatitis
d) hepatic damage
e) thrombophlebitis at injection sites.

Dysmorphogenicity
The mechanism of action of cytarabine makes it a potential dysmorphogen.

Idoxuridine

The main use of idoxuridine has been by local application in the treatment of herpes simplex infection of the conjunctivae and skin. However, it has also been used in treating herpes simplex encephalitis.

Chemistry

Idoxuridine (5-iodo-2'-deoxyuridine) has a molecular weight of 354.12. It is a white crystalline powder which is soluble in water.

Pharmacology

Biochemical Pharmacology

Idoxuridine has several actions which affect pyrimidine synthesis, nucleotide interconversion and DNA synthesis. The main effect of the drug arises from its metabolic conversion to a triphosphate derivative which is subsequently incorporated into DNA. It makes this DNA more susceptible to breakage and causes faulty transcription. Thus idoxuridine interferes with viral replication.

Pharmacodynamics

Idoxuridine has antiviral activity against viruses of the herpes group. Its spectrum of activity is similar to that of cytarabine.

Pharmacokinetics

Absorption and bioavailability: Idoxuridine is rapidly degraded by nucleotidase enzymes and hence must be injected if a systemic action is required.

Distribution: No detailed data are available.

Elimination: After intravenous injection idoxuridine disappears from the blood within 30 minutes. Only a small amount of the drug is excreted in urine. Probably the remainder of the dose is metabolised.

Plasma level correlations: No data are available.

Interactions

No definite interactions are known.

Toxicity

Idiosyncratic Toxicity

No well documented examples have been traced.

Dose-related Toxicity

Idoxuridine can inhibit DNA synthesis in mammalian cells as well as in viruses. Given intravenously it may cause bone marrow depression, stomatitis, alopecia and liver damage. It is a potential carcinogen.

Dysmorphogenicity

By virtue of its mode of action, idoxuridine is a potential dysmorphogen.

Treatment of Viral Infections of the Nervous System

Aseptic Meningitis

Viral aseptic meningitis is a self-limiting illness, requiring only symptomatic treatment once the diagnosis is established. Adequate analgesia should be provided and anti-emetics given if the patient is nauseated or vomiting. If vomiting is severe, parenteral fluid therapy may be required. Aseptic meningitis is discussed again on page 380.

Viral Panencephalitis

Unless the disorder is mild, intracranial pressure probably will be raised due to cerebral oedema. High dose steroids are then used (e.g. prednisolone or prednisone 150 to 200mg per day, or dexamethasone 16 to 24mg per day, given in 3 or 4 divided doses). Initially steroids are often given intravenously (e.g. a loading dose of 100mg prednisone or 8 to 12mg dexamethasone), with subsequent 4 to 6-hourly doses intravenously or intramuscularly till the patient can swallow. High steroid doses are continued till definite recovery is seen. Doses may then be reduced fairly rapidly e.g. by 50% every 3rd or 4th day. After a long course of steroids it may be advisable to stimulate adrenal function with several daily injections of tetracosactrin.

If a patient's condition deteriorates despite the use of steroids an additional attempt should be made to reduce intracranial pressure by using intravenous glycerol or mannitol (chapter II).

Apart from measures to reduce intracranial pressure, the management of viral panencephalitis comprises nursing care, maintenance of nutrition and hydration, sedation to control restlessness, and the use of anticonvulsants if epilepsy develops. During recovery and convalescence physiotherapy, occupational therapy and possibly speech therapy may be required.

Amantadine has been used at times in subacute sclerosing panencephalitis and in Jakob-Creutzfeld disease. Braham (1971) reported benefit from the drug in the latter disorder. Isoprinosine has also been used (Huttenlocher and Mattson, 1979).

Herpes Simplex Encephalitis

This disorder may present as a progressive temporal lobe mass lesion which, over several days, extends into a progressing diffuse encephalitis. In the focal mass lesion stage brain biopsy may permit aetiological diagnosis and possibly the neurosurgeon may then choose to remove the affected temporal lobe. The question of treatment has been discussed by Johnson (1972) and Liversedge (1976). The measures described above in treating panencephalitis may be employed *viz* steroids and various symptomatic treatments, if indicated. When the diagnosis has been proven, or on clinical grounds appears probable, some have used idoxuridine intravenously (100mg/kg/day) for 5 days, together with cytarabine (40mg/m²/day), also for 5 days. The results have not been particularly encouraging (Rappel et al., 1971), especially when the condition may sometimes undergo spontaneous recovery (Johnson et al., 1972). Recently adenine arabinoside has produced better results (Taber et al., 1977).

Poliomyelitis

Thanks to immunisation, poliomyelitis has largely disappeared from contemporary neurological practice. No specific pharmacological measures are available for the acute stages of the disorder.

Herpes Zoster

In the acute stage of the illness the treatment of herpes zoster involves the provision of pain relief and attempts to avoid infection in the skin lesions. The later problem of post-herpetic neuralgia was discussed in chapter VII.

Rickettsial Infections

In general rickettsial infections are a local regional problem and rarely present as primary neurological illnesses (of encephalitic type). Tetracyclines appear to be the drugs of first choice in their treatment, and chloramphenicol may be useful.

Bacterial, Protozoal and Fungal Infections

Bacterial and fungal infection of the nervous system may involve diffuse spread through the CSF to produce meningitis. Bacterial infection may also be localised, causing extradural, subdural or brain abscess. Infection with Hansen's bacillus selectively involves peripheral nerves. Localised fungal lesions may occur. Protozoal infections generally involve the nervous system widely. There are a number of patterns of neurological involvement which are characteristic of neurosyphilis (Merritt et al., 1946).

Disordered Mechanisms

Meningitis

Bacterial meningitis involves widespread infection of the meninges which provide an extensive absorptive surface for entry into the general circulation of bacterial toxins and products of inflammation. As well, bacterial infection may impair the secretory function of choroid plexus cells and may also interfere with CSF absorption through the arachnoid villi, increase CSF secretion and thus cause raised CSF pressure. Moreover there is also histological evidence of inflammation in, and damage to, the cerebral and cerebellar cortices in cases of meningitis. In some forms of meningitis, notably tuberculous, bacterial toxins may cause arteritis or cerebral venous thrombosis, leading to brain infarction. If treatment directed at the causative organism is delayed, or is otherwise inadequate, adhesions may have time to form in the subarachnoid space. If appropriately situated, these adhesions may obstruct the flow of CSF and produce obstructive hydrocephalus. Brain abscesses may form in association with the meningitis. These events are depicted schematically in figure 12.1.

Fungal meningitis generally runs a more protracted course than bacterial meningitis. Meningitis produced by spirochaetal infection is usually mild but, particularly in syphilis, there is a considerable tendency for arteritis to occur.

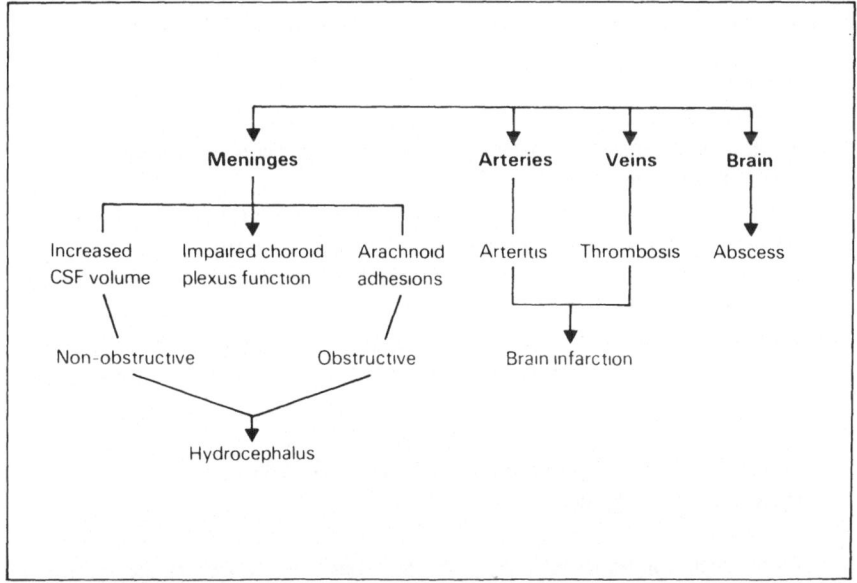

Fig. 12.1. Patterns of spread and consequences of nervous system infection.

Abscess

Abscess in the brain, or in the subdural or epidural space, produces the manifestations of a local mass lesion, added to the manifestations of localised bacterial infection. Such abscesses may arise from blood-borne infection, or from extension of local infection (e.g. from the middle ear or nasal accessory sinuses).

In Hansen's disease, peripheral nerves are involved directly by *Mycobacterium leprae*.

Correction of Disordered Mechanisms

Meningitis

The primary aim of therapy in bacterial, protozoal or fungal infection of the nervous system is to overcome the causative infection by using the appropriate antimicrobial agent, or agents. In general, the later the appropriate antimicrobial chemotherapy is given the greater is the risk of complications of the infection. The use of corticosteroids, in moderate dosage, may diminish arachnoid adhesion formation. In overwhelming infection (e.g. meningococcal septicaemia) steroids in high dosage may be needed to combat shock, and in this circumstance cortisol itself may be more appropriate therapy than glucocorticoids, because additional mineralocorticoid activity may be necessary. Should delayed or inadequate chemotherapy allow obstructive hydrocephalus to develop, some form of surgical drainage of CSF may be necessary.

Abscess

In intracranial abscess the surgical drainage of pus is necessary, as well as the use of appropriate antibiotic agents.

In treating either meningitis or intracranial abscess it may also be necessary to consider dealing with the source of the infection to prevent relapse or recurrence. On many occasions the antibiotic therapy given for the cranial infection will coincidentally serve this purpose. However, if there is, for example, a fistula between the subarachnoid space and the nasal cavity, following a fracture of the frontal bones of the skull, surgical closure of this fistula will be needed to prevent later reinfection.

Drugs Used in the Treatment of Bacterial Infections of the Nervous System

Many effective antimicrobial drugs are now marketed. In view of the relative infrequency of infection of the nervous system in contemporary neurological practice it would be out of keeping with the general attitude of this book to discuss all these drugs in detail. Therefore it has been decided to consider only those drugs which are used as primary therapy in the common forms of bacterial, protozoal and fungal meningitis and brain abscess. Information on other antibiotics may be obtained from works such as Goodman and Gilman (1975), Tolhurst et al. (1972) or Ball et al. (1978).

Penicillins

The natural and semisynthetic penicillins are widely used as antibacterial agents.

Chemistry

Chemically, the structure of the penicillins comprises a thiazolidine ring (α), joined to a β-lactam ring (β), to which is attached a side-chain (R) which determines the antibacterial and pharmacological characteristics of the derivative (fig. 12.2).

In the representative penicillins under consideration here, R has the configurations depicted in figure 12.3; the corresponding properties are also indicated. The various penicillins are acids with pKa values in the range 2.5 to 3.0.

Pharmacology

Biochemical Pharmacology

The penicillins inhibit the trans-peptidation reaction which produces cross linkages between the glycopeptide molecules that form part of the skeleton of bac-

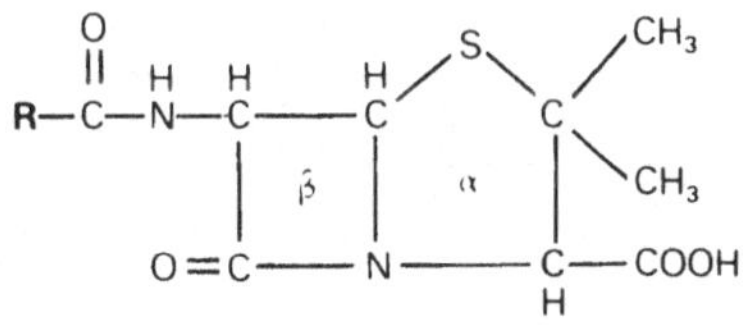

Fig. 12.2. The penicillin nucleus.

terial cell walls. In the absence of these linkages newly forming bacteria have cell walls which lack normal rigidity. Such bacteria are abnormally prone to osmotic injury. Human cells are not so affected, as their cell walls do not contain the relevant glycopeptides.

Pharmacodynamics

The penicillins exert their antibiotic action only while newly formed bacterial cells are synthesising their cell walls. Penicillins do not act on bacteria whose cell walls are already formed. Antibiotics which inhibit bacterial division, if given at the same time as a penicillin, may therefore prevent the penicillin exerting its actions. The antibacterial spectrum of benzylpenicillin includes mainly the following Gram-positive organisms: streptococci; staphylococci (unless they produce penicillinase); *Bacillus anthracis;* Corynebacteria; Listeria; *Myocytogenes erysipelothrix;* Clostridia; and among Gram-negative organisms *Neisseria meningitidis* and *Neisseria gonorrhoeae.* Benzylpenicillin also has an antibiotic effect in relation to Actinomyces species and to the spirochaete *Treponema pallidum.*

Cloxacillin is active against penicillinase-producing staphylococci, but its activity against other Gram-positive organisms is less than that of benzylpenicillin. Am-

	MW	R =	Antibiotic spectrum	Acid stability	Penicillinase resistance
Benzylpenicillin (Penicillin G)	334.38	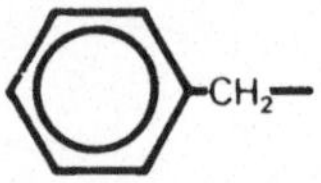	narrow	no	no
Cloxacillin	435.88	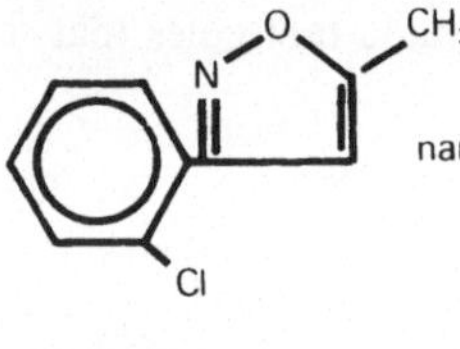	narrow	yes	yes
Ampicillin	349.42	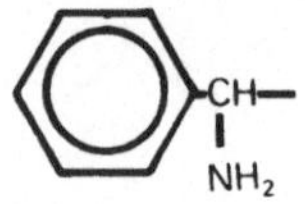	broad	yes	no
Carbenicillin	378.42	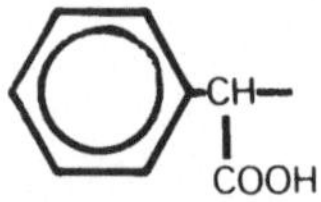	gram negative	no	no

Fig. 12.3. R side-chain configurations and properties of some penicillins.

picillin is a broad spectrum penicillin which is less active against Gram-positive organisms (apart from *Streptococcus faecalis* and *Listeria monocytogenes*) than is benzylpenicillin, and is inactive against penicillinase-producing staphylococci. However, ampicillin is active against many Gram-negative organisms including Salmonellae, Shigellae, most strains of *Haemophilus influenzae*, and some strains of *Escherichia coli*, Proteus and Klebsiella. Carbenicillin has antibacterial activity against Pseudomonas and some Proteus and Serratia species.

Pharmacokinetics

This subject is reviewed by Barza and Weinstein (1976).

Absorption and bioavailability: After *oral administration* benzylpenicillin is rapidly destroyed at gastric pH. In favourable circumstances up to one-third of an oral dose may be absorbed. Absorption occurs mainly from the duodenum and peak blood concentrations occur 30 to 60 minutes after ingestion. Because of the extent of its intragastric destruction benzylpenicillin is rarely given by mouth.

Cloxacillin and ampicillin are acid stable. Cloxacillin is 30 to 50 % bioavailable but ampicillin is well absorbed after oral administration. Whyatt et al. (1976) showed that 17 different ampicillin preparations had similar bioavailabilities. Peak plasma levels of ampicillin occur about 2 hours after ingestion.

Carbenicillin, not being acid stable, has too low and variable a bioavailability to be given by mouth in clinical practice.

After *intramuscular injection* peak blood levels of benzylpenicillin occur in 30 minutes, and peak levels of ampicillin and carbenicillin in 1 hour.

Because they achieve low concentrations in CSF if given orally or parenterally, penicillins may need to be injected *intrathecally*. The doses are much lower than the corresponding parenteral doses. Overdosage can be very dangerous, as penicillins act as convulsants if they achieve sufficient concentration in the brain.

Distribution: The apparent volumes of distribution of the four penicillins under consideration are: benzylpenicillin 0.3L/kg, ampicillin 0.39L/kg, cloxacillin 0.3L/kg and carbenicillin 0.17L/kg. Thus all four drugs are probably distributed throughout extracellular water, with the first three also distributing to some extent in intracellular water.

The plasma protein bindings of the drugs are, respectively, benzylpenicillin 65 %, cloxacillin 95 %, ampicillin 23 %, carbenicillin 50 %. By analogy with many other drugs, CSF concentrations of the various penicillins might have been expected to be similar to their plasma water concentrations. However CSF concentrations of benzylpenicillin are only 1 to 6 % of serum concentrations, ampicillin concentrations are 10 to 50 %, and no carbenicillin appears in the CSF of people who do not have meningitis. This apparent relative failure of penicillins to penetrate into the CSF has been ascribed to a blood-CSF barrier effect. This barrier effect breaks down in bacterial meningitis, when CSF penicillin concentrations are appreciably higher in relation to serum levels than they are when the meninges are not inflamed. However, it has been suggested that penicillins may be actively secreted out of CSF by the acid-secreting mechanism that exists in choroid plexus cells; this mechanism can be blocked by probenecid (Fishman, 1966; Walters et al., 1976). If so, the low levels of penicillins that occur in CSF when the meninges are not inflamed may reflect active extrusion of the drugs from CSF and not restricted entry of drugs into the CSF. The higher CSF penicillin levels in meningitis may be due to bacterial toxins inactivating the choroid plexus mechanism for removing organic acids from CSF.

Elimination: The half-life of benzylpenicillin is 0.5 hours, that of cloxacillin 25 minutes, that of ampicillin approximately 1 to 1.5 hours (Dittert et al., 1969), and that of carbenicillin 1 ± 0.25 hours (Hoffman et al., 1970). The fractions of a parenteral dose excreted unchanged in urine are benzylpenicillin 60 to 90% cloxacillin 78% (Cole et al., 1973); ampicillin 90 ± 7.5% (Jusko and Lewis, 1973), 92.4 ± 7.6% (Jusko et al., 1973), 79% (Cole et al., 1973) or 41.3% (Kunin and Finkelberg, 1970); carbenicillin 81.5 ± 8.6% (Cole et al., 1973). Thus the elimination of the absorbed penicillins occurs chiefly by renal excretion. This involves both glomerular filtration and active tubular transport. The latter mode of elimination can be competitively inhibited by administration of probenecid. Penicillin elimination is likely to be significantly reduced in the presence of renal insufficiency.

Some penicillin is excreted via the bile, though there is the possibility of an enterohepatic circulation of the drug. A little is lost in human milk and saliva.

Although bacterial penicillinase inactivates the drug by producing hydrolytic cleavage of the C-N bond in the β-lactam ring of the penicillin molecule, the resultant penicilloic acids do not appear to account for a significant amount of penicillin excretion in man, in relation to the magnitude of the doses used therapeutically.

Plasma level correlations: In treating bacterial meningitis the more relevant consideration is the CSF concentration of a penicillin, rather than its plasma concentration. As explained earlier, the quantitative relation between CSF and plasma concentrations is unpredictable in meningitis, and may vary during the course of the patient's illness. In intracranial abscess, plasma levels of the penicillin are more relevant. In therapy, penicillin concentrations well above the bactericidal threshold are usually attained. Therefore despite the rapid elimination of the penicillins, effective antibacterial plasma and tissue concentrations can usually be maintained with 6 or 8-hourly parenteral administration of the drug, if the organism in question is penicillin sensitive.

Interactions
Pharmacodynamic interactions: Penicillins may interact additively with other bactericidal antibiotics which damage bacteria by other biochemical mechanisms (e.g.

aminoglycosides, which interfere with ribosomal function). The bactericidal effect of penicillins may be reduced if they are given with bacteriostatic drugs (e.g. tetra-cyclines, erythromycin, chloramphenicol) since the latter prevent bacterial multiplica-tion, and the effect of the penicillins occurs only during cell wall synthesis in newly forming bacteria.

Pharmacokinetic interactions: Antacids may increase the ionisation of penicillins given orally, and hence delay their absorption. However, this effect tends to be offset by the antacid-induced decrease in gastric acidity. This local decrease in acidity tends to reduce the breakdown of acid-labile penicillins. Concurrent neomycin administration may produce a malabsorption syndrome which interferes with the ab-sorption of orally administered penicillins.

Probenecid inhibits renal tubular secretion of penicillins and therefore delays penicillin elimination, thus raising plasma and tissue penicillin levels. This action is sometimes used therapeutically.

Toxicity

Idiosyncratic Toxicity

Hypersensitivity reactions to penicillins are not rare, and there is cross-sen-sitivity between the various penicillins, so that patients who react to one penicillin are liable to react to the others. Immediate allergic reactions can occur within 20 minutes of penicillin administration in sensitised persons. The reaction may vary in severity from pruritus and urticaria to laryngeal spasm, hypotension and death. Drug fever or eosinophilia may occur. Delayed maculo-papular rashes are particularly common with ampicillin, especially in patients who have glandular fever.

Rarely, nephritis occurs after prolonged high dosage penicillin (particularly methicillin) therapy. It is not conclusively established that this is a hypersensitivity reaction.

Haemolytic anaemia is a rare complication of penicillin therapy.

Dose-related Toxicity

High dosages with sodium or potassium penicillin salts, particularly in persons with renal insufficiency, may produce electrolyte imbalance.

Excessive intrathecal penicillin dosage, or high systemic dosage in the presence of a defective blood-brain barrier, as in persons with uraemia, can lead to neurotoxic manifestations including convulsions, myoclonic jerking, coma and death.

Oral therapy with a penicillin may alter the bacterial flora of the alimentary tract and produce manifestations such as stomatitis, glossitis and diarrhoea. Use of penicillins may also lead to the emergence of bacterial strains resistant to these anti-biotics.

Dysmorphogenicity
There is no good evidence that the penicillins cause fetal abnormalities.

Aminoglycoside Antibiotics

This group of antibiotics includes streptomycin, gentamicin, kanamycin, tobramycin and neomycin. Only streptomycin and gentamicin will be considered here.

Streptomycin and Gentamicin

Streptomycin is used chiefly in tuberculous infections and gentamicin in severe Gram-negative infections including septicaemias.

Chemistry

Streptomycin (MW 581.58) and gentamicin are polar polycationic drugs which are water-soluble. The pKa of gentamicin is 8.2. It is a mixture of three closely related molecules, gentamicins C_1, C_2 and C_{1A}.

Pharmacology

Biochemical Pharmacology
Aminoglycoside antibiotics act on bacterial ribosomes to inhibit protein biosynthesis and impair the translation of the genetic code. In some way, as yet not adequately understood, this action on protein synthesis seems to account for the bactericidal effects of these drugs.

Pharmacodynamics
Streptomycin is bactericidal against many strains of *Mycobacterium tuberculosis*, against Shigella, Brucella, Erysipelothrix, *Listeria monocytogenes*, *Haemophilus ducreyi*, Nocardia and some Pasturella and Pseudomonas types. Strains of some other species exhibit widely varying sensitivities to streptomycin e.g. *Streptococcus pneumoniae*, Salmonellae, *Escherichia coli*, *H. influenzae*, Neisseria, *Proteus vulgaris*, *Staphylococcus aureus* and streptococci. Streptomycin is no longer a first-line antibiotic, except in the treatment of tuberculosis.

Gentamicin is highly bactericidal against *Pseudomonas aeruginosa*, *E. coli*, Klebsiella and Enterobacter. Many staphylococci, Group A streptococci, *H. influ-*

enzae and Bacteroides are sensitive, as are some Proteus strains and *M. tuberculosis.* Other organisms such as Neisseria and Clostridia are relatively resistant to the drug.

Bacterial resistance can develop to aminoglycoside antibiotics.

Pharmacokinetics

Absorption and bioavailability: The aminoglycosides are too polar to be absorbed well after oral administration. They are therefore given parenterally if a systemic action is required. After intramuscular injection peak streptomycin and gentamicin levels occur in 1 to 2 hours.

Distribution: At therapeutic concentrations in plasma some 20 to 30% of streptomycin and 70 to 80% of gentamicin are protein-bound. The apparent volumes of distribution of the drugs are 0.26 and 0.28L/kg respectively. Apparently both drugs distribute through extracellular water and enter cellular water to some extent. Streptomycin enters pleural, peritoneal and pericardial fluid and crosses the placenta. Very little enters CSF in the absence of meningitis, but CSF concentrations are higher if the meninges are inflamed. The distribution of gentamicin is generally similar, but even in meningitis entry into CSF is likely to be so poor that intrathecal and perhaps intraventricular therapy is required. Both antibotics are found in bile after their parenteral administration.

Elimination: The half-life of streptomycin is 2.72 ± 0.47 hours (Boxer et al., 1948) or 1.92 hours (Zintel et al., 1945), while that of gentamicin is 2 hours (Lockwood and Bower, 1973; Rodriguez et al., 1970) or 1.7 to 2.3 hours (Cutler et al., 1972).

A mean of 65% (Adcock and Hettig, 1946) or 66% (Zintel et al., 1945) of a streptomycin dose is excreted unchanged in urine. Corresponding figures for gentamicin are 81% (Regamey et al., 1973) or 69.8% (Gyselynek et al., 1971). Thus both these aminoglycoside antibiotics are eliminated chiefly by renal excretion. No metabolites of either drug are known. Elimination of these drugs is significantly slowed in persons with renal insufficiency.

Plasma level correlations: An intramuscular injection of 1g streptomycin produces peak plasma streptomycin levels of 25 to 30µg/ml. Highly sensitive bacteria are inhibited by less than 10µg/ml of streptomycin, and moderately sensitive ones by levels of 10 to 100µg/ml. Sensitive organisms are likely to respond to gentamicin concentrations below 5µg/ml. A gentamicin dose of 1mg/kg given by intramuscular injection is likely to produce a peak plasma gentamicin level in the region of 4µg/ml, and effective concentrations persist for 6 to 8 hours after dosage. Gentamicin serum levels in excess of 10µg/ml are likely to be ototoxic.

Interactions

Pharmacodynamic interactions: Aminoglycoside antibiotics can produce a degree of neuromuscular blockade. This can increase the actions of muscle relaxants which act by impairing neuromuscular transmission e.g. succinylcholine.

Aminoglycosides are ototoxic, and the risk of this effect is increased if the diuretic ethacrynic acid, another ototoxic substance, is given simultaneously. Gentamicin and cephalosporin antibiotics are said to have additive nephrotoxic effects.

Pharmacokinetic interactions: Carbenicillin, if mixed with gentamicin *in vitro*, is said to inactivate the latter drug. Prolonged oral aminoglycoside use can inhibit the growth of bacteria in the gut so that their production of vitamin K decreases. This can cause hypoprothrombinaemia.

Toxicity

Idiosyncratic Toxicity

Streptomycin may cause skin rashes, eosinophilia, fever, blood dyscrasias, angioneurotic oedema, exfoliative dermatitis, stomatitis and anaphylactic shock. Hypersensitivity to gentamicin is not common.

Dose-related Toxicity

Local reactions may occur at injection sites.

Ototoxicity: The aminoglycosides are ototoxic. The danger of ototoxicity is increased if ordinary therapeutic doses are used in persons with impaired renal function. Vestibular function is more severly affected than hearing. Ototoxicity is related not only to height of plasma levels of the drug but to duration of therapy.

Neuromuscular transmission block: The aminoglycosides tend to block neuromuscular transmission. This can lead to a dangerous situation if aminoglycosides are given to patients with untreated myasthenia.

Nephrotoxicity: Proteinuria, haematuria and urea retention may occur in a few patients. This side effect is not clearly dose-related.

Streptomycin is said to have occasionally caused optic neuritis and, if given intrathecally, spinal arachnoiditis.

Dysmorphogenicity

Streptomycin does not appear to be dysmorphogenic. The situation regarding gentamicin is not yet clear and the drug is best avoided in pregnant women.

Chloramphenicol

Chloramphenicol is an effective bacteriostatic agent with a rather wide spectrum of antibacterial activity. However, because of the risk of its inducing aplastic anaemia, chloramphenicol is now used mainly in serious infections for which no other appropriate antibiotic is available. The drug is still sometimes used to treat meningitis, and therefore is considered here.

Chemistry

Chloramphenicol (MW 323.14) is a stable white powder which is slightly soluble in water.

Pharmacology

Biochemical Pharmacology

Chloramphenicol inhibits protein synthesis in bacteria. It acts on the 50 S ribosomal subunit and suppresses the activity of the enzyme peptidyl transferase, so that ribosomal translocation becomes uncoupled from synthesis of peptide bonds.

The drug may also inhibit protein synthesis in mammalian cells, though the mechanisms involved in the inhibition may not be quite the same as those that apply in bacteria. This effect in mammalian cells may be responsible for producing aplastic anaemia.

Pharmacodynamics

Chloramphenicol is primarily a bacteriostatic antibiotic which, in fairly low concentrations, inhibits the growth of many Gram-negative species e.g. *Enterobacter aerogenes, E. coli, K. pneumoniae, Bordetella pertussis, H. influenzae,* Pasteurella, Bacteroides, *Salmonella typhi,* some proteus strains, Neisseria, Shigella, Brucella and *Vibrio cholerae.* At moderate concentrations it inhibits Actinomyces, *Bacillus anthracis, Corynebacterium diphtheriae,* Clostridium, Listeria, Bartonella and Leptospirae, and at higher concentrations some streptococci and staphylococci. It is also active against rickettsiae, Chlamydia and Mycoplasma. These *in vitro* responses are in general paralleled by the effects of chloramphenicol in animal infections with the relevant organisms.

Pharmacokinetics

Absorption and bioavailability: Chloramphenicol is well absorbed after oral administration. Peak plasma levels occur at about 2 hours. Different preparations may differ in bioavailability (Glazko et al., 1968; Bell et al., 1971).

Distribution: The apparent volume of distribution of chloramphenicol is 0.57L/kg i.e. body water approximately. The drug enters normal CSF readily, where its concentrations are 10 to 60% of those in whole plasma. Between 25 and 60% of the chloramphenicol in plasma is protein-bound, the percentage bound increasing with drug concentration. These figures suggest that plasma water and CSF chloramphenicol are probably in equilibrium. Chloramphenicol enters bile and milk and crosses the placenta.

Elimination: The half-life of chloramphenicol is 1.7 to 2.8 hours (Azzollini et al., 1972) or 1.6 to 3.3 hours (Kunin et al., 1959). Some 5 to 15% of a dose is excreted unchanged in urine (Kunin et al., 1959). The remainder is eliminated after biotransformation, which occurs in the liver and involves glucuronide formation, or hydrolysis. Unmetabolised chloramphenicol is excreted by glomerular filtration, but the metabolic products are secreted into urine by the renal tubule cells.

Plasma level correlations: After a dose of 4g, peak plasma chloramphenicol levels are in the range 20 to 40μg/ml. The minimum inhibitory concentration for chloramphenicol-sensitive bacteria which cause meningitis is often in the range 8 to 10μg/ml.

Interactions

Pharmacodynamic interactions: Chloramphenicol may potentially interfere with the antibacterial action of penicillins. Chloramphenicol inhibits bacterial synthesis of proteins, and unless proteins are synthesised for bacterial cell walls the penicillin cannot exert its effect by damaging the cell walls. This interaction rarely appears clinically significant.

Chloramphenicol may appear to interfere with the action of certain haematinics (e.g. iron, vitamin B_{12}, folic acid) possibly because chloramphenicol interferes with protein synthesis in red cell precursors.

Pharmacokinetic interactions: The antibacterial effects of chloramphenicol on the gut flora may cause decreased intestinal synthesis of vitamin K, leading to hypoprothrombinaemia (Christensen and Skovsted, 1969).

Chloramphenicol appears to inhibit the biotransformation of phenytoin (Ballek et al., 1973), bishydroxycoumarin (Christiansen and Skovsted, 1969), tolbutamide (Christiansen and Skovsted, 1969) and chlorpropamide (Petitpierre and Fabre, 1970), raising the plasma concentrations and prolonging the pharmacological activities of these drugs.

Toxicity

Idiosyncratic Toxicity

Occasionally chloramphenicol may cause rashes, drug fever, angioneurotic oedema, acute severe haemorrhage from the alimentary and vesical mucosae and atrophic glossitis. If used to treat syphilis, brucellosis or typhoid it may precipitate a Herxheimer reaction.

Bone marrow aplasia with pancytopenia is an uncommon complication of chloramphenicol therapy. The disorder has a very high mortality. The reaction is associated with prolonged chloramphenicol therapy and particularly with exposure to the drug on more than one occasion. However the marrow hypoplasia does not appear related to the size of the daily chloramphenicol dosage.

Dose-related Toxicity

Chloramphenicol may cause nausea, vomiting, diarrhoea and perineal irritation. Blurred vision, paraesthesiae of the digits, optic neuritis, and chromosomal abnormalities have been reported.

Chloramphenicol inhibits iron uptake into normoblasts. The risk of iron deficiency anaemia from chloramphenicol is related to drug dose. When plasma chloramphenicol levels exceed 25 µg/ml anaemia is likely. Recovery occurs about 2 weeks after cessation of therapy.

After 2 to 9 days of therapy neonates given chloramphenicol may develop a 'grey baby syndrome' with vomiting, refusal to feed, irregular rapid respiration, abdominal distension, periods of cyanosis, and the passage of loose green stools. Affected neonates become flaccid and hypothermic and appear ashen grey after 24 to 48 hours of the illness. There is a substantial mortality. This side effect is due to accumulation of unchanged chloramphenicol because of a poor biotransformation capacity in the neonate and a limited capacity for renal excretion of chloramphenicol itself.

Dysmorphogenicity

The effects of chloramphenicol on protein synthesis make it an undesirable drug for use during pregnancy.

Isoniazid

Chemistry

Isonicotinic acid hydrazide (isoniazid, INAH) is a basic drug with a molecular weight of 137.15; its structural formula is shown in figure 12.4. Isoniazid is a polar compound which is moderately soluble in water.

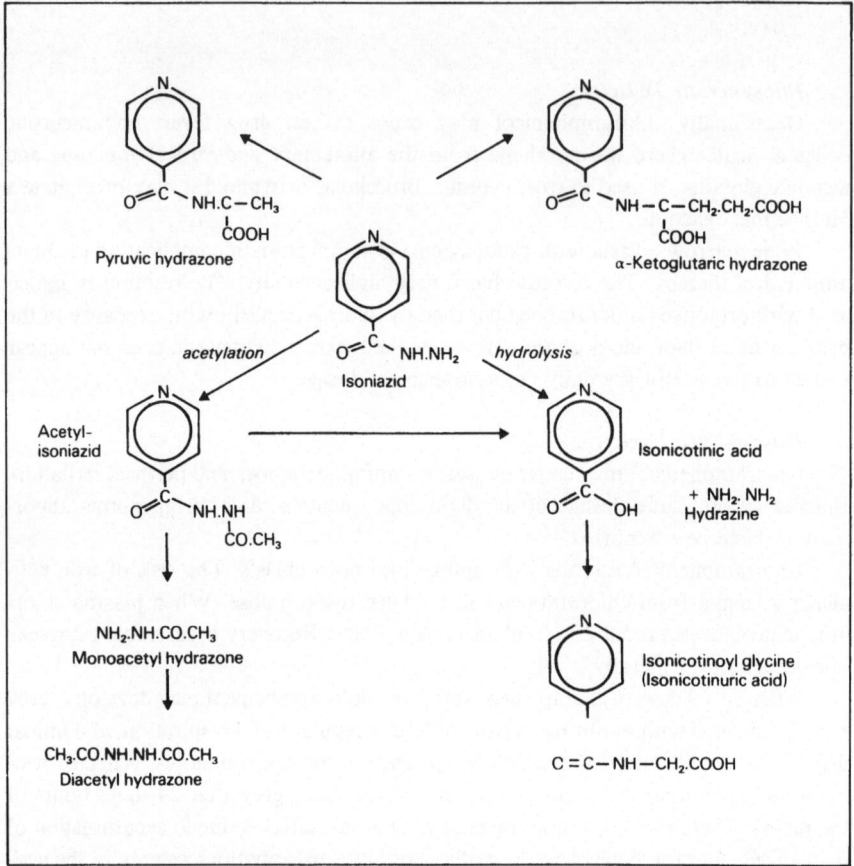

Fig. 12.4. Metabolic pathways of isoniazid.

Pharmacology

Biochemical Pharmacology

The biochemical mechanisms involved in the antituberculous effects of isoniazid are uncertain. Effects on bacterial lipids, on biosynthesis of nucleic acids, or on glycolysis have been suggested.

Pharmacodynamics

Isoniazid has bacteriostatic effects against *M. tuberculosis*, and also bactericidal effects when the organism is dividing.

Pharmacokinetics

Absorption and bioavailability: Isoniazid is readily absorbed after oral administration, with peak plasma concentrations 1 to 2 hours after dosage. Gelber et al. (1960) found no bioavailability differences between 6 oral formulations of the drug.

Distribution: The apparent volume of distribution of isoniazid is 0.6L/kg (Boxenbaum and Reigelman, 1976), suggesting a distribution throughout body water. The drug diffuses readily into all body fluids and cells. Some 50% of the isoniazid in plasma is bound to proteins (Tiitinen, 1969a). CSF concentrations are about 20% of those in whole plasma.

Elimination: Acetylation by liver enzymes is an important elimination pathway for isoniazid. A given population falls into two groups — slow and fast acetylators, determined by genetic factors (Ellard, 1976). For rapid acetylators figures for the half-life of isoniazid are 1.03 ± 0.16 hours (Peters and Levy, 1971), 1.33 ± 0.02 hours (Tiitinen, 1969b), and 0.67 to 1.33 hours (Jenne, 1964): for such persons $37 \pm 1\%$ of a dose is excreted unchanged in urine (Tiitinen, 1969). For slow acetylators half-life figures are 3.38 ± 0.12 hours (Acocella et al., 1972a), 3.52 ± 0.38 hours (Peters and Levy, 1971), 2.93 ± 0.05 hours (Tiitinen, 1969) and 2.33 to 3.33 hours (Jenne, 1964), while about 57% (Acocella et al., 1972a) or $66 \pm 1\%$ (Tiitinen, 1969) of an isoniazid dose is excreted unchanged. The biotransformation of isoniazid is not inducible (Ellard, 1976).

The major metabolic pathways for isoniazid (after Ellard and Gammon, 1975; Boxenbaum and Riegelman, 1976) are shown in figure 12.4. Aminosalicylic acid reduces the acetylation of isoniazid and causes increased plasma concentrations of the latter.

Plasma level correlations: In general plasma isoniazid concentrations in rapid acetylators are 20 to 50% of those of slow acetylators who receive the same isoniazid dose expressed on a body weight basis. Plasma isoniazid levels greater than 1 µg/ml 24 hours after the last dose are associated with a risk of toxic manifestations.

Interactions

Pharmacodynamic interactions: Isoniazid is usually combined with other antituberculous agents to provide enhanced antibacterial effects and to reduce the risks of resistant strains developing. An interaction between disulfiram and isoniazid has been reported (Whittington and Grey, 1969). It has been suggested that disulfiram may inhibit the enzyme dopamine-β-hydroxylase, while isoniazid inhibits monoamine oxidase. In consequence increased amounts of dopamine may accumulate or be converted to methylated catechol metabolites because of unaltered catechol-0-methyltransferase activity. This altered pattern of dopamine metabolism may produce mental changes and incoordination.

Pharmacokinetic interactions: The biotransformation of isoniazid is increased by ethyl alcohol, and slowed by *p*-aminosalicylic acid (Tiitinen, 1969a). Isoniazid, particularly in slow acetylators, reduces the elimination of phenytoin (Kutt et al., 1966) and may enhance the elimination of rifampicin (Leader, 1972).

Toxicity

Idiosyncratic Toxicity

Hypersensitivity to isoniazid is rare. It may cause fever, various types of skin rash, hepatitis, vasculitis, arthritic symptoms and different patterns of blood disorder (eosinophilia, thrombocytopenia, anaemia, agranulocytosis).

Dose-related Toxicity

Dose-related toxicity is more likely to occur in slow acetylators of the drug. The nervous system is often affected. Manifestations include peripheral neuropathy, epilepsy, optic neuritis (and optic atrophy), a toxic encephalopathy and various patterns of mental dysfunction (Adams and White, 1965). Pyridoxine administration can prevent the peripheral neuropathy and may also prevent the other neurological disturbances.

Isoniazid may cause hepatic necrosis, particularly in older persons and in slow acetylators. Other reported side effects include dry mouth, epigastric distress, urine retention in men, tinnitus and methaemoglobin formation. Isoniazid may worsen anaemia due to pyridoxine deficiency.

Dysmorphogenicity

Isoniazid is not usually considered a dysmorphogen, though if the drug is given in pregnancy it might be wise to ensure that pyridoxine deficiency does not develop.

Ethambutol

Chemistry

Ethambutol (MW 204.31) is a water soluble basic substance with pKa values of 6.6 and 9.5. The *d*-isomer is used clinically and is 200 times more potent as an antituberculous agent than the *l*-isomer.

Pharmacology

Biochemical Pharmacology

The exact mechanism of action of ethambutol is unknown.

Pharmacodynamics

Ethambutol inhibits many strains of *M. tuberculosis*, including strains resistant to streptomycin and isoniazid. The drug does not inhibit other bacteria.

Pharmacokinetics

Absorption and bioavailability: Some 75 to 80 % of an oral dose of ethambutol is said to be absorbed. Peak plasma levels occur 4 hours from dosage (Peets et al., 1965).

Distribution: Less than 40 % of the drug in plasma is protein-bound. Ethambutol enters red cells readily and achieves higher concentrations in these cells than in plasma. The drug does not pass through normal meninges into the CSF.

Elimination: The mean half-life of ethambutol is 4.17 hours, with 12.9 to 74.2 % (mean 46.2 %) of the dose being excreted unchanged in urine (Dume et al., 1971). Metabolites include an aldehyde and a dicarboxylic acid derivative (Peets et al., 1965).

Plasma level correlations: A single 25mg/kg dose of ethambutol produces a peak plasma level of the drug of about 5µg/ml some 2 hours after dosage.

Interactions

Pharmacodynamic interactions: Ethambutol interacts additively in respect to antituberculous effects if given with streptomycin and isoniazid.

Pharmacokinetic interactions: No well documented examples have been traced.

Toxicity

Idiosyncratic Toxicity

Skin rashes, joint pains, alimentary disturbances, fever, headache, dizziness and confusion may occur. Anaphylaxis, leucopenia and peripheral neuropathy are rare side effects.

Dose-related Toxicity

Optic neuritis, often reversible and related both to dosage and duration of therapy, may occur. It is unlikely with doses below 25mg/kg/day.

Ethambutol therapy causes raised plasma urate levels in about 50 % of patients given the drug, possibly because the drug decreases renal urate excretion.

Dysmorphogenicity

Ethambutol does not appear to be a known dysmorphogen.

Rifampicin

Rifampicin is an antibacterial agent with a very broad spectrum of action. In particular, it is used as an antituberculosis agent.

Chemistry

Rifampicin (MW 822.96) is a zwitterion (pKa 1.7 and 7.9) which is slightly soluble in water at acid pH and in organic solvents.

Pharmacology

Biochemical Pharmacology
The drug inhibits the bacterial enzyme DNA-dependent RNA polymerase, but does not affect this enzyme in mammalian cells.

Pharmacodynamics
Rifampicin inhibits the growth of *M. tuberculosis*. It also inhibits the growth of most Gram-positive bacteria, and some Gram-negative bacteria e.g. *E. coli*, Pseudomonas, Proteus and Klebsiella. It is very active against *Neisseria meningitidis* and inhibits the growth of certain viruses. Bacteria can develop resistance to the drug.

Pharmacokinetics
Absorption and bioavailability: Peak plasma levels occur 1 to 2 hours after oral dosage (Furesz et al., 1967). Absorption is slowed by the concurrent administration of *p*-aminosalicylic acid.

Distribution: The apparent volume of distribution of the drug is 0.93L/kg. Some 84 to 91% of the drug in plasma is protein-bound. The drug enters the various organs and body fluids, including CSF, readily. Its presence in urine, faeces, saliva, sputum, tears and sweat may colour these orange-red. Rifampicin crosses the placenta.

Elimination: Figures for the half-life of rifampicin are 2.80 ± 0.22 hours (Acocella et al., 1972b), 3.66 hours on the first day of therapy and 2.17 hours on the 21st day (Curci et al., 1972), 4.2 hours on the first day and 1.9 hours on the 30th day (Nitti et al., 1972), and 3.69 ± 0.51 hours on the first day and 2.40 ± 0.29 hours on the sixth day (Acocella et al., 1971). The percentage of the dose excreted unchanged in urine is 12% (Acocella, 1972b) or 12.5% (Furesz et al., 1967). The drug is biotransformed by acetylation. Rifampicin and its metabolite (which is also an antibacterial agent) are secreted into bile and undergo an enterohepatic circulation. However the acetyl metabolite is not as well absorbed from the alimentary tract as the parent drug, so that part of the metabolite produced is lost in faeces. Concentrations of the acetyl metabolite in urine are similar to concentrations of unmetabolised rifampicin in this fluid. The shortening of the rifampicin half-life with repeated dosage is due to increasing acetylation efficiency. Hepatic dysfunction slows the elimination of rifampicin. Isoniazid therapy, in slow acetylators of isoniazid, may speed the elimination of rifampicin (Leader, 1972).

Plasma level correlations: A single oral rifampicin dose of 600mg produces a mean peak plasma drug concentration of about 7µg/ml.

Interactions

Pharmacodynamic interactions: Rifampicin increases the *in vitro* antituberculous activity of streptomycin and isoniazid, but not that of ethambutol.

Pharmacokinetic interactions: These interactions have been reviewed by Zilly et al. (1977).

Aminosalicylic acid inhibits the absorption of rifampicin from the alimentary tract, as a result of absorption of the rifampicin by bentonite, an excipient in the aminosalicylate preparation. Rifampicin therapy is said to increase the dosage of anticoagulants required to maintain anti-clotting activity. The biochemical mechanisms involved in this interaction are not understood. Metabolism of the contraceptive pill, of oral hypoglycaemic agents and digitoxin is increased by rifampicin administration. It is believed that the combination of rifampicin and isoniazid increases the hazard of liver toxicity, particularly in persons who are slow acetylators or who have pre-existing liver disease.

Enzyme induction due to concurrent phenobarbitone therapy may cause a fall in plasma rifampicin levels, and probenecid therapy in some subjects may raise serum rifampicin levels, possibly by decreasing hepatic uptake of rifampicin.

Toxicity

Idiosyncratic Toxicity

Fever, pruritus, urticaria, skin rashes, eosinophilia, soreness of mouth and tongue, haemolysis, haematuria and renal insufficiency have been reported, as well as leucopenia, thrombocytopenia and anaemia.

Dose-related Toxicity

Nausea, vomiting, diarrhoea, abdominal pain, lethargy, drowsiness, headache, dizziness, confusion, diffuse weakness and numbness may occur. The drug is hepatotoxic. It may cause immunoglobulin light-chain proteinuria.

Dysmorphogenicity
It is not known whether rifampicin is a dysmorphogen.

Sulphone Drugs

These drugs, in particular dapsone, are used to treat Hansen's disease.

Chemistry

Dapsone (4,4'-diaminodiphenylsulphone — MW 248.30) is an acidic drug with a pKa of 1.2. It is practically insoluble in water but dissolves in ethyl alcohol.

Pharmacology

Biochemical Pharmacology
The antibacterial action of the sulphones is similar to that of the sulphonamides. These drugs are competitive antagonists of *p*-aminobenzoic acid and prevent this substance being incorporated into folic acid.

Pharmacodynamics
Sulphones are bacteriostatic for *M. tuberculosis* and for *M. leprae*.

Pharmacokinetics
Absorption and bioavailability: Dapsone is absorbed slowly but reasonably completely after oral administration, with peak plasma levels 1 to 3 hours after dosage.

Distribution: The drug is said to be distributed throughout body water. Some 72 to 80% of the drug in plasma is protein-bound. Sulphones tend to bind to skin and muscle, liver and kidney. They undergo an enterohepatic circulation.

Elimination: The half-life of dapsone is 17 to 21 hours, with 7.9 to 11.3% of a dose being excreted unchanged in urine (Gelber et al., 1971). The drug is biotransformed by acetylation, the rate of which depends on the acetylation capacity of the subject. Glucuronide formation also occurs and the rate of excretion of the glucuronide can be reduced by concurrent probenecid therapy.

Plasma level correlations: Little information is available.

Interactions
Pharmacodynamic interactions: No data are available.

Pharmacokinetic interactions: Probenecid therapy delays the renal excretion of dapsone and raises its plasma levels.

Toxicity

Idiosyncratic Toxicity

Drug fever, haematuria, pruritus, and skin rashes may occur. Lepromatous leprosy may exacerbate in a 'lepra reaction' which develops some 4 to 6 weeks after sulphone therapy is instituted. There may be fever, exfoliative dermatitis, jaundice, hepatic necrosis, lymphadenopathy, methaemoglobinaemia and anaemia.

Dose-related Toxicity

Anorexia, nausea and vomiting may occur. Occasionally headache, nervousness, insomnia, visual blurring and a reversible peripheral neuropathy (Rapoport and Guss, 1972) have occurred. The neuropathy, which predominantly affects motoneurones, may be a consequence of slow acetylation of the drug (Gutmann et al., 1976). A degree of haemolysis is common in patients receiving dapsone, as is methae-moglobinaemia.

Dysmorphogenicity

No information is available.

Amphotericin

Amphotericin is used in the local and systemic treatment of certain fungal infections. Its chief use in neurology is for cryptococcal meningitis.

Chemistry

Amphotericin (MW 924.11) is an amphoteric, unstable, water-soluble compound (at pH below 2 or above 11) with pKa values of 5.5 and 10.0

Pharmacology

Biochemical Pharmacology

Amphotericin appears to bind to a steroid moiety in the membrane of sensitive fungi. This binding causes increased membrane permeability.

Pharmacodynamics

Amphotericin has fungistatic, or in higher concentrations, fungicidal effects against *Cryptococcus neoformans, Histoplasma capsulatum, Coccidioides immitis,* Candida spp. *Blastomyces dermatidis* and other fungi. It has no clinically useful effect on bacteria, rickettsiae or viruses.

Pharmacokinetics

Absorption and bioavailability: After oral administration amphotericin is very poorly absorbed. Hence for systemic fungal infection it is necessary to give the drug intravenously and sometimes, in meningitis, intrathecally.

Distribution: Little is known of the distribution of this drug. About 10% of the drug in plasma is protein-bound, and little enters the CSF.

Elimination: The half-life is 0.92 to 1.88 days, and 2 to 5% of a dose is excreted unchanged in urine (Bindschadler and Bennett, 1969). Details of the drug's metabolism are not available.

Plasma level correlations: Usual therapeutic regimens produce plasma amphotericin levels in the range 2 to 4µg/ml, and these levels tend to persist in a fairly stable manner over a 24 hour dosage interval, because of the slow elimination of the drug.

Interactions

Pharmacodynamic interactions: Amphotericin therapy may cause hypokalaemia, and this can potentiate digoxin toxicity. Concurrent use of amphotericin and corticosteroids enhances the hypokalaemia.

Pharmacokinetic interactions: No examples can be traced.

Toxicity

Idiosyncratic Toxicity

Anaphylaxis, thrombocytopenia, flushing, diffuse pain and convulsions appear to be hypersensitivity reactions.

Dose-related Toxicity

Intravenous amphotericin may cause fever, phlebitis, headache, anorexia and anaemia. Hepatic damage may occur, with jaundice. Decreased renal function, with proteinuria, is common. There may be mild renal tubular acidosis with hypokalaemia and hypomagnesaemia. The milder degrees of renal damage appear to be reversible.

Intrathecal injection of amphotericin can cause nerve root pain, headache, dysaesthesiae, chemical meningitis and nerve palsies.

Dysmorphogenicity
Amphotericin is not a known dysmorphogen.

Flucytosine

Flucytosine is used as an antifungal agent (Zylstra, 1974).

Chemistry

Flucytosine (5-fluorocytosine) is a pyrimidine analogue with a MW 129.09. It is moderately soluble in water, and has pKa values of 2.90 and 10.71 (manufacturer's literature).

Pharmacology

Biochemical Pharmacology
In fungal cells flucytosine is transformed to 5-fluorouracil, which is then incorporated in nucleotides. The exact mode of antifungal activity is as yet uncertain.

Pharmacodynamics
Flucytosine inhibits the multiplication of *Cryptococcus neoformans*, *Aspergillus fumigatus*, *Sporotrichum schenkii* and some Candida strains. Minimum inhibitory concentrations are usually in the range 0.03 to 12.5μg/ml. Resistance to the drug can develop during the therapy of Candida and Cryptococcus infections.

Pharmacokinetics
Absorption and bioavailability: Flucytosine is rapidly and well absorbed after oral administration. Peak plasma levels occur about 2 hours after dosage.

Distribution: The drug is distributed throughout body water. Some 48 to 49% of the drug in plasma is bound to plasma protein (Davis and Reeves, 1971). CSF levels of the drug are 65 to 90% of those in plasma. Flucytosine crosses the placenta in rats (Chaube and Murphy, 1969).

Elimination: The half-life of flucytosine has a mean value of 5.6 hours (Dawborn et al., 1973), 2.89 hours (Schonebeck, 1973) or 3.91 ± 0.41 hours (Wade and Sudlow, 1972). Some 90% of a dose is excreted unchanged in urine (Koechlin et al., 1966). Since elimination of the drug is chiefly by renal excretion, flucytosine should be given with particular caution in patients with renal insufficiency.

Plasma level correlations: The usual single oral dose of 12.5 to 37.5mg/kg yields peak plasma flucytosine levels of about 30μg/ml. The subsequent time course of the plasma levels is highly dependent on renal function.

Interactions

Pharmacodynamic interactions: There is a mild additive antifungal interaction between flucytosine and amphotericin.

Pharmacokinetic interactions: Renal damage from concurrently administered amphotericin or other nephrotoxic drugs may raise plasma flucytosine levels, since the latter substance is eliminated almost exclusively by renal excretion.

Toxicity

Idiosyncratic Toxicity
No well documented instances have been traced.

Dose-related Toxicity
Flucytosine may cause:

1) skin rashes
2) nausea, vomiting and diarrhoea
3) bone marrow depression with anaemia, leucopenia and/or thrombocytopenia
4) biochemical evidence of hepatotoxicity and, rarely, overt jaundice
5) confusion, hallucinations, headache, drowsiness and vertigo.

Dysmorphogenicity
Data for man are not yet available, but in rats the drug causes fetal abnormalities (Chaube and Murphy, 1969).

Chloroquine

Cerebral malaria is likely to be an uncommon presenting neurological event, except in the tropics. Hence only one antimalarial agent, chloroquine, will be considered here.

Chloroquine is used to treat acute attacks of malaria and as a malaria prophylactic. It is also used to treat intestinal amoebiasis, rheumatoid arthritis and discoid lupus erythematosus.

Chemistry

Chloroquine (MW 319.89) is a water-soluble basic substance with pKa values of 8.4 and 10.8. It is usually given as its diphosphate.

Pharmacology

Biochemical Pharmacology

The antimalarial action of chloroquine appears related to its ability to combine strongly with double-stranded DNA. It inhibits DNA polymerase and, to a lesser extent, RNA polymerase. These effects on nucleic acids appear to occur in all cells, but the relative specificity of the antimalarial action of chloroquine may relate in part to preferential accumulation of the drug in parasitised red blood cells.

Pharmacodynamics

Chloroquine is active against asexual erythrocytic forms of *Plasmodium vivax, P. falciparum* and *P. malariae* and against gametocytes of *P. vivax*. Certain South American and Southeast Asian falciparum strains are now resistant to the drug. Chloroquine rapidly controls the parasitaemia and clinical symptoms in acute malarial attacks. Used prophylactically it lengthens the intervals between vivax malaria relapses.

Pharmacokinetics

Absorption and bioavailability: Chloroquine is absorbed rapidly and almost completely after oral administration. Parenteral preparations are needed only for patients who cannot swallow.

Distribution: About 55% of chloroquine in plasma is protein-bound (Berliner et al., 1948). The drug is widely distributed in the body and undergoes very substantial binding to many tissues, including parasitised red cells in which levels may be 100 times the plasma chloroquine level. Skin levels of chloroquine may be 30 to 60 times the plasma drug level (Olatunde, 1971). The apparent volume of distribution is about 30 to 40L/kg.

Elimination: The half-life of the drug is relatively long, about 72 hours. Some 70% of a dose is excreted unchanged in urine. The excretion of unchanged drug decreases in alkaline urine.

Biotransformation yields mono- and di-*N*-desethyl derivatives, a carboxylic acid derivative and other, as yet unidentified, minor metabolites.

The tight and extensive tissue binding of the drug causes small amounts to appear in urine for months after chloroquine dosage ceases.

Plasma level correlations: A daily chloroquine dose of 300mg produces mean steady-state plasma drug levels around 125ng/ml. With a 500mg dose once weekly, peak levels are in the range 150 to 250ng/ml, and fall to about 20 to 40ng/ml by the time the next dose is due.

Interactions

Pharmacodynamic interactions: None appear to be recorded, apart from additive effects when chloroquine is given with other antimalarial agents.

Pharmacokinetic interactions: Antimalarials such as amodiaquine, hydroxy-chloroquine and pamaquine, inhibit the biotransformation of chloroquine and raise its plasma levels (Gaudette and Coatney, 1961).

Toxicity

Idiosyncratic Toxicity
These reactions appear to be rare.

Dose-related Toxicity
In the doses used to treat acute attacks of malaria chloroquine may cause mild headache, gastrointestinal upset, visual disturbance and itching.

Chronic use may cause reversible lichenoid skin lesions and occasionally a vacuolar myopathy (Eadie and Ferrier, 1966). Use of 250 to 750mg daily for many months may lead to retinopathy (which is irreversible and causes loss of central vision).

Dysmorphogenicity
Chloroquine therapy may cause severe cochlear and vestibular damage to the fetus (Hart and Naunton, 1964).

Treatment of Nervous System Infection

Meningitis

The diagnosis of meningitis is confirmed by examination of the CSF. The cytology and glucose concentration will nearly always provide a good indication as to whether the meningitis is of bacterial or non-bacterial origin. If the meningitis is bacterial or fungal, microscopy with the use of appropriate stains may provide a rapid indication of the causative organism but definitive identification almost always requires bacteriological culture.

Bacterial Meningitis (Non-tuberculous)

General Measures
In patients with bacterial meningitis an attempt should be made to identify the source of the infection. The antibiotic used to treat the meningitis, if prescribed in ac-

cordance with bacteriological sensitivity studies, is likely to be effective against the primary source of infection also. However, the nature of the primary source of infection may make additional measures necessary to effect its cure. Thus a lung abscess may require surgical drainage or excision, a communication between the CSF and nasal accessory sinuses may require surgical closure, and bacterial endocarditis may need protracted antibiotic therapy.

The patient with meningitis, if conscious, is likely to be restless and to suffer from severe headache. He may therefore require sedation (e.g. diazepam) and analgesics (e.g. aspirin, pentazocine orally, or parenterally if there is vomiting). If he is vomiting, or if his level of consciousness is too depressed for him to maintain an adequate oral fluid intake, intravenous fluids will be necessary. Unless acute meningitis is very mild, it is often an advantage to set up an intravenous infusion and to deliver at least the initial doses of antibiotic by this route. It is also convenient to have an intravenous infusion inserted should a sudden complication (e.g. a convulsion) occur so that appropriate therapy can be given promptly into the patient's circulation.

Specific Antibiotic Therapy

Causative organism not identified: Not infrequently in meningitis the causative organism has not been identified before antibacterial therapy must be given. In this circumstance therapy should be chosen to cover infection with at least the three most common causes of pyogenic meningitis *viz Haemophilus influenzae, Neisseria meningitidis* and *Streptococcus pneumoniae*. The single most suitable antibiotics are ampicillin and chloramphenicol. These drugs may be given alone or in combination, the theoretical objection to combining a bactericidal and bacteristatic drug in practice not adversely affecting survival rates (Wehrle et al., 1967).

The dose of ampicillin should be at least 150mg/kg/day. The drug is preferably given intravenously, at least at first, and continued parenterally till the patient is well on the way to recovery, when the drug may be given orally. Chloramphenicol should be given in a dose of 100mg/kg/day, intravenously at first. Oral chloramphenicol therapy is used when the patient is well enough to swallow. The total daily dose of each of these antibiotics may be given in divided doses, 6-hourly. For each drug the initial loading dose is twice the 6-hourly dose.

When the causative organism has been identified the most appropriate antibiotics are as follows (unless sensitivity tests indicate otherwise).

Haemophilus influenzae: Both chloramphenicol and ampicillin are likely to be effective, though there have been some reports of failures of ampicillin therapy. This risk may be lessened by using intravenous ampicillin doses of 200 to 400mg/kg/day. Therapeutic failure may be due to the poor entry of ampicillin into CSF. This is not a limitation with chloramphenicol and, were it not for the small risk of producing aplastic anaemia, chloramphenicol might be the preferred drug. Hambleton and

Davies (1974) mentioned a possibility of residual toxicity if high intravenous doses of ampicillin were used to treat haemophilus meningitis. Thus each antibiotic may have its disadvantages in the circumstances.

Neisseria meningitidis: Benzylpenicillin is the antibiotic of choice, in 4 or 6-hourly intravenous dosage to a total of 400mg/kg/day. Intramuscular therapy in similar dosage may be used when the patient is well enough to do without intra-venous fluids. Oral ampicillin (150mg/kg/day in 4 divided doses) could reasonably be used as an alternative in the late stages of treatment when the patient is well on the way to recovery.

The question of prophylaxis against *N. meningitidis* in contacts may arise. Till re-cently sulphonamides were thought to be the drugs of choice, but now rifampicin is advised, in a single daily dose of 600mg on 4 consecutive days in adults (Beam et al., 1971). Children may be given rifampicin in a dose of 10mg/kg/day (Khuri-Bulos, 1973).

Streptococcus pneumoniae: Benzylpenicillin and ampicillin are the antibiotics of choice. Dosage of benzylpenicillin is as for meningococcal meningitis. Ampicillin doses are indicated above.

Streptococci: Benzylpenicillin, in dosage as above, is likely to be the most ap-propriate treatment.

Staphylococci: Cloxacillin 50mg/kg/day or methicillin 100mg/kg/day, divided in 4 or 6 intravenous doses each 24 hours is usually the most appropriate therapy. Methicillin is more likely to cause renal damage than cloxacillin.

Other bacteria: Particularly in the newborn, and in persons with hydrocephalus, other organisms, often Gram-negative, may sometimes cause meningitis. Hence in-travenous ampicillin 100 to 200mg/kg/day together with gentamicin in a dose up to 7.5mg/kg/day are likely to provide adequate therapy, unless sensitivity testing sug-gests that other antibiotics are more appropriate or the clinical response to the initial therapy is inadequate. It may be necessary to introduce aminoglycoside antibiotics directly into the lumbar or ventricular CSF should meningitis due to sensitive organ-isms fail to respond adequately to parenteral therapy. Gentamicin, for instance, penetrates very poorly into the CSF.

Duration of Therapy
Antibacterial therapy in pyogenic meningitis should be continued till the patient has very definitely recovered, as assessed clinically. The risks of overtreatment are usually very much less than the risks of undertreatment. Intravenous therapy is generally desirable initially, and it is often more comfortable for the patient to receive

his antibiotics intravenously, rather than intramuscularly, until he is well enough to take them orally and his meningitis is greatly improved clinically. When meningitis is treated early in its course improvement can sometimes be quite definite by the second or third day of therapy and the patient may be reasonably well by the end of a week. By this stage he might have been receiving oral therapy for the past 2 or 3 days. Sometimes recovery, though definite, is slower, particularly when the acute illness has been more severe, or when it has been treated late and perhaps treated with marginally adequate antibiotic doses. Here repeat CSF examination may be judged necessary, but if this is done it should be remembered that it takes several days for the CSF cell count and protein level to return to normal after infection is cured. A diminishing CSF polymorph count and a normal CSF glucose level, with the absence of organisms, suggests that the therapy is appropriate.

In general, antibacterial therapy for meningitis should continue for at least a week, even in cases who recover rapidly and fully, and it may be employed for much longer periods. There have been suggestions that antibiotic doses should increase as therapy progresses and the condition improves, since as meningeal irritation lessens many antibiotics enter the CSF less adequately. In practice such dosage increases rarely seem necessary.

Complications of Bacterial Meningitis

Consequences of delayed, inadequate therapy: When appropriate therapy has been delayed, meningeal inflammation may have become very severe and there may be active ventriculitis and acute cerebral cortical inflammation. In these circumstances larger than usual doses of the appropriate antibiotics given by intravenous administration may be desirable. It may be necessary to consider intrathecal administration of those antibacterial drugs which do not enter CSF readily, though one must be careful not to use too large an intrathecal dose. Penicillins, for instance, are convulsants if they gain access to the cerebral cortex in sufficient concentration. Intrathecal therapy may be given by the lumbar route or, particularly if there is a question of infection being loculated in the ventricles, may be given by an Ommaya reservoir connected surgically to a lateral ventricle. Antibiotics which may have to be given intrathecally, with their appropriate dosages, are: benzylpenicillin 8 to 25mg; carbenicillin 10 to 20mg; cloxacillin 3 to 10mg and gentamicin 2 to 10mg (the lower doses of all drugs are for infants, the higher for adults).

Intrathecal antibiotic therapy is ordinarily continued once or twice daily till clinical improvement begins. Such therapy carries some risk of complications (e.g. arachnoiditis, nerve palsies, convulsions). However, in the circumstances in which intrathecal therapy must be used, these risks appear acceptable. The risks may be reduced by avoiding excessive intrathecal dosage of the drugs.

Shock: Peripheral circulatory failure may occur in severe meningitis. It may be treated by the intravenous use of plasma volume expanders (e.g. human serum albumin) and high doses of cortisol (e.g. 100 to 200mg every 4 hours) as well as by appropriate antibacterial therapy. At present there is some tendency to use very high doses of glucocorticoids (e.g. 12mg dexamethasone IV 4-hourly).

Brain oedema: Brain oedema may occur from cerebral cortical inflammation or from cerebral infarction due to endarteritis, venous thrombosis or thrombophlebitis. High dose glucocorticoids (e.g. dexamethasone 4 to 8mg 4 times a day) may be helpful.

Obstruction of CSF flow: In acute meningitis, pus, and in later stages adhesions, may obstruct the CSF circulation and cause hydrocephalus. Treatment involves eradication of infection, if necessary by intraventricular antibiotic administration, and surgical drainage of obstructed CSF. If the hydrocephalus persists when the infection is overcome, surgical measures to bypass the obstruction definitively may be needed.

Local collections of pus or fluid: Bacterial meningitis may lead to loculated collections of pus, or of sterile fluid, in the ventricles or subarachnoid (or adjacent) spaces. It may also cause cerebral abscess. In these circumstances, as well as antibiotic therapy, surgical drainage is required.

Cranial nerve palsies: These may be due to direct implication by meningeal inflammation or to consequences of brain displacement as a result of hydrocephalus.

Tuberculous Meningitis

Tuberculous meningitis is usually a subacute illness which may sometimes reach a fairly advanced stage before the diagnosis is made. When a patient with a meningitis has a dominantly mononuclear pleocytosis and reduced glucose content in the CSF, and no acid-fast bacilli are seen, the differential diagnosis often rests between tuberculous and cryptococcal meningitis, meningitis due to recurrent infected emboli, and meningeal carcinomatosis. In these circumstances it is often wise to treat the patient for tuberculous meningitis till further investigation clarifies the aetiology.

The general management of tuberculous meningitis is similar to that of bacterial meningitis. Intravenous fluids and intravenous antibiotic therapy are necessary only in the more seriously ill patients.

In the past streptomycin and isoniazid were the mainstay of antituberculous therapy, but now studies such as that of Chandra (1976) have shown that better results are obtained with a combination of:

streptomycin — 1g daily by IM injection
isoniazid — 300mg daily, divided into 4 doses (8 to 10mg/kg/day)

rifampicin — 600mg daily, divided into 4 doses, and
ethambutol — 25mg/kg daily, as a single dose.

Therapy is continued until the meningitis is fully recovered. This is ascertained by serial CSF examinations. When the patient is clinically well, the CSF glucose is normal and the CSF pleocytosis is lessening, therapy may be reduced to, for example, oral isoniazid (e.g. 5mg/kg/day) and ethambutol (e.g. 15 to 25mg/kg/day) taken as an outpatient. However it may still be wise to re-examine and culture the CSF once or twice at monthly or 2-monthly intervals. The total duration of therapy is usually determined by the state of the extraneural (often pulmonary) disease, but treatment generally lasts 1.5 to 2 years.

Patients with tuberculous meningitis are customarily given oral glucocorticoids (e.g. prednisone 10 to 15mg 4 times a day or dexamethasone 2 to 3mg 4 times a day) to diminish the risk of CSF adhesion formation which subsequently causes hydrocephalus. Oral pyridoxine 50mg 2 or 3 times a day is given to protect against isoniazid neurotoxicity.

Cryptococcal Meningitis

In some parts of the world, and in patients whose immune mechanisms are depressed by disease or by chemotherapy, cryptococcal infection is a relatively frequent cause of subacute or chronic meningitis.

General principles of treatment are as for bacterial meningitis, but the course of the illness, and the duration of its treatment, are prolonged.

Till the introduction of flucytosine, the only treatment was amphotericin B. Amphotericin has to be administered in a daily intravenous infusion in 500ml glucose, given over several hours. For adults the initial daily dose is 0.25mg/kg. Doses are slowly increased to a maximum of 1.0 to 1.5mg/kg per day. The infusion is often accompanied by fever, anorexia and nausea, though these symptoms may be alleviated by a dose of a phenothiazine (e.g. 25 or 50mg thioridazine orally or parenterally) or by 4mg dexamethasone. It is important to monitor renal function every few days. Should any evidence of nitrogen retention occur, it is necessary to reduce the dosage or suspend treatment for a time, to avoid irreversible renal damage. The patient's clinical state may not provide a reliable guide to the progress of his illness, because the side effects of the therapy complicate the situation. Therefore CSF examination at intervals is necessary to see if the meningitis is coming under control. If the patient can tolerate the therapy and the CSF becomes clear of evidence of infection, treatment may be discontinued. However the CSF should still be examined once or twice at 1 or 2-monthly intervals to ensure that the infection does not relapse. If cryptococcal meningitis is not being controlled by intravenous amphotericin, or if renal toxicity is limiting dosage, it may be useful to give amphotericin intrathecally. The drug may be given by the lumbar route or intraventricularly, via an Ommaya reservoir, particularly if there is obstructive hydrocephalus. The intrathecal dose is 0.5mg, dissolved in 5mls CSF. The drug is given intrathecally 2 or 3 times a week till CSF examination indicates that the meningitis is being controlled, or till a total of 15mg is given. Sometimes maximal tolerated amphotericin doses will only partly suppress cryptococcal meningitis. Nevertheless, this partial control may enable the patient to live, as it were in symbiosis with his yeast, in reasonably good health for a very long time without further therapy.

Now that flucytosine is available this drug may be used as an alternative to amphotericin, or in conjunction with it. Flucytosine is given orally every 6 hours, in a daily dose of 50 to 150mg per kg. In the absence of prohibitive side effects, therapy continues till CSF examination indicates the infection is cured. Doses should be reduced if renal insufficiency develops as a result of concurrent amphotericin therapy.

The chief complication of cryptococcal meningitis is obstructive hydrocephalus, which may require surgical drainage as a temporary measure, and operative shunting as a more definitive one, when the infection is coming under control.

Extraneural cryptococcal lesions may occur (e.g. in the lung) where they may require local surgical excision.

Aseptic Meningitis

The aseptic meningitides are a group of self-limiting conditions usually due to one of a number of viruses. All that is required in their treatment are the general measures used in treating meningitis (e.g. analgesia, sedation, maintenance of fluid intake, and relief of vomiting) prescribed for a few days until spontaneous recovery occurs. No specific measures are available, or necessary.

Abscess

Abscess formation may occur in the brain or in the cranial or spinal subdural or epidural spaces. The clinical presentation of abscess usually involves a mixture of mass lesion and infective effects, though some more chronic brain abscesses can present purely as mass lesions.

Therapy of the mass lesion aspects of abscess involves measures to reduce intracranial pressure (chapter II) together with surgical drainage of the pus. Appropriate antibacterial therapy should be prescribed along the lines indicated in the treatment of meningitis. Antibiotic therapy is continued till the patient is clinically well and there is no evidence of a residual mass lesion.

Sometimes, in the more chronic forms of brain abscess, no organisms are found on culture. There is an increasing realisation that in these circumstances the infection may have been from anaerobic organisms which are not detected by routine culture techniques (De Louvois et al., 1977a, b). Agents such as metronidazole may be useful here (Ingram et al., 1977).

An attempt should be made to find the primary source of infection responsible for an intracranial abscess, in case this source requires special treatment in its own right, apart from the antibiotic therapy given for the organisms present in the abscess.

Neurosyphilis

Syphilitic infection of the nervous system is now a considerable rarity, a very different situation to that which applied 20 years ago. The treatment of choice is benzylpenicillin, usually given as procaine penicillin in a daily intramuscular dose of 600mg for 2 to 3 weeks. In patients allergic to penicillin a tetracycline may be used (e.g. IM rolitetracycline 250 to 375mg daily for 2 weeks). Parenteral antibiotics are preferred because of the possibility that the patient may omit oral therapy; however oral tetracycline 0.5g 4 times a day for 3 weeks is a satisfactory treatment.

The effect of treatment in controlling neurosyphilis is assessed by serial CSF examination at 3-monthly intervals. If the CSF pleocytosis is not clearing after 3 months — and is not gone by 6 months — or if the CSF protein level is not falling by one year after the antibiotic therapy, a further course of treatment is indicated. The titre of the serological test for syphilis should have fallen when measured one year after therapy. In general the CSF cell count is the best guide to therapeutic progress.

Penicillin therapy, when first given in neurosyphilis, may activate a Herxheimer reaction with fever, headache, muscle and joint pain, and enlargement of syphilitic lesions. Corticosteroid therapy may limit the severity of this reaction.

Hansen's Disease

Leprosy is an uncommon neurological disorder in temperate climates but occurs frequently in tropical countries.

Since dapsone is a very slowly eliminated drug it needs to be taken (by mouth) only twice a week, so long as the dosage is sufficient. Therapy begins with 25 or 50mg of dapsone twice weekly, and the dose is gradually increased to 100mg or 200mg twice weekly. Therapy is generally continued for many months, or years.

About 4 to 6 weeks after sulphone therapy is begun a 'lepra reaction', akin to the Herxheimer reaction, may occur. If severe enough to require treatment, the reaction can be suppressed by glucocorticoid administration.

Cerebral Malaria

Cerebral (falciparum) malaria is a disorder which carries a high mortality. Once the diagnosis is made by examination of peripheral blood, intravenous fluids should be given, together with high dosage glucocorticoids (e.g. 12mg dexamethasone phosphate) with further 8mg dexamethasone doses 4-hourly at first and then at decreasing intervals (Woodruff and Dickinson, 1968). Chloroquine (a total of 200mg of the base) should be given by intramuscular injection immediately (into two different sites); further 200mg chloroquine doses should be given 6-hourly to a maximum of 800mg in the first 24 hours.

Once the patient recovers enough to swallow, oral chloroquine can be used. After one or two daily 500mg doses, the patient may then receive 500mg chloroquine weekly as a prophylactic. Steroid therapy is rapidly reduced once the patient recovers consciousness.

Chapter XIII

Toxic and Deficiency Disorders

Principal Disorders and Drugs Discussed

Thiamine deficiency
Thiamine

Nicotinic acid deficiency
Nicotinic acid

Pyridoxine deficiency
Pyridoxine

Vitamin B$_{12}$ deficiency
Vitamin B$_{12}$

Folic acid deficiency
Folic acid

The intake of a number of toxic substances may produce disturbances of function of various parts of the nervous system. In general the treatment of these disorders is based on withdrawal of the toxic substance. There is usually no specific antidote (apart from the agents used to treat heavy metal poisoning p.136). Sometimes symptomatic therapy is necessary. On the other hand, deficiency of several of the vitamins can disturb neurological function, for which deficiency states specific therapy is available.

Thiamine Deficiency

Disturbed Mechanisms

Thiamine deficiency is most often of dietary origin, and generally occurs in chronic alcoholics, though it may be a complication of prolonged vomiting from any cause. A state reminiscent of the effects of chronic thiamine deficiency on the central nervous system occurs in Leigh's syndrome, though here there is no deficiency in thiamine intake. Thiamine deficiency may lead to one or more of the following:

1) Acute dysmnesic syndrome (Korsakoff's psychosis)
2) Wernicke's encephalopathy
3) Peripheral neuropathy

Thiamine (as its pyrophosphate) is the co-enzyme involved in the decarboxylation of pyruvate to acetate, prior to the entry of the latter into the tricarboxylic acid
cycle. Thiamine deficiency therefore restricts the amount of energy available for the
metabolic needs of cells. Virtually all the energy produced in neurones is ultimately
derived from glucose. For practical purposes there are no alternative sources of
energy. Therefore, in thiamine deficiency the function of nerve cells tends to become
deranged sooner than that of other body cells, which have other metabolic sources of
input of two carbon fragments into the Krebs cycle. Probably neurones with the
greatest metabolic requirement are those which are first affected in thiamine deficiency.

Correction of Disordered Mechanism

Thiamine, in sufficient dosage, can halt the progress of neurological damage
from thiamine deficiency and may completely, or partially, reverse the effects of previous damage if this damage has not been present too long, and is not too severe.

Drugs Used in Treatment

Thiamine

Thiamine is used in the treatment of actual, and potential, thiamine deficiency.

Chemistry

Thiamine is usually given as the hydrochloride (MW 337.28). The vitamin is
destroyed by alkalis, and by oxidising and reducing agents.

Pharmacology

Biochemical Pharmacology
Within cells thiamine reacts with adenosine triphosphate to form thiamine
pyrophosphate, which is the co-enzyme for the decarboxylation of pyruvate to acetate, and of α-ketoglutaric acid to glutamic acid.

Pharmacodynamics

In healthy persons thiamine, in ordinary doses, has no pharmacodynamic action. In persons with thiamine deficiency it can reverse the hyperkinetic circulatory state and cardiomyopathy, and help restore function in damaged peripheral and central neurones.

Pharmacokinetics

Absorption and bioavailability: Thiamine absorption from the alimentary tract is often incomplete, and limited to a maximum of 8 to 15mg per day. Absorption of the vitamin from the duodenum and small intestine is partly an active process and partly passive (Rindi and Ventura, 1972). Absorption of the vitamin from intramuscular injection sites is rapid and complete.

Distribution: After absorption thiamine is distributed through the various body cells till all thiamine stores are saturated with the vitamin.

Elimination: The body normally degrades about 1mg thiamine daily, forming pyrimidine which is excreted in urine. As more thiamine is given, proportionately more of the excess of dose over metabolic requirement is excreted unchanged in urine. Thus the body's capacity to split the thiamine molecule appears limited.

Plasma level correlations: No data are available.

Interactions

None appear to have been reported.

Toxicity

Apart from rare hypersensitivity reactions, thiamine preparations are non-toxic.

Treatment of Thiamine Deficiency

In clinical neurological practice thiamine deficiency nearly always occurs in association with chronic alcoholism. The deficiency state is treated with large doses of thiamine. These doses are probably well in excess of therapeutic requirements, but overdosage appears to have no adverse effects in man. In the acute stages of thiamine deficiency, which affects central or peripheral nervous system function, the vitamin is usually given parenterally at first to obtain a rapid effect. Parenteral administration obviates problems of uncertain absorption of the vitamin if the patient is vomiting, and ensures that the patient receives at least some thiamine, in case he goes on another drinking bout. The initial one or two doses of 100mg thiamine may be given intravenously 6 to 12 hours apart. After this, 100mg is given daily by intramuscular injection till the patient is clearly recovering and any vomiting has ceased. Thereafter thiamine is given orally in a dose of 50 to 100mg 3 times a day though the greater proportion of this dose is almost certainly unnecessary.

More severely ill patients often have other consequences of chronic alcoholism as well (e.g. cardiomyopathy, liver disease) which may also require treatment. If an alcoholic with Wernicke's encephalopathy or Korsakoff's psychosis is given glucose (possibly intravenously) without being given thiamine his neurological state may worsen and coma, if not already present, may ensue.

After maximum neurological recovery has been achieved it is usually wise to prescribe regular oral thiamine and to continue this unless it becomes clear that the patient is abstaining from all alcohol.

Nicotinic Acid Deficiency

Disordered Mechanisms

Nicotinic acid deficiency, of dietary origin, causes pellagra, which may be associated with other vitamin deficiency states. In the body nicotinic acid is incorporated in nicotinamide adenine dinucleotide (NAD) and its phosphate (NADP), which are the co-enzymes for various dehydrogenases, including those of the Krebs cycle and mitochondrial oxidation pathway. Deficiency of NAD and NADP, consequent on nicotinic acid deficiency, will disturb energy metabolism throughout the body. The clinical effects are most obvious in the skin, the gastrointestinal tract and the nervous system (where deficiency produces mood and memory changes, dementia and possibly peripheral neuropathy).

Correction of Disordered Mechanisms

The manifestations of pellagra, if not too long established, may be relieved by nicotinic acid.

Drugs Used in Treatment

Nicotinic Acid

Nicotinic acid has three major uses in contemporary practice:

1) The treatment of actual or potential nicotinic acid deficiency
2) The treatment of hyperlipidaemia
3) As a peripheral vasodilator.

Chemistry

Nicotinic acid (MW 123.11) is a water-soluble acidic substance with a pKa of 4.85. The structural formula of nicotinic acid is seen in figure 13.1.

Pharmacology

Biochemical Pharmaoclogy
In the body nicotinic acid is metabolically converted to NAD and NADP, the functions of which are mentioned above.

Pharmacodynamics
As well as correcting the consequences of its deficiency, nicotinic acid produces peripheral vasodilatation (with flushing and itching). Nicotinic acid may activate peptic ulcer and can cause a fall in plasma cholesterol and triglyceride levels if given in large doses for a long time.

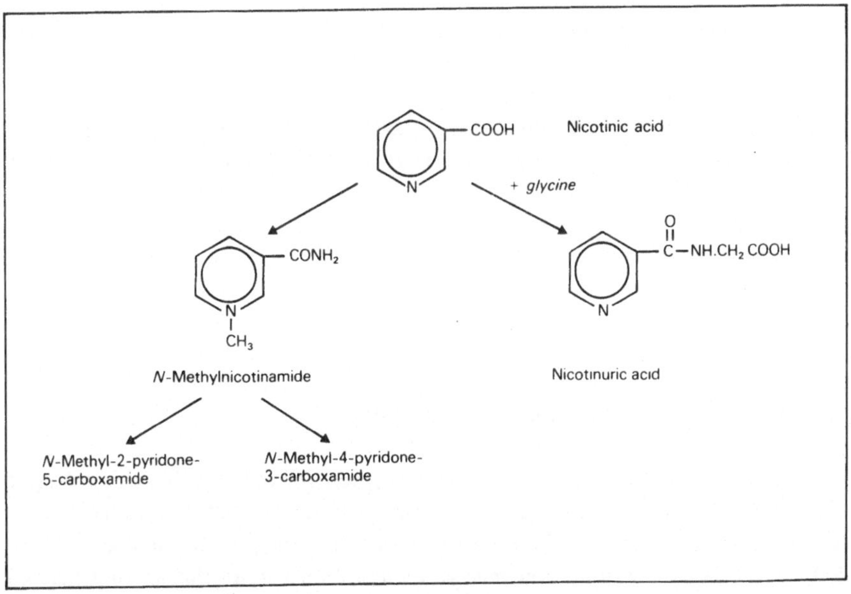

Fig. 13.1. The biotransformation of nicotinic acid.

Pharmacokinetics

Absorption and bioavailability: Nicotinic acid is well absorbed after oral or intramuscular administration.

Distribution: Nicotinic acid becomes distributed throughout cells in all tissues.

Elimination: Little unchanged nicotinic acid is found in urine after therapeutic doses of the vitamin, but as higher doses are given, increasing proportions of the dose are excreted unaltered. The biotransformation of nicotinic acid, apart from its conversion to NAD and NADP, is thought to follow the two main pathways set out in figure 13.1.

Plasma level correlations: Svedmeyr et al. (1969) showed that doses of nicotinic acid which raised plasma levels of the vitamin by 0.1 to 0.3µg/ml produced increased blood flow in skin and muscle.

Interactions

No interactions appear to be recorded.

Toxicity

Idiosyncratic Toxicity

No idiosyncratic reactions have been traced.

Dose-related Toxicity

Flushing, pruritus, gastrointestinal disturbance, activation of peptic ulcer and hepatotoxicity may occur when the drug is given in high dosage.

Dysmorphogenicity

Nicotinic acid is not a known dysmorphogen.

Treatment of Nicotinic Acid Deficiency

Pellagra responds rapidly to nicotinic acid given, for example, in an oral dose of 50mg 2 or 3-hourly. Nicotinic acid requirement is inversely related to the tryptophan content of the diet. Once nicotinic acid deficiency is cured, an oral intake of 25mg daily should be ample to prevent relapse, though 2 or 3 times this amount may be given to provide a margin of safety.

Pyridoxine Deficiency

Disordered Mechanisms

Pyridoxine deficiency in man may cause hypsarrhythmic epilepsy (West's syndrome) in infants, and peripheral neuropathy. A small outbreak of hypsarrhythmia followed the feeding of infants with a powdered milk preparation lacking in pyridoxine, and other cases have been reported (French et al., 1965). Since this experience it has seemed reasonable to give pyridoxine to hypsarrhythmic infants without waiting to prove the presence of pyridoxine deficiency by biochemical tests. Peripheral neuropathy due to isoniazid or hydrallazine therapy can be prevented by giving pyridoxine. Isoniazid inhibits the enzyme pyridoxal kinase which catalyses the conversion of pyridoxal to pyridoxal phosphate, which is the co-enzyme in several decarboxylation reactions.

Correction of Disordered Mechanisms

Administration of pyridoxine will prevent, or reverse, the consequences of pyridoxine deficiency, so long as they are not too long established.

Pyridoxine

Pyridoxine is used to correct actual or potential pyridoxine deficiency, and is also used as an anti-emetic, particularly in pregnancy.

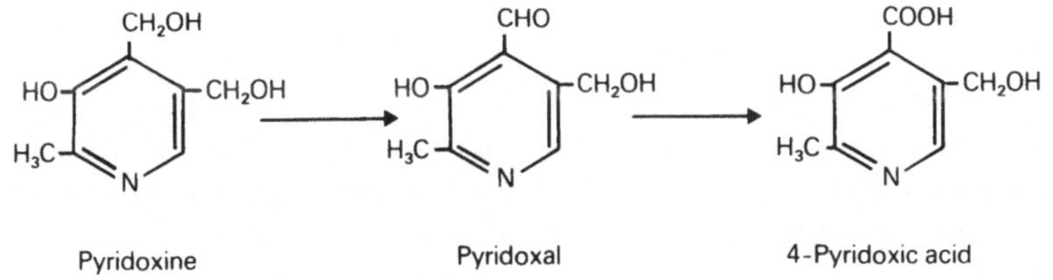

Fig. 13.2. The metabolism of pyridoxine.

Chemistry

Pyridoxine hydrochloride (MW 205.64) is a water soluble vitamin; the structural formula is seen in figure 13.2.

Pharmacology

Biochemical Pharmacology

In the body pyridoxine is converted to its aldehyde derivative pyridoxal. This is then converted to pyridoxal phosphate which is the co-enzyme in a number of decarboxylation reactions including those which form dopamine from dopa, and γ-aminobutyric acid (GABA) from glutamic acid.

Pharmacodynamics

Apart from correcting manifestations associated with its deficiency, pyridoxine in ordinary doses has no pharmacological action, except possibly for an anti-emetic effect.

Pharmacokinetics

Absorption and bioavailability: Pyridoxine is well absorbed after oral administration.

Distribution: Pyridoxine is widely distributed within cells.

Elimination: The data of Johansson et al. (1966) suggest that pyridoxine elimination is bi-exponential in man. It has a half-life of 40 to 228 days. The major metabolite, formed from pyridoxal by the action of hepatic aldehyde oxidase, is 4-pyridoxic acid (fig. 13.2).

Plasma level correlations: No data are available.

Interactions

Pharmacodynamic interactions: None appears to be recorded.

Pharmacokinetic interactions: Pyridoxine, given to relieve nausea produced by levodopa therapy for Parkinsonism, may so increase the peripheral decarboxylation of levodopa so that the therapeutic effect of this substance is impaired. Chronic intake of levodopa enhances the conversion of pyridoxine to its phosphate (Mars, 1975).

Toxicity

For practical purposes pyridoxine in therapeutic doses is non-toxic.

Treatment of Pyridoxine Deficiency

As a prophylactic agent against isoniazid neuropathy and neurotoxicity, and in infants with hypsarrhythmia, pyridoxine is given in an oral dose of 50mg 3 times a day. If the patient cannot swallow, it may be given by intramuscular injection. Hypsarrhythmia should be treated concurrently with steroids or tetracosactrin. If improvement occurs, it may be difficult to know whether the vitamin or the steroid is responsible, therefore the pyridoxine should be continued till the course of steroids is completed and then resumed if the hypsarrhythmia relapses.

Vitamin B_{12} Deficiency

Disordered Mechanisms

Vitamin B_{12} deficiency may cause subacute combined degeneration of the spinal cord. This illness includes peripheral neuropathy, dementia, and perhaps optic nerve injury, as well as spinal cord damage. It is likely to be associated with megaloblastic anaemia of some degree. The cause, in the great majority of instances, is a failure to absorb dietary vitamin B_{12} because of a lack of the 'intrinsic' factor which is produced in the stomach. Intrinsic factor is necessary for absorption of vitamin B_{12} at ileal level. Local ileal disease is a rare cause of the deficiency.

There have been suggestions that Leber's hereditary optic atrophy may be due to a genetically determined sensitivity to cyanide or cyanogens, and that tobacco amblyopia may be due to chronic cyanide toxicity (Wilson et al., 1971). Both disorders may show some response to hydroxycobalamin but not to cyanocobalamin (Chisholm et al., 1967; Foulds et al., 1968). Possibly vitamin B_{12} metabolism is altered in both these conditions.

Vitamin B_{12} is required for the hydrogen transfer and isomerisation which converts methylmalonate to succinate, though it is not clear how decreased activity in this mechanism leads to nervous system damage. The vitamin is also necessary to retain various sulphydryl groups in enzymes in the reduced form which is necessary for their biological activity. Impairment of this action may help explain neurological damage from vitamin B_{12} deficiency.

Correction of Disordered Mechanisms

Unlike the haematological effects of vitamin B_{12} deficiency, the neurological effects cannot be reversed by administration of folic acid. The treatment of subacute combined degeneration requires vitamin B_{12} itself, and the vitamin should be given parenterally to avoid the possibility of failure of its absorption from the alimentary tract.

Drugs Used in Treatment

Vitamin B$_{12}$

Vitamin B$_{12}$ is used in the treatment of clinical or subclinical vitamin B$_{12}$ deficiency.

Chemistry

Vitamin B$_{12}$ (cyanocobalamin) is a red, water-soluble neutral crystalline material with a molecular weight of 1355.42. It is stable at the temperatures of ordinary cooking. Cyanocobalamin is one of a number of cobalamins, complex chemical structures; hydroxocobalamin, in which the cyano (CN) group is replaced by a hydroxy (OH) is also used therapeutically, and in many instances interchangably, with cyanocobalamin.

The term vitamin B$_{12}$ is used here to embrace the whole family of cobalamins.

Pharmacology

Biochemical Pharmacology

Cobalamins are required for nucleic acid synthesis, and hence are necessary for normal growth, haematopoiesis and the maintenance of myelin. Cyanocobalamin, the co-enzyme form (i.e. 5'-deoxyadenosyl cobalamin) is required for:

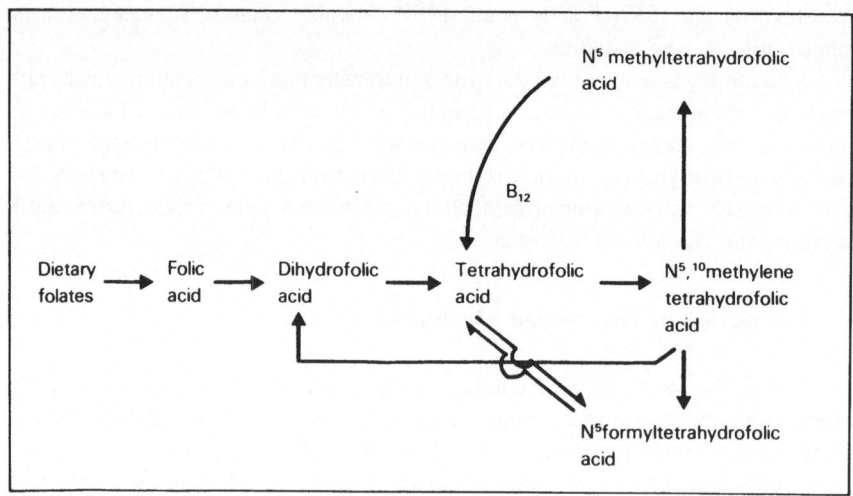

Fig. 13.3. The role of vitamin B$_{12}$ in folate metabolism.

1) The conversion of methylmalonate to succinate, in the sequence, proprionate → methylmalonate → succinate

2) The maintenance of -SH groups in reduced form in enzymes (e.g. co-enzyme A). Thus it may increase methionine formation by decreasing the oxidation of the methyl acceptor homocysteine.

Methylcobalamine (in which -CN in the cobalamin formula is $-CH_3$) is required to convert homocysteine to methionine. It appears likely that cyanocobalamin is required to convert methyltetrahydrofolate to tetrahydrofolate (fig. 13.3). Thus cyanocobalamin deficiency leads to folate deficiency in the presence of an adequate folate intake, and the effects of B_{12} deficiency on DNA synthesis (and thus on haematopoiesis) are probably due to such tetrahydrofolate deficiency. Folic acid therapy can correct the haematopoietic effects of vitamin B_{12} deficiency, but not the neurological effects, which appear related to effects of vitamin B_{12} apart from its actions on folate metabolism.

Pharmacodynamics

Vitamin B_{12} administration will reverse the biochemical and haematological evidence of its deficiency in man and halt neurological deterioration. The vitamin appears to have no effect if given in therapeutic dosage to persons not deficient in it.

Pharmacokinetics

Absorption and bioavailability: There are two absorption mechanisms for vitamin B_{12} in man, when the substance is taken orally. The first depends on the presence of gastric intrinsic factor (a glycoprotein, MW 50,000) which promotes the absorption of B_{12} at ileal level. This mechanism is saturated by a load of 1.5 to 3µg of B_{12}. The second mechanism does not depend on intrinsic factor and appears to allow significant absorption of the vitamin, possibly by simple diffusion, when enough B_{12} is given by mouth. However the intrinsic factor mechanism is the main one involved in B_{12} absorption and, if deficient, may lead to pernicious anaemia and other consequences of B_{12} deficiency. Thus for practical purposes adequate vitamin B_{12} absorption after oral administration depends on the availability of intrinsic factor.

After subcutaneous or intramuscular injection cyanocobalamin is rapidly and completely absorbed. Hydroxycobalamin and 5'-deoxyadenosylcobalamin are more protein-bound and less readily absorbed.

Distribution: Vitamin B_{12} becomes widely distributed in the body but 50 to 90% of the adult body's content of the vitamin is found in the liver. In the liver cyanocobalamin or hydroxycobalamin is converted into the co-enzyme form. Vitamin B_{12} binds to a specific globulin, and to glycoproteins, in blood. Only 1 to 10% of the vitamin in plasma is not bound to protein. Vitamin B_{12} crosses the placenta.

Elimination: The half-life of intravenously administered cyanocobalamin is about 6 days (Adams, 1963). Vitamin B_{12} undergoes an enterohepatic circulation. Some 3 to 8µg daily is secreted into bile from the liver, and in the normal adult all but approximately 1 µg is reabsorbed by the intrinsic factor mechanism. Normally 0.25µg of vitamin B_{12} is excreted in urine each day. In the presence of a B_{12} load (e.g. after injection) B_{12} excretion is determined by glomerular filtration rate.

Plasma level correlations: Normal serum vitamin levels are about 450pg/ml (range 200 to 900pg/ml). Clinical deficiency is not detectable till B_{12} levels are below 100pg/ml.

Interactions
Pharmacodynamic interactions: Chloramphenicol, possibly because of its effect on protein synthesis, is said to interfere with the effect of vitamin B_{12} in correcting megaloblastic anaemia.

Pharmacokinetic interactions: Aminosalicylic acid and neomycin impair the absorption of vitamin B_{12}. Tobacco smoke, with its high cyanide content, increases urine excretion of vitamin B_{12}, and tobacco smoking tends to lower serum vitamin B_{12} levels (Linnell et al., 1968).

Toxicity

Idiosyncratic Toxicity
Idiosyncratic reactions to vitamin B_{12} are very rare.

Dose-related Toxicity
Vitamin B_{12} is essentially non-toxic.

Dysmorphogenicity
Vitamin B_{12} is not known to be a dysmorphogen.

Treatment of Vitamin B_{12} Deficiency

Vitamin B_{12} is virtually non-toxic, and to allow a wide margin of safety, neurological manifestations of vitamin B_{12} deficiency are treated with doses of cyanocobalamin that are far in excess of those necessary to correct the deficit. A daily intramuscular injection of cyanocobalamin 1000µg (i.e. 1mg) is often given for 7 days. This is sufficient to restore depleted body stores of the vitamin and, if there has been anaemia, a reticulocyte response should be apparent. Neurological deterioration should halt, though neurological recovery is likely to occur slowly, over months, and may be incomplete. After the initial period of B_{12} replenishment, cyanocobalamin is usually given once a month, in a dose of 1mg, by injection, for the remainder of the patient's life. One would be very reluctant to rely on oral vitamin B_{12} therapy once neurological damage from vitamin B_{12} deficiency had occcurred.

Tobacco amblyopia, and Leber's optic atrophy, may be treated with parenteral hydroxocobalamin 1mg daily for 2 weeks, and then 1mg monthly.

Folic Acid Deficiency

Whether folic acid deficiency causes neurological disorder is arguable, but the vitamin is often enough used in neurological practice to warrant discussion.

Disordered Mechanisms

Folate deficiency may be of dietary origin, or may be due to various malabsorption syndromes or to therapy with agents which block the enzyme dihydrofolate reductase. In neurological practice folate deficiency is most often seen in patients receiving long term therapy with the anticonvulsants phenytoin, phenobarbitone and primidone. In these circumstances plasma folate levels are frequently reduced, but megaloblastic anaemia is considerably less common. The mechanism of the folate deficiency is not certain. There are suggestions that the anticonvulsants may impair folate absorption from the alimentary tract (Hoffbrand and Necheles, 1968) and also suggestions that these drugs induce the hepatic microsomal enzymes, which then consume increased amounts of folate (Maxwell et al., 1972).

There are suggestions that folate deficiency affords some protection against epilepsy (Reynolds, 1968) and that it may produce some mental dullness and even psychotic reactions. However, these matters are disputed. There has been a recent report that folate deficiency may cause a neurological disorder that is clinically similar to subacute combined degeneration, though serum vitamin B_{12} levels are normal (Manzoor and Runcie, 1976).

Correction of Disturbed Mechanisms

The effects of folate deficiency can be corrected by giving sufficiently large doses of folate orally.

Drugs Used in Treatment

Folic Acid

Folic acid is used to treat clinical or subclinical folate deficiency.

Chemistry

Folic acid (pteroylglutamic acid) is a slightly water-soluble substance with a molecular weight of 441.49.

Pharmacology

Biochemical Pharmacology

Folic acid itself is biologically inactive. Within the body it is reduced in stages to 5, 6, 7, 8 tetrahydrofolic acid, which is the co-enzyme form and which serves as an acceptor for one-carbon units at the 5 or the 10 position, forming other folate co-enzymes. These are involved in:

1) Purine synthesis
2) Pyrimidine nucleotide biosynthesis
3) Interconversion of serine and glycine
4) Catabolism of histidine to glutamic acid
5) Conversion of homocysteine to methionine (which also requires vitamin B_{12})
6) The generation of formate.

The more important pathways of folate metabolism are set out in figure 13.4. In folate deficiency, or block in tetrahydrofolate synthesis, the various reactions which require folate co-enzymes are depressed. The consequence is megaloblastic anaemia.

Pharmacodynamics

Folic acid therapy relieves the haematological manifestations of folate deficiency, unless there is inhibition of the enzyme dihydrofolate reductase. In the latter case the manifestations can be relieved by giving folinic acid. Folic acid has no effect if given to persons who are not folate deficient.

Pharmacokinetics

Absorption and bioavailability: After oral administration folic acid is well absorbed, mainly in the proximal small intestine. There are probably specific absorption mechanisms in the intestinal wall, but at higher folic acid doses absorption appears to occur chiefly by passive diffusion. Doses of folic acid of up to 15mg per day are fully absorbed. Dietary folate conjugates are less adequately absorbed, as they must be deconjugated prior to absorption. Folate absorption is decreased when the in-

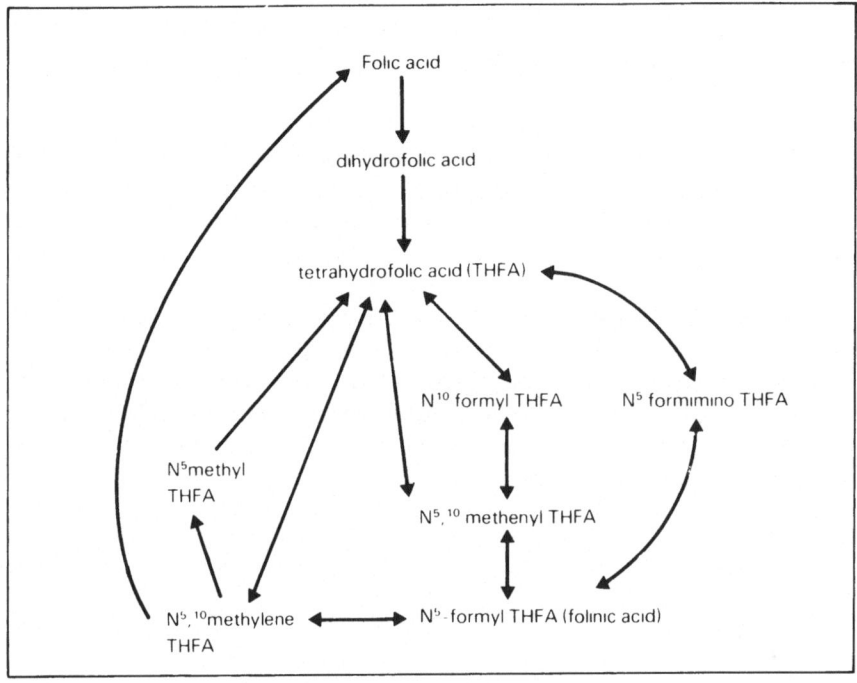

Fig. 13.4. The more important pathways of folate metabolism.

traluminal environment of the small intestine is made more alkaline (Benn et al., 1971). In sprue there may be very little absorption of dietary folate but very adequate absorption of folic acid.

Distribution: Some two-thirds of the folate in plasma is protein-bound (Johns et al., 1961). Folate is distributed to all tissues of the body. Entry of folic (and folinic) acids into cells probably depends on specific uptake mechanisms in cell membranes. The mechanisms are controlled by vitamin B_{12}. Some 50 % of the folate in the body (5 to 10mg) is found in the liver, mainly as 5-methyltetrahydrofolate. Folate is selectively concentrated in CSF, so that CSF folate (probably 5-methyltetrahydrofolate) levels are about 3 times higher than those in plasma (Chanarin et al., 1974).

Elimination: About half a 5mg folic acid dose is excreted in urine, and up to 90 % of a 15mg dose. Most of the excretion occurs within 6 hours of dosage. After intravenous administration, the half-life is 6 to 10 minutes (Sheehy et al., 1963). There appears to be a specific renal tubular resorption mechanism for folate, with a T_m of 50mg/minute.

Plasma level correlations: Folate levels in plasma below 3.5pg/ml are likely to be associated with clinical folate deficiency.

Interactions

Pharmacodynamic interactions: Chloramphenicol, because of its effect on protein biosynthesis, may antagonise the anti-anaemic effect of folic acid. Folic acid may interfere with the action of pyrimethamine in inhibiting toxoplasma (but not malarial) dihydrofolate reductase.

Pharmacokinetic interactions: Folic acid therapy causes a fall in plasma phenytoin level, and long term therapy with phenytoin, phenobarbitone or primidone causes reduced plasma folate levels (chapter VI). In states of vitamin B_{12} deficiency, folic acid therapy can increase the neurological damage caused by B_{12} lack, possibly by diverting B_{12} from its myelin-maintaining function to catalysing more formation of tetrahydrofolate from methylfolate (p.392).

Toxicity

Idiosyncratic Toxicity
No instances of idiosyncratic toxicity have been traced.

Dose-related Toxicity
There have been suggestions that high folate doses may produce a convulsant effect but there is no real evidence that this occurs in man, except perhaps by producing a fall in plasma phenytoin level in patients taking that anticonvulsant.

Dysmorphogenicity
Folic acid deficiency is suspected of being responsible for fetal malformations, but folic acid itself is not.

Treatment of Folate Deficiency

Oral folate doses of 0.5 to 1.0mg daily should suffice to treat folate deficiency. Higher doses e.g. 5 to 15mg daily are often used but, in patients with folate deficiency due to anticonvulsants, may cause a fall in plasma anticonvulsant levels necessitating revision of anticonvulsant dosage. There may be a case for using the minimum folic acid dose that corrects folate deficiency when this is due to anticonvulsant therapy, in the hope that this policy will produce minimal disturbance in antiepilepsy medication. However, it has not been established that such a dosage policy is successful in practice.

Chapter XIV

Neoplasms

Principal Disorder and Drugs Discussed

Cerebral neoplasm
  Corticosteroids (see also chapter II)
  Antineoplastic drugs (see also chapter XI)

Disordered Anatomy and Physiology

The nature of the neoplastic process and its initiation are not yet completely understood. The neoplasms that involve the nervous system may be primary, arising from the substance of the nervous system or from other structures within the skull or vertebral column, or secondary, originating elsewhere. As neoplasms grow they may constitute a mass lesion and raise intracranial pressure, as discussed in chapter II. Oedema may develop in the substance of the tumour, and in the surrounding neural tissue. The function of the affected portion of the brain or spinal cord may be impaired, and local disinhibition of neurones around the tumour may produce focal (partial) epilepsy. Pituitary tumours may have endocrine effects.

Correction of Disordered Anatomy and Physiology

In the present state of knowledge it is impossible to correct the process which initiates neoplasia. The neoplastic process itself may be interrupted, or impeded, by the use of ionising radiations and/or by various antineoplastic chemicals which interfere more with metabolic processes in actively growing and dividing cells than in normal cells. Occasionally secondary tumours within the nervous system (e.g. breast carcinoma metastases) may be hormone dependent.

High dose glucocorticoids probably have two different beneficial effects on brain tumours. By restoring the integrity of the blood-brain barrier within tumours, steroids may reduce oedema in and around tumours. Further, there is a clinical impression, and some experimental evidence (see chapter II) that steroids actually diminish the rate of tumour growth by interfering with the neoplastic process.

Radiotherapy and chemotherapy are rarely capable of completely stopping tumour growth. Therefore, where possible, the tumour mass is removed surgically. It may be possible to remove benign tumours or solitary metastases *in toto*, but complete surgical removal of gliomas or of multiple metastases is rarely possible because of the extent of the neurological defect that would be produced.

Defects in neurological function caused by tumours can rarely be treated except by removing the tumour, or at least decreasing its bulk. However epilepsy due to the tumour can be treated with anticonvulsant drugs. Hormonal replacement therapy may be given if pituitary tumours cause hypopituitarism.

Drugs Used in Treating Nervous System Neoplasia

Corticosteroids and osmotically acting agents were discussed in chapter II, and certain of the better established antineoplastic agents in chapter XI. A number of other agents are undergoing evaluation in the treatment of brain tumour. Such agents are usually employed by oncologists rather than by neurologists, and since their place in the chemotherapy of nervous system tumours is not yet established they will not be considered in detail here.

Treatment of Nervous System Tumours

When nervous system tumour is diagnosed a decision is taken as to whether the tumour is amenable to surgery. If it is, prior to operation intracranial pressure is usually reduced by the use of steroids and/or osmotically acting agents, as discussed in chapter II. Postoperatively, except in the case of benign tumours which have been totally removed, the question of radiotherapy will be considered if the tumour is of a type that is thought to be radiosensitive. Radiotherapy should also be considered in the case of inoperable tumour, or tumours. During the course of radiotherapy, and afterwards, it may be necessary to continue the use of chemical agents to maintain control of intracranial pressure.

In the case of secondary tumours, any appropriate chemotherapy or hormonal therapy that appears possible will no doubt be prescribed, probably in consultation with an oncologist. Meningeal carcinomatosis may be treated with intrathecally administered antineoplastic agents such as cytarabine and methotrexate.

Some centres are now treating malignant gliomas with nitrosoureas, antineoplastic agents which are sufficiently lipid-soluble to cross the blood-brain barrier. Drugs in this family include carmustine (BCNU), lomustine (CCNU) and methyl lomustine (methyl CCNU or semustine). These are sometimes combined with other agents such as procarbazine and vincristine, and high dose steroids. Concurrent radiotherapy may be employed. On the whole the data seem to suggest that the length of survival is increased, and the quality of survival improved, by radiotherapy and by such chemotherapy. However the optimal chemotherapeutic regimens are not yet worked out. The antineoplastic drugs may have very serious unwanted effects, including bone marrow depression and hepatotoxicity. Further, not all studies have shown the nitrosoureas to be of benefit in patients with glioblastomas (Brisman et al., 1976)

The current state of non-surgical treatment of brain tumour has been reviewed by Posner and Shapiro (1975).

References

Aarli, J.A.: Changes in serum immunoglobulin levels during phenytoin treatment of epilepsy. Acta Neurologica Scandinavica 54: 423-430 (1976).

Aarskog, D.: Association between maternal intake of diazepam and oral clefts. Lancet 2: 921 (1975).

Acheson, J.; Danta, G. and Hutchinson, E.C.: Controlled trial of dipyridamole in cerebral vascular disease. British Medical Journal 1: 614-615 (1969).

Acocella, G.; Bonollo, P.; Garimoldi, M.; Mainardi, M.; Tenconi, L.T. and Nicolis, P.B.: Kinetics of rifampicin and isoniazid administered alone and in combination to normal subjects and patients with liver disease. Gut 13: 47-53 (1972a).

Acocella, G.; Lamarina, A.; Nicolis, F.B.; Pagani, V. and Segre, G.: Kinetic studies on rifampicin II. Multicompartment analysis of the serum, urine and bile concentrations in subjects treated for one week. European Journal of Clinical Pharmacology 5: 111-115 (1972b).

Acocella, G.; Pagani, V.; Marchetti, M.; Baroni, G.C. and Nicolis, F.B.: Kinetic studies on rifampicin I. Serum concentration analysis in subjects treated with different oral doses over a period of two weeks. Chemotherapy 16: 356-370 (1971).

Adams, G.F.; Merrett, J.D.; Hutchison, W.M. and Pollock, A.M.: Cerebral embolism and mitral stenosis: survival with and without anticoagulants. Journal of Neurology, Neurosurgery and Psychiatry 37: 378-383 (1974).

Adams, J.F.: Biological half-life of vitamin B_{12} in plasma. Nature 198: 200 (1963).

Adams, P. and White, C.: Isoniazid-induced encephalopathy. Lancet 1: 680-682 (1965).

Adamson, R.H.: Metabolism of anticancer agents in man. Annals of the New York Academy of Science 179: 432-441 (1971).

Ad Hoc Committee: Classification of headache. Archives of Neurology 6: 173-176 (1962).

Adcock, J.D. and Hettig, R.A.: Absorption, distribution and excretion of streptomycin. Archives of Internal Medicine 77: 179-195 (1946).

Aellig, W.H. and Nuesch, E.: Comparative pharmacokinetic investigations with tritium-labelled ergot alkaloids after oral and intravenous administration in man. International Journal of Clinical Pharmacology 15: 106-111 (1977).

Agarwal, S.P. and Blake, M.I.: Determination of the pKa value for 5,5-diphenylhydantoin. Journal of Pharmaceutical Sciences 57: 1434-1435 (1968).

Agnoli, A.; Casacchia, M.; Ruggieri, S.; Volante, F. and Accornero, N.: Parkinson's tremor, relief by an antiaminic drug (BC105). Zeitschrift fur Neurologie 202: 154-158 (1972).

Agurell, S.; Berlin, A.; Ferngren, H. and Hellstrom, B.: Plasma levels of diazepam after parenteral and rectal administration in children. Epilepsia 16: 277-283 (1975).

Agurell, S.V.; Boreus, L.O.; Gordon, E.; Lindgren, J.E.; Ehrnebo, M. and Lonroth, U.: Plasma and cerebrospinal fluid concentrations of pentazocine in patients: assay by mass fragmentography. Journal of Pharmacy and Pharmacology 26: 1-8 (1974).

Albert, K.S.; Hallmark, M.R.; Sakmar, E.; Weidler, D.J. and Wagner, J.G.: Pharmacokinetics of diphenhydramine in man. Journal of Pharmacokinetics and Biopharmaceutics 3: 159-170 (1975).

Albert, K.S.; Sedman, A.J.; Wilkinson, P.; Stoll, R.G.; Murray, W.J. and Wagner, J.G.: Bioavailability studies of acetaminophen and nitrofurantoin. Journal of Clinical Pharmacology 14: 264-270 (1974).

Alexanderson, B.: Pharmacokinetics of desmethylimipramine and nortriptyline in man after single and multiple oral doses — a cross-over study. European Journal of Clinical Pharmacology 5: 1-10 (1972).

Alexanderson, B. and Borga, O.: Urinary excretion of nortriptyline and five of its metabolites in man after single and multiple oral doses. European Journal of Clinical Pharmacology 5: 174-180 (1973).

Alexanderson, B.; Sjoqvist, F. and Price Evans, D.A.: Steady state plasma levels of nortriptyline in twins: influence of genetic factors and drug therapy. British Medical Journal 4: 764-768 (1969).

Almon, R.R. and Appel, S.H.: Serum acetylcholine-receptor antibodies in myasthenia gravis. Annals of the New York Academy of Science 274: 235-243 (1976).

Alvord, E.C.: Pathology of Parkinsonism; in Fields (Ed) Pathogenesis and Treatment of Parkinsonism, p.161-183 (Thomas, Springfield 1958).

Anden, N.E.; Carlsson, A.; Dahlstrom, A.; Fuxe, K.; Hillarp, N.A. and Larsson, K.: Demonstration and mapping out of nigro-neostriatal dopamine neurons. Life Sciences 3: 523-530 (1964).

Anden, N.E.; Corrodi, H.; Fuxe, K.; Hokfeldt, B.; Hokfeldt, T.; Rydin, C. and Svensson, T.: Evidence for a central noradrenaline receptor stimulation by clonidine. Life Sciences 9: 513-523 (1970).

Anderson, W.A.D. and Bethea, W.J. Jr.: Renal lesions following administration of hypertonic sucrose. Journal of the American Medical Association 114: 1983-1987 (1960).

Anderson, P.G.: Ergotamine headache. Headache 15: 118-121 (1975).

Anggard, E.; Jonsson, L.E.; Hogmark, A.L. and Gunne, L.M.: Amphetamine metabolism in amphetamine psychosis. Clinical Pharmacology and Therapeutics 14: 870-880 (1973).

Annegers, J.F.; Elveback, L.R.; Hauser, W.A. and Kurland, L.T.: Do anticonvulsants have a teratogenic effect? Archives of Neurology 31: 364-373 (1974).

Anthony, J.J.: Malignant lymphoma associated with hydantoin drugs. Archives of Neurology 22: 450-454 (1970).

Anthony, M.: Migrainous neuralgia — an allergic disorder? Hemicrania 4(3): 2-5 (1972).

Anthony, M. and Lance, J.W.: Monoamine oxidase inhibition in the treatment of migraine. Archives of Neurology 21: 263-268 (1969).

Anthony, M. and Lance, J.W.: Histamine and serotonin in cluster headache. Archives of Neurology 25: 225-231 (1971).

Anthony, M.; Lance, J.W. and Somerville, B.: A comparative trial of pindolol, clonidine and carbamazepine in the interval therapy of migraine. Medical Journal of Australia 1: 1343-1346 (1972).

Arguelles, A.E. and Rosner, J.: Diazepam and plasma-testosterone levels. Lancet 3: 607 (1975).

Arita, T.; Hori, R.; Ito, K.; Ichikawa, K. and Uesugi, T.: Transformation and excretion of drugs in biological systems II. Transformation of metoclopramide in rabbits. Chemical and Pharmaceutical Bulletin 18: 1663-1669 (1970b).

Arita, T.; Hori, R.; Ito, K. and Sekikawa, H.: Transformation and excretion of drugs in biological systems IV. Reabsorption of biliary metoclopramide-N⁴-glucuronide and -N⁴-sulfonate from rabbit intestine. Chemical and Pharmaceutical Bulletin 18: 1675-1679 (1970a).

Arnold, K. and Gerber, N.: The rate of decline of diphenylhydantoin in human plasma. Clinical Pharmacology and Therapeutics 11: 121-134 (1970).

Asberg, M.; Cronholm, B.; Sjoqvist, F. and Tuck, D.: Relationship between plasma level and therapeutic effect of nortriptyline. British Medical Journal 3: 331-334 (1971).

Ashby, P. and White, D.G.: 'Presynaptic' inhibition in spasticity and the effect of β(4-chlorophenyl) GABA. Journal of Neurological Sciences 20: 329-338 (1973).

Atkinson, A.J. and Shaw, J.M.: Pharmacokinetic study of a patient with diphenylhydantoin toxicity. Clinical Pharmacology and Therapeutics 14: 521-528 (1973).

Avery, G.S.: Drug Treatment. Principles and practice of clinical pharmacology and therapeutics. (Adis Press, Sydney 1976).

Aviram, A.; Czaczkes, J.W. and Rosenmann, E.: Acute renal failure associated with sulthiame. Lancet 1: 818 (1965).

Axelrod, J.: Studies on sympathomimetic amines II. The biotransformation and physiological disposition of D-amphetamine, D-p-hydroxyamphetamine and D-methamphetamine. Journal of Pharmacology and Experimental Therapeutics 110: 315-326 (1954).

Axelrod, L.: Glucocorticoid therapy. Medicine 55: 39-65 (1976).

Azzaro, A.J.; Gutrecht, J.A. and Smith, D.J.: Effect of diphenylhydantoin on the uptake and catabolism of L-(^{3}H) norepinephrine in vitro in rat cerebral cortical tissue. Biochemical Pharmacology 22: 2719-2729 (1973).

Azzaro, A.J. and Rutledge, C.O.: Selectivity of release of norepinephrine, dopamine and 5-hydroxytryptamine by amphetamine in various regions of rat brain. Biochemical Pharmacology 22: 2801-2813 (1973).

Azzolinni, F.; Gazzaniga, A.; Lodola, E. and Natangelo, R.: Elimination of chloramphenicol and thiamphenicol in subjects with cirrhosis of the liver. International Journal of Clinical Pharmacology 6: 130-134 (1972).

Babcock, R.B.; Dumper, C.W. and Scharfman, W.B.: Heparin-induced immune thrombocytopenia. New England Journal of Medicine 295: 237-241 (1976).

Bach, J.F. and Dardenne, M.: Serum immunosuppressive activity of azathioprine in normal subjects and patients with liver disease. Proceedings of the Royal Society of Medicine 65: 260-263 (1972).

Bagley, C.M.; Bostick, F.W. and De Vita, V.T.: Clinical pharmacology of cyclophosphamide. Cancer Research 33: 226-233 (1973).

Balasubramaniam, K.; Lucas, D.B.; Mawer, G.E. and Simons, P.J.: The kinetics of amylobarbitone metabolism in healthy men and women. British Journal of Pharmacology 39: 564-572 (1970).

Baldessarini, R.J. and Greiner, E.: Inhibition of catechol-O-methyl transferase by catechols and polyphenols. Biochemical Pharmacology 22: 247-256 (1973).

Ball, A.P.; Gray, J.A. and Murdoch, M.McC.: Antibacterial Drugs Today, 2nd edition (Adis Press, New York, 1978).

Ballek, R.E.; Reidenberg, M.M. and Orr, L.: Inhibition of diphenylhydantoin metabolism by chloramphenicol. Lancet 1: 150 (1973).

Barbeau, A.: L-Depa therapy in Parkinson's disease: a crucial review of nine years' experience. Canadian Medical Association Journal 101: 59-68 (1969).

Barchi, R.L.: Myotonia. An evaluation of the chloride hypothesis. Archives of Neurology 32: 175-180 (1975).

Barnett, H.L.; Simons, D.J. and Wells, R.E. Jr.: Nephrotic syndrome occurring during Tridione® therapy. American Journal of Medicine 4: 760-764 (1948).

Barrow, C.G. and Rischbieth, R.H.: A drug trial of tranylcypromine for multiple sclerosis. Medical Journal of Australia 1: 414-416 (1965).

Barrow, S.J.; Darcey, B.A. and Booker, H.E.: Metabolism and kinetics of methsuximide in man. Neurology 24: 386 (1974).

Bartholini, G.; Kuruma, I. and Pletscher, A.: The metabolic pathway of L-3-0-methyldopa. Journal of Pharmacology and Experimental Therapeutics 183: 65-72 (1972).

Barza, M. and Weinstein, L.: Pharmacokinetics of the penicillins in man. Clinical Pharmacokinetics 1: 297-308 (1976).

Baumel, I.P.; Gallagher, B.B. and Mattson, R.H.: Phenylethylmalonamide (PEMA). An important metabolite of primidone. Archives of Neurology 27: 34-41 (1972).

Baumrucker, J.F.: Drug interaction — propranolol and Cafergot. New England Journal of Medicine 288: 916-917 (1973).

Baylis, E.M.; Crowley, J.M.; Preece, J.M.; Sylvester, P.E. and Marks, V.: Influence of folic acid on blood-phenytoin levels. British Medical Journal 1: 62-64 (1971).

Beam, W.E.; Newberg, N.R.; Devine, L.F.; Pierce, W.E. and Davies, J.A.: The effect of rifampin on the nasopharyngeal carriage of Neisseria meningitis in a military population. Journal of Infectious Diseases 124: 39-46 (1971).

Beckett, A.H.; Kourounakis, P.; Vaughan, D.F. and Mitchard, M.: The absorption, blood concentration and excretion of pentazocine after oral, intramuscular or rectal administration to man. Journal of Pharmacy and Pharmacology 22 (Suppl): 169 (1970).

Beckett, A.H.; Salmon, J.A. and Mitchard, M.: The relation between blood levels and urinary excretion of amphetamine under controlled acidic and under fluctuating urinary pH using ^{14}C amphetamine. Journal of Pharmacy and Pharmacology 21: 251-258 (1969).

Beermann, B.; Hellstrom, K. and Rosen, A.: The gastrointestinal absorption of atropine in man. Clinical

Science 40: 95-106 (1971).

Beermann, B.; Hellstrom, K. and Rosen, A.: On the metabolism of propantheline in man. Clinical Pharmacology and Therapeutics 13: 212-220 (1972).

Bein, H.J.: Pharmacological differentiation of muscle relaxants; in Birkmayer (Ed) Spasticity — A Topical Survey, p.76-82 (Huber, Berne 1972).

Bell, H.; Johansen, H.; Lunde, P.K.M.; Andersgaard, H.A.; Finholt, P.; Midtvedt, T.; Holum, E.; Martinussen, B. and Aarnes, E.G.: Absorption and dissolution characteristics of 14 different oral chloramphenicol preparations tested on healthy human male subjects. Pharmacology 5: 108-120 (1971).

Benn, A.; Swan, C.H.J.; Cooke, W.T.; Blair, J.A.; Matty, A.J. and Smith, M.E.: Effect of intraluminal pH on the absorption of pteroylmonoglutamic acid. British Medical Journal 1: 148-150 (1971).

Berde, B.; Cerletti, A.; Dengler, H.J. and Zoglio, M.A.: Studies in the interaction between ergot alkaloids and xanthine derivatives; in Cochrane (Ed) Background to Migraine III. (Heinemann, London 1970).

Bergmann, S.; Curzon, G.; Friedel, J.; Godwin-Austen, R.B.; Marsden, C.D. and Parkes, J.D.: The absorption and metabolism of a standard oral dose of levodopa in patients with Parkinsonism. British Journal of Clinical Pharmacology 1: 417-424 (1974).

Berkowitz, B.: Influence of plasma levels and metabolism on pharmacological activity: pentazocine. Annals of the New York Academy of Science 179: 269-281 (1971).

Berkowitz, B.A.; Asling, J.H.; Shnider, S.M. and Way, E.L.: Relationship of pentazocine plasma levels to pharmacological activity in man. Clinical Pharmacology and Therapeutics 10: 320-328 (1969).

Berlin, A. and Dahlstrom, H.: Pharmacokinetics of the anticonvulsant drug clonazepam evaluated from single oral and intravenous doses and by repeated oral administration. European Journal of Clinical Pharmacology 9: 155-159 (1975).

Berlin, A.; Siwers, B.; Agurell, S.; Hiort, A.; Sjoqvist, F. and Strom, S.: Determination of bioavailability of diazepam in various formulations from steady state plasma concentration data. Clinical Pharmacology and Therapeutics 13: 733-744 (1972).

Berliner, R.W.; Earle, D.P. Jr.; Taggart, J.V.; Zubrod, C.G.; Welch, W.G.; Conan, N.J.; Bauman, E.; Scudder, S.T. and Shannon, J.A.: Studies on the chemotherapy of the human malarias VI. The physiological disposition, antimalarial activity and toxicity of several derivatives of 4-aminoquinoline. Journal of Clinical Investigation 27: 98-107 (1948).

Bernat, J.L.; Sadowsky, C.H.; Vincent, F.M.; Nordgren, R.D. and Margolis, G.: Sclerosing spinal pachymeningitis. A complication of intrathecal administration of Depo-Medrol for multiple sclerosis. Journal of Neurology, Neurosurgery and Psychiatry 39: 1124-1128 (1976).

Berry, K. and Olszewski, J.: Pathology of intrathecal phenol injection in man. Neurology 13: 152-154 (1963).

Bianchine, J.R.: Metabolism of methysergide (MS) in the rabbit and man. Federation Proceedings 27: 238 (1968).

Bianchine, J.R.; Calimlim, L.R.; Morgan, J.P.; Dujuvnet, C.A. and Lasagna, L.: Metabolism and absorption of L-3,4 dihydroxyphenyllalanine in patients with Parkinson's disease. Proceedings of the New York Academy of Science 179: 126-140 (1971).

Bianchine, J.R. and Friedman, A.P.: Metabolism of methysergide and retroperitoneal fibrosis. Archives of Internal Medicine 126: 252-254 (1970).

Bianchine, J.R. and Shaw, G.M.: Clinical pharmacokinetics of levodopa in Parkinson's disease. Clinical Pharmacokinetics 1: 313-338 (1976).

Bickerstaff, E.R. and Holmes, J.M.: Cerebral arterial insufficiency and oral contraceptives. British Medical Journal 2: 726-729 (1967).

Bigger, J.T. Jr.; Schmidt, D.H. and Kutt, H.: Relationship between the plasma level of diphenylhydantoin sodium and its cardiac antiarrhythmic effect. Circulation 38: 363-374 (1968).

Bigorie, B.; Aimez, P.; Soria, R.J.; Samama, F.; Dimaria, G.; Guy-Grand, B. and Bour, H.: L'association triacetyl oleandomycin — tartrate d'ergotamine. Est-elle dangereuse? Nouvelle Presse Medicale 4:

2723-2725 (1975).

Bindschadler, D.D. and Bennett, J.E.: A pharmacologic guide to the clinical use of amphotericin B. Journal of Infectious Diseases 120: 427-436 (1969).

Bird, E.D.; Mackay, A.V.P.; Rayner, C.N. and Iversen, L.L.: Reduced glutamic-acid-decarboxylase activity of post-mortem brain in Huntington's chorea. Lancet 2: 1090-1092 (1973).

Birket-Smith, E.: Abnormal involuntary movements induced by anticholinergic therapy. Acta Neurologica Scandinavica 50: 801-811 (1974).

Birket-Smith, E.: Abnormal involuntary movements in relation to anticholinergics and levodopa therapy. Acta Neurologica Scandinavica 52: 158-160 (1975).

Birket-Smith, E. and Krogh, E.: Motor nerve conduction velocity during diphenylhydantoin intoxication. Acta Neurologica Scandinavica 47: 265-271 (1971).

Birkmayer, W. and Hornykiewicz, O.: Der L-Dioxyphenylalanin (= dopa)-Effekt bei der Parkinson-Akinese. Wiener Klinische Wochenschrift 73: 787-788 (1961).

Bleidner, W.E.; Harmon, J.B.; Hewes, W.E.; Lynes, I.E. and Hermann, E.C.: Absorption, distribution and excretion of amantadine hydrochloride. Journal of Pharmacology and Experimental Therapeutics 150: 484-490 (1965).

Blonsky, E.R.; Ericsson, A.D.; McKinney, A.S.; Rix, A.; Wang, R.I.H. and Rimm, A.A.: Phase II multiclinic study of elantrine in Parkinsonism. Clinical Pharmacology and Therapeutics 15: 46-50 (1974).

Blum, M.R.; Riegelman, S. and Becker, C.E.: Altered protein binding of diphenylhydantoin in uraemic plasma. New England Journal of Medicine 286: 109 (1972).

Bochner, F.; Hooper, W.D.; Eadie, M.J. and Tyrer, J.H.: Decreased capacity to metabolize diphenylhydantoin in a patient with hypersensitivity to warfarin. Australian and New Zealand Journal of Medicine 5: 462-466 (1975).

Bochner, F.; Hooper, W.D.; Sutherland, J.M.; Eadie, M.J. and Tyrer, J.H.: Diphenylhydantoin concentrations in saliva. Archives of Neurology 31: 57-59 (1974).

Bochner, F.; Hooper, W.D.; Tyrer, J.H. and Eadie, M.J.: The effect of dosage increments on blood phenytoin concentrations. Journal of Neurology, Neurosurgery and Psychiatry 35: 873-876 (1972a).

Bochner, F.; Hooper, W.D. Tyrer, J.H. and Eadie, M.J.: Factors involved in an outbreak of phenytoin intoxication. Journal of Neurological Sciences 16: 481-487 (1972b).

Bochner, F.; Hooper, W.D.; Tyrer, J.H. and Eadie, M.J.: The renal handling of diphenylhydantoin and 5-(p-hydroxyphenyl)-5-phenylhydantoin. Clinical Pharmacology and Therapeutics 14: 791-796 (1973).

Booker, H.E.: Trimethadione and other oxazolidinediones. Relation of plasma levels to clinical control; in Woodbury, Penry and Schmidt (Eds) Antiepileptic Drugs, p.403-407 (Raven Press, New York 1972).

Booker, H.E. and Celesia, G.G.: Serum concentrations of diazepam in subjects with epilepsy. Archives of Neurology 29: 191-194 (1973).

Booker, H.E.; Chun, R.W.M. and Sanguino, M.: Myasthenia gravis syndrome associated with trimethadione. Journal of the American Medical Association 212: 2262-2263 (1970).

Booker, H.E.; Hosokowa, K.; Burdette, R.D. and Darcey, B.: A clinical study of serum primidone levels. Epilepsie 11: 395-402 (1970).

Borga, O.; Azarnoff, D.L.; Forshell, G.P. and Sjoquist, F.: Plasma protein binding of tricyclic antidepressants in man. Biochemical Pharmacology 18: 2135-2143 (1969).

Borgesen, S.E.; Nielsen, J.L. and Moller, C.E.: Prophylactic treatment of migraine with propranolol. A clinical trial. Acta Neurologica Scandinavica 50: 651-656 (1974).

Borofsky, L.G.; Louis, S.; Kutt, H. and Roginsky, M.: Diphenylhydantoin: efficacy, toxicity and dose-serum level relationships in children. Journal of Pediatrics 81: 995-1002 (1972).

Boschenstein, F.K.; Reilly, J.A.; Yahr, M.D. and Correll, J.W.: Effect of low molecular weight dextran on cortical blood flow. Archives of Neurology 14: 288-293 (1966).

Bowden, A.N.; Bowden, P.M.A.; Friedmann, A.I.; Perkin, G.D. and Rose, F.C.: A trial of corticotrophin gelatin injection in acute optic neuritis. Journal of Neurology, Neurosurgery, and Psychiatry 37: 869-873 (1974).

Bowen, F.P.; Kamienny, R.S.; Burns, M.M. and Yahr, M.D.: Parkinsonism: effect of levodopa treatment on concept formation. Neurology 25: 701-704 (1975).

Boxenbaum, H.G. and Riegelman, S.: Pharmacokinetics of isoniazid and some metabolites in man. Journal of Pharmacokinetics and Biopharmaceutics 4: 287-325 (1976).

Boxer, G.E.; Jelinek, V.C.; Tomsett, R.; Du Bois, R. and Edison, A.O.: Streptomycin in the blood: chemical determinations after single and repeated intramuscular injections. Journal of Pharmacology and Experimental Therapeutics 92: 226-285 (1948).

Boyer, P.A. Jr.: Anticonvulsant properties of benzodiazepines. A review. Diseases of the Nervous System 27: 35-42 (1966).

Bradshaw, P. and Brennan, S.: Trial of long-term anticoagulant therapy in the treatment of small stroke associated with a normal carotid arteriogram. Journal of Neurology, Neurosurgery and Psychiatry 38: 642-647 (1975).

Braham, J.: Jakob-Creutzfeld disease: treatment by amantadine. British Medical Journal 4: 212-213 (1971).

Brand, J.J. and Perry, W.L.M.: Drugs used in motion sickness. Pharmacological Review 18: 895-924 (1966).

Bretag, A.H.: A quantitative assessment of the membrane lesion in myotonia; in Kakulas (Ed) Basic Research in Myology, p.641-646 (Excerpta Medica, Amsterdam 1973).

Breyer, U.; Gaertner, H.J. and Prox, A.: Formation of identical metabolites from piperazine and dimethylamino substituted phenothiazine drugs in man, rat and dog. Biochemical Pharmacology 23: 313-322 (1974).

Brink, J.J. and Freeman, E.A.: Effect of 5-phenyl-oxazolidinedione on sodium-potassium-magnesium-activated adenosine triphosphatase activity in mouse brain. Journal of Neurochemistry 19: 1783-1788 (1972).

Brisman, R.; Housepian, E.M.; Chang, C.; Duffy, P. and Balis, E.: Adjuvant nitrosourea therapy for glioblastoma. Archives of Neurology 33: 745-750 (1976).

Brodie, B.B.; Baer, J.E. and Craig, L.C.: Metabolic products of the cinchona alkaloids in human urine. Journal of Biological Chemistry 188: 576-581 (1951).

Brogden, R.N.; Speight, T.M. and Avery, G.S.: Levodopa: a review of its pharmacological proterties and therapeutic uses with particular reference to Parkinsonism. Drugs 2: 262-400 (1971).

Brogden, R.N.; Speight, T.M. and Avery, G.S.: Pentazocine: a review of its pharmacological properties, therapeutic efficacy and dependence liability. Drugs 5: 6-91 (1973).

Brogden, R.N.; Speight, T.M. and Avery, G.S.: Baclofen: a preliminary report on its pharmacological properties and therapeutic efficacy in spasticity. Drugs 8: 1-14 (1974).

Brown, J.C. and Johns, R.J.: Diagnostic difficulties encountered in the myasthenic syndrome sometimes associated with carcinoma. Journal of Neurology, Neurosurgery, and Psychiatry 37: 1214-1224 (1974).

Browne, T.R.; Dreifuss, F.E.; Dyken, P.R.; Goode, D.J.; Penry, J.K.; Porter, R.J.; White, B.G. and White, P.I.: Ethosuximide in the treatment of absence (petit mal) seizures. Neurology 25: 515-524 (1975).

Bruetman, M.E.; Fields, W.S.; Crawford, E.S. and De Bakey, M.: Cerebral hemorrhage in carotid artery surgery. Archives of Neurology 9: 458-467 (1963).

Brunner, N.G.; Berger, C.L.; Namba, T. and Grob, D.: Corticotropin and corticosteroids in generalized myasthenia gravis: comparative studies and role in management. Annals of the New York Academy of Sciences 274: 577-595 (1976).

Brunner, N.G.; Namba, T. and Grob, D.: Corticosteroids in management of severe, generalised myasthenia gravis. Effectiveness and comparison with corticotrophin therapy. Neurology 22: 603-610 (1972).

Bruyn, G.S.: The biochemical basis of migraine: a critique, in Klawans (Ed) Clinical Neuropharmacology, p.185-213 (Raven Press, New York 1976).

Buchanan, R.A.: Ethosuximide toxicity; in Woodbury, Penry and Schmidt (Eds) Antiepileptic Drugs, p.449-454 (Raven Press, New York 1972).

Buchanan, R.A.; Fernandez, L. and Kinkel, A.W.: Absorption and elimination of ethosuximide in children. Journal of Clinical Pharmacology 9: 393-398 (1969).

Buchanan, R.A.; Kinkel, A.W.; Goulet, J.R., and Smith, T.C.: The metabolism of diphenylhydantoin (Dilantin) following once daily administration. Neurology 22: 126-130 (1972).

Buchanan, R.A.; Kinkel, A.W. and Smith, T.C.: The absorption and excretion of ethosuximide. International Journal of Clinical Pharmacology 7: 213-218 (1973).

Buchthal, F.; Svensmark, O. and Simonsen, H.: Relation of EEG and seizures to phenobarbital in serum. Archives of Neurology 19: 567-572 (1968).

Buchthal, F. and Lennox-Buchthal, M.A.: Phenobarbital. Relation of serum concentration to control of seizures; in Woodbury, Penry and Schmidt (Eds) Antiepileptic Drugs, p.335-343 (Raven Press, New York, 1972).

Buchthal, F. and Svensmark, O.: Aspects of the pharmacology of phenytoin (Dilantin) and phenobarbital relevant to their dosages in the treatment of epilepsy. Epilepsia 1: 373-384 (1959).

Bucknall, R.C.; Dixon, A. St.J.; Glick, E.N.; Woodland, J. and Zutshi, D.W.: Myasthenia gravis associated with penicillamine treatment for rheumatoid arthritis. British Medical Journal 1: 600-602 (1975).

Bucy, P.C.: Is there a pyramidal tract? Brain 80: 376-392 (1957).

Bunker, J.P. and Vandam, L.D.: Effect of anaesthesia on metabolism and cellular functions. Pharmacological Reviews 17: 183-263 (1965).

Burns, J.J.; Yu, T.F.; Ritterband, A.; Perel, J.M.; Gutman, A.B. and Brodie, B.B.: A potent new uricosuric agent, the sulfoxide metabolite of the phenylbutazone analogue, G-25671. Journal of Pharmacology and Experimental Therapeutics 119: 418-426 (1957).

Burrows, G.D.; Davies, B. and Scoggins, B.A.: Plasma concentrations of nortriptyline and clinical response in depressive illness. Lancet 2: 619-623 (1972).

Burstein, S. and Klaiber, E.L.: Phenobarbital induced increase in 6 beta-hydroxycortisol excretion: clue to its significance in human urine. Journal of Clinical Endocrinology and Metabolism 25: 293 (1965).

Burton, J.L. and Shuster, S.: Effect of 1-Dopa on seborrhoea of Parkinsonism. Lancet 2: 19-20 (1970).

Butler, T.C.: Metabolic demethylation of 3,5-dimethyl-5-ethyl 2,4-oxazolidinedione (paramethadione, Paradione®). Journal of Pharmacology and Experimental Therapeutics 113: 178-185 (1955).

Butler, T.C.: The metabolic hydroxylation of phenobarbital. Journal of Pharmacology and Experimental Therapeutics 116: 326-336 (1956).

Butler, T.C.; Kuroiwa, Y.; Waddell, W.J. and Poole, D.T.: Effects of 5,5-dimethyl-2,4-oxazolidinedione (DMO) on acid-base and electrolyte equilibria. Journal of Pharmacology and Experimental Therapeutics 152: 62-66 (1966).

Butler, T.C. and Waddell, W.J.: Metabolic conversion of primidone (Mysoline) to phenobarbital. Proceedings of the Society for Experimental Biology and Medicine 93: 544-546 (1956).

Butler, T.C. and Waddell, W.J.: N-methylated derivatives of barbituric acids, hydantoin and oxazolidine used in the treatment of epilepsy. Neurology 8 (Suppl.)1: 106-112 (1958).

Butler, T.C.; Waddell, W.J. and Poole, D.T.: Demethylation of trimethadione and metharbital by rat liver microsomal enzymes: Substrate concentration: yield relationships and competition between substrates. Biochemical Pharmacology 14: 937-942 (1965).

Butzer, J.F.; Silver, D.E. and Sahs, A.L.: Amantadine in Parkinson's disease. A double-blind, placebo-controlled, crossover study with long-term follow up. Neurology 25: 603-606 (1975).

Calne, D.B.: Clinical neuropharmacology of levodopa; in Gilliland and Peden (Eds) The Scientific Basis of

Medicine Annual Reviews, p.32-57 (Athlone Press, London 1973).

Calvey, T.N.; Williams, N.E.; Muir, K.T. and Barber, H.E.: Plasma concentrations of edrophonium in man. Clinical Pharmacology and Therapeutics 19: 813-820 (1976).

Candelise, L.; Colombo, A. and Spinnler, H.: Anti-oedema treatment of completed stroke. Lancet 1: 806 (1974).

Cantu, R.C. and Schwab, R.S.: Ceruloplasmin rise and PBI fall in serum due to diphenylhydantoin. Archives of Neurology 15: 393-396 (1966).

Carlsson, A.: The occurrence, distribution and physiological role of catecholamines in the nervous system. Pharmacological Reviews 11: 490-493 (1959).

Carter, A.B.: Prognosis of cerebral embolisms. Lancet 2: 514-519 (1965).

Carter, A.B.: Hypotensive therapy in stroke survivors. Lancet 1: 485-489 (1970).

Cartlidge, N.E.F.; Hudgson, P. and Weightman, D.: A comparison of baclofen and diazepam in the treatment of spasticity. Journal of Neurological Sciences 23: 17-24 (1974).

Cavazzuti, G.B.: Prevention of febrile convulsions with dipropylacetate (Depakine®). Epilepsia 16: 647-648 (1975).

Cawthorne, T. and Haynes, D.R.: Facial palsy. British Medical Journal 2: 1197-1200 (1956).

Celesia, G.G. and Barr, A.N.: Psychosis and other psychiatric manifestations of levodopa therapy. Archives of Neurology 23: 193-200 (1970).

Cereghino, J.J.; Brock, J.T.; Van Meter, J.C.; Penry, J.K.; Smith, L.D.; Fisher, P. and Ellenberg, J.: Evaluation of albutoin as an antiepileptic drug. Clinical Pharmacology and Therapeutics 15: 406-416 (1974).

Cereghino, J.J.; Van Meter, J.C.; Brock, J.T.; Penry, J.K.; Smith, L.D. and White, B.G.: Preliminary observations of serum carbamazepine concentration in epileptic patients. Neurology 23: 357-366 (1973).

Chadwick, D.; Reynolds, E.H. and Marsden, C.D.: Relief of action myoclonus by 5-hydroxytryptophan. Lancet 1: 111-112 (1974).

Chadwick, D.; Reynolds, E.H. and Marsden, C.D.: Anticonvulsant-induced dyskinesias: a comparison with dyskinesias induced by neuroleptics. Journal of Neurology, Neurosurgery and Psychiatry 39: 1210-1218 (1976).

Chakrabarti, A.K. and Samantaray, S.K.: Diabetic peripheral neuropathy: nerve conduction studies before, during and after carbamazepine therapy. Australian and New Zealand Journal of Medicine 6: 565-568 (1976).

Chamberlin, H.R.; Waddell, W.J. and Butler, T.J.: A study of the product of demethylation of Tridione in the control of petit mal epilepsy. Neurology 15: 449-454 (1965).

Chanarin, I.; Mollin, D.L. and Anderson, B.B.: Folic acid deficiency and the megaloblastic anaemias. Proceedings of the Royal Society of Medicine 51: 757 (1958).

Chanarin, I.; Perry, J. and Reynolds, E.H.: Transport of 5-methyltetrahydrofolic acid into the cerebrospinal fluid in man. Clinical Science and Molecular Medicine 46: 369-373 (1974).

Chandra, B.: The use of clonazepam in the treatment of tic douloureux (a preliminary report). Proceedings of the Australian Association of Neurologists 13: 119-122 (1976).

Chandra, B.: Some aspects of tuberculous meningitis in Surabaya. Proceedings of the Australian Association of Neurologists 13: 73-81 (1976).

Chang, T.; Okerholm, R.A. and Glazko, A.J.: Identification of diphenhydramine (Benadryl®) metabolites in human subjects. Research Communications in Chemical Pathology and Pharmacology 9: 391-404 (1974).

Chase, T.N.: Fusaric acid in Parkinson's disease. Neurology 26: 637-639 (1974).

Chase, T.N.; Katz, R.J. and Kopin, I.J.: Effect of anticonvulsants on brain serotonin. Transactions of the American Neurological Association 94: 236-238 (1969).

Chase, T.N.; Woods, A.C. and Glaubiger, G.A.: Parkinson disease treated with a suspected dopamine receptor agonist. Archives of Neurology 30: 383-386 (1974).

Chaube, S. and Murphy, M.L.: The teratogenic effects of 5-fluorocytosine in the rat. Cancer Research 29: 554-557 (1969).

Chen, G.; Weston, J.K. and Bratton, A.C. Jr.: Anticonvulsant activity and toxicity of phensuximide, methsuximide and ethosuximide. Epilepsia 4: 66-76 (1963).

Cherington, M.: Botulism. Ten-year experience. Archives of Neurology 30: 432-437 (1974).

Cherington, M.: Guanidine and germine in Eaton-Lambert syndrome. Neurology 26: 944-946 (1976).

Chisholm, I.A.; Bronte-Stewart, J. and Foulds, W.G.: Hydroxycobalamin versus cyanocobalmin in the treatment of tobacco amblyopia. Lancet 2: 450-451 (1967).

Choi, Y.; Thrasher, K.; Werk, E.E. Jr.; Sholiton, L.J. and Olinger, C.: Effect of diphenylhydantoin on cortisol kinetics in humans. Journal of Pharmacology and Experimental Therapeutics 176: 27-34 (1971).

Christiansen, J. and Dam, M.: Influence of phenobarbital and diphenylhydantoin on plasma carbamazepine levels in patients with epilepsy. Acta Neurologica Scandinavica 49: 543-546 (1973).

Christiansen, J. and Dam, M.: Drug interaction in epileptic patients; in Schneider, Janz, Gardner-Thorpe, Meinardi and Sherwin (Eds) Clinical Pharmacology of Antiepileptic Drugs. p.197-200 (Springer, Berlin 1975).

Christensen, L.K. and Skovsted, L.: Inhibition of drug metabolism by chloramphenicol. Lancet 2: 1397-1399 (1969).

Chung, D-K and Koenig, M.G.: Reversible cardiac enlargement during treatment with amphotericin B and hydrocortisone. Report of three cases. American Review of Respiratory Diseases 103: 831-841 (1971).

Ciesielski, L; Maitre, M.; Cash, C. and Mandel, P.: Regional distribution in brain and effect on cerebral mitochondrial respiration of the anticonvulsive drug n-dipropylacetate. Biochemical Pharmacology 24: 1055-1058 (1975).

Clark, K. and Einspruch, B.C.: Lowering of intracranial pressure with urea. Archives of Neurology 6: 414-418 (1962).

Clasen, R.A.; Cooke, P.M.; Pandolfi, S.; Carnecki, G. and Bryar, G.: Hypertonic urea in experimental cerebral edema. Archives of Neurology 12: 424-434 (1965).

Claveria, L.E.; Calne, D.B. and Allen, J.G.: 'On-off' phenomenon related to high plasma levodopa. British Medical Journal 2: 641-643 (1973).

Cohan, S.L.; Pohlmann, J.L.W.; Mikszewski, J. and O'Doherty, D.S.: The pharmacokinetics of pyridostigmine. Neurology 26: 536-539 (1976).

Cohan, S.L.; Dretchen, K.L. and Neal, A.: Malabsorption of pyridostigmine in patients with myasthenia gravis. Neurology 27: 299-301 (1977).

Cohen, B. and De Jong, J.M.B.V.: Meclizine and placebo in treating vertigo of vestibular origin. Archives of Neurology 27: 129-135 (1972).

Cohn, R.: A neuropathological study of a case of petit mal epilepsy. Electroencephalography and Clinical Neurophysiology 24: 282 (1968).

Colburn, W.A.; Sibley, C.R. and Buller, R.H.: Comparative serum prednisone and prednisolone concentrations following prednisone or prednisolone administration to beagle dogs. Journal of Pharmaceutical Sciences 65: 997-1001 (1976).

Cole, M.; Kenig, M.D. and Hewitt, V.A.: Metabolism of penicillins to penicilloic acids and 6-aminopenicillanic acid in man and its significance in assessing penicillin absorption. Antimicrobial Agents and Chemotherapy 3: 463-468 (1973).

Connard, G.J.; Haavik, C.O. and Finger, K.F.: Binding of 5,5-diphenyl-hydantoin and its major metabolite to human and rat plasma proteins. Journal of Pharmaceutical Sciences 60: 1642-1646 (1971).

Conney, A.H.: Pharmacological implications of microsomal enzyme induction. Pharmacological Review 19: 317-366 (1967).

Connors, T.A.; Cox, P.J.; Farmer, P.B.; Foster A.B. and Jarman, M.: Some studies of the active intermediates formed in the microsomal metabolism of cyclophosphamide and isophosphamide. Biochemical Pharmacology 23: 115-129 (1974).

Connolly, M.E.: Clonidine (Catapres) in hypertension; in Walker (Ed) Ninth Symposium on Advanced Medicine p.192-201 (Pitman Medical, London 1973).

Consolo, S.; Ladinsky, H.; Peri, G. and Garattini, S.: Effect of diazepam on mouse whole brain and brain area acetylcholine and choline levels. European Journal of Pharmacology 27: 266-268 (1974).

Cooper, J.R.; Bloom, F.E. and Roth, R.H.: The Biochemical Basis of Neuropharmacology, 3rd Edition (Oxford, New York 1978).

Cope, C.L.: Adrenal steroids and disease, 2nd Edition (Pitman, London 1972).

Coppen, A.; Metcalfe, M.; Carroll, J.D. and Morris, J.G.L.: Levodopa and l-tryptophan therapy in Parkinsonism. Lancet 1: 654-658 (1972).

Costa, E. and Guidotti, A.: Molecular mechanisms in the receptor action of benzodiazepines. Annual Review of Pharmacology and Toxicology 19: 531-545 (1979).

Cotter, L.M.; Eadie, M.J.; Hooper, W.D.; Lander, C.M.; Smith, G.A. and Tyrer, J.H.: The pharmacokinetics of carbamazepine. European Journal of Clinical Pharmacology 12: 451-456 (1977).

Cotzias, G.C.: Parkinsonism and dopa. Journal of Chronic Diseases 22: 279-301 (1969).

Cotzias, G.C.; Papavasiliou, P.S. and Gellene, R.: Modification of Parkinsonism — chronic treatment with L-dopa. New England Journal of Medicine 280: 337-345 (1969).

Couch, J.R.; Ziegler, D.K. and Hassanein, R.: Amitriptyline in the prophylaxis of migraine. Neurology 26: 121-127 (1976).

Couper-Smartt, J.: Lithium in spasmodic torticollis. Lancet 2: 741-742 (1973).

Court, J.E. and Kase, C.S.: Treatment of tic douloureux with a new anticonvulsant (clonazepam). Journal of Neurology, Neurosurgery, and Psychiatry 39: 297-299 (1976).

Cowan, D.A.; Huizing, G. and Beckett, A.H.: Identification of four new metabolic products of metoclopramide using mass spectrometry. Xenobiotica 6: 605-616 (1976).

Cowger, M.L. and Labbe, R.F. The inhibition of terminal oxidation by porphyrinogenic drugs. Biochemical Pharmacology 16: 2189-2199 (1967).

Coyle, J.T. and Snyder, S.H.: Antiparkinson drugs: inhibition of dopamine uptake in the corpus striatum as a possible mechanism of action. Science 166: 899-901 (1969).

Craig, C.R. and Shideman F.E.: Metabolism and anticonvulsant properties of mephobarbital and phenobarbital in rats. Journal of Pharmacology and Experimental Therapeutics 176: 35-41 (1971).

Cucinell, S.A.; Conney, A.H.; Sansur, M. and Burns, J.J.: Drug interactions in man I. Lowering effect of phenobarbital on plasma levels of bishydroxycoumarin (Dicumarol) and diphenylhydantoin (Dilantini®). Clinical Pharmacology and Therapeutics 6: 420-429 (1965).

Curci, G.; Bergamini, N.; Veneri, V.D.; Ninni, A. and Nitti, V.: Half-life of rifampicin after repeated administration of different doses in humans. Chemotherapy 17: 373-381 (1972).

Curran, D.A.; Hinterberger, H. and Lance J.W.: Total plasma serotonin, 5-hydroxyindoleacetic acid and p-hydroxy-m-methoxymandelic acid excretion in normal and migrainous subjects. Brain 88: 997-1010 (1965).

Curry, S.H.: Action and metabolism of chlorpromazine; in Davies and Prichard (Eds) Biological Effects of Drugs in Relation to their Plasma Concentrations, p.201-210 (Macmillan, London 1973).

Curry, S.H.; Davis, J.M.; Janowsky, D.S. and Marshall, J.H.L.: Factors affecting chlorpromazine plasma levels in psychiatric patients. Archives of General Psychiatry 22: 209-215 (1970b).

Curry, S.H.; D'Mello, A. and Mould, G.P.: Destruction of chlorpromazine during absorption by rat intestine in vitro. British Journal of Pharmacology 40: 538-539 (1970a).

Curtis, D.R.; Game, C.J.A.; Johnston, G.A.R. and McCulloch, R.M.: Central effects of β-(p-chlorophenyl)-γ-aminobutyric acid. Brain Research 70: 493-499 (1974).

Curzon, G.: Involuntary movements other than Parkinsonism: biochemical aspects. Proceedings of the Royal Society of Medicine 66: 873-876 (1973).

Curzon, G.; Barrie, M. and Wilkinson, M.I.P.: Relationships between headache and amine changes after administration of reserpine to migrainous patients. Journal of Neurology, Neurosurgery and Psychiatry 32: 555-561 (1969).

Curzon, G.; Friedel, J.; Grier, L.; Marsden, C.D.; Parkes, J.D.; Shipley, M. and Zilkha, K.J.: Sustained-released levodopa in Parkinsonism. Lancet 1: 781 (1973).

Cutler, R.E.; Gyselynck, A.M.; Fleet, W.P. and Forrey, A.W.; Correlation of serum creatinine concentration and gentamycin half-life. Journal of the American Medical Association 219: 1037-1041 (1972).

Dalton, C.; Crowley, H.J.; Sheppard, H. and Schallek, W.: Regional cyclic nucleotide phosphodiesterase activity in cat central nervous system: effects of benzodiazepine (37820). Proceedings of the Society for Experimental Biology and Medicine New York 145: 407-410 (1974).

Dam, M.: The density and ultrastructure of the Purkinje cells following diphenylhydantoin treatment in animals and man. Acta Neurologica Scandinavica 49 (Suppl.): 1-65 (1972).

Daniel, P.M.; Moorhouse, S.R. and Pratt, O.E.: Do changes in blood levels of other aromatic aminoacids influence levodopa therapy? Lancet 1: 95 (1976).

Danks, D.M.; Barry, J.E. and Sheffield, L.J.: Digital hypoplasia and anticonvulsants during pregnancy. Journal of Pediatrics 85: 877 (1974).

Dasberg, H.H.; van der Kleijn, E.; Guelen, P.J.R. and van Praag, H.M.: Plasma concentrations of diazepam and of its metabolite N-desmethyl-diazepam in relation to anxiolytic effect. Clinical Pharmacology and Therapeutics 15: 473-483 (1974).

Davies, J.E.; Edmundson, W.F.; Carter, C.H. and Barquet, A.: Effect of anticonvulsant drugs on dicophane (D.D.T.) residues in man. Lancet 2: 7-9 (1969).

Davis, J.P. and Lennox, W.G.: A comparison of paradione and tridione in the treatment of epilepsy. Journal of Pediatrics 34: 273-278 (1949).

Davis, R.E. and Woodliff, H.J.: Folic acid deficiency in patients receiving anticonvulsant drugs. Medical Journal of Australia 2: 1070-1072 (1971).

Davis, R.R. and Reeves, D.S.: 5-Fluorocytosine and urinary candidiasis. British Medical Journal 1: 577-579 (1971).

Davison, C. and Smith, P.K.: The binding of salicylic acid and related substances to purified proteins. Journal of Pharmacology and Experimental Therapeutics 133: 161-170 (1961).

Dawborn, J.K.; Page, M.D. and Schiavone, D.J.: Use of 5-fluorocytosine in patients with impaired renal function. British Medical Journal 4: 382-384 (1973).

Day, R.O.; Paull, P.D.; Champion, G.D. and Graham, G.G.: Evaluation of an enteric coated aspirin preparation. Australian and New Zealand Journal of Medicine 6: 45-50 (1976).

Dayton, P.G.; Sicam, L.E.; Landrau, M. and Burns, J.J.: Metabolism of sulfinpyrazone (Anturane) and other thio-analogues of phenylbutazone in man. Journal of Pharmacology and Experimental Therapeutics 132: 287-290 (1961).

Decker, D.A. Jr. and Fincham, R.W.: Respiratory arrest in myasthenia gravis with colistimethate therapy. Archives of Neurology 23: 141-144 (1971).

De Lean, J.; Richardson, J.C. and Hornykiewicz, O.: Beneficial effects of serotonin precursors in postanoxic action myoclonus. Neurology 26: 863-868 (1976).

De Louvois, J.; Gortvai, P. and Hurley, R.: Bacteriology of abscesses of the central nervous system: a multicentre prospective study. British Medical Journal 2: 981-984 (1977a).

De Louvois, J.; Gortvai, P. and Hurley, R.: Antibiotic treatment of abscesses of the central nervous system. British Medical Journal 2: 985-987 (1977b).

Demoen, P.J.A.W.: Properties and analysis of haloperidol and its dosage forms. Journal of Pharmaceutical Sciences 50: 350-353 (1961).

Dencker, H.; Dencker, S.J.; Green, A. and Nagy, A.: Intestinal absorption, demethylation and enterohepatic circulation of imipramine. Clinical Pharmacology and Therapeutics 19: 584-586 (1976).

De Negri, M. and Lamedica, G.M.: ACTH therapy in infantile epilepsy. Paper presented to the European Study Group on Child Neurology, Kungah, cited by Brown, J.K.: Fits in childhood; in Laidlaw and Richens (Eds) A Textbook of Epilepsy, p.56-108 (Churchill-Livingstone, Edinburgh 1973).

Denny-Brown, D.: The Basal Ganglia and their Relation to Disorders of Movement (Oxford University Press, London 1962).

Dent, C.E.; Richens, A.; Rowe, D.J.F. and Stamp, T.C.B.: Osteomalacia with long-term anticonvulsant therapy in epilepsy. British Medical Journal 4: 69-72 (1970).

De Silva, J.A.F.; Koechlin, B.A. and Bader, G.: Blood level distribution patterns of diazepam and its major metabolite in man. Journal of Pharmaceutical Sciences 55: 692-702 (1966).

Diamond, S. and Levy, L.: Metabolic studies on a new anti-epileptic drug, Riker 594. Current Therapeutic Research 5: 325-330 (1963).

Diaz, P.M.: Interaction of pentylenetetrazole and trimethadione on the metabolism of serotonin in brain and its relation to the anticonvulsant action of trimethadione. Neuropharmacology 13: 615-621 (1974).

Dill, W.A.; Kazenko, A.; Wolf, L.M. and Glazko, A.J.: Studies on 5,5'-diphenylhydantoin (dilantin) in animals and man. Journal of Pharmacology and Experimental Therapeutics 118: 270-279 (1956).

Dill, W.A.; Peterson, L.; Chang, T. and Glazko, A.J.: Physiologic disposition of α-methyl-α-ethyl succinimide (ethosuximide; Zarontin®) in animals and man. American Chemical Society Abstracts 149th Annual Meeting, p30N (1965).

Dinovo, E.C.; Gottschalk, L.A.; Nandi, B.R. and Geddes, P.C.: GLC analysis of thioridazine, mesoridazine, and their metabolites. Journal of Pharmaceutical Sciences 65: 667-669 (1976).

Di Salle, E.; Pacifici, G.M. and Morselli, P.L.: Studies on plasma protein binding of carbamazepine. Pharmacology Research Communication 6: 193-202 (1974).

Dittert, L.W.; Griffin, W.O.; La Piana, J.C.; Shainfeld, F.J. and Doluisio, J.T.: Pharmacokinetic interpretation of penicillin levels in serum and urine after intravenous administration. Antimicrobial Agents and Chemotherapy 9: 42-48 (1969).

Dobkin, B.H.: Dexamethasone dosage suggested every 3-4 days in myasthenia gravis. Neurology 27: 202 (1977).

Dollery, C.T.; Davies, D.S.; Draffan, G.H.; Dargie, H.J.; Dean, C.R.; Reid, J.L.; Clare, R.A. and Murray, S.: Clinical pharmacology and pharmacokinetics of clonidine. Clinical Pharmacology and Therapeutics 19: 11-17 (1976).

Domek, N.S.; Barlow, C.F. and Roth, L.J.: An ontogenic study of phenobarbital-C[14] in cat brain. Journal of Pharmacology and Experimental Therapeutics 130: 285-293 (1960).

Dougan, D.; Wade, D. and Mearrick, P.: Effects of L-dopa metabolites at a dopamine receptor suggest a basis for 'on-off' effect in Parkinson's disease. Nature 254: 70-72 (1975).

Drachman, D.A.; Paterson, P.Y.; Schmidt, R.T. and Spehlmann, R.F.: Cyclophosphamide in exacerbations of multiple sclerosis. Therapeutic trial and a strategy for pilot drug studies. Journal of Neurology, Neurosurgery, and Psychiatry 38: 592-597 (1975).

Drachman, D.B.; Kao, I.; Pestronk, A. and Toyka, K.V.: Myasthenia gravis as a receptor disorder. Annals of the New York Academy of Sciences 274: 226-234 (1976).

Drachman, D.A., and Skom, J.H.: Procainamide — a hazard in myasthenia gravis. Archives of Neurology 13: 316-320 (1965).

Dreyfuss, J.; Bigger, J.T. Jr.; Cohen, A.I. and Schreiber, E.C.: Metabolism of procainamide in rhesus monkey and man. Clinical Pharmacology and Therapeutics 13: 366-371 (1972).

Dring, L.G.; Smith, R.L. and Williams, R.T.: The metabolic fate of amphetamine in man and other species. Biochemical Journal 116: 425-435 (1970).

Duby, S.E.; Cotzias, G.C.; Papavasiliou, P.S. and Lawrence, W.H.: Injected apomorphine and orally administered levodopa in Parkinsonism. Archives of Neurology 27: 474-480 (1972).

Dudley, K.H.; Bius, D.L. and Butler, T.C.: Metabolic fates of 3-ethyl-5-phenylhydantoin (ethotoin, peganone), 3-methyl-5-phenylhydantoin and 5-phenylhydantoin. Journal of Pharmacology and Experimental Therapeutics 175: 27-37 (1970).

Dudley, K.H.; Bius, D.L. and Waldrop, C.D.: Urinary metabolites of N-methyl-α-methyl-α-phenylsuccinimide (methsuximide) in the dog. Drug Metabolism and Disposition 2: 113-122 (1974).

Duggan, D.E.; Yeh, K.C.; Matalia, N.; Ditzler, C.A. and McMahon, F.G.: Bioavailability of oral dexamethasone. Clinical Pharmacology and Therapeutics 18: 205-209 (1975).

Duhm, B.; Maul, W.; Medenwald, H.; Patzchke, K. and Wegner, L-A.: Tierexperimentelle untersuchungen mit ³⁵S-markiertem N-(4'-sulfamylphenyl)-butansultam-(1,4). Zietschrift fur Natur-
forschung 18: 475-492 (1963).

Dume, T., Wagner, C. and Wetzels, E.: Zur Pharmakokinetic von Ethambutol bei Gesunden und
Patienten mit erminaler Niereninsuffizienz. Deutsche Medizinische Wochenschrift 96: 1430-1434
(1971).

Dunlop, D.: The therapeutics of migraine; in Smith (Ed) Background to Migraine, p.72-85 (Heinemann,
London 1969).

Dupont, E.; Hansen, H.J. and Dalby, M.A.: Treatment of benign essential tremor with propranolol. Acta
Neurologica Scandinavica 49: 75-84 (1973).

Duvoisin, R.C.; Lobo-Antunes, J. and Yahr, M.D.: Response of patients with postencephalitic Parkinsonism to levodopa. Journal of Neurology, Neurosurgery and Psychiatry 35: 487-495 (1972).

Dykes, M.H.M.: Evaluation of a muscle relaxant Dantrolene sodium (Dantrium). Journal of the
American Medical Association 231: 862-864 (1975).

Eadie, M.J.: The use of ergotamine in migraine. Medical Journal of Australia 2 (Suppl.): 26-29 (1972).

Eadie, M.J.: Plasma level monitoring of anticonvulsants. Clinical Pharmacokinetics 1: 52-66 (1976).

Eadie, M.J. and Ferrier, T.M.: Chloroquine myopathy. Journal of Neurology, Neurosurgery and Psychiatry 29: 331-337 (1966).

Eadie, M.J.; Lander, C.M.; Hooper, W.D. and Tyrer, J.H.: The effect of phenobarbitone dose on plasma
phenobarbitone levels in epileptic patients. Proceedings of the Australian Association of Neurologists 13: 89-96 (1976).

Eadie, M.J.; Lander, C.M.; Hooper, W.D. and Tyrer, J.H.: Factors influencing plasma phenobarbitone
levels in epileptic patients. British Journal of Clinical Pharmacology 4: 541-547 (1977).

Eadie, M.J. and Sutherland, J.M.: Arteriosclerosis in Parkinsonism. Journal of Neurology, Neurosurgery
and Psychiatry 27: 237-240 (1964).

Eadie, M.J. and Tyrer, J.H.: Anticonvulsant Therapy. Pharmacological Basis and Practice 2nd ed.
(Churchill-Livingstone, Edinburgh 1980).

Eadie, M.J.; Tyrer, J.H.; Bochner, F. and Hooper, W.D.: The elimination of phenytoin in man. Clinical
and Experimental Pharmacology and Physiology 3: 217-224 (1976).

Eadie, M.J.; Tyrer, J.H. and Hooper, W.D.: Diphenylhydantoin dosage. Proceedings of the Australian
Association of Neurologists 10: 53-59 (1973).

Eadie, M.J.; Tyrer, J.H.; Smith, G.A. and McKauge, L.: Pharmacokinetics of drugs used for petit mal absence epilepsy. Tyrer and Eadie (Eds) Proceedings of the Australian Association of Neurologists 14:
172-183 (Adis Press, New York 1977).

Eccles, J.C.: Physiology of Synapses (Academic Press, New York 1964).

Edelman, I.S.: Mechanism of action of steroid hormones. Journal of Steroid Biochemistry 6: 147-159
(1975).

Edwards, V.E.: Side effects of clonazepam therapy. Proceedings of the Australian Association of Neurologists 11: 199-202 (1974).

Edwards, V.E. and Eadie, M.J.: Clonazepam — a clinical study of its effectiveness as an anticonvulsant.
Proceedings of the Australian Association of Neurologists 10:61-66 (1973).

Ehrnebo, M.; Agurell, S.; Jalling, B. and Boreus, L.O.: Age differences in drug binding by plasma proteins: studies on human foetuses, neonates and adults. European Journal of Clinical Pharmacology
3: 189-193 (1971).

Eichelbaum, M.; Ekbom, K.; Bertilsson, L.; Ringberger, V.A. and Rane, A.: Plasma pharmacokinetics of
carbamazepine and its epoxide metabolite in man after single and multiple doses. European Journal
of Clinical Pharmacology 8: 337-341 (1975).

Eidelberg, E.; Neer, H.M. and Miller, M.K.: Anticonvulsant properties of some benzodiazepine derivatives. Possible use against psychomotor seizures. Neurology 15: 223-230 (1965).

Ehringer, H. and Hornykiewicz, O.: Verteilung von Noradrenalin und Dopamin (3-Hydroxytryptamin) im Gehirn des Menschen und ihr Verhalten bei Erkrankungen des extrapyramidalen Systems. Klinische Wochenschrift 38: 1236-1239 (1960).

Eisenberg, H.M.; Barlow, C.F. and Lorenzo, A.V.: Effect of dexamethasone on altered brain vascular permeability. Archives of Neurology 23: 18-22 (1970).

Ekbom, K.A.: Ergotamine tartrate orally in Horton's 'histaminic cephalgia' a new method of treatment. Acta Psychiatrica et Neurologica Scandinavica 46 (Suppl.): 105-113 (1947).

Ekbom, K.A.: Restless legs syndrome after partial gastrectomy. Acta Neurologica Scandinavica 42: 79-89 (1966).

Ekbom, K.: Carbamazepine in the treatment of tabetic lightning pains. Archives of Neurology 26: 374-378 (1972).

Ekbom, K.: Lithium in the treatment of chronic cluster headache. Headache 17: 39-40 (1977).

Ekbom, K.A. and Westerberg, C.E.: Carbamazepine in glossopharyngeal neuralgia. Archives of Neurology 14: 595-596 (1966).

Eldridge, R; Kanter, W. and Koerber, T.: Levodopa in dystonia. Lancet 2: 1027-1028 (1973).

Elion, G.B.: Significance of azathioprine metabolites. Proceedings of the Royal Society of Medicine 65: 257-260 (1972).

Ellard, G.A.: Variations between individuals and populations in the acetylation of isoniazid and its significance for the treatment of pulmonary tuberculosis. Clinical Pharmacology and Therapeutics 19: 610-625 (1976).

Ellard, G.A. and Gammon, P.T.: Pharmacokinetics of isoniazid metabolism in man. Journal of Pharmacokinetics and Biopharmaceutics 4: 83-113 (1976).

Ellis, K.O.; Butterfield, J.L.; Wessels, F.L. and Carpenter, J.F.: A comparison of skeletal, cardiac, and smooth muscle actions of dantrolene sodium — a skeletal muscle relaxant. Archives Internationales de Pharmacodynamie et de Therapie 224: 118-132 (1976).

Ellis, K.O. and Carpenter, J.F.: Mechanism of control of skeletal-muscle contraction by dantrolene sodium. Archives of Physical Medicine and Rehabilitation 55: 373-383 (1974).

Ellison, T.; Snyder, A.; Bolger, J. and Okun, R.: Metabolism of orphenadrine citrate in man. Journal of Pharmacology and Experimental Therapeutics 176: 284-295 (1971).

Elmquist, D.; Hofman, W.W.; Kugelberg, J. and Quastel, D.M.L.: An electrophysiological investigation of neuromuscular transmission in myasthenia gravis. Journal of Physiology 174: 417-434 (1964).

Engel, J.; Granerus, A.K. and Svanborg, A.: Piribedil in Parkinson's syndrome: a clinical study. European Journal of Clinical Pharmacology 8: 223-226 (1975).

Enger, E. and Boyesen, S.: Long-term Anticoagulant Therapy in Patients with Cerebral Infarction (Scandinavian University Books, 1966).

English, J.; Chakraborty, J.; Marks, V.; Trigger, D.J. and Thomson, A.G.: Prednisolone levels in the plasma and urine: a study of two preparations in man. British Journal of Clinical Pharmacology 2: 327-332 (1975).

Enmeads, J.; Hachinski, V.C. and Norris, J.W.: Ergotamine and the cerebral circulation. Hemicrania 7 (4): 6-10 (1976).

Ericsson, A.D.; McCann, D.; Sharpless, N. and Reveno, W.: Metabolic and clinical assessment of L-dopa in Parkinsonism. Neurology 20: 402 (1970).

Ericsson, A.L.: Potentiation of the l-Dopa effect in man by the use of catechol-O-methyltransferase inhibitors. Journal of Neurological Sciences 14: 193-197 (1971).

Erkkola, R. and Kanto, J.: Diazepam and breast feeding. Lancet 1: 1235-1236 (1972).

Escueta, A.V. and Appel, S.H.: Diphenylhydantoin and potassium transport in isolated nerve terminals. Journal of Clinical Investigation 50: 1977-1984 (1971).

Escueta, A.V. and Appel, S.H.: Brain synapses. An in vitro model for the study of seizures. Annals of Internal Medicine 129: 333-344 (1972).

Esplin, D.W.: Effect of diphenylhydantoin on synaptic transmission in cat spinal cord and stellate ganglion. Journal of Pharmacology and Experimental Therapeutics 120: 301-323 (1957).

Estes, J.W.; Pelikan, E.W. and Kruger-Thiemer, E.: A retrospective study of the pharmacokinetics of heparin. Clinical Pharmacology and Therapeutics 10: 329-337 (1969).

Eymard, P.; Simiand, J.; Tedule, R.; Polverelli, M.; Werbenec, J-P. and Brou, M.: Etude de la repartition et de la resorption du dipropylacetate de sodium marque au ^{14}C chez le rat. Journal of Pharmacology 2: 359-386 (1971).

Faero, O.; Kastrup, K.W.; Lykkegaard Nielsen, E.; Melchior, J.C. and Thorn, I.: Successful prophylaxis of febrile convulsions with phenobarbital. Epilepsia 13: 279-285 (1972).

Fahn, S. 'On-off' phenomenon with levodopa therapy in Parkinsonism. Clinical and pharmacologic correlations and the effect of intramuscular pyridoxine. Neurology 24: 431-441 (1974).

Fahn, S. and Isgreen, W.P.: Long-term evaluation of amantadine and levodopa combination in parkinsonism by double-blind crossover analysis. Neurology 25: 695-700 (1975).

Faigle, J.W.; Brechbuhler, S.; Feldmann, K.R. and Richter, W.J.: The biotransformation of carbamazepine; in Birkmayer (Ed) International Symposium on Epileptic Seizures — Behaviour — Pains, p.127-140 (Huber, Berne 1975).

Faigle, J.W. and Keberle, H.: The metabolism and pharmacokinetics of Lioresal; in Spasticity — a Topical Survey, p.94-100 (Huber, Berne 1973).

Falconer, M.A.: Place of vestibular nerve section in Meniere's disease. British Medical Journal 1: 269-273 (1965).

Fanchamps, A.: Pharmacodynamic principles of anti-migraine therapy. Headache 15: 79-90 (1975).

Fearnley, M.E.; Rainer, E.H.; Taverner, D.; Boyle, T. McM. and Miles, D.W.: Cervical sympathetic block in treatment of Bell's palsy. A controlled trial. Lancet 2: 725-727 (1964).

Fedrick, J.: Epilepsy and pregnancy: a report from the Oxford record linkage study. British Medical Journal 2: 442-448 (1973).

Fehr, H.U. and Bein, H.J.: Sites of action of a new muscle relaxant (baclofen, Lioresal, Ciba 34 647 — Ba). Journal of International Medical Research 2: 36-47 (1974).

Fennessy, M.R. and Lee, J.R.: The effect of benzodiazepines on brain amines of the mouse. Archives of Internal Pharmacodynamics 197: 37-44 (1972).

Ferngren, H. and Paalzow, L.: High frequency electro-shock seizures and their antagonism during postnatal development in the mouse. II. Effects of phenobarbital, sodium methobarbital, trimethadione, dimethadione, ethosuximide and acetazolamide. Acta Pharmacologica et Toxicologica 28: 477-483 (1969).

Fichman, M.P.; Kleeman, C.R. and Bethune, J.E.: Inhibition of antidiuretic hormone secretion by diphenylhydantoin. Archives of Neurology 22: 45-53 (1970).

Finucane, J.F. and Griffiths, R.S.: Effect of phenytoin therapy on thyroid function. British Journal of Clinical Pharmacology 3: 1041-1044 (1976).

Firemark, H.; Barlow, C.F. and Roth, L.J.: The entry, accumulation and binding of diphenylhydantoin-2-C^{14} in brain. Studies on adult, immature and hypercapnic cats. International Journal of Neuropharmacology 2: 25-38 (1963).

Firemark, H.M.; McIntyre, H.B.; Bodner, L.; Cho, A. and Jenden, D.: Amphetamine metabolism in hyperactive children. Neurology 27: 400 (1977).

Fischer, P.A.; Schneider, E.; Jacobi, P. and Maxion, H.: Effect of melanocyte-stimulating hormone-release inhibiting factor (MIF) in Parkinson's syndrome. European Neurology 12: 360-368 (1974).

Fishman, R.A.: Blood-brain and CSF barriers to penicillin and related organic acids. Archives of Neurology 15: 113-124 (1966).

Fleming, H.A. and Bailey, S.M.: Mitral valve disease, systemic embolism and anticoagulants. Postgraduate Medical Journal 47: 599-604 (1971).

Formby, B.: The in vivo and in vitro effect of diphenylhydantoin and phenobarbitone on K$^+$-activated phosphorohydrolase and (Na$^+$, K$^+$)-activated ATPase in particulate membrane fractions from rat brain. Journal of Pharmacy and Pharmacology 22: 81-85 (1970).

Forsman, A.; Martensson, E.; Nyberg, G. and Ohman, R.: A gas chromatographic method for determining haloperidol. A sensitive procedure for studying serum concentration and pharmacokinetics of haloperidol in patients. Naunyn-Schmiedeberg's Archives of Pharmacology 286: 113-124 (1974).

Forsmann, A. and Ohman, R.: On the pharmacokinetics of haloperidol. Nordisk Psykiatrisk Tidsskrift 28: 441-448 (1974).

Foster, L.B. and Frings, C.S.: Determination of diazepam (Valium) concentrations in serum by gas-liquid chromatography. Clinical Chemistry 16: 177-179 (1970).

Foulds, W.S.; Cant, J.S.; Chisholm, I.A.; Bronte-Stewart, J. and Wilson, J.: Hydroxycobalamin in the treatment of Leber's hereditary optic atrophy. Lancet 1: 896-897 (1968).

Fozard, J.R.: The animal pharmacology of drugs in the treatment of migraine; in Saxena (Ed) Migraine and Related Headaches, p.93-118 (Sandoz, Uden 1975).

Francini, F.; Santana, J.S. and Kitrosen, J.: La ciproeptadina, un antiistaminico e antiserotoninico con azione sul peso corporeo; rapporto preliminare. Minerva Medica 59: 3079-3082 (1968).

Frantzen, E.; Hansen, J.M.; Hansen, O.E. and Kristensen, M.: Phenytoin (Dilantin) intoxication. Acta Neurologica Scandinavica 43: 440-446 (1967).

French, J.H.; Grueter, B.B.; Druckman, R. and O'Brien, D.: Pyridoxine and infantile myoclonic seizures. Neurology 15: 101-113 (1965).

Frenkel, M.: Treatment of myasthenia gravis by ovulatory suppression. Archives of Neurology 11: 613-617 (1964).

Frey, H.H. and Hahn, I.: Untersuchungen uber die Bedeutung des durch Biotransformation gebildeten Phenobarbital fur die anticonvulsive Wirkung von Primidon. Archives of International Pharmocodynamics 128: 281-290 (1960).

Frey, H.H. and Schulz, R.: Time course of the demethylation of trimethadione. Acta Pharmacologica et Toxicologica 28: 477-483 (1970).

Frigerio, A.; Sossi, N.; Belvedere, G.; Pantarotto, C. and Garattini, S.: Identification of desmethylcyproheptadine-10, 11-epoxide and other cyproheptadine metabolites isolated from rat urine. Journal of Pharmaceutical Science 63: 1536-1540 (1974).

Frislid, K.; Berg, M.; Hansteen, V. and Lunde, P.K.M.: Comparison of the acetylation of procainamide and sulfadimidine in man. European Journal of Clinical Pharmacology 9: 433-438 (1976).

Fromm, G.H. and Killian, J.M.: Effect of some anticonvulsant drugs on the spinal trigeminal nucleus. Neurology 17: 275-280 (1966).

Fromm, G.H. and Landgren, S.: Effect of diphenylhydantoin on single cells in the spinal trigeminal nucleus. Neurology 13: 34-37 (1963).

Furesz, S.; Scotti, R.; Pallanza, R. and Mapelli, E.: Rifampicin: a new rifamycin. III Absorption, distribution and elimination in man. Arzneimittel-Forschung 17: 534-537 (1967).

Galbraith, A.W.: Treatment of acute herpes zoster with amantadine hydrochloride (Symmetrel). British Medical Journal 4: 493-495 (1973).

Galeazzi, R.L.; Benet, L.Z. and Sheiner, L.B.: Relationship between the pharmacokinetics and pharmacodynamics of procainamide. Clinical Pharmacology and Therapeutics 20: 278-289 (1976).

Gallagher, B.B. and Baumel, I.P.: Primidone. Absorption, distribution and excretion; in Woodbury, Penry and Schmidt (Eds) Anti-epileptic Drugs, p.357-359 (Raven Press, New York 1972).

Gallagher, B.B.; Smith, D.B. and Mattson, R.H.: The relationship of the anticonvulsant properties of primidone to phenobarbital. Epilepsia 11: 293-301 (1970).

Gamble, J.A.S.; MacKay, J.S. and Dundee, J.W.: Plasma levels of diazepam. British Journal of Anaesthesia 45: 1085 (1973).

Gamboa, E.T.; Isaacs, G. and Harter, D.H.: Chorea associated with oral contraceptive therapy. Archives of Neurology 25: 112-114 (1971).

Gardner, W.J. and Sava, G.A.: Hemifacial spasm: a reversible pathophysiologic state. Journal of Neurosurgery 19: 240-247 (1962).

Garfinkel, P.E.; Warsh, J.J.; Stancer, H.C.; Godse, D.D.; Brown, G.M. and Vranic, M.: The effect of a peripheral decarboxylase inhibitor (carbidopa) on monoamine and neuroendocrine function in man. Neurology 27: 443-447 (1977).

Garrettson, L.K. and Dayton, P.G.: Disappearance of phenobarbital and diphenylhydantoin from serum of children. Clinical Pharmacology and Therapeutics 11: 674-679 (1970).

Gastaut, H.: Clinical and electroencephalographical classification of epileptic seizures. Epilepsia 10 [Suppl. 2] (1969).

Gaudette, L.E. and Coatney, G.R.: A possible mechanism of prolonged antimalarial activity. American Journal of Tropical Medicine and Hygiene 10: 321-326 (1961).

Geets, W. and Pinon, A.: L'action metabolique et anti epileptique de l'Ospolot. Acta Neurologica et Psychiatrica Belgica 71: 164-172 (1971).

Gelber, R.; Jacobsen, P. and Levy, L.: A study of the availability of six commercial formulations of isoniazid. Clinical Pharmacology and Therapeutics 10: 841-848 (1969).

Gelber, R.; Peters, J.H.; Gordon, G.R.; Glazko, A.J. and Levy, L.: The polymorphic acetylation of dapsone in man. Clinical Pharmacology and Therapeutics 12: 225-238 (1971).

Gelenberg, A.J. and Poskanzer, D.C.: The effect of dantrolene sodium on spasticity in multiple sclerosis. Neurology 23: 1313-1315 (1973).

Gerardin, A.P.; Abadie, F.V.; Camperstrini, J.A. and Theobald, W.: Pharmacokinetics of carbamazepine in normal humans after single and repeated oral doses. Journal of Pharmacokinetics and Biopharmaceutics 4: 521-535 (1976).

Gerardin, A. and Hirtz, J.: The quantitative assay of carbamazepine in biological material and its application to basic pharmacokinetic studies; in Birkmayer (Ed) Epileptic Seizures — Behaviour — Pain, p.151-164 (Huber, Berne 1975).

Gerber, N. and Wagner, J.G.: Explanation of the dose-dependent decline of diphenylhydantoin plasma levels by fitting to the integrated form of the Michaelis-Menten equation. Research Communications in Chemical Pathology and Pharmacology 3: 455-466 (1972).

Gerlach, J.: Effect of CB J 54 (2-bromo-alpha-ergocryptine) on paralysis agitans compared with Madopar in a double-blind, cross-over trial. Acta Neurologica Scandinavica 53: 189-200 (1976).

German, J.; Kowal, A. and Ehlers, K.H.: Trimethadione and human teratogenesis. Teratology 3: 349-362 (1970).

Giardina, E-G.V.; Dreyfuss, J.; Bigger, J.T.; Shaw, J.M. and Schreiber, E.C.: Metabolism of procainamide in normal and cardiac subjects. Clinical Pharmacology and Therapeutics 19: 339-351 (1976).

Gibaldi, M. and Grundhofer, B.: Bioavailability of aspirin from commercial suppositories. Journal of Pharmaceutical Sciences 64: 1064-1066 (1975).

Gibaldi, M. and Perrier, D.: Pharmacokinetics (Marcel Dekker Inc., New York 1975).

Gibberd, F.B. and Small, E.: Interaction between levodopa and methyldopa. British Medical Journal 2: 90-91 (1973).

Gilbert, G.J.: Haloperidol in spasmodic torticollis. Lancet 2: 234-235 (1972a).

Gilbert, G.J.: The medical treatment of spasmodic torticollis. Archives of Neurology 27: 503-506 (1972b).

Gilbert, J.C. and Goldberg, L.I.: Characterization by cyproheptadine of the dopamine-induced contraction in canine isolated arteries. Journal of Pharmacology and Experimental Therapeutics 193: 435-442 (1975).

Gilbert, J.C.; Scott, A.K.; Galloway, D.B. and Petrie, J.C.: Ethosuximide: liver enzyme induction and D-glucaric acid excretion. British Journal of Clinical Pharmacology 1: 249-252 (1974).

Gilligan, B. and Hancock, R.: Enteric coated 1-Dopa (Prodopa). A new approach to 1-Dopa therapy in Parkinson's disease. Medical Journal of Australia 2: 824-826 (1975).

Giuditta, A.: The inhibition of a brain diaphorase by some hypnotics and nervous depressants. Journal of Neurochemistry 9: 329-334 (1962).

Glazko, A.J.: Antiepileptic drugs: biotransformation, metabolism and serum half-life. Epilepsia 16: 367-391 (1975).

Glazko, A.J.; Chang, T.; Baukema, J.; Dill, W.A.; Goulet, J.R. and Buchanan, R.A.: Metabolic disposition of diphenylhydantoin in normal human subjects following intravenous administration. Clinical Pharmacology and Therapeutics 10: 498-504 (1969).

Glazko, A.J. and Dill, W.A.: Other succinimides. Methsuximide and phensuximide; in Woodbury, Penry and Schmidt (Eds) Antiepileptic Drugs, p.455-464 (Raven Press, New York 1972).

Glazko, A.J.; Dill, W.A.; Young, R.M.; Smith, T.C. and Ogilvie, R.I.: Metabolic disposition of diphenhydramine. Clinical Pharmacology and Therapeutics 16: 1066-1076 (1974).

Glazko, A.J.; Kinkel, A.W.; Alegnani, W.C. and Holmes, E.L.: An evaluation of the absorption characteristics of different chloramphenicol preparations in normal human subjects. Clinical Pharmacology and Therapeutics 9: 472-483 (1968).

Glover, D. and Labadie, E.L.: Physiopathogenesis of subdural hematomas. Part 2. Inhibition of growth of experimental hematomas with dexamethasone. Journal of Neurosurgery 45: 393-397 (1976).

Glukov, B.N.; Jerusalimsky, A.P.; Canter, V.M. and Salganik, R.I.: Ribonuclease treatment of tick-borne encephalitis. Archives of Neurology 33: 596-603 (1976).

Godin, Y.; Heiner, L.; Mark, J. and Mandel, P.: Effects of di-n-propylacetate, an anticonvulsive compound, on GABA metabolism. Journal of Neurochemistry 16: 869-873 (1969).

Godwin-Austen, R.B.; Frears, C.C.; Bergmann, S.; Parkes, J.D. and Knill-Jones, R.P.: Combined treatment of Parkinsonism with l-Dopa and amantadine. Lancet 1: 383-385 (1970).

Godwin-Austen, R.B.; Kantamaneni, B.D. and Curzon, G.: Comparison of benefit from l-dopa in Parkinsonism with increase of amine metabolites in the C.S.F. Journal of Neurology, Neurosurgery and Psychiatry 34: 219-223 (1971).

Goldbaum, L.R. and Smith, P.K.: The interaction of barbiturates with serum albumin and its possible relation to their disposition and pharmacological actions. Journal of Pharmacology and Experimental Therapeutics 111: 197-209 (1954).

Goldberg, M.A.; Barlow, C.F. and Roth, L.J.: The effect of carbon dioxide on the entry and accumulation of drugs in the central nervous system. Journal of Pharmacology and Experimental Therapeutics 131: 308-318 (1961).

Goldberg, M.A. and Dorman, J.D.: Intention myoclonus: successful treatment with clonazepam. Neurology 26: 24-26 (1976).

Goldstein, A.; Aranow, L. and Kalman, S.M.: Principles of Drug Action (Wiley & Sons, New York 1974).

Gomersall, J.D. and Stuart, A.: Amitriptyline in migraine prophylaxis. Changes in pattern of attacks during a controlled clinical trial. Journal of Neurology, Neurosurgery, and Psychiatry 36: 684-690 (1973).

Goodall, J.A.D.; Kosmidis, J.C. and Geddes, A.M.: Effect of corticosteroids on course of Guillain-Barre syndrome. Lancet 1: 524-526 (1974).

Goodman, L.S. and Gilman, A.: The Pharmacological Basis of Therapeutics, 5th Edition (Macmillan, New York 1975).

Goodwin, F.K.; Murphy, D.L.; Brodie, H.K.H. and Bunney, W.E.: Levodopa. Alterations in behaviour. Clinical Pharmacology and Therapeutics 12: 383-396 (1971).

Graham, G. and Rowland, M.: Application of salivary salicylate data to biopharmaceutical studies of salicylates. Journal of Pharmaceutical Sciences 61: 1219-1222 (1972).

Gram, L.F. and Christiansen, J.: First-pass metabolism of imipramine in man. Clinical Pharmacology and Therapeutics 17: 555-563 (1975).

Gram, L.F. and Overo, K.F.: First-pass metabolism of nortriptyline in man. Clinical Pharmacology and Therapeutics 18: 305-314 (1975).

Green, J.R.; Troupin, A.S.; Halpern, L.M.; Friel, P. and Kanarek, P.: Sulthiame: evaluation as an anticonvulsant. Epilepsia 15: 329-349 (1974).

Green, L.N.: Dexamethasone in the management of symptoms due to herniated lumbar disc. Journal of Neurology, Neurosurgery and Psychiatry 38: 1211-1217 (1975).

Greenfield, J.G. and Bosanquet, F.D.: The brain-stem lesions in Parkinsonism. Journal of Neurology, Neurosurgery and Psychiatry 16: 213-226 (1953).

Griffiths, G.C.: Heparin osteoporosis. Journal of the American Medical Association 193: 91 (1965).

Growdon, J.H.; Shahani, B.T. and Young, R.R.: The effect of alcohol on essential tremor. Neurology 25: 259-262 (1975).

Growdon, J.H.; Young, R.H. and Shahani, B.T.: L-5-hydroxytryptophan in treatment of several different syndromes in which myoclonus is prominent. Neurology 26: 1135-1140 (1976).

Gubitz, R.H.; Akera, T. and Brody, T.M.: Comparative effects of substituted phenothiazines and their free radials on (NA$^+$, K$^+$)- activated adenosine triphosphatase. Biochemical Pharmacology 22: 1229-1235 (1973).

Guilleminault, C.; Raynal, D.; Takahashi, S.; Carskadon, M. and Dement, W.: Evaluation of short-term and long-term treatment of the narcolepsy syndrome with clomipramine hydrochloride. Acta Neurologica Scandinavica 54: 71-87 (1976).

Guilleminault, C.; Sigwald, J. and Castaigne, P.: Sleep studies and therapeutic trials with L-Dopa in a case of stiff man syndrome. European Neurology 10: 89-96 (1973).

Guisado, R. and Arieff, A.I.: Glycerol in cerebral oedema. Lancet 2: 183 (1975).

Guisado, R.; Arieff, A.I. and Massry, S.G.: Effects of glycerol administration on experimental brain oedema. Neurology 26: 69-75 (1976).

Gurcay, O.; Wilson, C.; Barker, M. and Eliason, J. Corticosteroid effect on transplantable rat glioma. Archives of Neurology 24: 266-269 (1971).

Guth, P.S. and Spirtes, M.A.: The phenothiazine tranquilizers: biochemical and biophysical actions; in Pfeiffer and Smythies (Eds) International Review of Neurobiology, Vol. 7, p.231-278 (Academic Press, New York 1964).

Gutmann, L.: Pathophysiologic aspects of human botulism. Archives of Neurology 32: 175-179 (1976).

Gutmann, L.; Martin, J.D. and Welton, W.: Dapsone motor neuropathy — an axonal disease. Neurology 26: 514-516 (1976).

Gyselynek, A.M.; Forrey, A. and Cutler, R.: Pharmacokinetics of gentamycin: Distribution and plasma and renal clearance. Journal of Infectious Diseases 124 (Suppl.): S70-S76 (1971).

Haerer, A.F. and Buchanan, R.A.: Effectiveness of single daily doses of diphenylhydantoin. Neurology 22: 1021-1025 (1972).

Hahn, T.J ; Hendin, B.A.; Scharp, C.R. and Haddad, J.G. Jr.: Effect of chronic anticonvulsant therapy on serum 25-hydroxycalciferol levels in adults. New England Journal of Medicine 287: 900-904 (1972).

Hambleton, G. and Davies, P.A.: Diagnosis and management of bacterial meningitis. Drugs 8: 15-53 (1974).

Hansen, J.M.; Kristensen, M. and Skovsted, L.: Sulthiame (Ospolot) as inhibitor of diphenylhydantoin metabolism. Epilepsia 9: 17-22 (1968).

Hansen, J.M.; Kristensen, M.; Skovsted, L. and Christensen, L.K.: Dicoumarol-induced diphenylhydantoin intoxication. Lancet 2: 265-266 (1966).

Hansen, J.M.; Sierskboek-Nielsen, A.; Kristensen, M.; Skovsted, L. and Christensen, L.K.: Effect of diphenylhydantoin on the metabolism of dicoumarol in man. Acta Medica Scandinavica 189: 15-19 (1971a).

Hansen, J.M.; Siersboek-Nielsen, K. and Skovsted, L.: Interaktion mellan difenylhydantoin och Karbamazepin; in Lidingo (Ed) Plasma Koncentrations bestamningar au Antiepileptika: Metodologiska och Kliniska Aspekter, p.48-50 (1971b).

Hansen, J.M.; Siersboek-Nielsen, K. and Skovsted, L.: Carbamazepine-induced acceleration of diphenylhydantoin and warfarin metabolism in man. Clinical Pharmacology and Therapeutics 12: 539-543 (1971c).

Hansen, J.M.; Siersboek-Nielsen, K.; Skvosted, L.; Kampmann, J.P. and Lumholtz, B.: Potentiation of warfarin by Co-trimoxazole. British Medical Journal 2: 684 (1975).

Hansen, S.E. and Feldberg, L.: Absorption and elimination of Zarontin. Danish Medical Bulletin 11: 54-55 (1964).

Hansten, P.D.: Drug Interactions. 2nd edition (Lea and Febiger, Philadelphia 1973).

Harbison, R.D. and Becker, B.A.: Relation of dosage and time of administration of diphenylhydantoin to its teratogenic effect in mice. Teratology 2: 305-312 (1969).

Harbison, R.D. and Becker, B.A.: Diphenylhydantoin teratogenicity in rats. Toxicology and Applied Pharmacology 22: 193-200 (1972).

Hare, L.E.; Yeh, K.C.; Ditzier, C.A.; McMahon, F.G. and Duggan, D.F.: Bioavailability of dexamethasone II. Dexamethasone phosphate. Clinical Pharmacology and Therapeutics 18: 330-337 (1975).

Hare, T.A.; Beasley, B.L.; Chambers, R.A.; Boehme, D.H. and Vogel, W.H.: Dopa and aminoacid levels in plasma and cerebrospinal fluid of patients with Parkinsons disease before and during treatment with L-Dopa. Clinica Chimica Acta 45: 274-280 (1973).

Harrison, M.J.G.; Marshall, J.; Meadows, J.C. and Ross Russell, R.W.: Effect of aspirin in amaurosis fugax. Lancet 2: 473-474 (1971).

Hart, C.W. and Naunton, R.F.: The ototoxicity of chloroquine phosphate. Archives of Otolaryngology 80: 407-412 (1964).

Hartshorn, E.A.: Handbook of Drug Interactions (Francke, Cincinnati 1970).

Harvey, D.J.; Glazener, L.; Stratton, C.; Nowlin, J.; Hill, R.M. and Horning, M.G.: Detection of a 5-(3,4-dihydroxy-1,5-cyclohexadiene-1-yl)-metabolite of phenobarbital and mephobarbital in rat, guinea pig and human. Research Communications in Chemical Pathology and Pharmacology 3: 557-566 (1972).

Harvey, P.K.P.: Some aspects of the neurochemistry of Epilim; in Legg (Ed) Clinical and Pharmacological Aspects of Sodium Valproate (Epilim) in the Treatment of Epilepsy, p.130-134 (MCS Consultants, Tunbridge Wells 1976).

Hass, W.K.: Occlusive cerebrovascular disease. Medical Clinics of North America 56: 1281-1297 (1972).

Hassall, C.; Feetam, C.L.; Leach, R.H. and Meynell, M.J.: Potentiation of warfarin by co-trimoxazole. British Medical Journal 2: 684 (1975).

Hassan, M.N.; Laljee, H.C.K. and Parsonage, M. J.: Experience in the treatment of resistant cases of epilepsy with sodium valproate (Epilim); in Legg (Ed) Clinical and Pharmacological Aspects of Sodium Valproate (Epilim) in the Treatment of Epilepsy, p.23-29 (MCS Consultants, Tunbridge Wells 1976).

Heckmatt, J.Z.; Houston, A.B.; Clow, D.J.; Stephenson, J.B.P.; Dodd, K.L.; Lealman, G.T. and Logan, R.W.: Failure of phenobarbitone to prevent febrile convulsions. British Medical Journal 1: 559-561 (1976).

Heller, G.L. and De Jong, R.N.: Treatment of the Guillain-Barre syndrome. Use of corticotropin and glucocorticoids. Archives of Neurology 8: 179-193 (1963).

Hernandez-Peon, R.: Anticonvulsive action of G32883. Proceedings of the Third Meeting of C.I.N.P. Munich, 303-311 (1962).

Heros, R.C.; Zervas, N.T. and Negoro, M.: Cerebral vasospasm. Surgical Neurology 5: 354-362 (1976).

Herskovits, E. and Blackwood, W.: Essential (familial) tremor — a case report. Journal of Neurology, Neurosurgery and Psychiatry 32: 509-511 (1969).

Heymann, W.: Nephrotic syndrome after use of trimethadione and Paradione in petit mal. Journal of the American Medical Association 202: 893-894 (1967).

Hichens, M. and Hogans, A.F.: Radioimmunoassay for dexamethasone in plasma. Clinical Chemistry 20: 266-271 (1974).

Hill, A.B.; Marshall, J. and Shaw, D.A.: Cerebrovascular disease trial of long-term anticoagulant therapy. British Medical Journal 2: 1003-1006 (1962).

Hillestad, L.; Hansen, T.; Melsom, H. and Drivenes, A.: Diazepam metabolism in normal man. 1 Serum concentrations and clinical effects after intravenous, intramuscular and oral administration. Clinical Pharmacology and Therapeutics 16: 479-484 (1974).

Hilton, B.: Blood platelets: a pathological difference between migrainous and control subjects. Hemicrania 3(2): 3-5 (1971).

Hilton, B.P. and Zilkha, K.J.: Effects of ergotamine and methysergide on blood platelet aggregation responses of migrainous subjects. Journal of Neurology, Neurosurgery and Psychiatry 37: 593-597 (1974).

Hinterberger, H.: The distribution of 3, 4-dihydroxyphenylalanine (DOPA) and of some of its metabolites in the blood of patients, during oral therapy with l-Dopa. Biochemical Medicine 5: 412-424 (1971).

Hishikawa, Y.; Ida, H.; Nakai, K. and Kaneko, Z.: Treatment of narcolepsy with imipramine (Tofranil) and desmethylimipramine (Pertofran). Journal of Neurological Sciences 3: 453-461 (1966).

Hitzemann, R.J. and Loh, H.H.: Effect of d-amphetamine on the turnover, synthesis and metabolism of brain phosphatidylcholine. Biochemical Pharmacology 22: 2731-2741 (1973).

Ho, D.W.H. and Frei, E.: Clinical pharmacology of l-D-arabinofuranosyl cytosine. Clinical Pharmacology and Therapeutics 12: 225-238 (1971).

Hoffbrand, A.V. and Necheles, T.F.: Mechanism of folate deficiency in patients receiving phenytoin. Lancet 2: 528-530 (1968).

Hoffman, T.A.; Cestero, R. and Bullock, W.E.: Pharmacodynamics of carbenicillin in hepatic and renal failure. Annals of Internal Medicine 73: 173-178 (1970).

Hokkanen, E.: Antibiotics in myasthenia gravis. British Medical Journal 1: 1111-1112 (1964).

Holden, K.R. and Freeman, J.M.: Neonatal seizures and their treatment. Clinics in Perinatology 2: 3-13 (1975).

Hollister, L.E.; Curry, S.H.; Derr, J.E. and Kanter, S.L.: Studies of delayed action medication V. Plasma levels and urinary excretion of four different dosage forms of chlorpromazine. Clinical Pharmacology and Therapeutics 11: 49-59 (1970).

Holmes, G.: On certain tremors in organic cerebral lesions. Brain 27: 327-375 (1904).

Hooper, W.O.; Bochner, F.; Eadie, M.J. and Tyrer, J.H.: Plasma protein binding of diphenylhydantoin. Clinical Pharmacology and Therapeutics 15: 276-282 (1974a).

Hooper, W.D.; Dubetz, D.K.; Bochner, F.; Cotter, L.M.; Smith, G.A.; Eadie, M.J. and Tyrer, J.H.: Plasma protein binding of carbamazepine. Clinical Pharmacology and Therapeutics 17: 433-440 (1975).

Hooper, W.D.; DuBetz, D.K.; Eadie, M.J. and Tyrer, J.H.: Preliminary observations on the clinical pharmacology of carbamazepine (Tegretol). Proceedings of the Australian Association of Neurologists 11: 189-198 (1974b).

Hooper, W.D.; Sutherland, J.M.; Bochner, F.; Tyrer, J.H.; and Eadie, M.J.: The effect of certain drugs on the plasma protein binding of diphenylhydantoin. Australian and New Zealand Journal of Medicine 3: 377-381 (1973).

Horn, A.S.; Cuello, A.C. and Miller, R.J.: Dopamine in the mesolimbic system of the rat brain: endogenous levels and the effect of drugs on the uptake mechanism and stimulation of adenylate cyclase activity. Journal of Neurochemistry 22: 265-270 (1974).

Horning, M.G.; Stratton, C.; Nowlin, J.; Harvey, D.J. and Hill, R.M.: Metabolism of 2-ethyl-2-methylsuccinimide (Ethosuximide) in the rat and human. Drug Metabolism and Distribution 1: 569-576 (1973).

Horning, M.G.; Zion, T.E. and Butler, C.M.: Metabolism of N-methyl-2-phenylsuccinamide (phensuximide) by the epoxide-diol pathway. Federation Proceedings 33: 525 (1974).

Horowitz, G. and Greenberg, J.: Pallido-pyramidal syndrome treated with levodopa. Journal of Neurology, Neurosurgery and Psychiatry 38: 238-240 (1975).

Horrocks, P.M.; Vicary, D.J.; Rees, J.E.; Parkes, J.D. and Marsden, C.D.: Anticholinergic withdrawal and benzhexol treatment in Parkinson's disease. Journal of Neurology, Neurosurgery and Psychiatry 36: 936-941 (1973).

Houghton, G.W. and Richens, A.: The effect of benzodiazepines and pheneturide on phenytoin metabolism in man. British Journal of Clinical Pharmacology 1: 344P-345P (1974).

Houghton, G.W.; Richens, A. and Leighton, M.: Effect of age, height, weight and sex on serum phenytoin concentration in epileptic patients. British Journal of Clinical Pharmacology 2: 251-256 (1975).

Howard, F.M.; Duane, D.D.; Lambert, E.H., and Daube, J.R.: Alternate-day prednisone: preliminary report of a double-blind controlled study. Annals of the New York Academy of Sciences 274: 596-607 (1976).

Huang, C.Y.; McLeod, J.G.; Sampson, D. and Hensley, W.J.: Clonazepam in the treatment of epilepsy. Proceedings of the Australian Association of Neurologists 10: 67-74 (1973).

Hubbe, P.: The prophylactic treatment of migraine with an antiserotonin pizotifen (BC105). Acta Neurologica Scandinavica 49: 108-114 (1973).

Hucker, H.B.; Stauffer, S.C. and Balletto, A.: Disposition and metabolic fate of cyproheptadine in rats dogs and cats. Federation Proceedings 32: 809 (1973).

Huffman, D.H.; Wan, S.H.; Azarnoff, D.L. and Hoogstraten, B.: Pharmacokinetics of methotrexate. Clinical Pharmacology and Therapeutics 14: 572-579 (1973).

Hughes, I.E.; Jellett, L.B. and Ilett, K.F.: The influence of various factors on the in vitro distribution of haloperidol in human blood. British Journal of Clinical Pharmacology 3: 285-288 (1976).

Hughes, R.C.; Polgar, J.G.; Weightman, D. and Walton, J.W.: Levodopa in Parkinsonism: the effects of withdrawal of anticholinergic drugs. British Medical Journal 2: 487-491 (1971).

Huisman, J.W.: Disposition of primidone in man: An example of autoinduction of a human enzyme system. Pharmaceutisch Weekblad 104: 799-802 (1969).

Huisman, J.W.; Van Heycop Ten Ham, M.W. and Van Zijl, C.W.H.: Influence of ethylphenacetamide on serum levels of other anti-epileptic drugs. Epilepsia 11: 207-215 (1970).

Hunter, J.: Effects of enzyme induction on vitamin D_3 metabolism in man; in Richens and Woodford (Eds) Anticonvulsant Drugs and Enzyme Induction, p.77-84 (Elsevier, Amsterdam 1976).

Hunter, J.; Maxwell, J.D.; Stewart, D.A.; Parsons, V. and Williams, R.: Altered calcium metabolism in epileptic children on anticonvulsants. British Medical Journal 4: 202-204 (1971).

Hutchinson, E.C.: Management of acute cerebral infarction; in Ross Russell (Ed) Cerebral Arterial Disease, p.158-180 (Churchill-Livingstone, Edinburgh 1976).

Huttenlocher, P.R. and Mattson, R.H.: Isoprinosine in subacute sclerosing panencephalitis. Neurology 29: 763-771 (1979).

Hvidberg, E.F. and Dam, M.: Clinical pharmacokinetics of anticonvulsants. Clinical Pharmacokinetics 1: 161-188 (1976).

Hyman, G.A., and Sommers, S.C.: The development of Hodgkins disease and lymphoma during anticonvulsant therapy. Blood 28: 416-427 (1966).

Imai, K.; Sugiura, M.; Tamura, Z.; Hirayama, K. and Narabayashi, H.: The plasma levels of Dopa and catecholamines after oral administration of L-DOPA. Chemical and Pharmaceutical Bulletin 19: 439-440 (1971).

Inaba, T.; Tang, B.K.; Endrenyi, L. and Kalow, W.: Amobarbital — a probe of hepatic drug oxidation in man. Clinical Pharmacology and Therapeutics 20: 439-444 (1976).

Ingham, H.R.; Selkon, J.B. and Roxby, C.M.: Bacteriological study of otogenic cerebral abscesses: chemotherapeutic role of metronidazole. British Medical Journal 2: 991-993 (1977).

Irvine, A.F.: Dangers of intrathecal hydrocortisone sodium succinate. Medical Journal of Australia 2: 690 (1975).

Iversen, L.L. and Johnston, G.A.R.: GABA uptake in rat central nervous system: comparison of uptakes in slices and homogenates and the effects of some inhibitors. Journal of Neurochemistry 18: 1939-1950 (1971).

Jackson, J.H.: A study of convulsions. Transactions of the Saint Andrews Medical Graduates Association 3: 162-204 (1870). Reprinted in Archives of Neurology 22: 184-188 (1970).

Jalling, B.; Boreus, L.O.; Rane, A. and Sjoqvist, F.: Plasma concentrations of diphenylhydantoin in young infants. Pharmacologica Clinica 2: 200-202 (1970).

James, O.; Lesna, M.; Roberts, S.H.; Pulman, L.; Douglas, A.P.; Smith, P.A. and Watson, A.J.: Liver damage after paracetamol overdose. Lancet 2: 579-581 (1975).

Jammes, J.L.: The treatment of cluster headaches with prednisone. Diseases of the Nervous System 36: 375-376 (1975).

Jarrell, M.A.; Greer, M. and Maren, T.H.: The effect of acidosis in hypokalemic periodic paralysis. Archives of Neurology 33: 791-793 (1976).

Jefferson, D.; Jenner, P. and Marsden, C.D.: Relationship between plasma propranolol concentration and relief of essential tremor. Journal of Neurology, Neurosurgery and Psychiatry 42: 831-837 (1979).

Jenkins, R.B. and Groh, R.H.: Mental symptoms in Parkinsonian patients treated with l-Dopa. Lancet 2: 177-180 (1970).

Jenne, J.W.: Pharmacokinetics and the dose of isoniazid and p-amino salicylic acid in the treatment of tuberculosis. Antibiotics and Chemotherapy 12: 407-432 (1964).

Jensen, B.N.: Trimethadione in the serum of patients with petit mal. Danish Medical Bulletin 9: 74-79 (1962).

Jensen, O. N. and Olesen, O.V.: Subnormal serum folate due to anticonvulsant therapy. A double-blind study of the effect of folic acid treatment in patients with drug-induced subnormal serum folates. Archives of Neurology 22: 181-182 (1970).

Johannessen, S.I.; Gerna, M.; Bakke, J.; Strandjord, R.E. and Morselli, P.L.: C.S.F. concentrations and serum protein binding of carbamazepine and carbamazepine-10, 11-epoxide in epileptic patients. British Journal of Clinical Pharmacology 3: 575-582 (1976).

Johannessen, S.I. and Strandjord, R.E.: The concentration of carbamazepine (Tegretol®) in serum and in cerebrospinal fluid in patients with epilepsy. Acta Neurologica Scandinavica 48 (Suppl.) 51: 445-446 (1972).

Johansson, S.; Lindstedt, S.; Register, U. and Wadstrom, L.: Studies on the metabolism of labelled pyridoxine in man. American Journal of Clinical Nutrition 18: 185-196 (1966).

Johns, D.G.; Sperti, S. and Burgen, A.S.V.: The metabolism of tritiated folic acid in man. Journal of Clinical Investigation 40: 1684-1695 (1961).

Johnson, K.P.; Rosenthal, M.S. and Lerner, P.I.: Herpes simplex encephalitis. The course in five virologically proven cases. Archives of Neurology 27: 103-108 (1972).

Johnson, R.T.: Treatment of herpes simplex virus encephalitis. Archives of Neurology 27: 97-98 (1972).

Johnson, W.H. and Ireland, P.E.: The control of vertigo by thiethylperazine. Archives of Otolaryngology 82: 261-266 (1965).

Johnsson, G. and Regardh, C-G: Clinical pharmacokinetics of β-adrenoceptor blocking drugs. Clinical Pharmacokinetics 1: 233-263 (1976).

Johnston, G.A.R.: L-Dopa and pyridoxal-5'-phosphate: tetrahydroisoquinoline formation. Lancet 1: 1068 (1971).

Jones, D.G.; Turnbull, M.J.; Lenman, J.A.R. and Robertson, M.A.H.: Effect of amantadine on the urinary excretion of some monoamines and metabolites in normal and Parkinsonian subjects. Journal of Neurological Sciences 17: 245-253 (1972).

Jones, R.E.; Burke, D.; Marosszeky, J.E. and Gillies, J.D.: A new agent for the control of spasticity. Journal of Neurology, Neurosurgery and Psychiatry 33: 464-468 (1970).

Jones, R.F. and Lance, J.W.: Baclofen (Lioresal) in the long-term management of spasticity. Medical Journal of Australia 1: 654-657 (1976).

Jordan, B.J.; Shillingford, J.S., and Steed, K.P.: Preliminary observations on the protein-binding and enzyme-inducing properties of sodium valproate (Epilim); in Legg (Ed) Clinical and Pharmacological Aspects of Sodium Valproate (Epilim) in the Treatment of Epilepsy, p.112-116 (MCS Consultants, Tunbridge Wells 1976).

Jorgensen, A. and Hansen, V.: Pharmacokinetics of amitriptyline infused intravenously in man. European Journal of Clinical Pharmacology 10: 337-341 (1976).

Jubiz, W.; Meikle, A.W.; Levinson, R.A.; Mizutani, S.; West, C.D. and Tyler, F.H.: Effect of phenytoin (diphenylhydantoin) on the metabolism of dexamethasone. New England Journal of Medicine 283: 11-14 (1970).

Julien, R.M.: Anticonvulsant action of diphenylhydantoin in mice with genetic cerebellar degeneration. Journal of Pharmacology and Experimental Therapeutics 180: 239-243 (1972).

Jusko, W.J. and Lewis, G.P.: Comparison of ampicillin and hetacillin pharmacokinetics in man. Journal of Pharmaceutical Sciences 62: 69-76 (1973).

Jusko, W.J.; Lewis, G.P. and Schmitt, G.W.: Ampicillin and hetacillin pharmacokinetics in normal and anephric subjects. Clinical Pharmacology and Therapeutics 14: 90-99 (1973).

Kadar, D.; Inaba, T.; Endrenyi, L.; Johnson, G.E. and Kalow, W.: Comparative drug elimination capacity in man — glutethimide, amobarbital, antipyrine and sulfinpyrazone. Clinical Pharmacology and Therapeutics 14: 552-560 (1973).

Kalser, S.C.: The fate of atropine in man. Annals of the New York Academy of Science 179: 667-683 (1971).

Kamenskaya, M.A.; Elmqvist, D. and Thesleff, S.: Guanidine and neuromuscular transmission I. Effect on transmitter release occuring spontaneously and in response to single nerve stimuli. Archives of Neurology 32: 505-508 (1975).

Kanto, J.; Kangas, L. and Siirtola, T.: Cerebrospinal fluid concentrations of diazepam and its metabolites in man. Acta Pharmacologica et Toxicologica 36: 328-334 (1975).

Kaplan, S.A.; Alexander, K.; Jack, M.L.; Puglisi, C.V.; de Silva, J.A.F.; Lee, T.L. and Weinfeld, R.E.: Pharmacokinetic profiles of clonazepam in dogs and humans and of flunitrazepam in dogs. Journal of Pharmaceutical Sciences 63: 527-532 (1974).

Kaplan, S.A.; Jack, M.L.; Alexander, K.; Puglisi, C.V.; de Silva, J.A.F.; Lee, T.L. and Weinfeld, R.E.: Pharmacokinetic profiles of diazepam in man following single intravenous and oral and chronic oral administration. Journal of Pharmaceutical Sciences 62: 1789-1796 (1973).

Karli, P. and Bergstrom, L.: Effect of baclofen on myotonia. Lancet 1: 1285-1286 (1974).

Karlin, J.M. and Kutt, H.: Acute diphenylhydantoin intoxication following halothane anesthesia. Journal of Pediatrics 76: 941-944 (1970).

Kartzinel, R. and Calne, D.B.: Studies with bromocryptine. Part I. 'On-off' phenomena. Neurology 26: 508-510 (1976).

Kaste, M.; Fogelholm, R. and Waltimo, O.: Combined dexamethasone and low-molecular-weight dextran in acute brain infarction: double-blind study. British Medical Journal 2: 1409-1410 (1976).

Kater, R.M.H.; Roggin, G.; Tobon, F.; Zieve, P. and Iber, F.L.: Increased rate of clearance of drugs from the circulation of alcoholics. American Journal of Medical Science 258: 35-39 (1969).

Kato, M. and Araki, S.: Paroxysmal kinesigenic choreoathetosis. Archives of Neurology 20: 508-513 (1969).

Kaul, P.N.; Whitfield, L.R. and Clark, M.L.: Chlorpromazine metabolism VIII: blood levels of chlorpromazine and its sulfoxide in schizophrenic patients. Journal of Pharmaceutical Science 65: 694-697 (1976).

Kauto, K. and Tammisto, P.: Comparison of two generically equivalent carbamazepine preparations. Annals of Clinical Research 6 (Suppl. 11): 21-25 (1974).

Kebabian, J.W.; Petzold, G.L. and Greengard, P.: Dopamine-sensitive adenyl cyclase in caudate nucleus of rat brain, and its similarity to the 'dopamine receptor'. Proceedings of the National Academy of Science, U.S.A. 69: 2145-2149 (1972).

Kelly, R.E. and Jellinek, E.H.: Intrathecal tuberculin in disseminated sclerosis. A controlled trial. British Medical Journal 2: 421-424 (1961).

Khuri-Bulos, N.: Meningococcal meningitis following rifampin prophylaxis. American Journal of Diseases of Children 126: 689-691 (1973).

Killian, J.M. and Fromm, G.H.: Carbamazepine in the treatment of neuralgia. Archives of Neurology 19:

129-136 (1968).

Kiloh, L.G.; Smith, J.S. and Williams, S.E.: Antiparkinson drugs as causal agents in tardive dyskinesia. Medical Journal of Australia 2: 591-593 (1973).

Kimball, O.P.: The treatment of epilepsy with sodium diphenyl hydantoinate. Journal of the American Medical Association 112: 1244-1245 (1939).

Kinkel, A.: Unpublished data, 1971. Cited by Glazko, A.J. and Dill, W.A.: Other succinimides; in Woodbury, Penry and Schmidt (Eds) Antiepileptic Drugs, p.455-464 (Raven Press, New York 1972).

Kiorboe, E.; Paludan, J.; Trolle, E. and Overvad, E.: Zarontin (ethosuximide) in the treatment of petit mal and related disorders. Epilepsia 5: 83-89 (1964).

Kirk, L.; Baastrup, P.C. and Schou, M.: Propranolol treatment of lithium-induced tremor. Lancet 2: 1086-1087 (1973).

Klatzko, I.: Neuropathological aspects of brain oedema. Journal of Neuropathology and Experimental Neurology 26: 1-14 (1967).

Klawans, H.L. Jr.: A pharmacologic analysis of Huntington's chorea. European Neurology 4: 148-163 (1970).

Klawans, H.L. Jr.: The pharmacology of tardive dyskinesias. American Journal of Psychiatry 130: 82-86 (1973a).

Klawans, H.L. Jr.: The Pharmacology of Extrapyramidal Movement Disorders (Karger, Basel 1973b).

Klawans, H.L.; Goetz, C. and Bergen, D.: Levodopa-induced myoclonus. Archives of Neurology 32: 332-334 (1975).

Klawans, H.L. and Moskovitz, C.: Cyclizine-induced chorea. Observations on the influence of cyclizine on dopamine-related movement disorders. Journal of Neurological Science 31: 237-244 (1977).

Klawans, H.L. and Rubovits, R.: Effect of cholinergic and anticholinergic agents on tardive dyskinesia. Journal of Neurology, Neurosurgery and Psychiatry 27: 941-947 (1974).

Klawans, H.L.; Topel, J.L. and Bergen, D.: Deanol in the treatment of levodopa-induced dyskinesias. Neurology 25: 290-293 (1975).

Klawans, H.L. and Weiner, W.J.: Attempted use of haloperidol in the treatment of l-dopa induced dyskinesias. Journal of Neurology, Neurosurgery and Psychiatry 37: 427-430 (1974a).

Klawans, H.L. and Weiner, W.J.: The effect of d-amphetamine on choreiform movement disorders. Neurology 24: 312-318 (1974b).

Klotz, U.; Antonin, K. -H. and Bieck, P.R.: Pharmacokinetics and plasma binding of diazepam in man, dog, rabbit, guinea pig and rat. Journal of Pharmacology and Experimental Therapeutics 199: 67-73 (1976).

Knop, H.J.; Van Der Kleijn, E. and Edmunds, L.C.: The determination of clonazepam in plasma by gas-liquid chromatography. Pharmaceutisch Weekblad 110: 297-309 (1975).

Knop, H.J.; Van Der Kleijn, E. and Edmunds, L.C.: Pharmacokinetics of clonazepam in man and laboratory animals; in Schneider, Janz, Gardner-Thorpe, Meinardi and Sherwin (Eds) Clinical Pharmacology of Antiepileptic Drugs, p.247-259 (Springer, Berlin 1975).

Knutsson, E.; Lindblom, U. and Martensson, A.: Plasma and cerebrospinal fluid levels of baclofen (Lioresal®) at optimal therapeutic responses in spastic paresis. Journal of Neurological Science 23: 473-484 (1974).

Kobayashi, K., Iwata, Y. and Mukawa, J.: Preferential action of Tegretol (G-32883) to limbic seizures. Clinical and experimental analysis. Brain and Nerve 19: 999-1005 (1967).

Kochar, M.S. and Itskovitz, H.D.: Treatment of idiopathic orthostatic hypotension (Shy-Drager syndrome) with indomethacin. Lancet 1: 1011-1014 (1978).

Koch-Weser, J.: Pharmacokinetics of procainamide in man. Annals of the New York Academy of Science 179: 370-382 (1971).

Koch-Weser, J. and Klein, S.W.: Procainamide dosage schedules, plasma concentrations and clinical effects. Journal of the American Medical Association 215: 1454-1460 (1971).

Koechlin, B.A.; Rubio, F.; Palmer, S.; Gabriel, T. and Duschinsky, R.: The metabolism of 5-fluorocytosine 2-^{14}C in the rat and the disposition of 5-fluorocytosine in man. Biochemical Pharmacology 15: 435-446 (1966).

Kolakowska, T.; Franklin, M. and Alapin, B.: Effect of long-term phenothiazine treatment on drug metabolism. British Journal of Clinical Pharmacology 2: 25-28 (1975).

Korkis, F.B.: Treatment of recent Bell's palsy by cervical sympathetic block. Lancet 1: 255-257 (1961).

Kragh-Sorensen, P.; Asberg, M. and Eggert-Hansen, C.: Plasma-nortriptyline levels in endogenous depression. Lancet 1: 113-115 (1973).

Kristensen, M.; Hansen, J.M. and Skovsted, L.: The influence of phenobarbital on the half-life of diphenylhydantoin in man. Acta Medica Scandinavica 185: 347-350 (1969).

Krupp, P.: The effect of Tegretol® on some elementary neuronal mechanisms. Headache 2: 42-46 (1969).

Kudrow, L.: Lithium prophylaxis for chronic cluster headache. Headache 17: 15-18 (1977).

Kuhara, T. and Matsumoto, J.: Metabolism of branched medium chain length fatty acids. 1-Omega oxidation of sodium dipropylacetate in rats. Biomedical Mass Spectrometry 1: 291-294 (1974).

Kunin, C.M. and Finkelberg, Z.: Oral cephalexin and ampicillin: Antimicrobial activity, recovery in urine, and persistence in blood of uremic patients. Annals of Internal Medicine 72: 349-356 (1970).

Kunin, C.M.; Glazko, A.J. and Finland, M.: Persistence of antibiotics in blood of patients with acute renal failure II. Chloramphenicol and its metabolic products in the blood of patients with severe renal disease or hepatic cirrhosis. Journal of Clinical Investigation 38: 1498-1508 (1959).

Kupferberg, H.J. and Yonekawa, W.: The metabolism of 3 methyl 5 ethyl 5 phenylhydantoin (mephenytoin) to 5 ethyl 5 phenylhydantoin (Nirvanol) in mice in relation to anticonvulsant activity. Drug Metabolism and Disposition 3: 26-29 (1975).

Kuruma, I.; Bartholini, G.; Tissot, R. and Pletscher, A.: The metabolism of L-3-O-methyldopa, a precursor of dopa in man. Clinical Pharmacology and Therapeutics 12: 678-682 (1971).

Kutt, H.: Biochemical and genetic factors regulating Dilantin® metabolism in man. Annals of the New York Academy of Science 179: 704-722 (1971).

Kutt, H.; Haynes, M.; Verebely, K. and McDowell, F.: The effect of phenobarbital on plasma diphenylhydantoin level and metabolism in man and in rat liver microsomes. Neurology 19: 611-616 (1969).

Kutt, H. and Louis, S.: Anticonvulsant drugs. II Clinical pharmacological and therapeutic aspects. Current Therapeutics 13: 59-82 (1972).

Kutt, H. and McDowell, F.: Management of epilepsy with diphenylhydantoin sodium. Journal of the American Medical Association 203: 969-972 (1968).

Kutt, H.; Winters, W.; Kokenge, R. and McDowell, F.: Diphenylhydantoin metabolism, blood levels, and toxicity. Archives of Neurology 11: 642-648 (1964).

Kutt, H.; Winters, W. and McDowell, F.H.: Depression of parahydroxylation of diphenylhydantoin by antituberculosis chemotherapy. Neurology 16: 594-602 (1966).

Ladd, H.; Oist, C. and Johnsson, B.: The effect of Dantrium® on spasticity in multiple sclerosis. Acta Neurologica Scandinavica 50: 397-408 (1974).

Lader, M.: Plasma concentrations of tricyclic antidepressant drugs. British Journal of Clinical Pharmacology 1: 281-283 (1974).

Laitinen, L.V.: Slowly absorbed L-Dopa preparation in the treatment of Parkinsonism. Acta Neurologica Scandinavica 49: 331-338 (1973).

Lambert, E.H. and Elmquist, D.: Quantal components of end-plate potentials in the myasthenic syndrome. Annals of the New York Academy of Science 183: 183-199 (1971).

Lance, J.W.: The Mechanism and Management of Headache, 2nd edition (Butterworths, London 1973).

Lance, J.W.; Anthony, M. and Somerville, B.: Comparative trial of serotonin antagonists in the management of migraine. British Medical Journal 2: 327-330 (1970).

Lance, J.W.; De Gail, P. and Preswick, G.: Short-term controlled trial of tranylcypromine in multiple sclerosis. Medical Journal of Australia 1: 410-413 (1965).

Landau, W.M.: Spasticity: the fable of a neurological demon and the emperor's new therapy. Archives of

Neurology 31: 217-219 (1974).

Lander, C.M.; Eadie, M.J. and Tyrer, J.H.: Interactions between anticonvulsants. Proceedings of the Australian Association of Neurologists 12: 111-116 (1975).

Lander, C.M.; Eadie, M.J. and Tyrer, J.H.: Factors influencing plasma carbamazepine concentrations. Proceedings of the Australian Association of Neurologists 14: 184-193 (1977).

Lander, C.M.; Edwards, V.E.; Eadie, M.J. and Tyrer, J.H.: Plasma anticonvulsant concentrations during pregnancy. Neurology 27: 128-131 (1977).

Larsen, P.R.; Atkinson, A.J. Jr.; Wellman, H.N. and Goldsmith, R.E.: The effect of diphenylhydantoin on thyroxine metabolism in man. Journal of Clinical Investigation 49: 1266-1279 (1970).

Lascelles, P.T.; Kocen, R.S. and Reynolds, E.H.: The distribution of plasma phenytoin levels in epileptic patients. Journal of Neurology, Neurosurgery and Psychiatry 33: 501-505 (1970).

Laterre, E.C. and Fortemps, E.: Deanol in spontaneous and induced dyskinesias. Lancet 1: 1301 (1975).

Leader: Council on drugs — Evaluation of a new antituberculous agent rifampin (Rifadin, Rimactone). Journal of the American Medical Association 220: 414-415 (1972).

Lechat, P.: Toxicological and pharmacological properties of chlormethiazole. Acta Psychiatrica Scandinavica Supplement 192: 15-22 (1966).

Leclercq, R. and Copinschi, G.: Patterns of plasma levels of prednisolone after oral administration in man. Journal of Pharmacokinetics and Biopharmaceutics 2: 175-187 (1974).

Legg, N.J.: Rebound migraine. British Medical Journal 2: 331 (1974).

Lehrer, G.M.; Maker, H.S. and Weissbarth, S.: Brain uptake of methylprednisolone acetate from the cerebrospinal fluid and systemic sites. Archives of Neurology 28: 324-328 (1973).

Leibowitz, M. and Lieberman, A.: Comparison of dopa decarboxylase inhibitor (carbidopa) combined with levodopa and levodopa alone on the cardiovascular system of patients with Parkinson's disease. Neurology 25: 917-921 (1975).

Lerman, P. and Nussbaum, E.: The use of sulthiame in myoclonic epilepsy of childhood and adolescence. Acta Neurologica Scandinavica 60 (Suppl): 7-12 (1975).

Leterrier, F.; Riegler, F. and Mariaud, J.F.: Comparative study of the action of phenothiazine and para-fluorobutyrophenone derivations on rat brain membranes using the spin label technique. Journal of Pharmacology and Experimental Therapeutics 186: 609-615 (1973).

Levi, A.J.; Sherlock, S. and Walker, D.: Phenylbutazone and isoniazid metabolism in patients with liver disease in relation to previous drug therapy. Lancet 2: 1275-1279 (1968).

Levine, S.B. and Leopold, I.H.: Advances in ocular corticosteroid therapy. Medical Clinics of North America 57: 1167-1177 (1973).

Levy, G.: Pharmacokinetics of salicylate elimination in man. Journal of Pharmaceutical Sciences 54: 959-967 (1965).

Levy, G. and Tsuchiya, T.: Salicylate accumulation kinetics in man. New England Journal of Medicine 287: 430-432 (1972).

Levy, G.; Tsuchiya, T. amd Amsel, L.P.: Limited capacity for salicyl phenolic glucuronide formation and its effect on the kinetics of salicylate elimination in man. Clinical Pharmacology and Therapeutics 13: 258-268 (1972).

Lewis, G.P.; Jusko, W.J.; Burke, C.W. and Graves, L.: Prednisolone side-effects and serum-protein levels. Lancet 2: 778-781 (1971).

Lewis, P.D. and Harrison, M.J.G.: Involuntary movements in patients taking oral contraceptives. British Medical Journal 4: 404-405 (1969).

Lieberman, A.; Goodgold, A.; Jonas, S. and Leibowitz, M.: Comparison of dopa decarboxylase inhibitor (carbidopa) combined with levodopa and levodopa alone in Parkinson's disease. Neurology 25: 911-916 (1975).

Lieberman, A.; Miyamoto, T.; Battista, A.F. and Goldstein, M.: Studies on the antiparkinsonian efficacy of lergotrile. Neurology 25: 459-462 (1975).

Lieberman, A.N. and Shupack, J.L.: Levodopa and melanoma. Neurology 24: 340-343 (1974).

Linnell, J.C.; Smith, A.D.M.; Smith, C.L.; Wilson, J. and Matthews, D.M.: Effects of smoking on metabolism and excretion of vitamin B12. British Medical Journal 2: 215-216 (1968).

Liversedge, L.A.: Herpes simplex encephalitis. Current ideas and treatment. Plans for the future. Proceedings of the Royal Society of Medicine 69: 193-194 (1976).

Liversedge, L.A.; Yuill, G.M.; Wilkinson, I.M.S. and Hughes, J.A.: Benefit from adrenocorticotrophin in myasthenia gravis. Journal of Neurology, Neurosurgery and Psychiatry 37: 412-415 (1974).

Livingstone, S.: Comprehensive Management of Epilepsy in Infancy, Childhood and Adolescence (Thomas, Springfield 1972).

Livingstone, S.; Villamater, C.; Sakata, Y. and Pauli, L.L.: Use of carbamazepine in epilepsy. Results in 87 patients. Journal of the American Medical Association 200: 116-120 (1967).

Lloyd, K.G. and Hornykiewicz, O.: Occurrence and distribution of aromatic L-aminoacid (L-Dopa) decarboxylase in the human brain. Journal of Neurochemistry 19: 1549-1559 (1972).

Lloyd, K.G. and Hornykiewicz, O.: L-glutamic acid decarboxylase in Parkinson's disease: effect of L-dopa therapy. Nature 243: 521-523 (1973).

Lockwood, W.R. and Bower, J.D.: Tobramycin and gentamycin concentrations in the serum of normal and anephric patients. Antimicrobial Agents and Chemotherapy 3: 125-129 (1973).

Lodge, A.B.: Thiopentone sensitivity and dystrophia myotonica. British Medical Journal 1: 1043-1044 (1958).

Loeb, C. and Priano, A.: Preliminary evaluation on the effects of clonazepam of Parkinsonian tremor. European Neurology 15: 143-145 (1977).

Loga, S.; Curry, S. and Lader, M.: Interactions of orphenadrine and phenobarbitone with chlorpromazine: plasma concentrations and effects in man. British Journal of Clinical Pharmacology 2: 197-208 (1975).

Loiseau, P.; Brachet, A. and Henry, P.: Concentration of dipropylacetate in plasma. Epilepsia 16: 609-615 (1975).

Loo, T.L.; Phil, D.; Luce, J.K.; Sullivan, M.P. and Frei, E.. Clinical pharmacologic observations on 6-mercaptopurine and 6-methylthiopurine ribonucleoside. Clinical Pharmacology and Therapeutics 9: 180-194 (1968).

Loong, S.C. and Ong, Y.Y.: Paroxysmal kinesigenic choreoathetosis. Report of a case relieved by L-dopa. Journal of Neurology, Neurosurgery and Psychiatry 36: 921-924 (1973).

Lou, H.O.C.: Oxazepam in the treatment of psychomotor epilepsy. Neurology 18: 986-990 (1968).

Lous, P.: Blood serum and cerebrospinal fluid levels and renal clearance of Phenemal in treated epileptics. Acta Pharmacologica et Toxicologica 10: 166-177 (1954).

Love, W.C.; Cashell, A.; Reynolds, M. and Callaghan, N.: Linoleate and fatty-acid patterns of serum lipids in multiple sclerosis and other diseases. British Medical Journal 3: 18-21 (1974).

Lovelace, R.E. and Horwitz, S.J.: Peripheral neuropathy in long-term diphenylhydantoin therapy. Archives of Neurology 18: 69-77 (1968).

Lovenberg, W.; Weissbach, H. and Udenfriend, S.: Aromatic l-aminoacid decarboxylase. Journal of Biological Chemistry 237: 89-93 (1962).

Ludvigsson, J.: Propranolol used in prophylaxis of migraine in children. Acta Neurologica Scandinavica 50: 109-115 (1974).

Lund, L.; Berlin, A. and Lunde, P.K.M.: Plasma protein binding of diphenylhydantoin in patients with epilepsy. Agreement between the unbound fraction in plasma and the concentration in the cerebrospinal fluid. Clinical Pharmacology and Therapeutics 13: 196-200 (1972).

Lund, L.; Lunde, P.K.; Rane, A.; Borga, O. and Sjoquist, F.: Plasma protein binding, plasma concentrations, and effects of diphenylhydantoin in man. Annals of the New York Academy of Science 179: 723-728 (1971).

Lund, M.; Sjo, O. and Hvidberg, E.: Plasma concentrations of ethotoin in epileptic patients; in Schneider, Janz, Gardner-Thorpe, Meinardi and Sherwin (Eds) Clinical Pharmacology of Anti-epileptic Drugs, p.111-114 (Springer, Berlin 1975).

Lunde. P.K.M.; Rane. A.; Yaffe. S.J.; Lund. L. and Sjoquist. F.: Plasma protein binding of diphenylhydantoin in man. Interaction with other drugs and the effect of temperature and plasma dilution.
Clinical Pharmacology and Therapeutics 11: 846-855 (1970).

Lundquist. G.: The risk of dependence on chlormethiazole. Acta Psychiatrica Scandinavica Supplement
192: 203-207 (1966).

Magnussen. I.; Dupont. E.; Prange-Hansen. A. and De Fine Olivarius. B.: Palatal myoclonus treated with
5-hydroxytryptophan and a decarboxylase inhibitor. Acta Neurologica Scandinavica 55: 251-253
(1977).

Mahon. W.A.; Inaba. T.; Umeda. T.; Tsutsumi. E. and Stone. R.: Biliary elimination of diazepam in man.
Clinical Pharmacology and Therapeutics 19: 443-450 (1976).

Maickel. R.P.; Cox. R.H. Jr.; Miller. F.P.; Segal. D.S. and Russell. R.W.: Correlation of brain levels of
drugs with behavioural effects. Journal of Pharmacology and Experimental Therapeutics 165:
216-224 (1969).

Maj. J.; Baran. L.; Grabowska. M. and Sowinska. H.: Effects of clonidine on the 5-hydroxytryptamine
and 5-hydroxyindoleacetic acid brain levels. Biochemical Pharmacology 22: 2679-2683 (1973).

Malaviya. A.N.; Many. A. and Schwartz. R.S.: Treatment of dermatomyositis with methotrexate. Lancet
2: 485-488 (1968).

Mandelli. M.; Morselli. P.L.; Nordio. S.; Pardi. G.; Sereni. F. and Tognoni. G.: Placental transfer of
diazepam and its disposition in the newborn infant. Clinical Pharmacology and Therapeutics 17:
564-572 (1975).

Mann. J.D.; Johns. T.R.; Campa. J.F. and Muller. W.H.: Long-term prednisone followed by thymectomy
in myasthenia gravis. Annals of the New York Academy of Science 274: 608-622 (1976).

Manninen. V.; Apejalahti. A.; Melin. J. and Karesoja. H.: Altered absorption of digoxin in patients given
propantheline and metoclopramide. Lancet 1: 398-400 (1973).

Mantle. T.J.; Tipton. K.F. and Garrett. N.J.: Inhibition of monoamine oxidase by amphetamine and related compounds. Biochemical Pharmacology 25: 2073-2077 (1976).

Manzoor. M. and Runcie. J.: Folate-responsive neuropathy: report of 10 cases. British Medical Journal 1:
1176-1178 (1976).

Mark. L.C.: Metabolism of barbiturates in man. Clinical Pharmacology and Therapeutics 4: 504-530
(1963).

Mars. H.: Levodopa. carbidopa. and pyridoxine in Parkinson disease. Archives of Neurology 30: 444-447
(1974).

Mars, H.: Effect of chronic levodopa treatment on pyridoxine metabolism. Neurology 25: 263-266
(1975).

Marsden. C.D. and Parkes. J.D.: 'On-off' effects in patients with Parkinson's disease on chronic levodopa
therapy. Lancet 1: 292-296 (1976).

Marshall. J.: The Management of Cerebrovascular Disease. 3rd edition (Blackwell Scientific Publications,
Oxford 1976).

Marshall. J. and Reynolds. E.H.: Withdrawal of anticoagulants from patients with transient ischaemic
cerebrovascular attacks. Lancet 1: 5-6 (1965).

Marshall. J. and Shaw. D.A.: Anticoagulant therapy in acute cerebrovascular accidents. A controlled trial.
Lancet 1: 995-998 (1960).

Martin. J.P.: Remarks on the functions of the basal ganglia. Lancet 1: 999-1005 (1959).

Martinex. G. and Snyder. R.D.: Transplacental passage of primidone. Neurology 23: 381-383 (1973).

Marucci. F.; Mussini. E.; Arioldi. L.; Fanelli. R.; Frigerio. A.; De Nadai. F.; Bizzi. A.; Rizzo. M.; Morselli. P.L. and Garattini. S.: Analytical and pharmacokinetic studies on butyrophenones. Clinica
Chimica Acta 34: 321-332 (1971).

Mathew. N.T.; Meyer. J.S.; Rivera. V.M.; Charney. J.Z. and Hartmann. A.: Double-blind evaluation of
glycerol therapy in acute cerebral infarction. Lancet 2: 1327-1329 (1972).

Maulding. H.V. and Zoglio. M.A.: Physical chemistry of ergot alkaloids and derivatives. I Ionisation constants of several medicinally active bases. Journal of Pharmaceutical Sciences 59: 700-701 (1970).

Maxwell, J.D.; Carrella, M.; Parkes, J.D.; Williams, R.; Mould, G.P. and Curry, S.H.: Plasma disappearance and cerebral effects of chlorpromazine in cirrhosis. Clinical Science 43: 143-151 (1972).

Maxwell, J.D.; Hunter, J.; Stewart, D.A.; Ardeman, S. and Williams, R.: Folate deficiency after anti-convulsant drugs: an effect of hepatic enzyme induction? British Medical Journal 1: 297-299 (1972).

Maynert, E.W.: Phenobarbital, Mephobarbital and Metharbital. Absorption, distribution and excretion; in Woodbury, Penry and Schmidt (Eds) Antiepileptic Drugs, p.303-310 (Raven Press, New York 1972).

McArdle, B.: Adynamia episodica hereditaria and its treatment. Brain 85: 121-148 (1962).

McDowell, F.; McDevitt, E. and Wright, I.S.: Anticoagulant therapy. Five years experience with the patient with an established cerebrovascular accident. Archives of Neurology 8: 209-214 (1963).

McGeachy, T.E. and Bloomer, W.E.: The phenobarbital sensitivity syndrome. American Journal of Medicine 14: 600-604 (1953).

McGeer, P.L.; McGeer, E.G. and Wada, J.A.: Glutamic acid decarboxylase in Parkinson's disease and epilepsy. Neurology 21: 1000-1007 (1971).

McGilveray, I.J. and Mattok, G.L.: Some factors affecting the absorption of paracetamol. Journal of Pharmacy and Pharmacology 24: 615-619 (1972).

McKenzie, S.A.; Selley, J.A. and Agnew, J.E.: Secretion of prednisolone into breast milk. Archives of Disease in Childhood 50: 894-896 (1975).

McKissock, W.; Richardson, A. and Walsh, L.: Primary intracerebral haemorrhage. Results of surgical treatment in 244 consecutive cases. Lancet 2: 683-686 (1959).

McLellan, D.L.: Co-contraction and stretch reflexes in spasticity during treatment with baclofen. Journal of Neurology, Neurosurgery and Psychiatry 40: 30-38 (1977).

McQueen, E.G.: New Zealand committee on adverse drug reactions. Eleventh annual report. New Zealand Medical Journal 84: 450-453 (1976).

McQuillen, M.P.; Gross, M. and Johns, R.J.: Chlorpromazine-induced weakness in myasthenia gravis. Archives of Neurology 8: 286-290 (1963).

Mechelse, K.; Goor, G.; Huizing, E.H.; Hammelburg, E.; Van Bolhuis, A.H.; Staal, A. and Verjaal, A.: Bell's palsy: prognostic criteria and evaluation of surgical decompression. Lancet 2: 57-60 (1971).

Meier, J. and Schreier, E.: Human plasma levels of some anti-migraine drugs. Headache 16: 96-104 (1976).

Meikle, W.A.; Weed, J.A. and Tyler, F.H.: Kinetics and interconversion of prednisolone and prednisone studied with new radioimmunoassays. Journal of Clinical Endocrinology and Metabolism 41: 717-721 (1972).

Meinardi, H.: Other antiepileptic drugs. Carbamazepine; in Woodbury, Penry and Schmidt (Eds) Antiepileptic Drugs, p.487-496 (Raven Press, New York 1972).

Meinardi, H.: Discussion; in Legg (Ed) Clinical and Pharmacological Aspects of Sodium Valproate (Epilim) in the Treatment of Epilepsy, p.48 (MCS Consultants, Tunbridge Wells 1976).

Meinardi, H.; Van Der Kleijn, E.; Meijer, J.W.A. and Van Rees, H.: Absorption and distribution of antiepileptic drugs. Epilepsia 16: 353-365 (1975).

Melchior, J.C.; Buchthal, F. and Lennox-Buchthal, M.A.: The ineffectiveness of diphenylhydantoin in preventing febrile convulsions in the age of greatest risk, under three years. Epilepsia 12: 55-62 (1971).

Melchior, J.C.; Svensmark, O. and Trolle, D.: Placental transfer of phenobarbitone in epileptic women, and elimination in newborns. British Medical Journal 2: 860-861 (1967).

Melzack, R. and Wall, P.D.: On the nature of cutaneous sensory mechanisms. Brain 85: 331-356 (1962).

Mendez, J.S.; Cotzias, G.C.; Mena, I. and Papavasilou, P.S.: Diphenylhydantoin. Blocking of levodopa effects. Archives of Neurology 32: 44-46 (1975).

Merritt, H.H.; Adams, R.D. and Solomon, H.C.: Neurosyphilis (Oxford University Press, New York 1946).

Meritt, H.H. and Putnam, T.J.: Sodium diphenyl hydantoinate in the treatment of convulsive disorders. Journal of the American Medical Association 111: 1068-1073 (1938).

Messiha, F.S. and Morgan, J.P.: Imipramine-mediated effects on levodopa metabolism in man. Biochemical Pharmacology 23: 1503-1507 (1974).

Meunter, M.D. and Tyce, G.M.: L-dopa therapy of Parkinson's disease: plasma L-dopa concentrations, therapeutic response, and side-effects. Mayo Clinic Proceedings 46: 231-239 (1971).

Meyer, J.S.; Charney, J.Z.; Rivera, V.M. and Mathew, N.T.: Treatment with glycerol of cerebral oedema due to acute cerebral infarction. Lancet 2: 993-997 (1971).

Meyer, J.S.; Shimazu, K.; Ohuchi, T.; Okamoto, S.; Koto, A.; Fukuuchi, Y. and Ericsson, A.D.: Cerebral metabolic effects of glycerol infusion in diabetics with stroke. Journal of Neurological Sciences 21: 1-22 (1974).

Michalek, H.: Inhibition of cholinesterase and acetylcholinesterase in vitro by butyrophenone neuroleptics. Biochemical Pharmacology 22: 1067-1074 (1973).

Michelson, M.J. and Danilov, A.F.: Synaptic vesicles, synaptic granules, autopharmacology. 5.1 Cholinergic transmission; in Bacq (Ed) Fundamentals of Biochemical Pharmacology, p.221-253 (Pergamon Press, Oxford 1971).

Miekle, A.W.; Jubiz, W.; Matsakura, S.; West, C.D. and Tyler, F.H.: Effect of diphenylhydantoin on the metabolism of metyrapone and the release of ACTH in man. Journal of Clinical Endocrinology and Metabolism 29: 1553-1558 (1969).

Millar, J.H.D.; Rahman, R.; Vas, C.J.; Noronha, M.J.; Liversedge, L.A. and Swinburn, W.R.: Effect of withdrawal of corticotrophin in patients on long-term treatment for multiple sclerosis. Lancet 1: 700-701 (1970).

Millar, J.H.D.; Vas, C.J.; Noronha, M.J.; Liversedge, L.A. and Rawson, M.D.: Long-term treatment of multiple sclerosis with corticotrophin. Lancet 1: 429-431 (1967).

Millar, J.H.D.; Zilkha, K.J.; Langman, M.J.S.; Wright, H.P.; Smith, A.D.; Belin, J. and Thompson, R.H.S.: Double-blind trial of linoleate supplementation of the diet in multiple sclerosis. British Medical Journal 1: 765-768 (1973).

Miller, E.: Deanol in the treatment of levodopa-induced dyskinesias. Neurology 24: 116-119 (1974).

Miller, E.M. and Nieburg, H.A.: L-Tryptophan in the treatment of levodopa induced psychiatric disorder. Diseases of the Nervous System 35: 20-23 (1974).

Miller, E.M. and Wiener, L.: Ro4-4602 and levodopa in the treatment of Parkinsonism. Neurology 24: 482-486 (1974).

Miller, H.G.; Foster, J.B.; Newell, D.J.; Barwick, D.D. and Brewis, R.A.L.: Multiple sclerosis: therapeutic trials of chloroquine, soluble aspirin, and gammaglobulin. British Medical Journal 2: 1436-1439 (1963).

Miller, H.; Newell, D.J. and Ridley, A.: Multiple sclerosis. Trials of maintenance treatment with prednisolone and soluble aspirin. Lancet 1: 127-129 (1961a).

Miller, H.; Newell, D.J. and Ridley, A.: Multiple sclerosis. Treatment of acute exacerbations with corticotrophin (ACTH). Lancet 2: 1120-1122 (1961b).

Miller, H.G.; Newell, D.J.; Ridley, A.R. and Schapira, K.: Therapeutic trials in multiple sclerosis. Final reports on effects of intrathecal injection of tuberculin (PPD). British Medical Journal 1: 1726-1728 (1962).

Millichap, J.G. and Ortiz, W.R.: Nitrazepam in myoclonic epilepsies. American Journal of Diseases of Childhood 112: 242-248 (1966).

Mirkin, B.L.: Diphenylhydantoin: placental transport, fetal localization, neonatal metabolism and possible teratogenic effects. Journal of Pediatrics 78: 329-337 (1971).

Mohammed, Y.S. and Mahfouz, M.M.: Inhibition of rat brain and heart monoamine oxidase by atropine. Biochemical Pharmacology 26: 871-874 (1977).

Mohr, P.D.: Allergic reactions to tetracosactrin. British Medical Journal 4: 162 (1975).

Moller, J. and Rosen, A.: Comparative studies on intramuscular and oral effective doses of some anticholinergic drugs. Acta Medica Scandinavica 184: 201-209 (1968).

Monster, A.W.; Herman, R.; Meeks, S. and McHenry, J.: Co-operative study for assessing the effects of a pharmacological agent on spasticity. American Journal of Physical Medicine 52: 163-188 (1973).

Montanari, C.; Ferrari, F. and Bavazzano, A.: Urinary excretion of amantadine by the elderly. European Journal of Clinical Pharmacology 8: 349-350 (1975).

Moore, R.G.; Robertson, A.V.; Smyth, M.P.; Thomas, J. and Vine, J.: Metabolism and urinary excretion of chlormethiazole in humans. Xenobiotica 5: 687-696 (1975b).

Moore, R.G.; Triggs, E.J.; Shanks, C.A. and Thomas, J.: Pharmacokinetics of chlormethiazole in humans. European Journal of Clinical Pharmacology 8: 353-357 (1975a).

Morgan, J.P.; Bianchine, J.R.; Spiegel, H.E.; Rivera-Calimlim, L. and Hersey, R.M.: Metabolism of levodopa in patients with Parkinson's disease. Archives of Neurology 25: 39-44 (1971).

Morgan, J.P.; Rivera-Calimlim, L.; Messiha, F.; Sundaresan, P.R. and Trabert, N.: Imipramine-mediated interference with levodopa absorption from the gastrointestinal tract in man. Neurology 25: 1029-1034 (1975).

Morrell, F.; Bradley, W. and Ptashne, M.: Effect of diphenylhydantoin on peripheral nerve. Neurology 8: 140-144 (1958).

Morris, J.G.L.; Parsons, R.L.; Trounce, J.R. and Groves, M.J.: Plasma dopa concentrations after different preparations of levodopa in normal subjects. British Journal of Clinical Pharmacology 3: 983-990 (1976).

Morselli, P.L.; Biandrate, P.; Frigerio, A. and Garattini, S.: Pharmacokinetics of carbamazepine in rats and humans. European Journal of Clinical Investigation 2: 297 (1972).

Morselli, P.L.; Bossi, L. and Gerna, M.: Pharmacokinetic studies with carbamazepine in epileptic patients in Birkmayer (Ed) International Symposium on Epileptic Seizures — Behaviour — Pain, p.141-150 (Huber, Berne 1975).

Morselli, P.L.; Gerna, M.; De Maio, D.; Zanda, G.; Viani, F. and Garattini, S.: Pharmacokinetic studies on carbamazepine in volunteers and in epileptic patients; in Schneider, Janz, Gardner-Thorpe, Meinardi and Sherwin (Eds) Clinical Pharmacology of Antiepileptic Drugs. p.166-179 (Springer, Berlin 1975).

Morselli, P.L.; Gernal, M. and Garattini, S.: Carbamazepine plasma and tissue levels in the rat. Biochemical Pharmacology 20: 2043-2047 (1971).

Morselli, P.L.; Rizzo, M. and Garattini, S.: Effect of sulthiame on blood and brain levels of diphenylhydantoin in the rat. Biochemical Pharmacology 19: 1846-1847 (1970).

Morselli, P.L.; Rizzo, M. and Garattini, S.: Interaction between phenobarbital and diphenylhydantoin in animals and in epileptic patients. Annals of the New York Academy of Science 179: 88-107 (1971).

Mosforth, J. and Taverner, D.: Physiotherapy for Bell's palsy. British Medical Journal 2: 675-677 (1958).

Mountain, K.R.; Hirsch, J. and Gallus, A.S.: Neonatal coagulation defect due to anticonvulsant drug treatment in pregnancy. Lancet 1: 265-268 (1970).

Mouridsen, H.T.; Faber, O. and Skovsted, L.: The metabolism of cyclophosphamide. Dose dependency and the effect of long-term treatment with cyclophosphamide. Cancer 37: 665-670 (1976).

Mouridsen, H.T. and Jacobsen, E.: Pharmacokinetics of cyclophosphamide in renal failure. Acta Pharmacologica et Toxicologica 36: 409-414 (1975).

Muller, W. and Wollert, U.: Characterization of the binding of benzodiazepines to human serum albumin. Nauryn-Schmiedelberg's Archives of Pharmacology 280: 229-237 (1973).

Munsat, T.L.: Therapy of myotonia. A double-blind evaluation of diphenylhydantoin, procainamide and placebo. Neurology 17: 359-369 (1967).

Mustard, J.F. and Packham, M.A.: Drugs inhibiting platelet function. Biochemical Pharmacology 22: 3151-3156 (1973).

Mutani, R. and Fariello, R.: Azione del nuovo antiepilettico Ro 5/4023 sull attivita del focus epilettogeno cortico moterio da allumina. Bollettino dell Societa Italiana di Biologia Sperimentale 47: 127-129 (1971).

Naestoft, J.; Lund, M.; Larsen, N.E. and Hvidberg, E.: Assay and pharmacokinetics of clonazepam in humans. Acta Neurologica Scandinavica 49: 103-108 (1973).

Nahorski, S.R.: Biochemical effects of the anticonvulsants trimethadione, ethosuximide and chlordiazepoxide in rat brain. Journal of Neurochemistry 19: 1937-1946 (1972).

Nakamura, K. and Bernheim, F.: Effects of some drugs on the γ-aminobutyric acid transaminase and the succinic semialdehyde dehydrogenase of rat brain. Japanese Journal of Pharmacology 11: 37-45 (1961).

Nathan, P.W.: Intrathecal phenol to relieve spasticity in paraplegia. Lancet 2: 1099-1102 (1959).

Nathan, P.W.: The action of diazepam in neurological disorders with excessive motor activity. Journal of Neurological Science 10: 33-50 (1970).

Nathan, P.W. and Wall, P.D.: Treatment of post-herpetic neuralgia by prolonged electrical stimulation. British Medical Journal 3: 645-647 (1974).

Nelson, E. and Morioka, T.: Kinetics of the metabolism of acetaminophen in humans. Journal of Pharmacological Science 52: 864-868 (1963).

Neuvonen, P.J. and Penttila, O.: Interaction between doxycycline and barbiturates. British Medical Journal 1: 535-536 (1974).

Newkirk, T.A.; Tourtelotte, W.W. and Reinglass, J.L.: Prolonged control of increased intracranial pressure with glycerin. Archives of Neurology 27: 95-96 (1972)

Nimmerfall, F. and Rosenthaler, J.: Ergot alkaloids; hepatic distribution and estimation of absorption by measurement of total radioactivity in bile and urine. Journal of Pharmacokinetics and Biopharmaceutics 4: 57-66 (1976).

Nitti, V.; Veneri, F.D.; Ninni, A. and Medla, G.: Rifampicin blood serum levels and half-life during prolonged administration in tuberculous patients. Chemotherapy 17: 121-129 (1972).

Noach, E.L.; Woodbury, D.M. and Goodman, L.S.: Studies on the absorption, distribution, fate and excretion of 4-C¹⁴-labelled diphenylhydantoin. Journal of Pharmacology and Experimental Therapeutics 122: 301-314 (1958).

Nora, J.J.; Nora, A.H. and Way, G.L.: Cardiovascular maldevelopment associated with maternal exposure to amantadine. Lancet 2: 607 (1975).

Noronha, M.J. and Bevan, P.L.T.: A literature review of unwanted effects of treatment with Epilim; in Legg (Ed) Clinical and Pharmacological Aspects of Sodium Valproate (Epilim) in the Treatment of Epilepsy, p.61-65 (MCS Consultants, Tunbridge Wells 1976).

Norris, F.H.; Calanchini, P.R.; Fallat, R.J.; Panchari, S. and Jewett, B.: The administration of guanidine in amyotrophic lateral sclerosis. Neurology 24: 721-728 (1974).

Norris, F.H. Jr.; Eaton, J.M. and Mielke, C.H.: Depression of bone marrow by guanidine. Archives of Neurology 30: 184-185 (1974).

Norris, J.W.: Steroid therapy in acute cerebral infarction. Archives of Neurology 33: 69-71 (1976).

Norwood, C.W.: A review of recent advances in vascular smooth muscle pharmacology. Surgical Neurology 7: 91-94 (1977).

Odar-Cederlof, I. and Borga O.: Kinetics of diphenylhydantoin in uraemic patients: consequences of decreased plasma protein binding. European Journal of Clinical Pharmacology 7: 31-37 (1974).

Olatunde, I.A.: Chloroquine concentrations in the skin of rabbits and man. British Journal of Pharmacology 43: 334-340 (1971).

Olesen, O.V.: Disulfiram (Antabuse) as inhibitor of phenytoin metabolism. Acta Pharmacologica et Toxicologica 24: 317-322 (1966).

Olesen, O.V.: Determination of sultiam (Ospolot) in serum and urine by thin-layer chromatography: serum levels and urinary output in patients under long term treatment. Acta Pharmacologica et Toxicologica 26: 22-28 (1968).

Olesen, O.V. and Dam, M.: The metabolic conversion of primidone (Mysoline) to phenobarbitone in patients under long-term treatment. Acta Neurologica Scandinavica 43: 348-356 (1967).

Olesen, O.V. and Jensen, O.N. Drug-interaction between sulthiame (Ospolot) and phenytoin in the treatment of epilepsy. Danish Medical Bulletin 16: 154-158 (1969).

Olesen, O.V. and Jensen, O.N.: The influence of folic acid on phenytoin (DPH) metabolism and the 24-hours fluctuation in urinary output of 5-(p-hydroxyphenyl)-5 phenyl-hydantoin (HPPH). Acta Pharmacologica et Toxicologica 28: 265-269 (1970).

Olsen, G.D.; Bennett, W.M. and Porter, G.A.: Morphine and phenytoin binding to plasma proteins in renal and hepatic failure. Clinical Pharmacology and Therapeutics 17: 677-684 (1975).

Olsson, P.; Lagergren, H. and Ek, S.: The elimination from plasma of intravenous heparin. Acta Medica Scandinavica 173: 619-630 (1963).

O'Malley, K.; Stevenson, I.H. and Turnbull, M.J.: Amantadine and drug metabolism. Lancet 1: 685 (1972).

Ordonez, L.A.; Arbrus, M.; Boyson, S.; Goodman, M.N.; Ruderman, N.B. and Wurtman, R.J.: Skeletal muscle: reservoir for exogenous L-Dopa. Journal of Pharmacology and Experimental Therapeutics 190: 187-191 (1974).

O'Rielly, R.A.: Studies on the optical enantimorphs of warfarin in man. Clinical Pharmacology and Therapeutics 16: 348-354 (1974).

Orme, M.; Breckenridge, A. and Brooks, R.V.: Interactions of benzodiazepines with warfarin. British Medical Journal 3: 611-614 (1972).

Orton, T.C. and Nicholls, P.J.: Effect in rats of subacute administration of ethosuximide, methsuximide and phensuximide on hepatic microsomal enzymes and porphyrin turnover. Biochemical Pharmacology 21: 2253-2261 (1972).

Oxbury, J.M.: Diseases of the nervous system; treatment of stroke. British Medical Journal 4: 450-452 (1975).

Packam, H.A.; Warrior, E.S.; Glynn, M.F.; Senyi, A.S. and Mustard, J.F.: Alteration of the response of platelets to surface stimuli by pyrazole compounds. Journal of Experimental Medicine 126: 171-188 (1967).

Palmer, K.N.V.: Polyradiculopathy (Guillain-Barre syndrome) treated with 6-mercaptopurine. Lancet 1: 733-734 (1965).

Palmer, L.; Bertilsson, L.; Collste, P. and Rawlins, M.: Quantitative determination of carbamazepine in plasma by mass fragmentography. Clinical Pharmacology and Therapeutics 14: 827-832 (1973).

Pappas, G.D.: Some morphological considerations of the blood-brain barrier. Journal of Neurological Science 10: 241-246 (1970).

Parke, D.: The Biochemistry of Foreign Compounds (Pergamon, Oxford 1968).

Parkes, D.: Amantadine. Advances in Drug Research 8: 11-81 (1974).

Parkes, J.D.: Bromocriptine in the treatment of Parkinsonism. Drugs 17: 365-382 (1979).

Parkes, J.D.; Zilkha, K.J.; Marsden, P.; Baxter, R.C.H. and Knill-Jones, R.P.: Amantadine dosage in treatment of Parkinson's disease. Lancet 1: 1130-1133 (1970).

Patten, B.M.; Mendell, J.; Bruun, B.; Curtin, W. and Carter, S.: Double-blind study of the effects of dexamethasone on acute stroke. Neurology 22: 377-383 (1972).

Pearce, J.M.S.; Gubbay, S.S. and Walton, J.N.: Long-term anticoagulant therapy in transient cerebral ischaemic attacks. Lancet 1: 6-9 (1965).

Pearce, L.A.; Waterbury, L.D. and Green, H.D.: Amantadine hydrochloride: alteration in peripheral circulation. Neurology 24: 46-48 (1974).

Peets, E.A.; Sweeney, W.M.; Place, V.A. and Buyske, D.A.: The absorption, excretion and metabolic fate of ethambutol in man. American Review of Respiratory Diseases 91: 51-58 (1965).

Penry, J.K.; Porter, R.J. and Dreifuss, F.E.: Ethosuximide. Relation of plasma levels to clinical control; in Woodbury, Penry and Schmidt (Eds) Antiepileptic Drugs. p.431-441 (Raven Press, New York 1972).

Perry, T.L.; Hansen, S. and Kloster, M.: Huntington's chorea. Deficiency of γ-aminobutyric acid in brain. New England Journal of Medicine 288: 337-342 (1973).

Peters, J.H. and Levy, L.: Dapsone acetylation in man: Another example of polymorphic acetylation. Annals of the New York Academy of Science 179: 660-666 (1971).

Peterson. H. De C.: Association of trimethadione therapy and myasthenia gravis. New England Journal of Medicine 274: 506-507 (1966).

Peterson. R.E.: The miscible pool and turnover rate of adrenocortical steroids in man. Recent Progress in Hormone Research 15:231-261 (1959).

Peterson. R.E.; Pierce. C.E.; Wyngaarden. J.B.; Bunim. J.J. and Brodie. B.B.: The physiological disposition and metabolic fate of cortisone in man. Journal of Clinical Investigation 36: 1301-1312 (1957).

Petitpierre. B. and Fabre. J.: Chlorpropamide and chloramphenicol. Lancet 1: 789 (1970).

Petruch. F.; Schuppel. R.V.A. and Steinhilber. G.: Effect of diphenylhydantoin on hepatic drug hydroxylation. European Journal of Clinical Pharmacology 7: 281-285 (1974).

Pilling. J.B.; Baker. J.; Iversen. L.L.; Iversen. S.D. and Robbins. T.: Plasma concentrations of l-Dopa and 3-methoxydopa and improvement in clinical ratings and motor performance in patients with Parkinsonism treated with l-dopa alone or in combination with amantadine. Journal of Neurology. Neurosurgery and Psychiatry 38: 129-135 (1975).

Pincus, J.H.: Diphenylhydantoin and ion flux in lobster nerve. Archives of Neurology 26: 4-10 (1972).

Pincus, J.H.; Grove. I.; Marino. B.B. and Glaser. G.E.: Studies on the mechanism of action of diphenylhydantoin. Archives of Neurology 22: 566-571 (1970).

Pinder. R.M.; Brogden. R.N.; Sawyer. P.R.; Speight. T.M. and Avery. G.S.: Levodopa and decarboxylase inhibitors: a review of their clinical pharmacology and use in the treatment of Parkinsonism. Drugs 11: 329-377 (1976).

Pinder. R.M.; Brogden. R.N.; Sawyer. P.R.; Speight. T.M. and Avery. G.S.: Metoclopramide: a review of its pharmacological properties and uses in therapeutics and diagnosis. Drugs 12: 81-131 (1976a).

Pinder. R.M.; Brogden. R.N.; Speight. T.M. and Avery. G.S.: Clonazepam: a review of its pharmacological properties and therapeutic efficacy in epilepsy. Drugs 12: 321-361 (1976b).

Pinder. R.M.; Brogden. R.N.; Speight. T.M. and Avery. G.S.: Dantrolene sodium. A review of its pharmacological properties and therapeutic efficacy in spasticity. Drugs 13: 3-23 (1977a).

Pinder. R.M.; Brogden. R.N.; Speight. T.M. and Avery. G.S.: Sodium valproate: a review of its pharmacological properties and therapeutic efficacy in epilepsy. Drugs 13: 81-123 (1977b).

Pinelli. P.; Tonali. P. and Scoppetta. C.: Long-term treatment of myasthenia gravis with alternate-day prednisone. European Neurology 12: 129-141 (1974).

Piper. D.W.; Glover. W.E. and Anthony. M.: Cimetidine. Current Therapeutics 18: 11-16 (1977).

Pitlick. W.H.; Levy. R.H.; Troupin. A.S. and Green. J.R.: Pharmacokinetic model to describe self-induced decreases in steady-state concentrations of carbamazepine. Journal of Pharmaceutical Sciences 65: 462-463 (1976).

Pletscher. A.; Brossi. A. and Gey. K.F.: Benzoquinolizine derivatives: a new class of monoamine decreasing drugs with psychotropic action. International Review of Neurobiology 4: 275-306 (1962).

Porter. R.J.; Penry. J.K.; Lacy. J.R.; Newmark. M.E. and Kupferberg. H.J.: The clinical efficacy and pharmacokinetics of phensuximide and methsuximide. Neurology 27: 375 (1977).

Posner. J.B. and Shapiro. W.R.: Brain tumor. Current state of treatment and its complications. Archives of Neurology 32: 781-784 (1975).

Powell. L. and Axelsen. E.: Corticosteroids in liver disease: studies on the biological conversion of prednisone to prednisolone and plasma protein binding. Gut 13: 690-696 (1972).

Prescott. L.F.; Roscoe. P.; Wright. N. and Brown. S.S.: Plasma-paracetamol half-life and hepatic necrosis in patients with paracetamol overdosage. Lancet 1: 519-522 (1971).

Prichard. J.W.: Effect of phenobarbital on a leech neuron. Neuropharmacology 11: 589-590 (1972).

Prockop. L.D.: The pharmacology of increased intracranial pressure; in Klawans (Ed) Clinical Neuropharmacology. p.147-171 (Raven Press. New York 1976).

Pscheidt. G.R.: Monoamine oxidase inhibitors; in Pfeiffer and Smythies (Eds) International Review of Neurobiology. Vol.7. p.191-229 (Acadmic Press. New York 1964).

Pynnonen. S. and Sillanpaa. M.: Carbamazepine and mother's milk. Lancet 2: 563 (1975).

Rafal. R.D.; Gummow. L. and Grimm. R.J.: Treatment of progressive supranuclear palsy with methysergide; neuropsychologic improvement in five patients. Neurology 27: 351 (1977).

Rajput. A.H.; Kazi. R.H. and Rozdilsky. B.: Striatonigral degeneration response to levodopa therapy. Journal of Neurological Sciences 16: 331-341 (1972).

Rallison. M.L.; Carlisle. J.W.; Lee. R.E.; Vernier. R.L. and Good. R.A.: Lupus erythematosus and Stevens-Johnson syndrome. American Journal of Diseases of Children 101: 725-738 (1961).

Randall. L.O. and Schallek. W.: Pharmacological activity of certain benzodiazepines; in Efron (Ed) Psychopharmacology: A Review of Progress 1957-1967. p.153-184 (Public Health Service Publication No. 1836. 1968).

Rane. A.; Bertilsson. L. and Palmer. L.: Disposition of placentally transferred carbamazepine (Tegretol®) in the newborn. European Journal of Clinical Pharmacology 8: 283-284 (1975).

Rane. A.; Hojer. B. and Wilson. J.T.: Kinetics of carbamazepine and its 10. 11-epoxide metabolite in children. Clinical Pharmacology and Therapeutics 19: 276-283 (1976).

Rane. A.; Lunde. P.K.M.; Jalling. B.; Yaffe. S.J. and Sjoqvist. F.: Plasma protein binding of diphenylhydantoin in normal and hyperbilirubinemic infants. Journal of Pediatrics 78: 877-882 (1971).

Rapoport. A.M. and Guss. S.B.: Dapsone-induced peripheral neuropathy. Archives of Neurology 27: 184-185 (1972).

Rappel. M.; Dubois-Dalcq. M.; Sprecher. S.; Thiry. L.; Lowenthal. A.; Pelc. S. and Thus. J.P.: Diagnosis and treatment of herpes encephalitis. A multidisciplinary approach. Journal of Neurological Sciences 12: 443-458 (1971).

Rausing. A. and Trell. F.: Malignant lymphogranulomatosis and anticonvulsant therapy. Acta Medica Scandinavica 189: 131-136 (1971).

Rawlins. M.D.; Collste. P.; Bertilsson. L. and Palmer. L.: Distribution and elimination kinetics of carbamazepine in man. European Journal of Clinical Pharmacology 8: 91-96 (1975).

Rawlins. M.D.; Henderson. D.B. and Hijab. A.R.: Pharmacokinetics of paracetamol (acetaminophen) after intravenous and oral administration. European Journal of Clinical Pharmacology 11: 283-286 (1977).

Rawson. M.D. and Liversedge. L.A.: Treatment of retrobulbar neuritis with corticotrophin. Lancet 2: 222 (1969).

Regamey. C.; Gordon. R.C. and Kirby. W.M.: Comparative pharmacokinetics of tobramycin and gentamycin. Clinical Pharmacology and Therapeutics 14: 396-403 (1973).

Rehbinder. D. and Deckers. W.: Untersuchungen zur Pharmakokinetic und zum Metabolismus des 2-(2.- 6-dichlorophenylamino)-2-imidazoline hydrochloride (S.T.155). Arzneimittel-Forschung 19: 169-176 (1969).

Reid. J.L.; Calne. D.B.; Vakil. S.D.; Allen. J.G. and Davies. C.A.: Plasma concentration of levodopa in Parkinsonism before and after inhibition of peripheral decarboxylase. Journal of Neurological Sciences 17: 45-51 (1972).

Reinglass. J.L.: Dose response curve of intravenous glycerol in the treatment of cerebral oedema due to trauma. Neurology 24: 743-747 (1974).

Reynolds. E.H.: Mental effects of anticonvulsants. and folic acid metabolism. Brain 91: 197-214 (1968).

Reynolds. E.H.: Discussion; in Wink (Ed) Tegretol in Epilepsy. p.118-122 (Nicholls. Manchester 1973).

Reynolds. E.H.; Fenton. G.; Fenwick. P.; Johnson. A.L. and Laundy. M.: Interaction of phenytoin and primidone. British Medical Journal 2: 594-595 (1975).

Richardson. S.G.N.; Fletcher. D.J. and Jeavons. P.M.: Sodium valproate and platelet function; in Legg (Ed) Clinical and Pharmacological Aspects of Sodium Valproate (Epilim) in the Treatment of Epilepsy. p.119-122 (MCS Consultants. Tunbridge Wells. 1976).

Richens. A.: Drug estimation in the treatment of epilepsy. Proceedings of the Royal Society of Medicine 67: 1227-1229 (1974).

Richens. A.: A study of the pharmacokinetics of phenytoin (diphenylhydantoin) in epileptic patients. and the development of a nomogram for making dose increments. Epilepsia 16: 627-646 (1975).

Richens, A.: Drug Treatment of Epilepsy (Henry Kimpton, London 1976).

Richens, A. and Dunlop, A.: Serum-phenytoin levels in management of epilepsy. Lancet 2: 247-248 and 2: 1305-1306 (1975).

Richens, A. and Houghton, G.S.: Phenytoin intoxication caused by sulthiame. Lancet 2: 1442-1443 (1973).

Richens, A. and Rowe, D.J.F.: Disturbance of calcium metabolism by anticonvulsant drugs. British Medical Journal 4: 73-76 (1970).

Richens, A.; Scoular, I.T.; Ahmad, S. and Jordan, B.J.: Pharmacokinetics and efficacy of Epilim in patients receiving long-term therapy with other antiepileptic drugs; in Legg (Ed) Clinical and Pharmacological Aspects of Sodium Valproate (Epilim) in the Treatment of Epilepsy, p.78-88 (MCS Consultants, Tunbridge Wells 1976).

Rieder, J.: Plasma levels and derived pharmacokinetic parameters of unchanged nitrazepam in man. Arzneimittel-Forschung 23: 212-218 (1973).

Rieder, J. and Wendt, G.: Pharmacokinetics and metabolism of the hypnotic nitrazepam. Symposium on Benzodiazepines, Milan 1-11-71 to 4-11-71 (1971).

Riegelman, S.; Rowland, M. and Epstein, W.L.: Griseofulvin-phenobarbital interaction in man. Journal of the American Medical Association 213: 426-431 (1970).

Rindi, G. and Ventura, U.: Thiamine intestinal transport. Physiological Reviews 52: 821-827 (1972).

Rinne, U.K.; Laaksonen, H.; Riekkinen, P. and Sonninen, V.: Brain glutamic acid decarboxylase activity in Parkinson's disease. European Neurology 12: 13-19 (1974).

Rinne, U.K.; Sonninen, V. and Siirtola, T.: Plasma concentrations of levodopa in patients with Parkinson's disease. Response to administration of levodopa alone or combined with a decarboxylase inhibitor and clinical correlations. European Neurology 10: 301-310 (1973).

Rivera-Calimlim, G.; Castaneda, L. and Lasagna, L.: Effects of mode of management on plasma chlorpromazine in psychiatric patients. Clinical Pharmacology and Therapeutics 14: 978-986 (1973).

Rivera-Calimlim, L.; Dujovne, C.A.; Morgan, J.P.; Lasagna, L. and Bianchine, J.R.: L-Dopa treatment failure: explanation and correction. British Medical Journal 4: 93-94 (1970).

Rizzo, M.; Biandrate, P.; Tognoni, G. and Morselli, P.L.: Amantadine in depression: relationship between behavioural effects and plasma levels. European Journal of Clinical Pharmacology 5: 226-228 (1973).

Roberts, J.B.; Thomas, B.H. and Wilson, A.: Excretion and metabolism of oral ^{14}C-neostigmine in the rat. Biochemical Pharmacology 15: 71-75 (1966).

Robins, A.H.: Melanocyte-stimulating hormone and Parkinsonism. Lancet 1: 727 (1973).

Rockoff, M.A.; Marshall, L.F. and Shapiro, H.M.: High dose barbiturate therapy in humans: a clinical review of 60 patients. Annals of Neurology 6: 194-199 (1979).

Rodriguez, V.; Stewart, D. and Bodley, G.P.: Gentamycin sulphate distribution in body fluids. Clinical Pharmacology and Therapeutics 11: 275-281 (1970).

Roos, A.: Intracellular pH and intracellular buffering power of the cat brain. American Journal of Physiology 209: 1233-1246 (1965).

Roseman, E.: Dilantin toxicity. A clinical and electroencephalographic study. Neurology 11: 912-921 (1961).

Rosen, A.D. and Vastola, E.F.: Clinical effects of cyclophosphamide in Guillain-Barre polyneuritis. Journal of Neurological Sciences 30: 179-187 (1976).

Rosen, J.A.: Paroxysmal choreoathetosis. Archives of Neurology 11: 385-387 (1964).

Roses, A.D. and Appel, S.H.: Muscle membrane protein kinase in myotonic muscular dystrophy. Nature 250: 245-248 (1974).

Ross Russell, R.W.: Transient cerebral ischaemia; in Ross Russell (Ed) Cerebral Arterial Disease, p.125-145 (Churchill-Livingstone, Edinburgh 1976).

Rothermich, N.O.: Diphenylhydantoin intoxication. Lancet 2: 640 (1966).

Rowland. M.: Amphetamine blood and urine levels in man. Journal of Pharmaceutical Science 58: 508-509 (1969).

Rowland. M.; Riegelman. S.; Harris. P.A. and Sholkoff. S.D.: Absorption kinetics of aspirin in man following oral administration of an aqueous solution. Journal of Pharmaceutical Science 61: 379-385 (1972).

Rowsell. A.; Neylan. C. and Wilkinson. M.: Ergotamine-induced headache in migrainous patients. Headache 13: 65-67 (1973).

Rudman. D.; Bixler. T.J. II and Del Rio. A.E.: Effect of free fatty acids on binding of drugs by bovine serum albumin. by human serum albumin and by rabbit serum. Journal of Pharmacology and Experimental Therapeutics 176: 261-272 (1971).

Rushworth. G.: Muscle tone and the muscle spindle in clinical neurology: in Williams (Ed) Modern Trends in Neurology. Vol. 3. p.36-56 (Butterworths. London 1962).

Ryan. R.E. Sr.; Diamond. S. and Ryan. R.E. Jr.: Double blind study of clonidine and placebo for the prophylactic treatment of migraine. Headache 15: 202-206 (1975).

Saad. S.F.; El Masey. A.M. and Scott. P.M.: Influence of certain anticonvulsants on the concentration of γ aminobutyric acid in the cerebral hemispheres of mice. European Journal of Pharmacology 17: 386-392 (1972).

Saariskoski. S. and Seppala. M.: Immunosuppression during pregnancy: transmission of azathioprine and its metabolites from mother to fetus. American Journal of Obstetrics and Gynecology 115: 1100-1106 (1973).

Sakalis. G.; Curry. S.H.; Mould. G.P. and Lader. M.H.: Physiologic and clinical effects of chlorpromazine and their relationship to plasma level. Clinical Pharmacology and Therapeutics 13: 931-946 (1972).

Saltzstein. S.L. and Ackerman. L.V.: Lymphadenopathy induced by anticonvulsant drugs and mimicking clinically and pathologically malignant lymphomas. Cancer 12: 164-182 (1959).

Salzman. N.P. and Brodie. B.B.: Physiological disposition and fate of chlorpromazine and method for its estimation in biological material. Journal of Pharmacology and Experimental Therapeutics 118: 46-54 (1956).

Sandler. M.: Migraine: a pulmonary disease? Lancet 1: 618-619 (1972).

Sandler. M.; Fellows. L.E.; Calne. D.B. and Findley. L.J.: Oxprenolol and levodopa in Parkinsonian patients. Lancet 1: 168 (1975).

Sandler. M.; Ruthven. C.R.J.; Goodwin. B.L.; Hunter. K.R. and Stern. G.M.: Variation of levodopa metabolism with gastrointestinal absorption site. Lancet 1: 238-240 (1974).

Sandler. M.; Youdim. M.B.H. and Hanington. E.: A phenylethylamine oxidising defect in migraine. Nature 250: 335-337 (1974).

Santagostino. G.; Facino. R.M. and Pirillo. D.: Urinary excretion of amitriptyline-N-oxide in humans. Journal of Pharmaceutical Science 63: 1690-1692 (1974).

Sapeika. N. and Kaplan. E.R.: Effect of the antiepileptic drug sodium valproate on induction of hepatic microsomal P_{450}. Research Communications in Chemical Pathology and Pharmacology 10: 767 (1975).

Satoyoshi. E.; Murakami. K. and Okazaki. T.: Triamterene in the treatment of myasthenia gravis. Lancet 1: 741-742 (1964).

Sattes. H.: Treatment of delirium tremens with chlormethiazole. Acta Psychiatrica Scandinavica 192 (Suppl.): 139-143 (1966).

Saunders. L.: The Absorption and Distribution of Drugs (Balliere Tindall. London 1974).

Savitz. M.H. and Malis. L.I.: Intractable pain treated with intrathecal isotonic iced saline. Journal of Neurology. Neurosurgery. and Psychiatry 36: 417-420 (1973).

Sawaya. M.C.B.; Horton. R.W. and Meldrum. B.S.: Effects of anticonvulsant drugs on the cerebral enzymes metabolizing GABA. Epilepsia 16: 649-655 (1975).

Scatton. B.; Cheramy. A.; Besson. M.J. and Glowinski. J.: Increased synthesis and release of dopamine in the striatum of the rat after amantadine treatment. European Journal of Pharmacology 13: 131-133 (1970).

Schaefer, A.; Seregi, A. and Pfeifer, A.K.: Effects of tetrabenazine and of chlorpromazine on sub-mitochondrial adenosine triphosphatases of rat brain in the presence of the soluble fraction. Biochemical Pharmacology 22: 2375-2379 (1973).

Schafer, H.R.: Some problems concerning the quantitative assay of primidone and its metabolites; in Schneider, Janz, Gardner-Thorpe, Meinardi and Sherwin (Eds) Clinical Pharmacology of Antiepileptic Drugs, p.124-129 (Springer, Berlin 1975).

Schallek, W. and Kuehn, A.: Effects of trimethadione, diphenylhydantoin and chlordiazepoxide on afterdischarges in brain of cat. Proceedings of the Society for Experimental Biology and Medicine 112: 813-817 (1963).

Schmidt, R. and Fanchamps, A.: Effect of caffeine on intestinal absorption of ergotamine in man. European Journal of Clinical Pharmacology 7: 213-216 (1974).

Schmidt, R.P. and Wilder, B.J.: Epilepsy (Davis and Co., Philadelphia 1968).

Schmidt, R.T.; Lee, R.H. and Spehlmann, R.: Comparison of dantrolene sodium and diazepam in the treatment of spasticity. Journal of Neurology, Neurosurgery and Psychiatry 39: 350-356 (1976).

Schobben, E.; Van Der Kleijn, E. and Gabreels, F.J.M.: Pharmacokinetics of di-N-propylacetate in epileptic patients. European Journal of Clinical Pharmacology 8: 97-105 (1975).

Schonebeck, J.; Polak, A.; Fernex, M. and Schoular, H.J.: Pharmacokinetic studies on the oral antimycotic agent 5-fluorocytosine in individuals with normal and impaired kidney function. Chemotherapy 18: 321-336 (1973).

Schroeder, P.L.; Peters, H.A. and Dahl, D.S.: Polymyositis and penicillamine. Archives of Neurology. 27: 456-457 (1972).

Schussler, G.C.: Diazepam competes for thyroxine binding sites. Journal of Pharmacology and Experimental Therapeutics 178: 204-209 (1971).

Schwab, R.S.; England, J.C. Jr.; Poskanzer, D.C. and Young, R.R.: Amantadine in the treatment of Parkinson's disease. Journal of the American Medical Association 208: 1168-1170 (1969).

Schwartz, A.; Lindenmayer, G.E. and Allen, J.C.: The sodium-potassium adenosine triphosphatase: pharmacological, physiological and biochemical aspects. Pharmacological Reviews 27: 3-134 (1975).

Schwartz, D.E.; Bruderer, H.; Rieder, J. and Brogsi, A.: Metabolic studies of tetrabenazine, a psychotrophic drug in animals and man. Biochemical Pharmacology 15: 645-655 (1966).

Schwartz, D.E.; Jordan, J.C. and Ziegler, W.H.: Pharmacokinetics of the decarboxylase inhibitor benserazide in man: its tissue distribution in the rat. European Journal of Clinical Pharmacology 7: 39-45 (1974).

Schwartz, D.E.; Koechlin, B.A.; Postma, E.; Palmer, S. and Krol, G.: Metabolites of diazepam in rat, dog and man. Journal of Pharmacology and Experimental Therapeutics 149: 423-435 (1965).

Schwartz, I.L.; Breed, E.S. and Maxwell, M.H.: Comparison of the volume of distribution, renal and extrarenal clearances of inulin and mannitol in man. Journal of Clinical Investigations 29: 517-520 (1950).

Sears, S.S.: Nonketotic hyperosmolar hyperglycemia during glycerol therapy for cerebral edema. Neurology 26: 89-94 (1976).

Sehgal, A.D. and Gardner, W.J.: Place of intrathecal methylprednisolone acetate in neurological disorders. Transactions of the American Neurological Association 88: 275-276 (1963).

Sehgal, A.D.; Tweed, D.C.; Gardner, W.J. and Foote, M.K.: Laboratory studies after intrathecal corticosteroids. Determination of corticosteroids in plasma and cerebro-spinal fluid. Archives of Neurology 9: 64-68 (1963).

Sellers, E.M. and Koch-Weser, J.: Kinetics and clinical importance of displacement of warfarin from albumin by acidic drugs. Annals of the New York Academy of Sciences 179: 213-225 (1971).

Senior, B. and Loridan, L.: Studies of liver glycogenoses with particular reference to the metabolism of intravenously administered glycerol. New England Journal of Medicine 279: 958-965 (1968).

Sevitt, S.: Fat Embolism (Butterworth, London 1962).

Seybold, M.E. and Drachman, D.B.: Gradually increasing doses of prednisone in myasthenia gravis. New England Journal of Medicine 290: 81-84 (1974).

Shahani, B.T. and Young, R.R.: Physiological and pharmacological aids in the differential diagnosis of tremor. Journal of Neurology, Neurosurgery and Psychiatry 39: 772-783 (1976).

Shapiro, S.; Slone, D.; Hartz, S.C.; Rosenberg, L.; Siskind, V.; Monson, R.P.; Mitchell, A.A.; Heinonen, O.P.; Idanpaan-Heikkila, J.; Haro, S. and Saxen, L.: Anticonvulsants and parental epilepsy and the development of birth defects. Lancet 1: 272-275 (1976).

Shapiro, W.R. and Posner, J.B.: Corticosteroid hormones. Effects in an experimental brain tumor. Archives of Neurology 30: 217-221 (1974).

Shaw, K.M.; Hunter, K.R. and Stern, G.M.: Medical treatment of spasmodic torticollis. Lancet 1: 1339 (1972).

Sheehy, T.W.; Santini, R. Jr.; Guerra, R.; Angel, R. and Plough, I.C.: Tritiated folic acid as a diagnostic aid in folic deficiency. Journal of Laboratory and Clinical Medicine 61: 650-659 (1963).

Sherwin, A.L.: General Discussion; in Schneider, Janz, Gardner-Thorpe, Meinardi and Sherwin (Eds) Clinical Pharmacology of Antiepileptic Drugs, p.145 (Springer, Berlin 1975).

Sherwin, A.L. and Robb, J.P.: Ethosuximide: Relation of plasma level to clinical control; in Woodbury, Penry and Schmidt (Eds) Antiepileptic Drugs, p.443-448 (Raven Press, New York 1972).

Shibasaki, H.; Tabira, T.; Inoue, N.; Goto, I. and Kuroiwa, Y.: Carbamazepine for painful crises in Fabry's disease. Journal of Neurological Science 18: 47-51 (1973).

Shoeman, D.W. and Azarnoff, D.L.: The alteration of plasma proteins in uremia as reflected in their ability to bind digitoxin and diphenylhydantoin. Pharmacology 7: 169-177 (1972).

Shoulson, J.; Kartzinel, R. and Chase, T.N.: Huntington's disease: treatment with dipropylacetic acid and gamma-aminobutyric acid. Neurology 26: 61-63 (1976).

Sicuteri, F.M.D.: Headache as a possible expression of deficiency of brain 5-hydroxytryptamine (central denervation supersensitivity). Headache 12: 69-72 (1972).

Sicuteri, F.; Del Bianco, P.L. and Anselmi, B.: Migraine as a cyclic disease with latent and overt components — effects with an antiaminic drug. Headache 10: 53-62 (1970).

Sicuteri, F.; Franchi, G. and Del Bianco, P.L.: An antiaminic drug, BC105, in the prophylaxis of migraine. International Archives of Allergy and Applied Immunology 31: 78-93 (1967).

Silberberg, D.; Lisak, R. and Zweiman, B.: Multiple sclerosis unaffected by azathioprine in a pilot study. Archives of Neurology 28: 210-212 (1973).

Sillanpaa, M.: Clonidine prophylaxis of childhood migraine and other vascular headache. A double blind study of 57 children. Headache 17: 28-31 (1977).

Silverman, G. and Braithwaite, R.A.: Benzodiazepines and tricyclic antidepressant plasma levels. British Medical Journal 3: 18-20 (1973).

Simon, D. and Penry, J.K.: Sodium di-n-propylacetate (DPA) in the treatment of epilepsy. Epilepsia 16: 549-573 (1975).

Simon, H.E.: Myasthenia gravis: Effect of treatment with anterior pituitary extract. Journal of the American Medical Association 104: 2065-2066 (1935).

Simonsen, N.; Olsen, P.Z.; Kuhl, V.; Lund, M. and Wendelboe, J.: A double blind study of carbamazepine and diphenylhydantoin in temporal lobe epilepsy. Acta Neurologica Scandinavica 60 (Suppl.): 39-42 (1975).

Simpson, J.A.: An evaluation of thymectomy in myasthenia gravis. Brain 81: 112-144 (1958).

Simpson, J.A.: Myasthenia gravis: a new hypothesis. Scottish Medical Journal 5: 419-436 (1960).

Simpson, J.R.: 'Collagen disease' due to carbamazepine (Tegretol). British Medical Journal 2: 1434 (1966).

Sims, K.L.; Davis, G.A. and Bloom, F.E.: Activities of 3, 4-dihydroxy-L-phenylalanine and 5-hydroxy-L-tryptophan decarboxylases in rat brain: assay characteristics and distribution. Journal of Neurochemistry 20: 449-464 (1973).

Sjo, O.; Hvidberg, E.F.; Naestoft, J. and Lund, M.: Pharmacokinetics and side-effects of clonazepam and its 7-amino-metabolite in man. European Journal of Clinical Pharmacology 8: 249-254 (1975).

Sjoholm, I.; Kober, A.; Odar-Cederlof, I. and Borga, O.: Protein binding of drugs in uremic and normal serum: the role of endogenous binding inhibitors. Biochemical Pharmacology 25: 1205-1213 (1976).

Sjoqvist, F.: A pharmacokinetic approach to the treatment of depression; in Teorell, Dedrick and Condliffe (Eds) Pharmacology and Pharmacokinetics, p.315-320 (Plenum Press, New York 1974).

Sjoqvist, F.; Alexanderson, B.; Asberg, M.; Bertilsson, L.; Borga, O.; Hamberger, B. and Tuck, D.: Pharmacokinetics and biological effects of nortriptyline in man; in Proceedings of the Symposium on Biological and Pharmaceutical Aspects of Pharmacokinetics and Therapeutics. Acta Pharmacologica et Toxicologica 29 (Suppl. 3): 255-280 (1971).

Skeith, M.D.; Healey, L.A. and Cutler, R.E.: Urate excretion during mannitol and glucose diuresis. Journal of Laboratory and Clinical Medicine 70: 213-220 (1967).

Skou, J.C.: Enzymatic basis for active transport of Na$^+$ and K$^+$ across cell membrane. Physiology Review 45: 596-617 (1965).

Sloan, L.L. and Gilger, A.P.: Visual effects of Tridione®. American Journal of Ophthalmology 30: 1387-1405 (1947).

Smith, B.: Brain damage after intrathecal methotrexate. Journal of Neurology, Neurosurgery and Psychiatry 38: 810-815 (1975).

Smith, M.J.H. and Smith, P.K.: The salicylates. A critical bibliographic review (Interscience, New York 1966).

Smith, S.E. and Rawlins, M.D.: Variability in Human Drug Response (Butterworth, London 1973).

Smythe, G.A. and Lazarus, L.: Suppression of human growth hormone secretion by melatonin and cyproheptadine. Journal of Clinical Investigation 54: 116-121 (1974).

Snaith, R.P. and Warren, H. de B.: Treatment of Huntington's chorea with tetrabenazine. Lancet 1: 413-414 (1974).

Solomon, H.M.; Reich, S.; Spirt, N. and Abrams, W.B.: Interactions between digitoxin and other drugs in vitro and in vivo. Annals of the New York Academy of Sciences 79: 362-369 (1971).

Solomon, H.M. and Schrogie, J.J.: The effect of phenyramidol on the metabolism of diphenylhydantion. Clinical Pharmacology and Therapeutics 8: 554-556 (1967).

Somani, S.M.; Roberts, J.B. and Wilson, A.: Pyridostigmine metabolism in man. Clinical Pharmacology and Therapeutics 13: 393-399 (1972).

Somerville, B.W.: Estrogen-withdrawal migraine I. Duration of exposure required and attempted prophylaxis by premenstrual estrogen administration. Neurology 25: 239-244 (1975a).

Somerville, B.W.: Estrogen-withdrawal migraine II. Attempted prophylaxis by continuous estradiol administration. Neurology 25: 245-250 (1975b).

Sorell, T.C.; Forbes, I.J.; Burness, P.R. and Rischbieth, R.H.C.: Depression of immunological function in patients treated with phenytoin sodium (sodium diphenylhydantoin). Lancet 2: 1233-1235 (1971).

Sourkes, T.L.: Possible new metabolites mediating actions of L-Dopa. Nature 229: 413-414 (1971).

Spector, R.G.: The influence of anticonvulsant drugs on formyl tetrahydrofolic acid stimulation of rat brain respiration in vitro. Biochemical Pharmacology 21: 3198-3201 (1972).

Speight, T.M. and Avery, G.S.: Pizotifen (BC-105): a review of its pharmacological properties and its therapeutic efficacy in vascular headaches. Drugs 3: 159-203 (1972).

Staples, R.E.: Teratology; in Woodbury, Penry and Schmidt (Eds) Antiepileptic Drugs, p.55-62 (Raven Press, New York 1972).

Starreveld-Zimmerman, A.A.E.; Van Der Kolk, W.J.; Meinardi, H. and Elshove, J.: Are anticonvulsants teratogenic. Lancet 2: 48-49 (1973).

Stein, S. and Pembrook, R.C.: Cross-sensitivity to Dilantin (diphenylhydantoin) and Celontin (methsuximide). Journal of Pediatrics 66: 799-801 (1965).

Steiner, J.A.; Low, P.A.; Huang, C.Y.; West, M.; Uther, J.B.; Allsop, J.L. and Chalmers, J.P.: L-Dopa and the Shy-Drager syndrome. Medical Journal of Australia 2: 133-136 (1974).

Steiner, J.C; Winkelman, A.C. and de Jesus, P.V. Jr.: Pentazocine-induced myopathy. Archives of Neurology 28: 408-409 (1973).

Stensrud, P. and Sjaastad, O.: Clonidine (Catapresan)-double blind study after long term treatment with the drug in migraine. Acta Neurologica Scandinavica 53: 233-236 (1976).

Stensrud, P. and Sjaastad, O.: Short-term clinical trial of propranolol in racemic form (Inderal), d-propranolol and placebo in migraine. Acta Neurologica Scandinavica 53: 229-232 (1976a).

Stoll, A.: Recent investigations on ergot alkaloids. Chemical Reviews 47: 197-218 (1950).

Stoll, A. and Hofmann, A.: The ergot alkaloids; in Manske and Holmes (Ed) The Alkaloids — Chemistry and Physiology, Vol. 8, p.725-783 (Academic Press, New York 1965).

Strandjord, R.E. and Johannessen, S.I.: One daily dose of diphenylhydantoin (DPH) to patients with epilepsy. Acta Neurologica Scandinavica 48 (Suppl. 51): 499-500 (1972).

Strang, R.R.: The symptom of restless legs. Medical Journal of Australia 1: 1211-1213 (1967).

Strickland, G.T.: Febrile penicillamine eruption. Archives of Neurology 26: 474 (1972).

Sturm, G.; Weseman, W. and Schollmeyer, J.D.: Pharmacokinetics and synaptic effects of adamantanimines in the rat — a study by GC-MS. Clinical Chemistry 21: 1027 (1975).

Sugita, E.T. and Niebergall, P.J.: Prednisone; in 'The Bioavailability of Drug Products', p36-38. American Pharmaceutical Association, Washington (1973).

Sutherland, J.M. and Eadie, M.J.: Cluster headache; in Research and Clinical Studies in Headache, Vol. 3 p.92-125 (Karger, Basel 1972).

Sutherland, J.M.; Hooper, W.D.; Eadie, M.J. and Tyrer, J.H.: Buccal absorption of ergotamine. Journal of Neurology, Neurosurgery and Psychiatry 37: 1116-1120 (1974).

Svedin, C-O.: Side effects of chlormethiazole therapy. Acta Psychiatrica Scandinavica 192 (Suppl.): 199-201 (1966).

Svedmeyr, N.; Harthon, L. and Lundholm, L.: The relationship between the plasma concentration of free nicotinic acid and some of its pharmacologic effects in man. Clinical Pharmacology and Therapeutics 10: 559-570 (1969).

Svendsen, T.L.; Kristensen, M.B.; Hansen, J.M. and Skovsted, L.: The influence of disulfiram on the half-life and metabolic clearance rate of diphenylhydantoin and tolbutamide in man. European Journal of Clinical Pharmacology 9: 439-441 (1976).

Svensmark, O. and Buchthal, F.: Diphenylhydantoin and phenobarbital. Serum levels in children. American Journal of Diseases in Children 108: 82-87 (1964).

Swank, R.L.: Multiple sclerosis: twenty years on low fat diet. Archives of Neurology 23: 460-474 (1970).

Swash, M.; Roberts, A.H.; Zakko, H. and Heathfield, K.W.G.: Treatment of involuntary movement disorders with tetrabenazine. Journal of Neurology, Neurosurgery and Psychiatry 35: 186-191 (1972).

Sweet, R.D.; Blumberg, J.; Lee, J.E. and McDowell, F.H.: Propranolol treatment of essential tremor. Neurology 24: 64-67 (1974).

Sweet, R.D.; Lee, J.E. and McDowell, F.H.: Methyldopa as an adjunct to levodopa treatment of Parkinson's disease. Clinical Pharmacology and Therapeutics 13: 23-27 (1972).

Sweet, R.D. and McDowell, F.H.: Plasma dopa and functional oscillations after chronic treatment of Parkinson's disease. Neurology 24: 358 (1974).

Sweet, R.D. and McDowell, F.H.: Plasma dopa concentrations and the 'on-off' effect after chronic treatment of Parkinson's disease. Neurology 24: 953-956 (1974a).

Sweet, R.D.; McDowell, F.H.; Wasterlain, C.G. and Stern, P.H.: Treatment of 'on-off' effect with a dopa decarboxylase inhibitor. Archives of Neurology 32: 560-563 (1975).

Sweet, R.D.; Solomon, G.E.; Wayne, H.; Shapiro, E. and Shapiro, A.K.: Neurological features of Gilles de la Tourette's syndrome. Journal of Neurology, Neurosurgery and Psychiatry 36: 1-9 (1973).

Sweet, R.D.; Wasterlain, C.G. and McDowell, F.H.: Piribedil, a dopamine agonist, in Parkinson's disease. Clinical Pharmacology and Therapeutics 16: 1077-1082 (1974).

Swinburn, W.R. and Liversedge, L.A.: Long-term treatment of multiple sclerosis with azathioprine. Journal of Neurology, Neurosurgery and Psychiatry 36: 124-126 (1973).

Symonds, C.P.: A particular variety of headache. Brain 79: 217-232 (1956).

Taber, L.H.; Greenberg, S.B.; Perez, F.I. and Couch, R.B.: Herpes simplex encephalitis treated with Vidarabine (adenine arabinoside). Archives of Neurology 34: 608-610 (1977).

Takamori, M.: Caffeine, calcium and Eaton-Lambert syndrome. Archives of Neurology 27: 285-291 (1972).

Tanner, A.; Bochner, F.; Caffin, J.; Halliday, J. and Powell, L.W.: Dose-dependent prednisolone kinetics. Clinical Pharmacology and Therapeutics 25: 571-578 (1979).

Tarsy, D.; Leopold, N. and Sax, D.S.: Physostigmine in choreiform movement disorders. Neurology 24: 28-33 (1974).

Tarsy, D.; Parkes, J.D. and Marsden, C.D.: Metoclopramide and pimozide in Parkinson's disease and levodopa-induced dyskinesias. Journal of Neurology, Neurosurgery and Psychiatry 38: 331-335 (1975).

Taverner, D.: Alleviation of post-herpetic neuralgia. Lancet 2: 671-673 (1960).

Taverner, D.; Cohen, S.B. and Hutchinson, B.C.: Comparison of corticotrophin and prednisolone in treatment of idiopathic facial paralysis (Bell's palsy). British Medical Journal 4: 20-22 (1971).

Taverner, D.; Kemble, F. and Cohen, S.B.: Prognosis and treatment of idiopathic facial (Bell's) palsy. British Medical Journal 4: 581-582 (1967).

Taylor, K.M. and Laverty, R.: The effect of chlordiazepoxide, diazepam and nitrazepam on catecholamine metabolism in regions of the rat brain. European Journal of Pharmacology 9: 296-301 (1969).

Teravainen, H.; Larsen, A. and Fogelholm, R.: Comparison between the effects of pindolol and propranolol on essential tremor. Neurology 27: 439-442 (1977).

Teychenne, P.F.; Park, D.M.; Findley, L.J.; Rose, F.C. and Calne, D.B.: Nomifensine in Parkinsonism. Journal of Neurology, Neurosurgery and Psychiatry 39: 1219-1221 (1976).

Theobald, W. and Kunz, H.A.: Zur Pharmakologie des Antiepilepticums 5-Carbamyl-5H-dibenzo (b, f) azepin. Arzneimittel-Forschung 13: 122-125 (1963).

Theobald, W.; Wilhelmi, G. and Krupp, P.: Analgesic and anticonvulsant activity of derivatives of dibenz (b, f) azepine; in Soulairac, Cahn and Charpentier (Eds) Pain, p.239-249 (Academic Press, London 1968).

Thompson, R.H.P.; Eddleston, A.L.W.F. and Williams, R.: Low plasma-bilirubin in epileptics on phenobarbitone. Lancet 1: 21-22 (1969).

Thorn, G.W.: Clinical considerations in the use of corticosteroids. New England Journal of Medicine 274: 775-781 (1966).

Tiitinen, H.: Modification by para-aminosalicylic acid and sulfamethazine of the isoniazid inactivation in man. Scandinavian Journal of Respiratory Diseases 50: 281-290 (1969a).

Tiitinen, H.: Isoniazid and ethionamide serum levels and inactivation in Finnish subjects. Scandinavian Journal of Respiratory Diseases 50: 110-124 (1969).

Tolhurst, A.C.; Buckle, G. and Williams, S.W.: Chemotherapy with Antibiotics and Allied Drugs. (Australian Government Publishing Service, Canberra 1972).

Tolosa, E.S. and Loewenson, R.B.: Essential tremor: treatment with propranolol. Neurology 25: 1041-1044 (1975).

Tolosa, E.S.; Martin, W.E.; Cohen, H.P. and Jacobson, R.L.: Patterns of clinical response and plasma dopa levels in Parkinson's disease. Neurology 25: 177-183 (1975).

Toman, J.E.P.; Swinyard, E.A. and Goodman, L.S.: Properties of maximal seizures and their alterations by anticonvulsant drugs and other agents. Journal of Neurophysiology 9: 231-240 (1946).

Toole, J.F.; Janeway, R.; Choi, K.; Cordell, R.; Davis, C.; Johnston, F. and Miller, H.S.: Transient ischaemic attacks due to atherosclerosis. A prospective study of 160 patients. Archives of Neurology 32: 5-12 (1975).

Tourtellotte, W.W. and Haerer, A.F.: Use of an oral corticosteroid in the treatment of multiple sclerosis. Archives of Neurology 12: 536-545 (1965).

Tourtellotte, W.W.; Reinglass, J.L. and Newkirk, T.A.: Cerebral dehydration action of glycerol. I. Historical aspects with emphasis on the toxicity and intravenous administration. Clinical Pharmacology and Therapeutics 13: 159-171 (1972).

Triedman, H.M.; Fishman, R.A. and Yahr, M.D.: Determination of plasma and cerebrospinal fluid levels of Dilantin in the human. Transactions of the American Neurological Association 85: 166-170 (1960).

Troupin, A.S. and Friel, P.: Anticonvulsant levels in saliva, serum and cerebrospinal fluid. Epilepsia 16: 223-227 (1975).

Troupin, A.S.; Ojemann, L.M. and Dodrill, C.B.: Mephenytoin: a reappraisal. Epilepsia 17: 403-414 (1976).

Tuchmann-Duplessis, H.: Drug Effects on the Fetus (Adis Press, New York 1975).

Tyrer, J.H.; Eadie, M.J.; Sutherland, J.M. and Hooper, W.D.: Outbreak of anticonvulsant intoxication in an Australian city. British Medical Journal 4: 271-273 (1970).

Vajda, F.J.E.; Merory, J. and Bladin, T.F.: Fluctuations of plasma phenytoin levels on single dose and twice daily dose regimes. Proceedings of the Australian Association of Neurologists 12: 61-64 (1975).

Vajda, F.; Morris, P.; Drummer, O. and Bladin, P.: Studies on sodium valproate — a new anticonvulsant; in Legg (Ed) Clinical and Pharmacological Aspects of Sodium Valproate (Epilim) in the Treatment of Epilepsy, p.92-100 (MCS Consultants, Tunbridge Wells, 1976).

Vajda, F.J.E.; Prineas, R.J. and Lovell, R.R.H.: Interaction between phenytoin and benzodiazepines. British Medical Journal 1: 346 (1971).

Vakil, S.D.; Critchley, E.M.R.; Philips, J.C.; Fahim, Y.; Haydock, C.; Cocks, A. and Dyer, T.: The effect of sodium valproate (Epilim) on phenytoin and phenobarbitone blood levels; in Legg (Ed) Clinical and Pharmacological Aspects of Sodium Valproate (Epilim) in the Treatment of Epilepsy, p.75-77 (MCS Consultants, Tunbridge Wells 1976).

Van Der Kleijn, E.: Kinetics of distribution and metabolism of diazepam in animals and humans. Archives of Internal Pharmacodynamics 182: 433-436 (1969).

Van Der Kleijn, E.; Guelen, P.J.M.; Van Wijk, C. and Baars, I.: Clinical pharmacokinetics in monitoring chronic medications with anti-epileptic drugs; in Schneider, Janz, Gardner-Thorpe, Meinardi and Sherwin (Eds) Clinical Pharmacology of Antiepileptic Drugs, p.11-33 (Springer, Berlin 1975).

Van Der Kleijn, E.; Van Rossum, J.M.; Muskens, E.T.J.M. and Rijntjes, N.V.M.: Pharmacokinetics of diazepam in dogs, mice and humans. Acta Pharmacologica et Toxicologica 29 (Suppl. 3): 109-127 (1971).

Van Meter, J.C.; Buckmaster, H.S. and Shelley, L.L.: Concurrent assay of phenobarbital and diphenylhydantoin in plasma by vapour-phase chromatography. Clinical Chemistry 16: 135-138 (1970).

Van Woert, M.H. and Sethy, V.H.: Treatment of post-anoxic intention myoclonus. Lancet 1: 1285 (1974).

Vardi, J.; Oberman, Z.; Rabey, I.; Streifler, M.; Ayalow, D. and Herzberg, M.: Weight loss in patients treated long-term with levodopa. Journal of Neurological Sciences 30: 33-40 (1976).

Verebely, K. and Inturrisi, C.E.: Disposition of propoxyphene and norpropoxyphene in man after a single oral dose. Clinical Pharmacology and Therapeutics 15: 302-309 (1974).

Vesell, E.S. and Page, J.G.: Genetic control of the phenobarbital-induced shortening of plasma antipyrine half-lives in man. Journal of Clinical Investigation 48: 2202-2209 (1969).

Vessman, J.; Alexanderson, B.; Sjoqvist, F.; Strindberg, B. and Sundwall, A.: Comparative pharmacokinetics of oxazepam and nortriptyline after single oral doses in man; Garattini, Mussini and Randall, (Eds) The Benzodiazepines, p.165-173 (Raven Press, New York 1973).

Vickers, S.; Stuart, E.K.; Bianchine, J.R.; Hucker, H.B.; Haffe, M.E.; Rhodes, R.E. and Vandenheuval, W.J.A.: Metabolism of carbidopa [L-(-)-2-hydrazino-3, 4-dihydroxy-α-methylhydrocinnamic acid monohydrate], an aromatic amino acid decarboxylase inhibitor, in the rat, dog, rhesus monkey and man. Drug Metabolism and Distribution 2: 9-22 (1974).

Vickers, S.; Stuart, E.K.; Hucker, H.B. and Vandenheuval, W.J.A.: Further studies on the metabolism of carbidopa (-)-L-α-hydrazino-3, 4-dihydroxy-β-methylbenzenepropanoic acid monohydrate, in the human, rhesus monkey, dog and rat. Journal of Medicinal Chemistry 18: 134-138 (1975).

Vidrio, H. and Hong, E.: Vascular tone and reactivity to serotonin in the internal and external carotid vascular beds of the dog. Journal of Pharmacology and Experimental Therapeutics 197: 49-56 (1976).

Viukari, M.N.A. and Salmimies, P.: Serum-thioridazine levels after different dosage forms. Lancet 2: 1271 (1973).

Volans, G.N.: The effect of metoclopramide on the absorption of effervescent aspirin in migraine. British Journal of Clinical Pharmacology 2: 57-63 (1975).

Volzke, E. and Doose, H.: Dipropylacetate (Depakine®, Ergenyl®) in the treatment of epilepsy. Epilepsia 14: 185-193 (1973).

Vose, C.W.; Ford, G.C.; Grigson, S.J.W.; Haskins, N.J.; Prout, M.; Stevens, P.M.; Rose, D.A.; Palmer, R.F. and Rudel, H.: Pharmacokinetics of propantheline bromide in normal man. British Journal of Clinical Pharmacology 7: 89-93 (1979).

Vroom, F.Q.; Jarrell, M.A. and Maren, T.H.: Acetazolamide treatment of hypokalaemic periodic paralysis. Probable mechanism of action. Archives of Neurology 32: 385-392 (1975).

Wade, D.N. and Sudlow, G.: The kinetics of 5-fluoro-cytosine elimination in man. Australian and New Zealand Journal of Medicine 2: 153-158 (1972).

Wagner, J.G.: Biopharmaceutics and Relevant Pharmacokinetics (Drug Intelligence Publications, Washington 1971).

Wagner, J.G.: Fundamentals of Clinical Pharmacokinetics (Drug Intelligence Publications, Washington 1975).

Wagner, J.G.; Welling, P.G. and Sedman, A.J.: Plasma concentrations of propoxyphene in man. II. Pharmacokinetics. Internationale Zeitschrift fur Klinische. Pharmakologie Therapie und Toxikologie 5: 381-388 (1972).

Wainscott, G.; Kaspi, T. and Volans, G.N.: The influence of thiethylperazine on the absorption of effervescent aspirin in migraine. British Journal of Clinical Pharmacology 3: 1015-1021 (1976).

Wallgren, H.; Nikander, P.; Boguslawsky, P.V. and Linkoia, J.: Effect of ethanol, tert-butanol and chlormethiazole on net movements of sodium and potassium in electrically stimulated cerebral tissue. Acta Physiologica Scandinavica 91: 83-93 (1947).

Wallis, W.; Kutt, H. and McDowell, F.: Intravenous diphenylhydantoin in treatment of acute repetitive seizures. Neurology 18: 513-525 (1968).

Walshe, F.M.R.: A critical analysis of the paralysis agitans syndrome; in Critchley (Ed) James Parkinson 1755-1824, p.245-268 (Macmillan, London 1955).

Walshe, J.M.: Copper chelation in patients with Wilson's disease. A comparison of penicillamine and triethylene tetramine. Quarterly Journal of Medicine 42: 441-452 (1973).

Walters, I.N.; Teychenne, P.F.; Claveria, L.E. and Calne, D.B.: Penicillin transport from cerebrospinal fluid. Neurology 26: 1006-1010 (1976).

Warmolts, J.K. and Engel, W.K.: Remarkable benefit from alternate-day prednisone treatment in myasthenia gravis. Lancet 2: 1198-1199 (1970).

Waters, W.E. and O'Connor, P.J.: Prevalence of migraine. Journal of Neurology, Neurosurgery and Psychiatry 38: 613-616 (1975).

Watts, J.C.: A fatal case of erythema multiforme exudativum (Stevens-Johnson syndrome) following therapy with Dilantin. Pediatrics 30: 592-594 (1962).

Weedon, A.P.: Diphenylhydantoin sensitivity. A syndrome resembling infectious mononucleosis with a morbili-form rash and cholestatic hepatitis. Australian and New Zealand Journal of Medicine 5: 561-563 (1975).

Wehrle, P.F.; Mathies, A.W.; Leedom, J.M. and Ivler, D.: Bacterial meningitis. Annals of the New York Academy of Sciences 145: 488-498 (1967)

Weikel, J.H. Jr.; Wheeler, A.G. and Joiner, P.D.: Metabolic fate and toxicology of methdilazine [10-(1-methyl-3-pyrrolidyl methyl) phenothiazine]. Toxicology and Applied Pharmacology 2: 68-82 (1960).

Weil, A.A.: EEG findings in a certain type of psychosomatic headache: dysrhythmic migraine. Electroencephalography and Clinical Neurophysiology 4: 181-186 (1952).

Weily, H.S. and Genton, E.: Pharmacokinetics of procainamide. Archives of Internal Medicine 130: 366-369 (1972).

Weiss, J.L.; Cohn, C.K. and Chase, T.N.: Reduction of catechol-O-methyl transferase activity by chronic L-Dopa therapy. Nature 234: 218-219 (1971).

Welling, P.G.; Lyons, L.L.; Tse, F.L.S. and Craig, W.A.: Propoxyphene and norpropoxyphene: influence of diet and fluid on plasma levels. Clinical Pharmacology and Therapeutics 19: 559-565 (1976).

Wells, C.E.: Trimethadione: its dosage and toxicity. Archives of Neurology and Psychiatry 77: 140-155 (1957).

Welton, D.G.: Exfoliative dermatitis and hepatitis due to phenobarbital. Journal of the American Medical Association 143: 232-234 (1950).

West, H.H.: Treatment of spasmodic torticollis with amantadine: a double-blind study. Neurology 27: 198-199 (1977).

Whittington, H.G. and Grey, L.: Possible interaction between disulfiram and isoniazid. American Journal of Psychiatry 125: 1725-1729 (1969).

Whittle, B.A.: Pre-clinical teratological studies on sodium valproate (Epilim) and other anticonvulsants; in Legg (Ed) Clinical and Pharmacological Aspects of Sodium Valproate (Epilim) in the Treatment of Epilepsy, p.105-110 (MCS Consultants, Tunbridge Wells 1976).

Whyatt, P.L.; Slywka, G.W.A.; Melikian, A.P. and Meyer, M.C.: Bioavailability of 17 ampicillin products. Journal of Pharmaceutical Sciences 65: 652-656 (1976).

Whyte, R.K.; Hunter, K.R.; Laurence, D.R.; Stern, G.M. and Armitage, P.: Levodopa and orphenadrine hydrochloride in Parkinsonism. European Journal of Clinical Pharmacology 4: 18-21 (1971).

Wiederholt, I.C.; Genco, M. and Foley, J.M.: Recurrent episodes of hypoglycaemia induced by propoxyphene. Neurology 17: 703-706 (1967).

Wilder, B.J. and Ramsay, R.E.: Oral and intramuscular phenytoin. Clinical Pharmacology and Therapeutics 19: 360-364 (1976).

Wilkinson, G.R. and Beckett, A.H.: Absorption, metabolism and excretion of the ephedrines in man. I The influence of urinary pH and urine volume output. Journal of Pharmacology and Experimental Therapeutics 162: 139-147 (1968).

Wilkinson, M.: Preliminary report on the use of clonidine (Boehringer Ingelheim) in the treatment of migraine. Research and Clinical Study on Headache 3: 315-320 (1972).

Willis, A.L.: An enzymatic mechanism for the antithrombotic and antihemostatic actions of aspirin. Science 183: 325-327 (1974).

Wilson, C.G.; Ssendagire, R.; May, C.S. and Paterson, J.W.: Measurement of plasma prednisolone in man. British Journal of Clinical Pharmacology 2: 321-325 (1975).

Wilson, J.; Linnell, J.C. and Matthews, D.M.: Plasma cobalamins in neuro-ophthalmological diseases. Lancet 1: 259-261 (1971).

Wilson, J.T.; Atwood, G.F. and Shand, D.G.: Disposition of propoxyphene and propranolol in children. Clinical Pharmacology and Therapeutics 19: 264-270 (1976).

Wirth, N.; Hoffmeister, F. and Sommer, S.: The pharmacology of Ospolot®. German Medical Monthly 6: 309-312 (1961).

Wise, B.L. and Chater, N.: Effect of mannitol on cerebrospinal fluid pressure. Archives of Neurology 4: 200-202 (1961).

Wold, J.S. and Fischer, L.J.: The tissue distribution of cyproheptadine and its metabolites in rats and mice. Journal of Pharmacology and Experimental Therapeutics 183: 188-196 (1972).

Wolf, S.M.: Effectiveness of daily phenobarbitol in the prevention of febrile seizure recurrences in 'simple' febrile convulsions and 'epilepsy triggered by fever'. Epilepsia 18: 95-99 (1977).

Wolf, S.M.; Wagner, J.H.; Davidson, S. and Forsythe, A.: Treatment of Bell's palsy with prednisone: a prospective randomized study. Neurology 28: 158-161 (1978).

Wolff, H.G.: Headache and Other Head Pain, 2nd Edition (Oxford University Press, New York 1963).

Woodbury, D.M.: Mechanism of action of anticonvulsants; in Jasper, Ward and Pope (Eds) Basic Mechanisms of Epilepsies, p.647-681 (Little, Brown and Co., Boston 1969).

Woodbury, D.M. and Kemp, J.W.: Some possible mechanisms of action of anti-epileptic drugs. Pharmakopsychiatry and Neuro-psychopharmakologie 3: 201-226 (1970).

Woodbury, D.M.; Penry, J.K. and Schmidt, R.P.: Antiepileptic Drugs (Raven Press, New York 1972).

Woodruff, A.W. and Dickinson, C.J.: Use of dexamethasone in cerebral malaria. British Medical Journal 3: 31-32 (1968).

Wyler, A.R.; Wilkus, R.J. and Troupin, A.S.: Methysergide in the treatment of narcolepsy. Archives of Neurology 32: 265-268 (1975).

Yang, H-Y. T. and Neff, N.H.: β-phenylethylamine: a specific substrate for type B monoamine oxidase of brain. Journal of Pharmacology and Experimental Therapeutics 187: 365-371 (1973).

Yatsu, F.M.: Stroke therapy: status of anti-platelet aggregation drugs. Neurology 27: 503-504 (1977).

Yonekawa, W.; Kupferberg, H.J. and Cantor, F.: A gas chromatographic method for the determination of ethotoin (3-ethyl-5-phenylhydantoin) in human plasma; in Schneider, Janz, Gardner-Thorpe, Meinardi and Sherwin (Eds) Clinical Pharmacology of Antiepileptic Drugs, p.115-121 (Springer, Berlin 1975).

Young, A.B.; Zukin, S.R. and Snyder, S.H.: Interaction of benzodiazepines with central nervous glycine receptors: possible mechanism of action. Proceedings of the National Academy of Science, U.S.A. 71: 2246-2250 (1974).

Yuill, G.M.; Swinburn, W.R. and Liversedge, L.A.: Treatment of polyneuropathy with azathioprine. Lancet 2: 854-856 (1970).

Zamis, E. and Hanington, E.: A possible pharmacological approach to migraine. Lancet 2: 298-300 (1969).

Ziegler, V.E.; Co, B.T.; Taylor, J.R.; Clayton, P.J. and Biggs, J.T.: Amitriptyline plasma levels and therapeutic response. Clinical Pharmacology and Therapeutics 19: 795-801 (1976).

Zilly, W.; Breimer, D.D. and Richter, E.: Pharmacokinetic interactions with rifampicin. Clinical Pharmacokinetics 2: 61-70 (1977).

Zilversmit, D.B. and McCandless, E.L.: Fate of intravenously administered glycerol. Proceedings of the Society for Experimental Biology and Medicine 95: 755-757 (1957).

Zintel, H.A.; Flippin, H.F.; Nichols, A.C.; Wiley, M.M. and Rhoads, J.E.: Studies on streptomycin in man. I Absorption, distribution, excretion and toxicity. American Journal of Medical Sciences 210: 421-430 (1945).

Zoglio, M.A. and Maulding, H.V.: Complexes of ergot alkaloids and derivatives. II Interaction of dihydroergotoxine with certain xanthines. Journal of Pharmaceutical Sciences 59: 215-219 (1970).

Zucker, M.B. and Peterson, J.: Inhibition of adenosine diphosphate-induced secondary aggregation and other platelet function by acetylsalicylic acid ingestion. Proceedings of the Society for Experimental Biology (N.Y.) 127: 547-551 (1968).

Zylstra, W.: Cryptococcosis and 5-fluorocytosine. Australian and New Zealand Journal of Medicine 4: 296-299 (1974).

Appendix I

Summary of pharmacokinetic data for drugs commonly used in clinical neurology

Drug	Properties			Absorption			Distribution		Elimination		
	MW	Acid/Base	pKa	$T_{1/2}$ (hours)	Fraction absorbed	T_{max} (hours)	V_D (litres/kg)	Protein binding (%)	$T_{1/2}$ (hours)	Excreted unchanged in urine (%)	Clearance (litres/kg/h)
Amantadine	151.26	B			~1.0	1-4	6.2		9-15:21	86	
Amitriptyline	277.39	B	9.4					82-96	17.1	5	
Amphetamine	135.20	B	9.93			2			7-34	17-73	
Amphotericin B	924.11	amphoteric	5.5:10.0		low			~10	22-45	2-5	
Ampicillin	349.42	A		~1.0				23	1-1.5	90	
Aspirin	180.15	A	3.5		<1.0-1.0				0.2-0.33		
Salicylic acid		A	3.0			2	0.1-0.18	50-90	2.9-22	14	
Azathioprine	277.29					2		30	3-5		
Baclofen	213.67	amphoteric	3.85:9.25		~1.0	1-2		30	3-4	80	
Benserazide	257.25				~0.7	<1	0.3		<2		
Benzylpenicillin	334.38	A			<0.3	0.5-1.0		65	0.5	60-90	
Carbamazepine	236.3	neutral		7.4	<1.0	<20	~1.0	75	28-39	<2	
Carbenicillin	378.42	A			low		0.17	50	1	82	
Carbidopa	244.25				0.4-0.7	0.5-5.0			2	15	
Chloramphenicol	323.14					2	0.57	25-60	2-3	5-15	
Chlormethiazole	161.66	B	3.2		0.15 (first-pass)		5.4	63	4	<5	1.4
Chloroquine	319.89	B	8.4:10.8		1.0		30-40	55	72	70	
Chlorpromazine	318.88	B			<1.0 (first-pass)	2-4	20	95-98	30	almost 0	
Clonazepam	315.72	B	1.5:10.5		~0.9	2-4	2.6	47	22-26	2	0.05
Clonidine	266.57	B			0.65-0.95	1.5	3.94	20	13	53	0.32
Cloxacillin	435.88	A			0.3-0.5		0.3	95	0.4	78	
Cyanocobalamin	1355.42							90-99	144		

Drug	MW	A/B	pKa		F			%	t½	
Cyclizine	266.37	B				1	~0.15	0-10	5	30
Cyclophosphamide	261.10	B			0.95	4-8				<20
Cyproheptadine	287.39				<0.2					
Cytarabine	243.22	B	4.5						1.85	7
Dantrolene	314.26	A			0.7	3-6	1.5			
Dapsone	248.30	A	1.2			1-3		72-80	8.7	1.0
Dexamethasone	392.45				0.78	1-3		77	17-21	8-11
Dextropropoxyphene	339.48	B	6.3			2-3			3-4.5	1.5
Diazepam	284.76	B	3.3		>0.9	1	0.7-2.6	90	6.5-8.0	
Dimercaprol	124.21					0.5-1.0			20-36	
Diphenhydramine	255.35	B		0.38	0.5 (first-pass)	2-4		<2	7	<1
Ergotamine	581.65	B	6.25		? low	2.1			?21	4
Ethambutol	204.31	B	6.6;9.5		0.75-0.80	4		<40	4.2	13-74
Ethosuximide	204.22	A	9.3		~1.0	1-4		0	60	19-30
Flucytosine	129.09		2.9;10.7			2	0.7	48-49	3.9	90
Folic acid	441.49	A			~1.0			67	0.1-0.16	
Gentamicin									2	50-90
Glycerol	92.09	neutral				1-2	0.15	70-80	0.5	varies with dose
Haloperidol	375.88	B	8.25		0.45	2-6	17-30	90-92	12.6-22.0	~1
Heparin	3000-37500	A					0.06	0	0.67-2.5	
Idoxuridine	354.12								<0.5	
Isoniazid	137.15					1-2	0.6	50	1-1.3[1]; 2.5-3.5[2]	37[1]; 57-66[2]
Levodopa	197.19	neutral	2.3;8.7; 9.9		variable	1-3		0	1-3	
Mannitol	182.17	neutral							1.1	<1.0
Meclozine	390.96	B					0.159			
Methdilazine	296.43	B			1.0 dose-related					~100
Methotrexate	454.46		4.3;5.5		?			25-50		
Methylphenobarbitone	246.26	A	7.6			<7	1.9		26	80
Methysergide	353.48	B	6.62			2		32	1.5-2.0	<5; <50

Drug	Properties			Absorption			Distribution		Elimination		
	MW	Acid/Base	pKa	$T_{1/2}$ (hours)	Fraction absorbed	T_{max} (hours)	V_D (litres/kg)	Protein binding (%)	$T_{1/2}$ (hours)	Excreted unchanged in urine (%)	Clearance (litres/kg/h)
Metoclopramide	299.81	B			< 0.10					low	
Neostigmine bromide	303.20										
Nicotinic acid	123.11	A	4.85								
Nitrazepam	281.26	B	3.4;10.8	0.32	> 0.85	2	2.1	55	25		
Orphenadrine	269.37	B			> 0.9				14	8	
Paracetamol	151.16	neutral		0.12	0.63-0.89		1.03	20-50	2-3	~2	
Penicillamine	149.21								7		
Pentazocine	285.44	B			~0.5 (first-pass)	1-3	3	30-40	2.5-6.0	8-24	
Phenindione	223.23	A					0.7	50	5-10	21	
Phenobarbitone	232.23	A	7.2		~1.0	6-18	0.6	~90	72-96	5	
Phenytoin	252.26	A	8.2		~1.0	3-12	2.0	57	22±9	40	
Pindolol	248.32	B	6.95	0.4	1.0		6.9	89	3-4		0.35
Pizotifen	295.45	B			< 1 and varies	5-7	0.8-1.3		22-26		
Prednisolone	360.44								3.5	10-30	
Prednisone	355.44				< 1 and varies	1			1		
Primidone	218.25	neutral			0.75-1.0	3	0.6	0	10-12		~0.35-0.7
Procainamide	271.79	B	9.2			1-2	2	15	2-3	40-80	
Promethazine	284.41	B	9.1		~0.10				9		
Propantheline bromide	448.42										
Propranolol	259.34	B			0.3 (first-pass)		3.6	93	2-3	<1	0.8-0.9

Pyridostigmine bromide	261.14			< 0.10	1.5-2.0				9.4
Pyridoxine hydrochloride	205.64							40-228	
Quinine	324.41	B	5.07;9.7		1-3		90	8.5	5
Rifampicin	822.96	B	1.7;7.9		1-2	0.93	84-91	2.8-4.0	12
Streptomycin	581.58	B			1-2		20-30	2.75	65
Sulphinpyrazone	404.48	A	2.8				98-99	4.3	
Tetrabenazine	317.41			< 1.0					< 100
Thiamine	337.28	B							
Troxidone	143.14	A	6.13	high	0.5	0.15-0.40	84-90	16	
Valproic acid	166.20	A	4.95		< 1			8-10	
Warfarin	308.32	A	5.05	~ 1.0		0.1	97	30-50	7

1 Fast acetylators.
2 Slow acetylators.
NB Where values are not shown data have not been traced.

Appendix II

Principal drugs considered, with some of their synonyms and proprietary names.

Drug	Synonym	Proprietary name(s)
Amantadine		'Symmetrel'
Amitriptyline		'Triptizol' 'Tryptanol'
Amphetamine		'Benzedrine'
Amphotericin	Amphotericin B	'Fungilin', 'Fungizone'
Ampicillin		'Penbritin'
Amylobarbitone		'Amytar'
Aspirin	Acetylsalicylic acid	
Atropine		
Azathioprine		'Imuran'
Baclofen		'Lioresal'
Benserazide	Serazide hydrochloride	'Madopar' (with levodopa)
Benzylpenicillin	Penicillin G	
Carbamazepine		'Tegretol'
Carbenicillin		
Carbidopa		'Sinemet' (with levodopa)
Chloramphenicol		
Chlormethiazole		'Heminevrin'
Chloroquine		
Chlorpromazine		'Largactil'
Clonazepam		'Rivotril', 'Clonopin'
Clonidine		'Catapres', 'Dixarit'
Cloxacillin		
Corticotrophin	ACTH	
Cyanocobalamin	Vitamin B_{12}	
Cyclizine		'Marzine'
Cyclophosphamide		'Endoxana'
Cyproheptadine		'Periactin'
Cytarabine	Cytosine arabinoside	

Drug	Synonym	Proprietary name(s)
Dantrolene		'Dantrium'
Dapsone		
Dexamethasone		
Dextropropoxyphene	Propoxyphene	
Diazepam		'Valium'
Dimercaprol	BAL	
Diphenhydramine		'Benylin' 'Benadryl'
Edrophonium		'Tensilon'
Ergotamine		
Ethambutol		
Ethosuximide		'Zarontin'
Flucytosine	5-Fluorocytosine	
Folic Acid		
Gentamicin		
Glycerol	Glycerin	
Guanidine	Carbamidine	
Haloperidol		'Serenace'
Heparin		
Idoxuridine	IDU	
Isoniazid		
Levodopa	Dopa, L-Dopa	
Mannitol		
Meclozine	Meclizine	
Methdilazine		'Dilosyn'
Methotrexate	Amethopterin	
Methylphenobarbitone		'Prominal'
Methysergide		'Deseril'
Metoclopramide		'Maxolon'
Neostigmine Bromide		'Prostigmine'
Nicotinic Acid		
Nitrazepam		'Mogadon'
Orphenadrine	Mephenamine	'Disipal'
Paracetamol	Acetaminphen	
Penicillamine		
Pentazocine		'Fortral', 'Talwin'
Phenindione		
Phenobarbitone		
Phenytoin	Diphenylhydantoin	'Dilantin' 'Epanutin'
Pindolol	Prindolol	'Visken'

Drug	Synonym	Proprietary name(s)
Pizotifen	Pizotyline	'Sandomigran'
Prednisolone		
Prednisone		
Primidone		'Mysoline'
Procainamide		'Pronestyl'
Promethazine		'Phenergan'
Propantheline bromide		'Pro-Banthine'
Propranolol		'Inderal'
Pyridostigmine bromide		'Mestinon'
Pyridoxine hydrochloride		
Quinine		
Rifampicin	Rifampin, rifaldazine	
Streptomycin		
Sulphinpyrazone	Sulfinpyrazone	'Anturan'
Sulthiame	Sultiamine	'Ospolot'
Tetrabenazine		'Nitroman'
Tetracosactrin		'Synacthen'
Thiamine	Vitamin B_1, aneurine hydrochloride	
Troxidone	Trimethadione	'Tridione'
Valproic acid	(sodium valproate)	'Epilim' 'Depakene'
Warfarin		

Subject Index

A

Abscess, brain 26
  treatment 250, 380
Acetazolamide
  periodic paralysis 80
Acetylcholine 50
Acetylcholinesterase inhibitors 49
Acetylsalicylic acid 233-238
  absorption and bioavailability 234
  acute migraine 259, 274
  biochemical pharmacology 233
  biotransformation 236
  chemistry 233
  childhood migraine 281
  distribution 235
  elimination 235
  interactions 237
  multiple infarcts 326
  pain relief 232
  pharmacodynamics 233
  plasma level correlations 236
  toxicity 237
  transient ischaemic attacks 325
ACTH
  see corticotrophin
Adenosine triphosphatase
  phenytoin activation 19
α-Adrenergic agonists
  migraine 260
β-Adrenergic blockers
  migraine 260, 279
Adynamia episodica hereditaria 80
Akathisia
  Ekbom's syndrome 152
Alcoholism
  thiamine 386
  thiamine deficiency and 385
Amantadine

chemistry 101
Jakob-Creutzfeldt disease 347
panencephalitis 347
Parkinsonism 110
pharmacology 102
spasmodic torticollis 141
toxicity 103
Ambenonium 49, 50
Aminoglycoside antibiotics 356
Amitryptiline
  chemistry 250
  contraction headache 255
  metabolites 251
  migraine 260, 279
  pharmacology 252
  toxicity 253
Amphetamine 20
  biotransformation 291
  cataplexy 296
  chemistry 290
  narcolepsy 295
  parasomnia 296
  pharmacology 291
  toxicity 293
  tremor from 145
Amphotericin
  chemistry 369
  cryptococcal meningitis 379
  pharmacology 369
  toxicity 370
Ampicillin 352
  see also penicillins
  bacterial meningitis 375
  Haemophilus influenzae 375
  Neisseria meningitidis 376
  Streptococcus pneumoniae 376
Amylobarbitone
  chemistry 192
  pharmacology 192

status epilepticus 226
toxicity 193
Anaesthesia
  myotonia: precautions 69
Anaesthetic, local
  brain infarction 322
Analgesics
  bacterial meningitis 375
  contraction headache 255
  migrainous neuralgia 284
  pain relief: short term 246
  peripheral neuropathy 288
  subarachnoid haemorrhage 309
Analgesic nephropathy
  migraine and 274
Antibacterial drugs 350-374
  abscess 380
  meningitis 375-378
    complications 377
Antibody suppression
  myasthenia 59
Anticholinergics
  incontinence 299
Anticholinergics, centrally acting 104-109
  chemistry 104
  Parkinsonism 111
  pharmacology 104-107
  toxicity 108
Anticholinesterases 51-55
  absorption and bioavailability 53
  distribution 54
  elimination 54
  interactions 55
  myasthenia 58
  pharmacodynamics 53
  pharmacology 51
  plasma level correlations 54
  retention, urinary 299
  toxicity 55
Anticoagulants
  brain infarction 323
  brain ischaemia 313
    progressive 324
  emboli 312
  thrombosis 311
    risks 320
  transient ischaemia 325
Anticonvulsants 168-179, 184-194
  basilar artery migraine 282
  epilepsy 168
    combinations 223
    loading doses 223
    long term therapy 223
    neonatal 224
    therapeutic levels 216
Antidepressants, tricyclic 20

Anti-emetics
  acute migraine 274
    ergotamine and 276
Antihistamines 156-159
  chemistry 157
  migraine 260, 266
  pharmacology 157
  toxicity 159
  vertigo 158, 161
Antineoplastic drugs 400
Antiserotinin drugs
  chemistry 267
  migraine 260, 266
    prevention 278
  pharmacology 268
  toxicity 269
Antithrombotic drugs
  transient ischaemia 325
Antiviral drugs 344-346
Apomorphine 20
  Parkinsonism 115
Arterial occlusion 312
Arterial spasm 312
Aspirin
  see acetylsalicylic acid
Asterixis 151
Athetosis 132
Atropine 20, 57, 105
  incontinence 300
Autoimmune disorders 331-341
  classification 331
  disordered mechanisms 331
    correction 332
  drugs used in 332-340
  treatment 340
Azathioprine
  autoimmune disease 341
  chemistry 332
  myasthenia 61
  pharmacology 332
  toxicity 334

                        B

Baclofen
  chemistry 72
  pharmacology 73
  toxicity 74
Bacterial infections
  see infections
Barbiturate coma
  raised intracranial pressure 45
Barbiturates 184-192
  absorption and bioavailability 186
  biochemical pharmacology 185

distribution 186
elimination 188
epilepsy 184, 221
interactions 190
pharmacodynamics 186
plasma level correlations 189
toxicity 191
Bell's palsy 78-80
disordered mechanisms 78
correction 79
treatment 79
Benserazide
chemistry 97
pharmacology 97
toxicity 101
Benzhexol 105
Benzodiazepines 200-207
absorption and bioavailability 202
biochemical pharmacology 201
chemistry 200
distribution 202
elimination 202
interactions 206
myoclonic epilepsy 220
pharmacodynamics 201
plasma level correlations 206
toxicity 207
Benztropine 105
Benzylpenicillin 352
see also penicillins
Neisseria meningitidis 376
neurosyphilis 381
Streptococcus pneumoniae 376
Betahistine 159
Betamethasone 35
Bethanechol 305
see also cholinergic drugs
Biperiden 105
Blood-brain barrier 18
Botulism 49
guanidine 56
Brain, disorders of
see individual disorders
Breast milk
anticonvulsants in 226
Bromocriptine
Parkinsonism 115
Butyrophenones 127-129
see haloperidol

C

Caffeine
Eaton-Lambert syndrome 61
Carbachol

see cholinergic drugs
Carbamazepine 179-184
absorption and bioavailability 181
biochemical pharmacology 179
biotransformation 180
chemistry 179
distribution 181
elimination 182
epilepsy 221
myoclonic 220
pregnancy 225
Fabry's disease 288
interactions 183
peripheral neuropathy 288
pharmacodynamics 179
plasma level correlations 182
tabetic pains 288
toxicity 183
trigeminal neuralgia 285
Carbamylcholine 49
Carbenicillin 352
see also penicillins
Carbidopa
biotransformation 100
chemistry 97
pharmacology 97
toxicity 101
Carbon dioxide
brain infarction 322
Carcinomatosis, meningeal
treatment 400
Carmustine
malignant glioma 400
Cataplexy 296
Causalgia 288
Cerebral dehydrating drugs
mode of action 30
osmotic 30
raised intracranial pressure 44
short term use 43
Chloramphenicol
bacterial meningitis 375
chemistry 359
Haemophilus influenzae 375
pharmacology 359
Rickettsial infection 348
toxicity 361
Chlorimipramine
cataplexy 296
Chlormethiazole
chemistry 213
metabolic pathways 214
pharmacology 214
status epilepticus 226
toxicity 215
Chloroquine

chemistry 372
  malaria 382
  pharmacology 373
  toxicity 374
Chlorpromazine
  see also phenothiazines
  acute migraine 273
Cholinergic crisis
  myasthenia 58
Cholinergic drugs
  chemistry 302
  pharmacology 303
  toxicity 304
Chorea 117-132
  contraceptives causing 117
  disordered mechanisms 117
    correction 118
  drugs used in 119-130
  levodopa-induced 132
  rheumatic: penicillins 132
  treatment 131
Choreoathetosis
  anticonvulsants 152
Clonazepam
  see also benzodiazepines
  biotransformation 205
  Lennox-Gastaut syndrome 219
  myoclonic epilepsy 219
  Parkinsonism 116
  status epilepticus 226
Clonidine
  chemistry 271
  migraine prophylaxis 279
  pharmacology 271
  toxicity 272
Cloxacillin 352
  see also penicillins
  staphylococci 376
Cluster headache 282-284
Coma, barbiturate
  raised intracranial pressure 45
Constipation, neurogenic
  treatment 305
Contraceptives, oral
  arterial occlusion and 312
  cause of chorea 117
  migraine and 277
Convulsions, febrile
  infancy 224
Corticosteroids 33-42
  absorption and bioavailability 37
  autoimmune disease 340
  Bell's palsy 79
  biochemical pharmacology 35
  brain infarction 322
  chemistry 34

distribution 38
  elimination 38
  encephalitis 329
  glucocorticoid functions 36
  Guillain-Barre polyneuritis 329
  half-lives 39
  hypsarrhythmia 391
  interactions 40
  migraine 281
  multiple sclerosis 328, 329
  myasthenia 49, 60
  myoclonic epilepsy 219
  myotonia 68
  neurology: use in 34
  neuromyelitis optica 329
  panencephalitis 347
  peripheral neuropathy 288
  pharmacodynamics 36
  plasma level correlations 40
  polymyositis 340
  polyneuropathy 340
  raised intracranial pressure 43
  toxicity 40
  viral infection 343
Corticotrophin 41
  multiple sclerosis 330
Cortisol 33, 35
Cortisone 33, 35
  see also corticosteroids
CSF
  drugs and 18
    active secretion 18
    passive diffusion 18
CSF examination
  meningitis 374, 378, 379
  neurosyphilis 381
CSF obstruction 378
Cyanocobalamin 392
  see also vitamin B_{12}
Cyclizine
  see also antihistamines
  acute migraine 273
Cyclophosphamide
  autoimmune disease 341
  biotransformation 336
  chemistry 334
  Guillain-Barre syndrome 341
  pharmacology 335
  toxicity 337
Cycrimine hydrochloride 105
Cyproheptadine 267
  see also antiserotonin drugs
  migraine prevention 278
Cytarabine
  chemistry 344
  herpes simplex 348

meningeal carcinomatosis 400
pharmacology 344
toxicity 345

D

Dantrolene
  chemistry 74
  pharmacology 75
  toxicity 75
Dapsone
  chemistry 368
  Hansen's disease 381
  pharmacology 368
  toxicity 369
Decarboxylase inhibitor
  dopamine levels: effect on 98
Deficiency disorders 383-398
Dehydrating drugs, cerebral
  see cerebral dehydrating drugs
Dementia
  multi-infarct 326
  vitamin B_{12} and 391
Demyelinating disease 327-341
  disordered mechanisms 327
    correction 328
  drugs used in 329
  treatment 330
Dermatomyositis
  methotrexate 341
Desipramine
  Parkinsonism 116
Desmethylimipramine
  sleep disorders 296
Dexamethasone 35, 45
  see also corticosteroids
  brain ischaemia 313
  nerve root compression 287
Dexamphetamine
  chemistry 290
  narcolepsy 295
  pharmacology 291
  toxicity 293
Dextrans
  vascular disease 319
Dextropropoxyphene
  chemistry 240
  pharmacology 241
  toxicity 242
Diazepam
  see also benzodiazepines
  acute migraine 273
  bacterial meningitis 375
  biotransformation 203

contraction headache 255
Ekbom's syndrome 152
status epilepticus 226
temporo-mandibular joint pain 288
tremor 145, 151
Diet
  emboli and 312
  folate deficiency and 395
  migraine: phenelzine and 270
  migraine prevention 277
  multiple sclerosis 328
  nicotinic acid and 386
Dimercaprol
  chemistry 139
  pharmacology 139
  toxicity 140
  Wilson's disease 142
Diphenhydramine 106
Dipyridamole
  transient ischaemia 325
  vascular disease 319
Distigmine bromide 50
Dopa-decarboxylase inhibitors 97-101
Dopamine deficiency
  see Parkinsonism
Drug absorption
  half-time 15
  inhalation 6
  intramuscular 5
  intravenous 5
  oral 2
  passive 3
  rectal 5
  subcutaneous 5
Drug action
  mechanisms of 18
Drug biotransformation 8
Drug clearance 16
Drug distribution 6
Drug elimination 8
Drug excretion
  bile 10
  faeces 10
  other routes 10
  urine 9
Drug interactions 11
  pharmacodynamic 12
  pharmacokinetic 11
Drugs and the nervous system
  entry into 16
Dystonias 135-142
  disordered mechanisms 135
    correction 136
  drugs used in 136-140
  treatment 140-142
Dyskinesias 81

E

Eaton-Lambert syndrome 49, 61
  guanidine 56
Edrophonium 49, 50, 51, 54, 57
Ekbom's syndrome 152
Elantrine
  Parkinsonism 116
Emboli 312
Encephalitis, myelinoclastic 330
  corticosteroids 329
Encephalopathy, spongioform 143
Ephedrine 49
  syncope 229
Epilepsy 163-226
  disordered mechanisms 163
    correction 166
  drugs used in 168-215
  limiting discharge spread 167
    anticonvulsants 168
  neonatal 224
  neuronal polarisation 167
  pregnancy 225
  prevention 217-224
    absences 217
    myoclonic 218
  treatment 215-226
    general principles 215
Epilepsy, generalised 165
Epilepsy, hypsarrhythmic
  pyridoxine deficiency and 389
Epilepsy, myoclonic 165
  childhood 219
  infancy 218
Epilepsy, partial 165
Ergotamine
  chemistry 260
  continuing therapy 281
  migraine
    acute 259, 273
    hemiparaesthetic 282
  migrainous neuralgia 283
  pharmacology 261
  structure 262
  toxicity 264
Ethambutol
  chemistry 364
  pharmacology 364
  toxicity 365
  tuberculous meningitis 379
Ethopropazine 106
  tremor 146
Ethosuximide
  chemistry 194
  epilepsy, myoclonic 220
  epilepsy, petit mal 217
  risks 218
  interactions 195
  metabolic pathways 196
  pharmacology 194
  toxicity 196
Ethotoin
  epilepsy 178
Ethyl alcohol
  tremor 146, 151

F

Fabry's disease 288
Flucytosine
  chemistry 371
  cryptococcal meningitis 380
  pharmacology 371
  toxicity 372
Fludrocortisone 35
  syncope 229
Folate deficiency
  disordered mechanisms 395
    correction 395
  treatment 398
Folic acid
  chemistry 396
  folate deficiency: use in 396
  metabolic pathways 397
  pharmacology 396
  toxicity 398
Fungal infections
  see infections

G

GABA
  concentrations: chorea and 118
  structure 72
GABA shunt 207
Gentamicin
  chemistry 356
  pharmacology 356
  toxicity 358
Gilles de la Tourette syndrome 152
Glioma, malignant
  treatment 400
Glucocorticoids 33
  autoimmune disease 340
  brain oedema 378
  brain tumour 399
  demyelinating disease 330
  malaria 381
  multiple sclerosis 330
  side effects 41

Glucose 30
  metabolism 18
Glutamic acid decarboxylase
  chorea and 118
Glycerol 30, 31
  brain infarction 322
  chemistry 32
  oral 44
  panencephalitis 247
  pharmacology 32
  toxicity 33
Guanidine 49
  chemistry 56
  pharmacology 56
  toxicity 56
Guillain-Barre syndrome
  treatment 330, 341
    corticosteroids 329

H

Haematoma 26
  extradural 308
  intracerebral 26, 309
  intracranial 307
    causes 307
  subdural 308
Haemorrhage, intracranial 306-310
  causes 306
  disordered mechanisms 306
    correction 307
  treatment 308-310
Haemorrhage, subarachnoid 26
  treatment 308, 309
Hallucinations, hypnagogic 296
Haloperidol 20
  chemistry 127
  chorea 131
  pharmacology 127
  spasmodic torticollis 141
  toxicity 129
  tremor 146
Hansen's disease 381
Headache 247-284
  see also migraine
Headache, contraction 247-255
  disordered mechanisms 248
    correction 249
  drugs used in 250-254
  treatment 249, 254
Heat treatment
  headache 249, 254
Hemiballismus 131, 132
  relief 119

Heparin
  brain infarction 323
  brain ischaemia 313
  chemistry 314
  pharmacology 314
  toxicity 315
Herpes simplex encephalitis 347
Herpes zoster 348
Herxheimer reaction
  penicillin-induced 381
Huntington's disease 132
Hydrocephalus, obstructive
  meningitis and 380
Hydrocortisone 33
  see also corticosteroids
5-Hydroxytryptamine 20
5-Hydroxytryptophan 20
  myoclonus 143
Hyoscine 105
Hypertension
  brain infarction and 326
  intracranial haematoma and 307
  progressive ischaemia and 324
Hypertonic saline 30
Hypsarrhythmia
  pyridoxine deficiency and 389
  treatment 218, 391

I

Idoxuridine
  chemistry 345
  herpes simplex 348
  pharmacology 346
Imipramine
  sleep disorders 294, 296
Incontinence, urinary 298-305
  disordered mechanisms 298
    correction 299
  drugs used in 299-304
  treatment 299, 304
Infarction, brain 310-326
  anticoagulants 323
  collateral circulation
    promotion 322
  disordered mechanisms 310
    correction 311
  pressure reduction 322
  treatment 320-324
    long term 326
    spasm 322
    thrombosis 320
Infarcts, multiple 325
Infections 342-382
Infections, bacterial 348-382

disordered mechanisms 349
  correction 350
drugs used in 350-374
Infections, fungal 348-382
  disordered mechanisms 349
  correction 350
Infections, protozoal 348-382
Infections, viral 342-348
  disordered mechanisms 342
  correction 343
  drugs used in 344-346
  treatment 347
Insomnia
  disordered mechanisms 289
  correction 290
  treatment 297
Intracranial pressure, raised 25-45
  barbiturate coma 45
  causes 26
  disordered mechanisms 26
  correction 27
  drugs used in 30-42
  treatment 42-45
    alternatives 29
    dehydrating agents 44
    indications 42
    long term 44
    primary causes 28
    secondary mechanisms 29
    short term 43
    steroids 43, 45
Ischaemia, brain 310-326
  causative process: correction 311
  collateral circulation promotion 313
  disordered mechanisms 310
  correction 311
  drugs used in 313-320
  persistent 324
  pressure reduction 313
  treatment 320-326
Ischaemic attacks, transient
  treatment 324
Isoniazid
  chemistry 362
  metabolic pathways 361
  pharmacology 362
  toxicity 363
  tuberculous meningitis 378
Isoproterenol 147

J

Jakob-Creutzfeldt disease
  amantadine 347
Joint pain, temporo-mandibular 288

L

Labyrinthitis
  vertigo and: treatment 160
Lacunes 325
Laxatives 305
Leber's optic atrophy
  hydroxocobalamin 395
Lennox-Gastaut syndrome 219
Leprosy 381
Lergotrile
  Parkinsonism 116
Leucotomy, prefrontal
  pain relief 232
Levodopa 20, 87-96
  absorption and bioavailability 90
  biochemical pharmacology 88
  chemistry 88
  distribution 91
  elimination 93
  failure of response 113
  interactions 94
  metabolic pathways 92
  on-off effect 114
  overdose: dystonia 135
  Parkinsonism 111-116
  pharmacokinetics 90
  plasma level correlations 93
  spasmodic torticollis 141
  torsion dystonia 142
  toxicity 95
  tremor 146
Levodopa-decarboxylase inhibitor
  Parkinsonism: dosage 112
Linoleic acid
  multiple sclerosis 328, 330
Lithium
  spasmodic torticollis 141
  tremor-inducing 145
Lomustine
  malignant glioma 400
Lymphorrhages
  myasthenia 59
Lysergic acid diethylamine 20

M

Malaria, cerebral 381
Mannitol 30, 31
  chemistry 32
  panencephalitis 347
  pharmacology 32
  toxicity 33
Meclozine
  see antihistamines

Melanocyte-stimulating hormone
  Parkinsonism 116
Meniere's disease
  vertigo and: treatment 160
Meningeal carcinomatosis 400
Meningitis, aseptic 347, 380
Meningitis, bacterial 26
  complications 377
  disordered mechanisms 349
  drugs used in 350-364
  treatment 350, 374-378
    duration 376
    general 374
    specific 375
Meningitis, cryptococcal 379
Meningitis, fungal 349
Meningitis, tuberculous 378
Mercaptopurine 333
Methadone 241
Methdilazine 267
  see also antiserotonin agents
  migraine prevention 278
Methoin
  epilepsy 178
Methotrexate
  autoimmune disease 340
  chemistry 337
  dermatomyositis 349
  meningeal carcinomatosis 400
  pharmacology 338
  toxicity 339
Methsuximide 193
  epilepsy 197
Methyl lomustine
  malignant gliomas 401
Methyldopa 97
Methylphenidate
  sleep disorders 294
Methylphenobarbitone
  see also barbiturates
  epilepsy 221
Methylprednisolone 35
Methysergide
  cerebral spasm 312
  chemistry 265
  migraine prophylaxis 280
  myoclonus and 143
  pharmacology 265
  toxicity 266
Metoclopramide
  acute migraine 275
  chemistry 129
  nausea and vomiting 162
  pharmacology 129
  toxicity 131
  vertigo 156

Metronidazole
  brain abscess 381
Migraine 255-282
  acute: correction 258
  aura 282
  basilar artery 282
  childhood 281
  continuing 281
  dehydration 274
  diet and 270
  disordered mechanisms 256
    correction 258
  drugs used in 260-273
  hemiparaesthetic 281
  mixed headache 280
  precipitating factors 257, 277
  prevention 259, 277
    non-pharmacological 277
  treatment 273-280
    acute 273-277
    alternatives 276
    continuous 278-280
Mineralocorticoids 33
Monoamine oxidase inhibitors
  migraine 260, 270
    prevention 280
    risks 270
Motor function disorders 46-152
  involuntary 81-152
  voluntary 46-80
Multiple sclerosis 328-331
  correction 328
  diet and 328
  drugs used in 329
  treatment 329
    alternatives 330
Myasthenia 47-62
  antibody suppression 59
  disordered mechanisms 47
    correction 48
  drugs to avoid 61
  drugs used in 49-56
  generalised 58
  localised 57
  management 57-62
  neonatal 61
  ocular 57
  plasmapheresis in 48
Myoclonus 20
  disordered mechanisms 143
    correction 144
  drugs used in 144
  types 143
Myotonia 62-69
  anaesthesia and 69
  corticosteroids 68

disordered mechanisms 62
    correction 62
drugs used in 63-68
treatment 68

N

Narcolepsy 20
    disordered mechanisms 289
        correction 290
    treatment 295
Nausea and vomiting 154-162
    disordered mechanisms 154
        correction 155
    drugs used in 156-159
    migraine and 259, 274
    treatment 162
Neck muscle spasm
    vertigo and: treatment 160
Neostigmine 49, 51
Neoplasm, nervous system 399-401
    disordered anatomy 399
        correction 399
    treatment
        chemotherapy 400
        radiotherapy 400
Nerve root compression
    treatment 287
Nerve section
    neuralgias 286
Neuralgias 282-287
    glossopharyngeal 286
    migrainous 282-284
    occipital 286
    post-herpetic 287
    supraorbital 286
    trigeminal 284-286
Neurological disease: treatment 21-24
    symptomatic 22-23
    underlying disease 21
Neuromyelitis optica 330
    steroids 329
Neuronal cell membranes 19
Neuropathy, peripheral
    pyridoxine deficiency and 389
    treatment 287
    vitamin B_{12} deficiency and 391
Neuropharmacology 1-24
Neurosyphilis 381
Nicotinic acid
    biotransformation 387
    chemistry 387
    pharmacology 387

    toxicity 388
Nicotinic acid deficiency
    disordered mechanism 386
        correction 386
    treatment 388
Nitrazepam
    see also benzodiazepines
    biotransformation 204
    insomnia 297
    myoclonic epilepsy 220
    sleep disorders 295
Nitrosoureas
    malignant glioma 400
Nomifensine
    Parkinsonism 116

O

Ocular imbalance 160
Oedema, brain 26
    glucocorticoids 378
    reduction 322
Orphenadrine 106
    spasmodic torticollis 141
Oxazolidinediones
    epilepsy 197
Oxprenolol
    Parkinsonism 116
    tremor 151
Oxytremorine
    tremor from 145

P

Pain 230-288
    disordered mechanisms 230
        correction 231
    drugs used for 232-246
    nerve root section 231
    tabetic 288
    treatment, general 246
        long term 247
        short term 246
Palsy 378
    pseudobulbar 326
Panencephalitis
    subacute 143
    viral 347
Papilloma, choroid plexus 26
Paracetamol
    chemistry 238
    childhood migraine 281
    pharmacology 238
    toxicity 240

Paramethasone 35
Paramyotonia congenita 80
Parasomnia 296
Parkinsonism 82-117
  disordered mechanisms 82
    correction 84
  drugs used in 87-109
  physical activity: role 116
  treatment 109-117
    surgery 116
Paroxysmal disorders 163-229
  see epilepsy, syncope
Peak plasma levels 15
Pellagra 388
Penicillamine
  chemistry 136
  pharmacology 137
  toxicity 138
  Wilson's disease 142
Penicillin
  CSF levels 18
Penicillins 351-356
  absorption and bioavailability 353
  biochemical pharmacology 351
  chemistry 351
  distribution 353
  elimination 354
  interactions 354
  nervous system infection 375, 376, 381
  pharmacodynamics 352
  plasma level correlations 354
  toxicity 355
Pentazocine
  acute migraine 273
  chemistry 244
  metabolic pathway 243
  pharmacology 244
  toxicity 245
Periodic paralysis 80
Peripheral neuropathy
  see neuropathy, peripheral
Pharmacodynamics
  nervous system 18
Pharmacokinetics
  principles 2-16
Phenelzine
  migraine 270
Phenindione
  chemistry 316
  pharmacology 316
  toxicity 318
Phenobarbitone
  see also barbiturates
  Ekbom's syndrome 152
  epilepsy 221
  febrile convulsions 225

  folate deficiency and 395
  metabolites 187
Phenothiazines 20, 121-126
  absorption and bioavailability 123
  biochemical pharmacology 121
  biotransformation 124
  chemistry 121
  chorea 131
  distribution 123
  dystonia and 135
  Ekbom's syndrome 152
  elimination 123
  interactions 125
  levodopa and 114
  nausea and vomiting 162
  pharmacodynamics 122
  plasma level correlations 125
  tardive dyskinesia 134
  toxicity 126
  vertigo 161
Phenothiazines, neuroleptic
  nausea and vomiting 156
  vertigo 156
Phensuximide 193
  epilepsy 197
Phentolamine
  cerebral spasm 312
Phenoxybenzamine
  cerebral arterial spasm 312
Phenytoin 168-178
  absorption and bioavailability 171
  adenosine triphosphatase and 19
  biochemical pharmacology 170
  chemistry 168
  distribution 171
  elimination 173
  epilepsy 220
    pregnancy 225
  Fabry's disease 288
  febrile convulsions 225
  folate deficiency and 395
  interactions 174-176
  metabolic pathways 169
  myotonia 68
  pharmacodynamics 170
  plasma level correlations 173
  toxicity 176-178
  trigeminal neuralgia 285
Physostigmine 49
Pindolol 146-150
  absorption and bioavailability 148
  biochemical pharmacology 148
  chemistry 147
  distribution 148
  elimination 149
  interactions 150

migraine prevention 279
pharmacodynamics 148
toxicity 150
tremor 151
Piribedil
    Parkinsonism 115
Pizotifen 267
    see also antiserotonin drugs
    migraine prevention 278
    tremor 146
Plasma drug levels 11
    time course 12
Plasma half-life 14
Poliomyelitis 348
Polymyositis
    corticosteroids 340
Polyneuropathy
    azathioprine 341
    corticosteroids 340
Potassium salts
    myasthenia 59
Potassium sulphide
    Wilson's disease 142
Prednisolone 35
    see also corticosteroids
    multiple sclerosis 329
Prednisone 35
    see also corticosteroids
    migrainous neuralgia 284
    multiple sclerosis 329
    myotonia 68
Pregnancy
    epilepsy 225
Primidone
    see also barbiturates
    biotransformation 188
    epilepsy 222
Procainamide
    chemistry 65
    metabolism 67
    myotonia 68
    pharmacology 65
    toxicity 67
Procarbazine
    neoplasms 401
Prochlorperazine
    see also phenothiazines
    acute migraine 273
Procyclidine 105
Promethazine
    see antihistamines
Propantheline 57
    chemistry 301
    incontinence 300, 304
    pharmacology 301
    toxicity 302

Propoxyphene
    see dextropropoxyphene
Propranolol 146-150
    absorption and bioavailability 148
    biochemical pharmacology 148
    biotransformation 149
    chemistry 147
    distribution 148
    Ekbom's syndrome 152
    elimination 149
    interactions 150
    Parkinsonism 116
    pharmacodynamics 148
    toxicity 150
    tremor 145, 151
Pyridostigmine 49, 51, 57
Pyridoxine
    chemistry 390
    dopamine levels: effect on 98
    hypsarrhythmia 219
    levodopa and 114
    metabolism 389
    toxicity 390
    tuberculous meningitis 379
Pyridoxine deficiency
    disordered mechanisms 389
        correction 389
    treatment 391

                        Q

Quinalbarbitone
    hemiparaesthetic migraine 282
Quinine
    chemistry 63
    myotonia 68
    pharmacology 63
    toxicity 64

                        R

Raised intracranial pressure
    see intracranial pressure, raised
Reserpine 20
Restless legs 152
Retention
    faecal 305
    urinary 298-305
Rheumatic chorea
    penicillins 132
Ricksettial infection 348
Rifampicin
    chemistry 368

pharmacology 366
toxicity 367
tuberculous meningitis 379

S

Salbutamol
    cerebral spasm 312
Schilder's disease
    corticosteroids 329
Serotonin
    cerebral spasm and 312
    structure 262
Shy-Drager syndrome 113, 229
Sleep disorders 289-297
    drugs used in 290-295
    treatment 295-297
Sleep paralysis 296
Sodium diocytlsulphosuccinate
    faecal retention 305
Sodium pump
    phenytoin activation 19
Sodium valproate
    see valproic acid
Somnambulism 296
Spasm, cerebral arterial 312
Spasticity 69-78
    disordered mechanisms 69
        correction 71
    drugs used in 72-76
    treatment 76
        local anaesthetic 77
        surgery 78
Sphincter disturbances 298-304
    treatment 304
Spironolactone 49
    myasthenia 59
Spongioform encephalopathy 143
Status epilepticus 226
Streptomycin
    chemistry 356
    pharmacology 356
    toxicity 358
    tuberculous meningitis 378
Striato-nigral degeneration 113
Succinimides 193, 194
Sucrose 30
Sulphinpyrazone
    transient ischaemia 325
    vascular disease 319
Sulphone drugs 368
    see also dapsone
Sulthiame
    chemistry 211
    epilepsy 222
        myoclonic 220

pharmacology 212
    toxicity 213
Sympathectomy, regional
    causalgia 288
Sympathomimetic drugs
    incontinence 299
    syncope 228
Synaptic function
    drug-induced modification 19
    transmitter molecules 19
Synaptic transmitters
    action at receptors 20
    molecular degradation 21
    storage and release 20
Syncope 227-229
    diagnosis 227
    disordered mechanisms 227
        correction 227
    drugs used in 228
    treatment 229

T

Tabetic pain
    carbamazepine 288
Tardive dyskinesia 133-135
    disordered mechanisms 133
        correction 134
    drugs used in 134
    treatment 134
Temporo-mandibular joint pain
    treatment 288
Tension headache
    see headache, contraction
Tetrabenazine 20
    chemistry 119
    chorea 132
    pharmacology 119
    toxicity 121
Tetracosactrin 41
    absorption 42
    half-life 42
    hypsarrhythmia 391
    panencephalitis 347
    side effects 42
Tetracyclines
    neurosyphilis 381
    Ricksettsial infection 348
Thalamotomy
    torsion dystonia 142
Therapeutic ranges 11
Thiamine
    alcoholism 386
    chemistry 384
    pharmacology 384

toxicity 385
Thiamine deficiency
  disturbed mechanisms 383
    correction 384
  treatment 385
Thiethylperazine
  see phenothiazines
Thioridazine
  see also phenothiazines
  chorea 131
  spasmodic torticollis 141
  tardive dyskinesia 134
Thrombosis 311
Thymectomy 48
  myasthenia 59
Thymoma 48, 58
Tic douloureux 284-286
Tics 152
Tobacco amblyopia
  hydroxocobalamin 395
Torsion dystonia 142
Torticollis, spasmodic 141
Toxic disorders 383
Tractotomy, spinothalamic
  pain relief 232
Transient ischaemic attacks 324
Tremor 144-151
  disordered mechanisms 145
    correction 145
  drugs used in 146-150
  essential 151
  treatment 150
    surgery 146
  types 145
Triamterene
  myasthenia 59
Triethylenetetramine
  Wilson's disease 142
Trifluoperazine
  see phenothiazines
Troxidone
  chemistry 198
  epilepsy 198
  pharmacology 198
  toxicity 199
Tryptophan 20

                U

Urea 30

                V

Valproic acid
  biotransformation 209

chemistry 208
chorea and 118
interactions 210
Lennox-Gastaut syndrome 219
myoclonic epilepsy 219
pharmacology 208
toxicity
Vascular disease 305-326
  see individual diseases
Vasodilating drugs
  brain ischaemia 313
Vertigo 153-162
  causative disorders 155, 160
  disordered mechanisms 153
    correction 155
  drugs used in 156-159
  treatment 160
  utricular positional 160
Vestibular neuronitis
  vertigo and: treatment 160
Vincristine
  neoplasms 401
Viral infections
  see infections
Vitamin B_{12}
  chemistry 392
  Leber's disease 391
  pharmacology 392
  tobacco amblyopia 391
  toxicity 394
Vitamin B_{12} deficiency
  disordered mechanisms 391
    correction 391
  treatment 394
Vitamin K_1
  brain infarction 323
Volume of distribution 15
Vomiting
  see also nausea
  meningitis and 347

                W

Warfarin
  brain infarction 323
  chemistry 316
  pharmacology 316
  toxicity 318
Wernicke's encephalopathy 155
West's syndrome
  pyridoxine and 389
  treatment 218
Wilson's disease 142